ALLE ZEIT WACH 1842

H. Manabe B.W. Zweifach K. Messmer (Eds.)

Microcirculation in Circulatory Disorders

With 283 Figures

Springer-Verlag
Tokyo Berlin Heidelberg New York London Paris

Hisao Manabe, M.D.
President of National Cardiovascular Center of Japan
Suita, Osaka, 565 Japan

Benjamin W. Zweifach, Ph.D.
Professor Emeritus of Bioengineering
University of California, San Diego
La Jolla, CA 92093, USA

Konrad Messmer, M.D.
Professor of Experimental Surgery
University of Heidelberg
D-6900 Heidelberg, Federal Republic of Germany

ISBN-13:978-4-431-68080-2 e-ISBN-13:978-4-431-68078-9
DOI: 10.1007/978-4-431-68078-9

Typesetting: Asco Trade Typesetting, Hong Kong/Fujicom, Tokyo

Preface

Nowadays, a knowledge of the microcirculation has become essential for a thorough understanding of the mechanism of organ disorders. In Osaka on 1-2 August 1987, a conference on microcirculatory disorders was held as the Satellite Symposium of the Fourth World Congress for Microcirculation and to mark the tenth anniversary of the National Cardiovascular Center of Japan. It was an opportune time for such a meeting, which drew the attendance of biomedical scientists and clinicians from many different parts of the world. The pathophysiological significance of the microcirculation in ischemia and disease was elucidated with lively presentations dealing with both experimental and clinical aspects.

The present volume summarizes the proceedings of that symposium. A review is made of recent advances in microvascular disorders, following which cerebral, myocardial, and peripheral tissue ischemia, multiple organ failure, gastroenterological disorders, and methodology are closely examined.

We wish to express our thanks to our contributors, who obliged us by submitting their manuscripts within the time limit. We are grateful to Prof. Masaharu Tsuchiya, President of the Fourth World Congress for Microcirculation, who generously allowed these proceedings to be published. We would also like to thank Dr. Syoten Oka, Dr. Hiroshi Abe, Dr. Teruo Omae, Prof. Takenobu Kamada, Dr. Hiroshi Sakakibara, Dr. Tohru Sawada, and other members of the organizing committee. We are also obliged to Drs. Nobuko Tsushima, Nobuhiro Sato, Hiroaki Naritomi, and Ryu Nakayama for organizing the session symposia. Thanks must finally go to Dr. Hideyuki Niimi, who substantially organized the meeting and assisted in the editing of this work.

We believe that this book will contribute much toward increasing our understanding of the early diagnosis and prevention of circulatory diseases.

July, 1988

Hisao Manabe
Benjamin W. Zweifach
Konrad Messmer

Table of Contents

Chapter 1
Recent Progress in Microcirculatory Disorders

Chapter 2
Multiple Organ Failure

Chapter 3
Gastroenterological Disorders

Chapter 5
Myocardial Ischemia

Chapter 7
Methodology for Microvascular Disorders

Chapter 1
Recent Progress in Microcirculatory Disorders

Microcirculation in Health and Disease

BENJAMIN W. ZWEIFACH[1]

Introduction

Although considerable information is available concerning the ultrastructure and histology of the terminal vascular bed for humans, our understanding of the dynamics of this system rests largely upon experimental studies in animals. In situ measurements of microvessel behavior in man have been made in superficial structures, such as the eye [1], the nailfold or the digits [2], or the skin in general and dealt in the main with structural alternations in particular vessels. The most meaningful measurements in patients that dealt with functional mechanisms were concerned with blood-tissue exchange [3].

Despite the limited scope of intravital studies, data on the retina and bulbar conjunctiva in man have been found to be especially valuable because it is possible to follow the entire hierarchy of microvessels [4]. The weakness of such observations stems from the fact that they are largely descriptive. Studies of the nailfold vessels of the digits provide dynamic information on a set of important exchange vessels [5], but their relevance to underlying mechanisms is difficult to ascertain on this basis alone. What is needed, because of the circumscribed nature of such observations, is a suitable frame of reference that deals with the functional effectiveness of the network in the same area.

Pathophysiology of the Microcirculation

The development of microvascular abnormalities is usually interpreted as a secondary manifestation of parenchymal cell disorders. There is increasing evidence, however, that the cellular constituents of the terminal vasculature—the endothelial cells and smooth muscle cells—are equally vulnerable and can develop structural and functional defects sufficient to undermine microvascular homeostatic adjustments.

The use of the direct observational approach to identify microvascular abberations has a number of distinct advantages as well as limitations. Obviously, it

[1] AMES-Bioengineering, M-005, University of California, San Diego, La Jolla, CA 92093, USA

cannot be claimed that the superficial structures used for human microcirculation studies are essential for life. Furthermore, their manifestations may not be an adequate representation of the microvascular dysfunction in other organs that are more directly involved in disease, such as the heart, brain, and kidneys. On the other hand, systemic diseases in general are consistently associated with striking microvascular changes, even in the skin [6] and conjunctival vessels [7], so that there is no reason to believe that modifications in microcirculatory appearance and design are organ specific. Examples of the various types of microvascular departures that have been reported are: vessel rarefaction, aneurysms (micropools), proliferation (retina), tortuosity (length, width), ischemia—arterial vasospasm and arteriosclerosis, hyperemia, hypertrophy of wall—connective tissue (hyperplasia) and smooth muscle (size and number), and basement membrane—thickening in capillaries. It appears likely that basic organizational features common to all microvascular beds are undermined in disease and that regional differences represent only a matter of degree of change.

Each microvascular bed has a structural design which meets the metabolic needs of that tissue under steady state conditions and provides for additional needs during functional work. Under normal circumstances, adjustments of microvessel caliber serve to modulate pressure and flow as nutritive exchange requirements fluctuate. On the other hand, under conditions of age or in systemic disease, blood tissue exchange may be compromised for a variety of reasons: Pressure can be subnormal or hypernormal, volume deficits can undermine regional delivery of blood, the flow properties of the blood may be altered, derangements of cell metabolism may exist, neuroendocrine imbalance may be present, etc. In each case, the end result is an impairment at the blood-tissue exchange level that requires a series of adjustments. Where a chronic imbalance develops, adjustments of vessel caliber by themselves cannot sustain local homeostasis and it becomes necessary for the microvasculature to undergo various degrees of structural realignment.

The aging process per se is associated with a series of structural modifications that resemble those reported for diseases such as hypertension or diabetes [1, 7]. In this regard, it should be recalled that during embryogenesis a nondescript mesh of capillary-sized vessels is remodeled by a process in which pathways with varying degrees of active flow are transformed into the hierarchy of muscular and nonmuscular channels characteristic of the adult microvascular bed. Although the degree of vascular remodeling is stabilized in the adult when parenchymal tissue needs have reached a plateau, the array of microvascular constituents retain their capacity for growth and continue to undergo appropriate realignment throughout life in a compensatory direction.

The remodeling process serves to maintain local homeostasis under steady state conditions but at the expense of the flexibility of the system, which becomes progressively limited with time. In the long run, continued restructuring of the network serves to compromise its capacity to meet both systemic and local needs for the redistribution of flow within the network.

The term "disease" implies either a structural abnormality or a functional imbalance. Adaptive measures include changes in arteriolar length or dimension to meet flow requirements; increased capillarization provides an increased sur-

Table 1. Incidence of selected microvascular abnormalities in bulbar conjunctiva of moderate and more severe forms of diabetes mellitus for patients of comparable age. After Ditzel [1]

	Group 2 ($n = 35$) without late diabetic manifestations (%)	Group 5 ($n = 60$) with late diabetic manifestations (%)
Vascular changes		
Arteriolar irregularities	6	32
Capillary elongation	74	87
Venular irregularities	66	93
Venular sacculations	17	25
Arteriolar/venular diameter ratio < 1:3	51	68
Perivascular changes		
Edema	26	72
"Hyaline" infiltration	51	68
Hemorrhage	6	3

Capillary and venular manifestations predominate

face for exchange; venular widening or tortuosity may be secondary to a change in transmural pressure or local blood volume, etc. Morphometric adaptation in this context usually appears well in advance of more striking microangiopathies and can be demonstrated by comparing successive microcirculatory segments [8].

The majority of studies in man list the incidence of abnormal manifestations and describe the lesions in general terms, e.g., ischemic trend versus hyperemic trend, hyperplastic versus atrophic network, on the assumption that there is a similar response throughout the network. Table 1 is taken from a paper by Ditzel [1] on diabetes with a higher incidence of the various lesions in individuals with a more severe form of the disease. Observations on various tissues, however, show that remodeling is not uniform throughout the network but develops focally in discrete portions of the microvascular bed and then spreads to other portions until more and more vessels are involved.

Much of the early interest in microcirculation in man was centered on its role in the inflammatory process. The demonstration that the fatal course of traumatic and hemorrhagic shock was associated with peripheral circulatory insufficiency led in the 1940s to a renewed interest in intrinsic microcirculatory control mechanisms. Our understanding of the functional properties of the various segments of the terminal vascular bed has, however, developed largely from intravital microscopy of animal tissues. Unfortunately, comparable studies in humans can be made only on a limited number of sites—in the skin and in the eye—so that the data base for disease remains largely inferential.

Even superficial inspection of the terminal vascular bed in flat tissues under low magnification makes it clear that the topography of the network has been modified under conditions of disease. The number of vessels and length and width of the capillaries and venules are increased, and as a consequence there is a maldistribution of blood within the network. In the bulbar conjunctiva of the eye, the normally white background shows evidence of infiltration and becomes mottled and dark with a trend for a more dense network[4].

An increased incidence of microangiopathy is seen, especially in venules, as systemic disease processes become more severe [5, 9]; an increased permeability is manifest by the leakage of labeled macromolecules from the capillaries and postcapillaries; this occurs against the background of a structural reorganization of the network topography.

Even in studies on the nailfold where the focus is on single capillary loops, the exchange vessels initially show structural abnormalities, and in turn an increased leakage of plasma proteins [5, 9]. It is interesting to note that the changes in the terminal vascular bed can occur independently of large blood vessel disease. When a population of control patients is surveyed, some 10%-15% show an atypical microvascular deployment in the bulbar conjunctiva. It is our impression that this small cohort is in fact a set of high-risk individuals who are in an early subclinical stage of disease and who should be followed closely.

A common failing associated with disease prior to evidence of any structural abnormality is an inability of local control mechanisms to readjust blood flow when the system is perturbed by a standard test, such as the hyperemic response following temporary microocclusion [9]. Substantial in vivo and in vitro evidence indicates that changes in the rheological properties of the blood can contribute to microcirculatory insufficiency [10]. Emphasis in the past was placed on the effect of aggregation of red blood cells on microvascular perfusion [11]. In recent years, the deformability of the leukocytes has also been found to be modified to the point where circulation through many capillaries is interrupted completely [12].

The fact that particular vascular alterations are associated consistently with different systemic diseases makes it plausible to assume that an important aspect of the pathophysiology of disease is a progressive impairment of microvascular efficiency. Because of the multifaceted nature of local homeostasis, the same end result can develop through any of a number of pathways.

Most of the observations in man represent circumstantial evidence that is difficult to relate to the severity of the disease process. The clinical significance of particular microvascular symptoms will remain limited until data are provided that relates them to specific facets of the functional behavior of the network.

Structural Remodeling

The venular channels are consistently involved in the adaptive response to both aging and disease [1, 4, 7], probably because any disturbance of pressure-flow relationships leads to an ineffective distribution of blood, which becomes further compounded on the low shear side of the network.

Striking modifications of the capillaries and postcapillaries are associated with both aging and disease. The fact that venular abnormalities are encountered even in the absence of capillary modifications [7, 8] suggests that the two are independent phenomena. A common finding during microcirculatory insufficiency is a redistribution of the circulating volume in the network with a larger fraction being shifted into the outflow side of the bed. As a consequence, there is a relative increase in outflow resistance and a disproportionately higher capillary pressure.

If we accept the premise that the principal function of the microvascular segment of the circulation is blood-tissue exchange, then the following compensatory adjustments, whether structural or functional, should contribute to the efficacy of the exchange process: Lumen dimensions, length, tortuosity, diameter of branch ratios, number of vessels, and wall thickness—hyperplasia and hypertrophy. In order to fulfill exchange requirements, changes in the design of the system must allow not only for the delivery of an increased or decreased volumetric flow rate, but also for the distribution of the apportioned volume within the meshwork of capillaries so as to provide an appropriate surface area for effective exchange. Transit time must be kept within limits, and pressures must be adjusted to conform to the constraints of the Starling constitutive equation for fluid exchange. It is obvious that a substantive analysis of microvascular remodeling cannot be achieved by following only one set of vessels, such as the capillaries.

Just how this sequence of autoregulatory features is maintained remains to be demonstrated. Inasmuch as the continuum of microvessels represents an organic unit, changes in any particular segment will have an influence on the function of the entire network and can lead to readjustments elsewhere in the terminal vascular bed. The adaptive process is thus an iterative sequence which is most effective under steady state conditions.

Microcirculatory Organization

The theory of design as applied to biological systems assumes in an evolutionary context that after numerous modifications over the years the organizational features are optimal with respect to a particular function served by that system.

Optimal design principles usually revolve around a basic functional attribute of a particular organic entity. In the case of the microvascular apparatus, a number of different approaches have been adopted. Mayrovitz and Roy [13], on the basis of an earlier concept by Marray [14], emphasized a design compatible with the work energy function of the network through the maintenance of an r^3 (radius) relationship to flow. Kamiya and Togawa [15] postulated that the design of the vascular system is optimized so as to keep the shear stress constant in the various segments of the network.

If one adopts a more direct point of view, the structural design of the microvascular network can be formulated in terms of an optimal relationship between the surface area available for exchange and volumetric flow levels.

The details of the structural remodeling will depend upon whether an imbalance is the result of a systemic derangement or is local in origin, e.g., why permeability is altered or vascular smooth muscle tone is impaired: Optimal design principles, vascular smooth muscle tone—setting and modulation, and endothelial cell transducer activity—arterial and capillary. The end result in either case should serve to restore optimal physical conditions for microvascular exchange. Local homeostasis is thus stabilized by a combination of structural and functional factors.

Although numerous examples of functional adaptation have been cited [16], structural adaptations have not been given adequate consideration. More subtle changes in microvascular deployment are difficult to recognize unless some type of morphometric analysis is used, so that emphasis is placed on extreme or distinctly pathological phenomena.

When the terminal vascular beds in different tissues are examined, it can be seen that a variety of adaptive processes are utilized to achieve the same end result, depending upon the physical constraints imposed by the architecture of the tissue, the level of metabolic activity, and the extremes in the range of functional activity.

Specific changes in individual vessels or in the realignment of the hierarchical array of microvessels are induced by different physical factors: Wall thickening reflects the uneven strain resulting from transmural pressure changes; increases in length and new vessel formation result from flow-related factors. Comparatively few data on modifications of the network pattern as a whole have been presented until quite recently despite its obvious importance for tissue homeostasis.

Conclusion

Attempts to utilize recent advances in our knowledge of the biology of cells that make up the microcirculation have been hampered by the fact that data on individual segments through intravital microscopy may not have the resolution needed to deal with the problem. In a similar context, we cannot deal adequately with macromeasurements for masses of tissue without knowledge of the contribution of the individual microvessels that make up the terminal vascular bed in that tissue. In neither case do we have enough information to extrapolate from one to the other. Either measurements at both the macro- and microlevels must be made concurrently during a set of test perturbations or a model based on firm structural information must be developed. Three-dimensional arrays of this kind are not as yet available for complete arterial-capillary-venular pathways.

Despite their limitations, in situ measurements of microvascular behavior in humans do offer a number of distinctive applications: Detection of high-risk individuals, index of disease severity, effectiveness of therapy, and disease etiology; they can serve as a measure of the effectiveness of a therapeutic regime and for the early detection of disease-related inroads on tissue homeostasis. Disease that is intrinsic to the microvascular constituents themselves remains a distinct possibility, but its indentification requires future methodological developments for the in situ measurement of the cellular constituents of the microvascular system.

References

1. Ditzel J (1967) The in vivo reactions of the small blood vessels to diabetes mellitus. Acta Med Scand [Suppl] 476: 123–134

2. Davis E, Landau J, Ivry M (1966) Clinical capillary microscopy. Thomas, Springfield
3. Parving HH (1975) Microvascular permeability to plasma proteins in hypertension and diabetes mellitus in man—on the pathogenesis of hypertensive and diabetic microangiopathy. Danish Med Bull 22: 217–233
4. Tsushima N, Nakayama R (1983) Microcirculation of bulbar conjunctive. In: Tsuchiya M, Wayland H, Oda M, Okazaki I (eds) Intravital observations of organ microcirculation. Excerpta Medica, Amsterdam, pp 15–28
5. Bollinger A, Frey J, Jager K, Furier J, Seglias J, Siegenthaler W (1982) Patterns of diffusion through skin capillaries in patients with long terms diabetes. N Engl J Med 307: 1305–1310
6. Ryan TJ (1977) The microcirculation of the skin in old age. Gereont Clin 8: 327–337
7. Fenton BM, Zweifach BW, Worthen DW (1979) Quantitative morphometry of conjunctival microcirculation in diabetes mellitus. Microvasc Res 18: 153–166
8. Zweifach BW, Chen PC, Kovalcheck S (1981) Digital image processing of the microcirculation in diabetes. Bibl Anat 20: 653–655
9. Fagrell B, Tooke J, Östergren J (1984) Vital capillaroscopy for evaluating skin microcirculation in humans. Prog Appl Microcirc 6: 129–140
10. Wells RE Jr (1964) Rheology of blood in the microvasculature N Engl J Med 270: 832–839
11. McMillan DE (1975) Deterioration of the microcirculation in diabetes. Diabetes 24: 944–957
12. Viollier AF, Senn JH (1978) Disorders in leukocyte function in diabetes mellitus. Schweiz Med Wschr 108: 1585–1587
13. Mayrovitz HN, Roy J (1983) Microvascular blood flow: evidence indicating a cubic dependence on arteriolar diameter. Am J Physiol 245: H1031–H1038
14. Murray CD (1926) The physiological principle of minimum work: I. The vascular system and cost of blood volume. Proc Natl Acad Sci USA 12: 207–214
15. Kamiya A, Togawa T (1972) Optimal branching of the vascular tree. Bull Math Biophys 34: 431–438
16. Davis E (1980) Clinical vasomicroscopy. In: Kaley G, Altura BM (eds) Microcirculation. University Park Press, Baltimore, pp 223–234

Microvascular Flow Disturbances: Rheological Aspects

PETER GAEHTGENS[1]

Introduction

Strongly nonhomogeneous distribution of blood flow represents one of the most characteristic features of the microcirculation under the various circulatory conditions which are associated with flow disturbances. It has been shown in numerous experimental studies both in isolated whole organs and individual microvascular beds that two phenomena dominate the perfusion under such circumstances.

First, reduction of perfusion pressure leads to an alteration of the distribution of segmental flow resistance. As shown by direct measurements, dilatation of precapillary arterioles [1] occurs presumably as a result of metabolic and/or myogenic relaxation of the smooth muscle cells. This causes the precapillary resistance to decrease. Conversely, an increase in flow resistance is found in postcapillary vessels [2], such that the pre- to postcapillary resistance ratio is usually decreased considerably (Fig. 1). It is thought that this readjustment of the resistance distribution serves to maintain capillary pressure at a relatively constant level.

Second, the number of perfused arteriovenous pathways is usually found to be reduced under conditions of low flow or decreased perfusion pressure. This is experimentally identified as a decrease of capillary surface area [8] or functional capillary density. Direct intravital microscopy may reveal that flow is reduced or even brought to a complete standstill in some vascular pathways, while others still show apparently unchanged perfusion. As a consequence of both the increased nonuniformity of spatial flow distribution and the complete exclusion of individual flow pathways from perfusion, the function of the microcirculation as an exchange system is compromized.

Microvascular Flow Disturbances

Among the various attempts to explain the occurrence of microvascular stasis in the face of positive driving pressures, closure of the precapillary arterioles was

[1]Department of Physiology, Freie Universität Berlin, Arnimallee 22, 1000 Berlin 33, Federal Republic of Germany

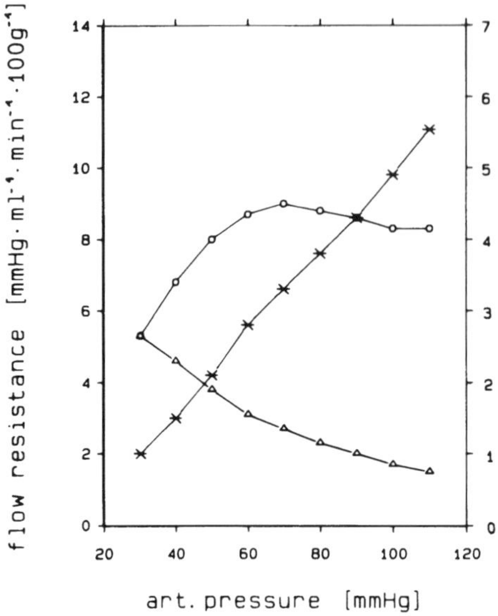

Fig. 1. Effect of reduction of arterial pressure on arterial and venous segmental resistances in skeletal muscle. The arteriovenous resistance ratio (*right ordinate*) decreases significantly with pressure reduction. Recalculated from Thulesius and Johnson [2]

long postulated until it became increasingly clear that progressive arteriolar dilatation occurs instead [1]. This may be due to both myogenic and metabolic mechanisms in a situation where both transmural pressures and blood flow are reduced, but this clearly rules out the possibility that capillary flow stop is due to precapillary closure. While in this respect intravital microscopic studies confirm whole-organ measurements of segmental resistance distribution, the occurrence of capillary stasis still remains to be unexplained.

For these and other reasons, the contribution of blood rheology to microcirculatory flow disturbances has been extensively discussed [3]. Such discussions are usually based on the fact that blood represents a strongly non-Newtonian fluid, which implies that its apparent viscosity increases significantly upon reduction of the shear rate, particularly below a level of approximately 50 s^{-1}. Furthermore, measurements obtained in large coaxial viscometers have been extrapolated to a yield value of shear stress at which the fluid turns into a solid and thus comes to a standstill because of the formation of red cell aggregates. Such aggregates have also been believed to resist the low shear stresses occurring at low driving pressures in a microvascular network, thus leading to what has been termed "rheological occlusion." Although this concept appears to be quite convincing, it still suffers from the fact that direct measurements of the rheological properties of blood under the conditions of low flow in the microcirculation are extremely difficult [9, 10] and have not yet been obtained to an extent which would allow precise predictions of their hemodynamic relevance during low flow states. Thus, most of the rheological discussion pertinent here is based on the theoretical application of data obtained in vitro to the hemodynamic situation in the microvascular system.

Blood Rheology

It must also be clearly pointed out that the present understanding of blood flow properties even under in vitro conditions of viscometric or tube flow is not complete. Several complicating factors need to be taken into account before the conventional shear stress-shear rate relationship obtained in vitro can be applied to blood flow in a cylindrical tube or vessel. It has long been known that overall blood viscosity, if determined in tubes whose diameter decreases below approximately 300 μm, decreases substantially and eventually approaches that of the suspending plasma at tube diameters in the range of 10–20 μm [11]. This Fahraeus-Lindqvist [12] effect is to some extent related to the dependence of tube hematocrit on tube diameter at a given and constant discharge hematocrit (Fahraeus effect) [13]. As a consequence, it must be expected that in the immediate pre- and postcapillary vessels, plasma viscosity is by far the most important rheological determinant of resistance, whereas hematocrit is of a lesser importance here than in the macrocirculation.

However, with regard to low-flow conditions, it is relevant to add that this interpretation is only based on experimental observations at very high rates of shear, i.e, in the absence of manifest red cell aggregation. More recent experimental evidence obtained in small tubes [4–6] indicates that the formation of red cell aggregates at low shear causes viscous resistance to fall (rather than to rise, as predicted by rotational viscometry), such that under low-shear flow the range of tube diameters in which the Fahraeus-Lindqvist effect becomes effective is greatly enlarged [14]. As a consequence, apparent blood viscosity at low shear is not only very similar in tubes of different size (between approximately 150 and 30 μm) but is also very low compared with its value at high shear.

Such observations suggest that the contribution of blood rheology to flow resistance in low-flow states is really much smaller than hitherto assumed and in fact does not suffice to explain the observed increase of resistance in the postcapillary venules nor the occurrence of stasis in an increasing number of arteriovenous pathways. This conclusion is substantiated by the fact that these in vitro studies also showed the absence of a yield point in the sense of complete standstill of flow despite the presence of positive driving pressures [14]. It must also be added that the in vitro data suggesting the existence of a yield point [15–17] do not agree quantitatively: Substantial differences in the magnitude of the observed yield pressures are noted, which calls for caution in the application of such findings to in vivo conditions. Furthermore, the arteriovenous pressure drops observed in vivo at the point of flow stagnation [1] are substantially greater than could be explained on the basis of rheological observations of a yield point. This goes to show that considerable uncertainty still exists with respect to the direct application of rheological knowledge to microcirculatory flow disturbances.

Blood Flow in Tubes

In discussing the rheological behavior of blood in tube flow, one additional phenomenon must be mentioned. Almost all of the data that have been obtained up to now were determined in horizontal flow systems, in which, in principle, the

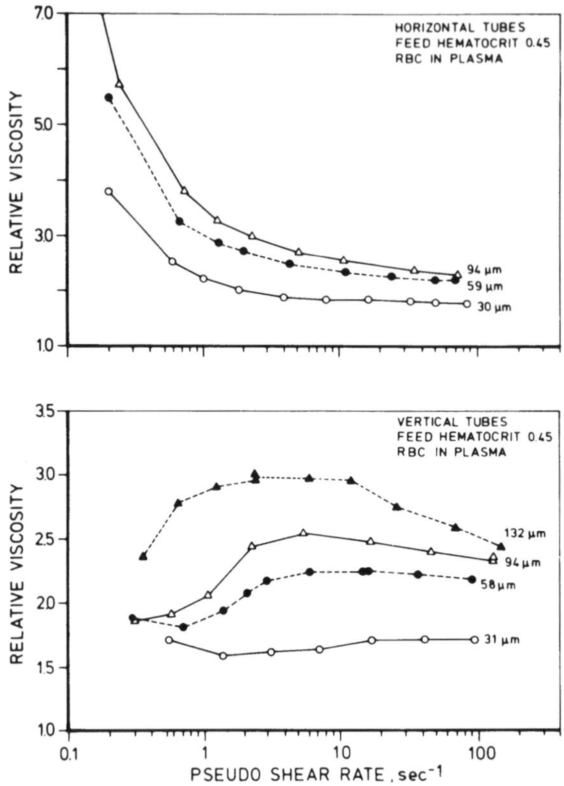

Fig. 2a, b. Variation of apparent blood viscosity with shear rate in **a** horizontal and **b** vertical tubes of different diameter. Data redrawn from Reinke et al. [5]

occurrence of sedimentation cannot be entirely ruled out. If blood rheological behavior is studied in vertical tubes [4], in which the effect of sedimentation is significantly reduced, an entirely different behavior is in fact observed: Upon reducing the shear rate from values of around 100 s^{-1} the apparent viscosity increases very slightly but then decreases again strongly (Fig. 2) as soon as red cell aggregation occurs and, therefore, a cell-free plasma layer is formed which reduces the frictional losses of pressure energy [5]. Again, these studies indicate that at very low shear rates (below approximately 1 s^{-1}) apparent viscosity in vertical tubes is very low and almost independent of tube diameter in the range studied. It is, therefore, fair to say that in contrast to the conclusions drawn from rotational viscometry, the manifestation of red cell aggregation in this system leads to a decrease rather than increase of viscous resistance. In horizontal tubes of the same diameter range, however, reduction of shear rate leads to a substantial increase of viscous resistance (Fig. 2), which must be attributed to the sedimentation of the aggregating red cells [14] and this in the horizontal tube leads to a nonsymmetric radial red cell distribution profile [5]. This pattern looks quite similar to the one seen in rotational viscometers, although it is brought about by a very different combination of phenomena. The increase of viscosity at very low shear notwithstanding, these recent studies with horizontal tubes have not confirmed the existence of a yield point in the sense of complete flow stagnation in the presence of positive driving pressures [5]. However, a proper description of the flow pattern existing at extremely low driving forces in such a system of fully developed axial nonuniformity of red cell concentration is not yet completed and needs further exploration. Therefore, a direct contribution of the rheological properties of blood to the observation of stasis in a microvascular network cannot at present be entirely assessed.

The conclusion from these findings clearly indicates that in the tube flow of blood, sedimentation plays a very important role in determining effective viscous resistance as a function of shear rate. It is clearly not possible to extrapolate these findings directly and quantify the rheological effects in the microcirculation, mainly because of two reasons: First, the effect of red cell sedimentation must be a function of vessel orientation and, obviously, of the ratio between red cell transit time and sedimentation velocity. Both single vessel orientation and transit time will vary considerably within any given microvascular network, such that the overall effect cannot easily be assessed. Second, the presence of consecutive bifurcations within a branching microvascular network introduces additional phenomena which are associated with the distribution and partition of plasma and red cells at the branch points. While some of the mechanisms underlying these partition phenomena have been studied both in vitro and in vivo [18, 19], the distribution of cellular and plasmatic flux in a complete network at low-flow rates cannot be derived even though the mechanisms at each single bifurcation may be well understood. This is due to the fact that radial asymmetry in any vessel segment feeding a bifurcation will dominate cell partition at the next bifurcation. Therefore, the complex sedimentation pattern within the segments of a network completely modifies not only local hematocrits, and thus the effective viscous resistance in each single vessel segment, but also the dispersion of transit pathways and transit times through this network.

Rheological Factors Causing Flow Stagnation

Even though it may at present not be possible to quantify the contribution of blood rheology as one of the factors causing flow stagnation, it is still possible that flow disturbances in microvascular networks are at least in part due to the rheological phenomena mentioned above. It appears, however, that red cell sedimentation has been underestimated within the group of rheological phenomena affecting microvascular flow. Strongly heterogeneous hematocrit distribution, which may follow from sedimentation in single vessel segments, represents a cause of strongly heterogeneous distribution of viscous resistance; this may eventually favor flow stagnation in single vessel segments and in the dependent parts of the network, while neighboring areas supplied by vessel segments receiving very much reduced hematocrit will show relative overperfusion. From a rheological point of view, the greatly increased heterogeneity of intranetwork perfusion and, thus, of substrate delivery is not so much the result of shear-dependent aggregation of red cells, but mainly a secondary consequence of cell sedimentation within vessel segments.

It appears quite remarkable that under normal perfusion conditions the heterogeneity of flow distribution is so relatively small. This is, of course, only possible because of the presence of metabolically controlled smooth muscle tone.

Reduction of flow due to reduction of driving pressure, therefore, primarily causes a reduction of resistance in the precapillary resistance vessels, where metabolic vessel dilatation dominates over any possible rheological effects. However, this is only true as long as the vasodilatory capacity is still present and can be actively recruited. If this is not the case, such as in postischemic hypoperfusion or in situations of prolonged flow reduction, the described rheological phenomena will take place, eventually limiting the possibility of effective microcirculatory reperfusion.

While the quantitative role of blood rheology for flow in the microcirculation in general is thus not completely clear, the possibilities of rheological obstruction of single capillaries by single blood cells appears to be better understood. A large body of literature has accumulated to describe, in quantitative terms, the micromechanical properties of blood cells which are relevant for passage through vascular channels whose diameters are smaller than those of resting blood cells. The normal microrheological properties of red cells which allow deformation, stable orientation, and tank treading motion of the cell membrane during capillary flow do not appear to represent a significant impediment for normal capillary passage. Although theoretically the possibility exists that under very low driving pressures single capillary channels are effectively obstructed due to red cell micromechanics [20–22], most of the present data would suggest that this phenomenon occurs at much lower pressures than are actually observed in vivo. This statement may, of course, have to be modified if substantial variations in capillary diameter exist very locally, thus escaping detection by the usual methodology of intravital microscopy. If such localized stenosis occurs to some extent, single red cells may indeed also cause capillary stasis [22], particularly in the case of compromised microrheology.

White Cells and Capillary Plugging

Under normal circumstances, however, white cells are much more likely to contribute to the flow disturbances seen in the capillary bed during low-flow states. Reports of capillary plugging by leukocytes [23–25] have shown that this phenomenon occurs whenever the perfusion pressure is significantly reduced under otherwise normal conditions. In contrast to the red cells, even the normal microrheology of white blood cells allows such an event to take place, because of their effectively much lower deformability [26]. Although this has never been experimentally verified, it is quite possible that the narrowest arteriovenous pathways in the microvessel network are the first to be excluded from flow by obstructing leukocytes. In order to understand the effects brought about by leukocyte plugging in a given microvascular network, it is therefore of great interest also to analyze the topology of such networks because of the possibility of white cell shunting under physiological flow conditions and redistribution of white cell flows in the case of low-flow perfusion. In the rat mesentery, white cell concentration has been found to increase systematically from the most proximal to the most distal capillaries within a given network [27]. This is largely due to the exclusion of leukocytes from proximal side branches because of their low relative flow rate. Obviously, the most distal capillaries belong to the longest

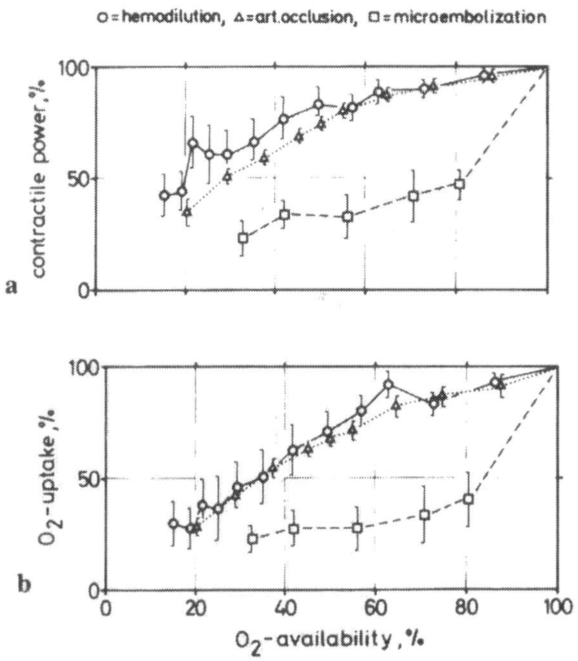

Fig. 3a, b. Effect of reduced O_2 supply on performance (**a**) and O_2 uptake (**b**) of exercising skeletal muscle. O_2 supply was modified by hemodilution, partial occlusion of the feeding artery, or intra-arterial injection of microspheres

arteriovenous pathways, which are therefore most prone to capillary plugging by white cells.

Although plugging of capillaries by white cells may not represent a permanent event, even transient but repetitive capillary occlusion is of great functional significance, since it very effectively reduces the period during which free supply to the dependent tissue is possible [28]. Due to the interrelationship between single blood cell micromechanics and the distribution of such cells within microvascular networks, it may well be that the functional consequences of capillary plugging by white cells will be different in different tissues in which different topologies of the microvascular network exist. In any case, a substantial increase in flow heterogeneity must be expected to occur. Since flow heterogeneity in turn leads to a reduction in the efficiency of exchange systems, it is quite understandable that the flow disturbances caused at the level of the microcirculation lead to a much greater functional deficit than the reduction of general oxygen supply at the level of the macrocirculation. This is illustrated in Fig. 3, in which data are compared that were obtained from skeletal muscle during systemic hemodilution, partial occlusion of the large supplying artery, and after intra-arterial injection of microspheres. It is evident that in the last case both function and O_2 consumption are most dramatically affected even though the total supply may be relatively well maintained. This documents the substantial reduction of efficiency which occurs in the microcirculation when flow heterogeneity is greatly enhanced. These experimental data may serve as a model of the effects brought about by white cell plugging of single capillaries and thus illustrate the potentially enormous relevance of blood rheology in this context.

The as yet unexplained observation of increased venous resistance upon reduction of perfusion pressure may also, at least in part, be due to the rheological behavior of white cells. Under a variety of conditions which lead to microcirculatory flow disturbances, white cells are seen to adhere to the vascular endothelium of postcapillary venules, a phenomenon also typical for any nonspecific inflammatory reaction. It has been shown in model studies [7] and supported by direct measurements in microvessels [9] that adhering white cells may cause a significant elevation of flow resistance by reducing the effective diameter of the vessel segment. Adhesion of white cells is, however, only possible if the cells have marginated as a result of rheological interaction with other blood cells in flow. The mechanisms of this rheological margination have been studied in detail [29–31]; clearly, any increase in red cell aggregation brought about by, e.g., reduction of flow or shear rates, will cause a displacement of white cells toward the vessel wall and thus favor margination and adhesion. This is a very potent mechanism demonstrating the close interrelation between rheological behavior and microvascular hemodynamics.

Conclusion

In summary, the complex architecture of the microvascular system as well as its responses to a local deficit of substrate supply do not permit at present a straightforward and simple application of general hemorheology to the analysis of microcirculatory flow disturbances. The bulk properties of the blood which are mostly described on the basis of in vitro viscometry may not be appropriate guidelines in the assessment of the contribution of rheology to such disturbances, and microrheological information on flow behavior of blood cell suspensions is still rather incomplete. However, individual mechanisms can be identified which clearly result from cellular micromechanics and interactions during flow and show pronounced effects on hydrodynamic resistance. This is most obvious for single vessel occlusion by single poorly deformable red or white cells, but it may also be true for the manifestation of increased heterogeneity of flow within the microvessel networks which is characteristic of most flow disturbances that are functionally relevant.

References

1. Reneman RS, Slaaf DW, Lindbom L, Tangelder GJ, Arfors KE (1980) Muscle blood flow disturbances produced by simultaneously elevated venous and total muscle tissue pressures. Microvasc Res 20: 307–318
2. Thulesius O, Johnson PC (1966) Pre- and postcapillary resistance in skeletal muscle. Am J Physiol 210: 869–872
3. Schmid-Schönbein H (1976) Critical closing pressure or yield shear stress as the cause of disturbed peripheral circulation? Acta Chir Scand Suppl 465: 10–19
4. Reinke W, Johnson PC, Gaehtgens P (1986) Effect of shear rate variation on apparent viscosity of human blood in tubes of 29 to 94 μm diameter. Circ Res 59: 124–132
5. Reinke W, Gaehtgens P, Johnson PC (1987) Blood viscosity in small tubes: effect of shear rate, red cell aggregation, and sedimentation. Am J Physiol 253: H540–H547
6. Gaehtgens P (1987) Tube flow of human blood at low shear: the effect of red cell

aggregation on apparent viscosity. Clin Hemorheol 7: 399 (Abstract)
7. Bagge U, Blixt A, Braide M (1986) Macromodel experiments on the effect of wall-adhering white cells on flow resistance. Clin Hemorheol 6: 365–372
8. Dahlberg B (1979) Transcapillary solute exchange in skeletal muscle after injury and during shock. Acta Physiol Scand [Suppl] 472: 1–82
9. Lipowsky HH, Usami S, Chien S (1980) In vivo measurement of "apparent viscosity" and microvessel hematocrit in the mesentery of the cat. Microvasc Res 19: 297–319
10. Lipowsky HH, Kovalcheck S, Zweifach BW (1978) The distribution of blood rheological parameters in the microvasculature of cat mesentery. Circ Res 43: 738–749
11. Gaehtgens P (1980) Flow of blood through narrow capillaries: rheological mechanisms determining capillary hematocrit and apparent viscosity. Biorheology 17: 183–189
12. Fahraeus R, Lindqvist T (1931) The viscosity of the blood in narrow capillary tubes. Am J Physiol 26: 562–568
13. Fahraeus R (1928) Die Strömungsverhältnisse und die Verteilung der Blutzellen im Gefäßsystem. Klin Wschr 7: 100–106
14. Gaehtgens P (1987) Tube flow of human blood at near zero shear. Biorheology 24: 367–376
15. Kiesewetter H, Radtke H, Schmid-Schönbein H (1981) The yield shear stress of blood in branched models of the microcirculation. Effect of hematocrit and plasma macromolecules. Bibl Haemat 47: 14–20
16. Merrill EW, Benis AM, Gilliland ER, Sherwood TK, Salzman EW (1965) Pressure-flow relation of human blood in hollow fibers at low flow rates. J Appl Physiol 20: 954–967
17. Meiselman HJ, Merrill EW, Salzman EW, Gilliland ER, Pelletier GA (1967) Effect of dextran on rheology of human blood: low shear viscometry. J Appl Physiol 22: 480–486
18. Klitzman B, Johnson PC (1982) Capillary network geometry and red cell distribution in hamster cremaster muscle. Am J Physiol 242: H211–H219
19. Fenton BM, Carr RT, Cokelet GR (1985) Nonuniform red cell distribution in 20–100 micron bifurcations. Microvasc Res 29: 103–126
20. Zarda PR, Chien S, Skalak R (1977) Interaction of viscous incompressible fluid with an elastic body. Comp Meth Fluid Struct Int Prob 26: 65–82
21. Secomb TW, Skalak R, Zkaya N, Gross JF (1986) Flow of axisymmetric red blood cells in narrow capillaries. J Fluid Mech 163: 405–423
22. Secomb TW (1987) Flow-dependent rheological properties of blood in capillaries. Microvasc Res 34: 46–58
23. Bagge U, Amundson B, Lauritzen C (1980) White blood cell deformability and plugging of skeletal muscle capillaries in hemorrhagic shock. Acta Physiol Scand 108: 159–163
24. Gaehtgens P, Ley K, Pries AR, Müller R (1985) Mutual interaction between leukocytes and microvascular blood flow. Progr Appl Microcirc 7: 15–28
25. Engler RL, Schmid-Schönbein GW, Pavelec RS (1983) Leukocyte capillary plugging in myocardial ischemia and reperfusion in the dog. Am J Pathol 111: 98–111
26. Bagge U (1976) Granulocyte rheology. Blood Cells 2: 481–490
27. Ley K, Pries AR, Gaehtgens P (1987) Distribution of leukocytes in microvascular networks. Pflügers Arch Ges Physiol [Suppl 1] 408: R21 (Abstract)
28. Gaehtgens P (1987) Pathways and interactions of white cells in the microcirculation. Progr Appl Microcirc 12: 51–66
29. Nobis U, Pries AR, Cokelet GR, Gaehtgens P (1985) Radial distribution of white cells during blood flow in small tubes. Microvasc Res 29: 295–304
30. Goldsmith HL, Spain S (1984) Margination of leukocytes in blood flow through small tubes. Microvasc Res 27: 204–222
31. Schmid-Schönbein GW, Usami S, Skalak R, Chien S (1980) The interaction of leukocytes and erythrocytes in capillary and postcapillary vessels. Microvasc Res 19: 45–70

Microvascular Regulation: Normal Function and Disturbance in Disease

Paul C. Johnson[1]

Introduction

An understanding of the disturbance of microvascular regulation requires first that we understand the normal state. Our current understanding of normal regulation has developed slowly over many years. The earliest view of the regulation of the peripheral circulation was that blood flow to the tissues was determined essentially by sympathetic constriction of arterial vessels and by arterial perfusion pressure. To the extent that the special needs of organs for increased blood flow were recognized (such as skeletal muscle in exercise), it was thought that neurally mediated local vasodilation was responsible. Shunting of flow among organs according to local needs was also hypothesized. For example, the vasoconstriction of skin blood vessels observed during mental activity was thought to increase total peripheral resistance by activation of the sympathetic nervous system, increasing arterial pressure, and, thereby, forcing more blood through the brain [1]. A few workers such as Roy and Brown [2] did suggest that locally produced metabolities such as carbon dioxide and hydrogen ions may cause vasodilation in special circumstances such as exercise and reactive hyperemia. But there was an overriding emphasis on the central regulation of all aspects of peripheral circulatory function.

Principal Features of Vascular Control

With the development of techniques for isolated organ perfusion, it became apparent that central control was, at best, a partial answer. For example, isolated organs such as skeletal muscle and myocardium [3] showed functional hyperemia during increased metabolic activity and exhibited basal vascular tone, which could not be attributed to the sympathetic nervous system since the organs were completely denervated. Moreover, the isolated organs showed a tendency to maintain constant blood flow as arterial pressure was altered (autoregulation) and exhibited reactive hyperemia after a period of flow stoppage [4]. At the

[1]Department of Physiology, University of Arizona College of Medicine, Tucson, AZ 85724, USA

same time, studies of blood flow in intact and isolated organs showed that neural control mechanisms did play a significant role in overall regulation of vascular resistance [5]. By the early 1960s, an overview of the control of the peripheral circulation would have incorporated the following essential features and mechanisms:

Principal features of vascular control:
a) Initial vascular tone
b) Decreased tone with reduced arterial perfusion pressure (autoregulation)
c) Decreased tone with increased functional activity (functional hyperemia)

Principal known mechanisms of vascular control:
a) Neural vasoconstriction (α-receptor stimulation)
b) Myogenic regulation (sensitivity to intravascular pressure)
c) Metabolic regulation (sensitivity to local metabolic conditions)

In the intact, innervated organ, initial vascular tone could be attributed in part to neural vasoconstrictor activity, but the latter could not, of course, explain that tone which remained after denervation. The residual tone after denervation, which was usually quite substantial, could be attributed to a myogenic mechanism, that is, a sensitivity to intravascular pressure [6]. The decreased tone with reduced arterial perfusion pressure (autoregulation) could be ascribed to the myogenic mechanism since the stimulus would be lost as pressure was lowered. But it could also be ascribed to a buildup of vasodilator metabolites subsequent to the fall in blood flow, reducing O_2 delivery and washout of metabolites.

The third principal feature, functional hyperemia, could be explained as a central mechanism involving loss of neural vasoconstriction to the organ except that it was seen in denervated preparations. The myogenic mechanism would not explain functional hyperemia except possibly in specialized circumstances of muscle contraction momentarily lowering transmural pressure in the blood vessels and would not be important overall in explaining functional hyperemia. On the other hand, metabolically produced vasodilator substances could readily explain functional hyperemia.

One approach to situations where multiple mechanisms may be involved is to invoke the law of physiological parsimony, that is, to explain phenomena with as few mechanisms as possible. And the mechanisms themselves should be as simple as we can imagine them, consistent with the observations. While I do not know how valid this law is, it is a useful starting point. Thus, for example, one aspect of the physiological parsimony approach would be to postulate that all vascular beds are essentially alike and all possess the same regulatory mechanisms even though the manifestation of control in various vascular beds is quite different. Skeletal muscle, for example, shows a 10- to 20-fold increase in blood flow during functional hyperemia and relatively low flow in the resting state. In other beds, such as the splanchnic region, blood flow is higher in the resting tissue and functional hyperemia is more limited [7]. A similarity principle can be invoked here as we note that metabolic activity in skeletal muscle increases much more during maximum activity than in other organs and thus the concentration of vasodilator metabolites may change much more in skeletal muscle than in other beds. Thus, it seems worth examining that there is a single set of controls for all vascular beds which expresses itself quantitively differently in different organs because the vasculature is exposed to a greater or lesser change in mediators.

It may also be postulated that a single vasodilator substance is released and causes functional hyperemia in all organs. The question of whether a single vasodilator substance mediated functional hyperemia has been studied by a number of investigators, considering adenosine as the universal vasodilator. Watkinson et al. [8] have produced evidence for adenosine as a physiological mediator of functional hyperemia in cardiac muscle and brain, but available evidence is less encouraging for adenosine as a mediator in skeletal muscle. Moreover, we also have to consider the possible importance of differences between metabolic schemes in the slow oxidative and fast glycolytic muscle. It has been suggested in skeletal muscle that a variety of substances play a role, with potassium believed to be important at the initiation of exercise and other vasodilator substances coming into play as exercise continues. If we consider functional hyperemia in other vascular beds, such as the salivary glands where bradykinin is believed to be important [7], the stomach where prostaglandins may play a role, and the intestine where cholecystokinin is thought to mediate functional hyperemia [7], we find a great diversity of mediators rather than physiological parsimony. Since these last-mentioned mediators, which operate in the gastrointestinal tract, are not products of oxidative metabolism their tie to functional hyperemia presumably is not by metabolic pathways. Thus, at the minimum, we have two principal ways in which functional hyperemia is brought about, namely through oxidative metabolism and through humoral agents released by an other process. If we consider K^+ released from the parenchymal cell as a separate pathway, there is a third type of chemical mediator of functional hyperemia. We can, however, see that the mediators fall into several categories, which makes understanding of the mechanisms a little more rational.

It appears, therefore, that we have to examine chemical mediators of functional hyperemia on an organ-by-organ basis and not assume that there is a single "generic" chemical control which can be understood from studies on one or two organs. One can hope, however, that several organs have similar control systems. In any case, the mechanism by which each of these controls works in a given organ will need to be analyzed in detail.

Local Mechanisms

With these general considerations as background, I would like now to consider several local control systems and be a little more specific as to how some of these systems may operate. I will use as my primary focus the role which local mechanisms play in blood flow autoregulation. It is clear that more than one mechanism is involved in autoregulation, depending upon the vascular bed.

Let us look first at the possible role of metabolic factors in blood flow autoregulation. Blood flow autoregulation is a rather ubiquitous phenomenon as shown in Fig. 1. It is quite pronounced in a number of vascular beds, the kidney, brain, and myocardium, where flow is essentially constant over a wide range of arterial pressures [4]. If we pursue the law of physiological parsimony, we might again propose that autoregulation has a single cause such as the metabolic control

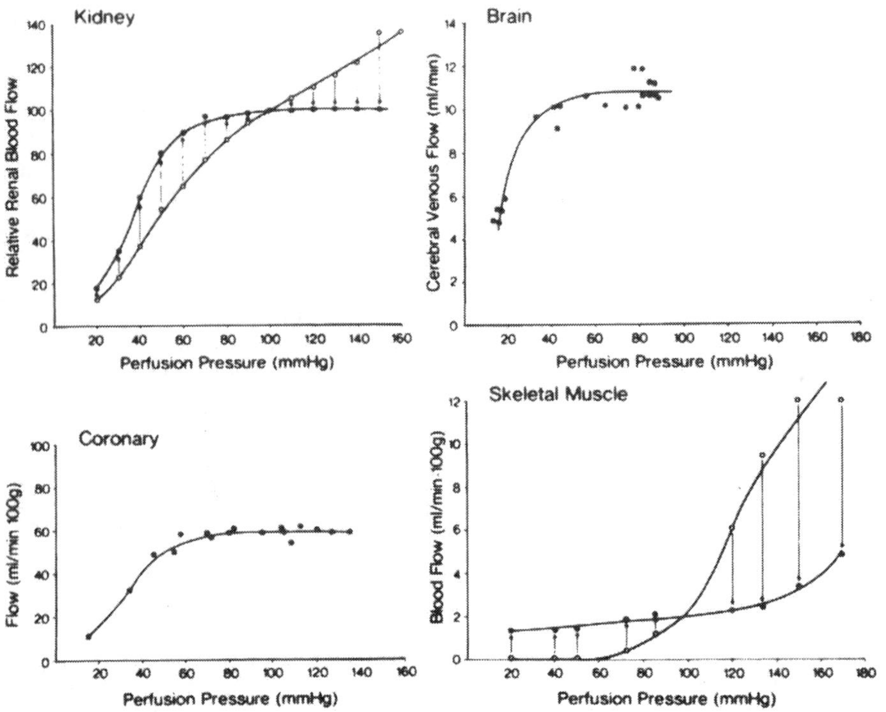

Fig. 1. Examples of blood flow autoregulation in four vascular beds. After Johnson (1980) with permission

mechanism. According to the metabolic hypothesis, vasodilator metabolites are produced constantly by the tissues under normal circumstances. When arterial pressure is reduced and flow falls, the concentration of metabolites increases, due to either reduced washout or an increased production of vasodilator metabolites as a secondary effect of reduced tissue PO_2. Since the latter possibility seems more likely, let us examine it further.

A hypothesis of blood flow autoregulation based upon tissue PO_2 is shown in Fig. 2 from the work of Granger and Shepherd [9]. As shown in this diagram, tissue PO_2 depends upon blood flow, which determines the rate of O_2 delivery, and capillary density, which determines the average diffusion distance from capillary to adjacent mitochondria in the parenchymal cell. It is also postulated that as the PO_2 falls in the vicinity of the mitochondria, a vasodilator substance is produced and diffuses to the precapillary sphincters, which relax and increase the number of capillaries with flow. This increased density reduces the diffusion distance and increases tissue PO_2. It is suggested that alteration of capillary density is the first line of defense so to speak when flow decreases, perhaps because the precapillary sphincter or its analog in skeletal muscle, the terminal arteriole, is more responsive to an increase in concentration of vasodilator metabolites.

The next line of defense is dilation of the arteriole, which will increase blood flow and, therefore, oxygen delivery. When tissue PO_2 falls further and blood is flowing in the capillaries, the concentration of vasodilator substances reaches

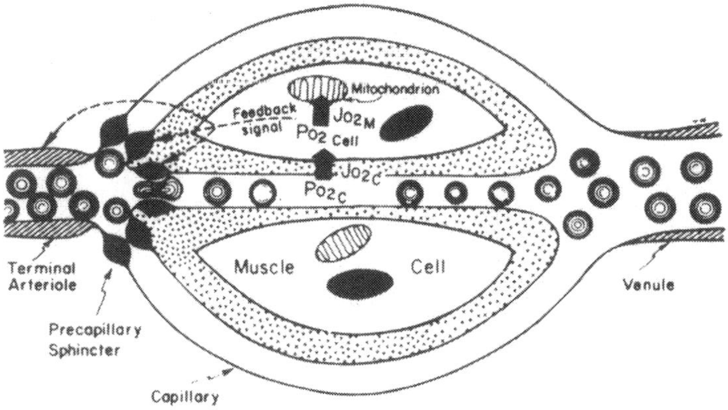

Fig. 2. Hypothesis of local blood flow regulation in which terminal arteriole regulates flow and flow distribution in the capillary bed by metabolic feedback mechanism. After Granger and Shepherd [9] with permission

such levels that the arterioles now begin to dilate. In these model studies, it can be shown that oxygen consumption is better maintained when both precapillary sphincter and resistance vessel mechanisms are present than when only one is present [9].

Our own studies on the role of metabolic factors in autoregulation have utilized the sartorius muscle of the cat, either completely isolated and perfused [10] or simply exteriorized.

To test the hypothesis that arteriolar tone during autoregulation in skeletal muscle is controlled by metabolic factors relating to oxygen delivery, we have examined autoregulation in the sartorius muscle during elevated tissue oxygen.

The surgically isolated sartorius muscle is mounted on the microscope stage and a clamp is placed on the arterial circuit to control arterial perfusion pressure. The muscle is transilluminated with a condensor and light source beneath the stage. A velocity-measuring system is incorporated into the microscope and a diameter-measuring device is used off-line to obtain readings of velocity and diameter as arterial pressure is reduced in a stepwise fashion. From arteriolar diameter and red cell velocity, volume flow can be calculated. Also, with repetitive replay, red cell velocity in a group of capillaries can be determined using the dual window.

When arterial pressure is reduced in a stepwise fashion, as shown in Fig. 3, flow becomes more continuous in the capillary network, suggesting a functional increase in capillary density. Also, the arterioles dilate and calculated volume flow is maintained in the arterioles, indicating good flow autoregulation [10].

To test the hypothesis that these changes in vascular diameter were due to a vasodilator produced in response to oxygen lack, we increased the ambient oxygen level over this muscle from 0% to 10% or 20% oxygen in nitrogen. As we will show subsequently, this procedure significantly increases tissue PO_2. If the hypothesis is correct, then providing oxygen from another source should reduce the tissue level of vasodilators and interrupt the vasodilator feedback loop.

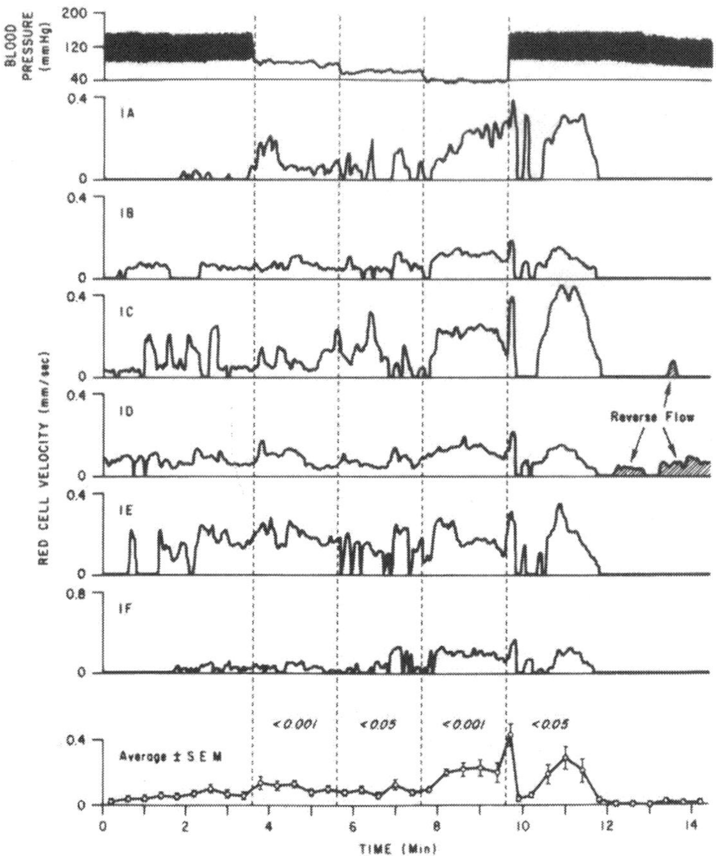

Fig. 3. Simultaneous flow in six adjacent capillaries in cat sartorius

To control the ambient PO_2 level, we enclosed the microscope stage in a clear plastic tent and ventilated the area over the muscle with pure nitrogen or a nitrogen–oxygen mixture. The surface of the muscle was covered with a thin layer of silicone fluid. We found that the arterioles constricted under elevated oxygen quite substantially, as would be expected if less vasodilator were being produced. We also found that all the arterioles dilated with pressure reduction except the largest first-order vessels, which seemed not to dilate with pressure reduction in this series of experiments (Fig. 4) [10]. This autoregulatory dilation was weakened under 10% oxygen in nitrogen and abolished under 20% O_2, indicating that perhaps a vasodilator is no longer produced when tissue PO_2 is elevated.

Subsequent to this study done by Sullivan and Johnson, a report appeared in the literature which suggested an alternative mode of action for oxygen, namely a direct effect on the arteriole. This work was reported by Jackson and Duling [11] using the hamster cheek pouch. By trimming away the tissue immediately surrounding a length of arteriole, they were able to eliminate any likely effect

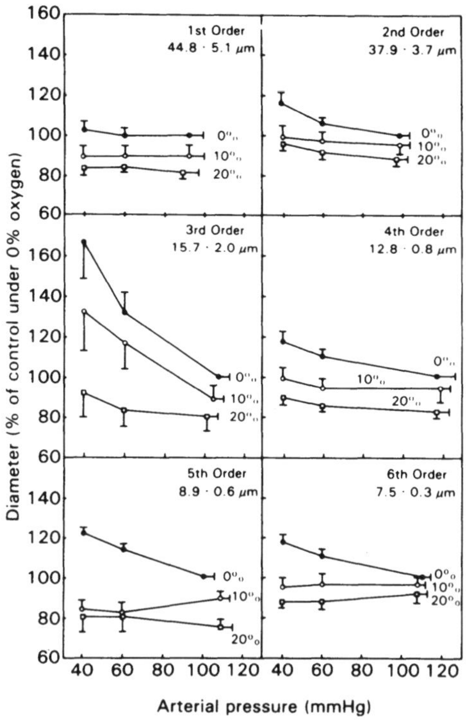

Fig. 4. Diameter changes in arterioles of cat sartorius muscle with stepwise reduction in arterial pressure in six orders of arterioles. Effects of increasing ambient O_2 level from 0% to 10 and 20% O_2 are shown. After Sullivan and Johnson [10] with permission

of vasodilator metabolites produced in the surrounding tissue. However, when the oxygen level over this preparation was altered they still observed constriction of the arteriole. This constriction was correlated with increased oxygenation of the blood in the arteriole. Thus, it appears that there is a direct constrictor effect of oxygen on the arteriole. They also found that an oxygen-induced vasoconstriction could be propagated along the arteriole to a region where tissue oxygen levels were not altered. These findings indicate that a direct action of oxygen on the arteriole must be considered in our overall assessment of the role of oxygen in autoregulation.

At this point, it is pertinent to consider the oxygen levels in the arteriole itself and how these levels might be affected by altering the ambient oxygen levels over the tissue. It was shown by Duling and Berne [12] that there is a very substantial oxygen loss along the length of the arterioles. If the PO_2 over the tissue is elevated, one would expect that this oxygen loss would be attenuated and the PO_2 in the most distal vessels would be most affected.

In our laboratory, we have recently utilized the Whalen oxygen electrode to measure PO_2 at various points in the sartorius muscle arteriolar and capillary network [13]. The findings are shown in Table 1. As indicated in this table, there is a gradual fall in periarteriolar PO_2 from the second to the fifth order arterioles under 0% O_2. Under 10% O_2, there is surprisingly no change in periarteriolar PO_2; we would have expected to see a rise. The reason for this absence of change is probably related to the vasoconstriction and associated fall in blood flow which occurs under oxygen. Since there is no rise in periarteriolar PO_2

(which is very nearly the same as intraluminal PO_2), it is likely that there is no local effect of elevated oxygen directly on the arteriole. There is, however, an increase in tissue PO_2 at the venous end of the capillary. This increase in tissue PO_2 could reduce the production of vasodilator metabolites and cause the arterioles to constrict. This rise in parenchymal PO_2 may also be responsible for the abolition of autoregulatory dilation as arterial pressure is reduced, since this tissue level would no longer be dependent upon oxygen delivery from the bloodstream. Definitive evidence that a change in PO_2 of the parenchymal cells is responsible for autoregulation requires additional experiments, in which PO_2 would be measured at various tissue sites during the autoregulatory response to reduced arterial pressure under different ambient PO_2 levels.

In passing, further comment should be made on the possible site or sites of production of vasodilator metabolites. If we consider the usual scheme of tissue PO_2 distribution, the lowest O_2 tension would be found at the venous end of the capillary network. Therefore, it would seem that this is the most likely site for production of metabolites. One caveat that should be entered, however, is that tissue PO_2 levels are generally well above the critical level for aerobic metabolism, which is generally thought to be of the order of 1 mmHg based on in vitro studies. In our studies, the average tissue level was above 20 mmHg. Of course, critical PO_2 may be different in the intact tissue or there may be oxygenases which have a higher k_m. Also, a few areas where tissue PO_2 is quite low may be critically important in controlling flow. A second consideration is that sites of low tissue PO_2 may be some distance from the arteriole which regulates flow to the region. Thus, the response time could be rather slow.

Let us now turn to the possible role of other mechanisms in autoregulation. We have seen in skeletal muscle that autoregulation can be completely abolished when ambient oxygen is increased—suggesting that metabolic mechanisms may completely explain the autoregulatory phenomenon. But autoregulation is also seen in the cat mesentery, where metabolic factors are of lesser importance [14]. In microcirculatory studies of the cat mesentery, the preparation is isolated and perfused from the animal in a manner analagous to that used for the sartorius muscle. When arterial pressure to the mesentery is reduced, the arterioles dilate and a calculated volume flow is well maintained (Fig. 5), demonstrating a pronounced autoregulation in this vascular bed. In the cat mesentery, there is evidence for a myogenic response or pressure sensitivity of the arterioles. Very simply put, the concept is that as intravascular pressure rises the arteriole is stimulated to contract. The most direct test of this hypothesis is to elevate pressure in the vascular bed in the absence of a change in flow. This can be done in several ways. One involves stopping flow completely in the isolated intestinal loop and connecting the arterial and venous extracorporeal circuits to a static pressure reservoir. The reservoir is then elevated to produce a step increase in intravascular pressure. This pressure increase causes sustained constriction of the arterioles, which begins to weaken somewhat in the 3rd min, possibly due to developing hypoxia of the preparation.

There is also evidence that tissue oxygen tension is not important in autoregulation. When the ambient PO_2 level over the mesentery is elevated, autoregulation is not altered significantly (Lang and Johnson, unpublished data).

It has been proposed that the myogenic response reflects a tendency of the

Table 1. Oxygen tension (mmHg) at sites in cat sartorius muscle

Ambient O_2 concentration	Suffusion solution	Periarteriolar oxygen tension: 2nd order arteriole	Periarteriolar oxygen tension: 3rd order arteriole	Periarteriolar oxygen tension: 5th order arteriole	Venous capillary
0%	16.1 ± 2.9	50.5 ± 3.3	51.2 ± 8.3	40.1 ± 2.4	22.8 ± 3.3
10%	66.2 ± 4.4	47.5 ± 3.2	50.0 ± 7.1	41.4 ± 3.5	35.2 ± 2.5
n	34	17	4	12	12

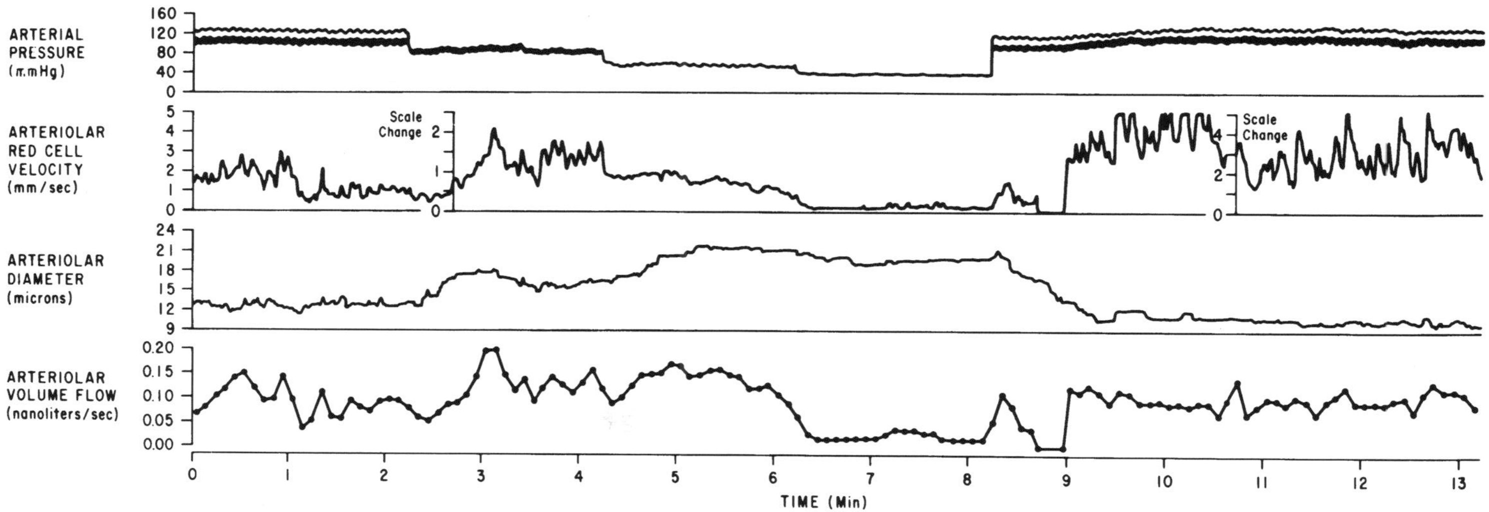

Fig. 5. Effect of stepwise reduction of arterial pressure on diameter and calculated volume flow in arterioles of cat mesentery. After Johnson and Intaglietta [13] with permission

smooth muscle cell to maintain a constant wall tension in the arteriole. It has also been suggested that, at least in brain arteries, the myogenic response is mediated by endothelial cells since removal of these cells abolishes the response [15]. Whatever the mechanism may prove to be, it is obvious that the myogenic response is an important control system in certain vascular beds.

Control Mechanism in Abnormal States

Let us turn now to consider how these control mechanisms may be altered in abnormal states.

In hemorrhagic hypotension, arterial pressure is reduced, which should induce an autoregulatory response and help to maintain blood flow. However, at the same time, sympathetic nerve activity increases, which should induce arteriolar constriction and reduce blood flow further. At the microcirculatory level, it has been observed that hemorrhage leads to arteriolar constriction in skeletal muscle, but the results are complex. In some studies, it has been noted that small arterioles dilate while larger arterioles constrict [16]. This is interpreted as due to a dominant effect of sympathetic activity on large arterioles, while the small arterioles appear to be more responsive to metabolic influences. It might also be suggested that the small arterioles lack sympathetic innervation. There are two reasons for thinking this is not the case. First, small arterioles constrict to the same degree (percentage) as large arterioles to sympathetic trunk stimulation. However, the constriction is not maintained: Vascular escape rapidly occurs. Second, when ambient PO_2 levels over muscle are elevated, the dilation of small arterioles during hemorrhage is suppressed. It remains to be determined why the small arterioles are more responsive to metabolic influences. Since large and small arterioles are embedded in the same tissue, it would appear that both should be subjected to the same metabolic influences. Perhaps the vascular smooth muscle in small arterioles is different from that in large arterioles. Alternatively, perhaps the intraluminal PO_2 plays a role, since it is higher in the large arterioles. Both of these possibilities deserve further study.

Since vascular resistance rises in skeletal muscle with hemorrhage it appears that the constriction of the large arterioles more than compensates for the dilation of the small arterioles. However, there are apparently concurrent changes in other areas of the microcirculation, which may contribute to the rise in resistance. It has been reported that white cells adhere to the venular wall during prolonged hypotension [16]. This effect would tend to increase vascular resistance, at least to a modest degree. Perhaps more importantly this phenomenon would tend to elevate capillary pressure. In extremely low-flow states, plasma volume tends to fall, whereas with moderate levels of hypotension fluid is reabsorbed from the tissue spaces and plasma volume rises, presumably because capillary pressure falls [17].

From a homeostatic point of view, the negation of autoregulation by the sympathetic nervous system during hemorrhage may be considered advantageous to the organism, since it allows diversion of cardiac output to more critical organs such as the brain and myocardium. The temporary suppression of autoregulation also assures that capillary pressure will fall, which will lead in turn to fluid reabsorption and restoration of plasma volume and filling pressure of the heart. Thus, the overriding influence of sympathetic control in vascular beds such as skeletal muscle is doubly important.

If systemic arterial pressure rises, the effects are the opposite of those seen with arterial pressure reduction: Sympathetic nerve activity decreases and local control mechanisms are completely dominant. In this instance, autoregulation plays a much different function, namely to protect the organ from overperfusion. The most deleterious aspect of overperfusion is probably not the elevated flow (although elevated tissue oxygen might lead to increased free radical formation), rather the elevation of capillary pressure might lead to capillary damage. In the case of the brain, this could lead to disruption of the blood-brain barrier and very serious consequences.

In considering these two examples it is clear that if the normal autoregulatory responses are compromised by disease, there could be serious consequences whenever blood pressure moves outside the normal range. A fall in arterial pressure would cause underperfusion in essential organs such as the brain and myocardium. The consequences would be less important in tissues such as skeletal muscle where central control mechanisms override local control. As noted above, a rise in arterial pressure without the buffering affect of autoregulation could lead to capillary damage.

Suppression of the autoregulatory response is seen when an organ is traumatized, and it is not uncommon in brain injury [18]. Two levels of effect are seen on the brain circulation in trauma. The first level is characterized by loss of the normal autoregulatory response. The second, more severe situation is the development of false autoregulation as capillary damage allows rapid outward movement of fluid from the blood in the tissue. In this instance, tissue pressure rises because the brain is encased in a rigid container. The tissue pressure then becomes a function of arterial pressure and constitutes a back pressure, which effectively offsets changes in arterial pressure. While this may seem desirable from the standpoint of flow regulation, it occurs at the expense of further aggravation of injury to the capillaries and disturbance of the normal fluid environment of the cerebral tissue. Thus, the presence of flow autoregulation is not a clear indicator that microcirculatory function is normal.

Acknowledgment. This research was supported by NIH grants HL AM 15390, HL 07249, and HL 17421.

References

1. Howell WH (1918) A Textbook of physiology. Saunders, Philadelphia, p 634
2. Roy CS, Brown GJ (1880) The blood pressure and in the variations in the arterioles, capillaries and smaller veins. J Physiol (Lond) 2: 323–359
3. Berne RM (1964) Regulation of coronary blood flow. Physiol Rev 44: 1–29
4. Johnson PC (1964) Review of previous studies and current theories of autoregulation. Circ Res 15 (Suppl 1): 2–9
5. Folkow B (1955) Nervous control of the blood vessels. Physiol Rev 35: 629–663
6. Folkow B (1952) A study of the factors influencing the tone of denervated blood vessels perfused at various pressures. Acta Physiol Scand 27: 99–117

7. Lundgren O (1978) Alimentary canal. In: Johnson PC (ed) Peripheral circulation. Wiley, New York
8. Watkinson WP, Foley DH, Rubio R, Berne RM (1979) Myocardial adenosine formation with increased cardiac performance in the dog. Am J Physiol 236 (Heart Circ Physiol 5): H13–H21
9. Granger HJ, Shepherd AP (1973) Intrinsic microvascular control of tissue oxygen delivery. Microvasc Res 5: 49–72
10. Sullivan SM, Johnson P (1981) Effect of oxygen on blood flow autoregulation in cat sartorius muscle. Am J Physiol 241 (10): H807–H815
11. Jackson WF, Duling BR (1983) The oxygen sensitivity of hamster cheek pouch arterioles: In vitro and in situ studies. Circ Res 53: 515–525
12. Duling BR, Berne RM (1970) Longitudinal gradients in periarteriolar oxygen tension. Circ Res 27: 669–678
13. Johnson PC, Intaglietta M (1976) Contributions of pressure and flow sensitivity to autoregulation in mesenteric arterioles. Am J Physiol 231: 1686–1698
14. Boegehold M, Johnson PC (1988) Periarteriolar and tissue PO_2 during sympathetic escape in skeletal muscle. Am J Physiol 254: H929–H936
15. Harder DR (1987) Pressure-induced myogenic activation of cat cerebral arteries is dependent on intact endothelium. Circ Res 60: 102–107
16. Eriksson E, Lisander B (1972) Low flow states in microvessels of skeletal muscle in cat. Acta Physiol Scand 6: 202–210
17. Lundvall J, Gustafsson D (1982) Impairment during marked hypotension of the plasma volume control in hemorrhage. Acta Physiol Scand 114: 371–378
18. Enevoldsen EM, Jensen FT (1977) "False" autoregulation of cerebral blood flow in patients with severe head injury. Acta Neurol Scand (Suppl) 64: 514–515
19. Johnson P (1980) The myogenic response. In: Bohr DF, Somlyo Ap, Sparks HV Jr (eds) Cardiovascular system. Handbook of Physiology, vol 2, chap 15. American Physiological Society, Bethesda, pp 409–442

Oxygen Delivery and Microcirculation in the Brain

DIETRICH W. LÜBBERS[1]

Introduction

When the oxygen pressure of the venous blood of the brain decreases below 20 Torr, the O_2 supply of the human brain becomes so insufficient that unconsciousness occurs [1], although at 20 Torr the blood still contains about one-third of the arterial O_2 concentration. However, because of its low oxygen pressure, this amount of oxygen is obviously useless for the O_2 supply. Opitz and Schneider [2] took these results as a sign for the brain tissue oxygen being mainly transported by diffusion and reported model calculations using Krogh's model of tissue oxygen supply.

Dissolved gases, like oxygen, are transported by diffusion if there is a local oxygen pressure difference. According to Henry's law, oxygen concentration, C_{O_2}, is proportional to oxygen pressure, P_{O_2}:

$$C_{O_2} = \alpha \cdot P_{O_2} \quad \text{or} \quad P_{O_2} = C_{O_2}/\alpha \tag{1}$$

$$\alpha = C_{O_2}/P_{O_2} \tag{2}$$

The proportionality constant, α, denotes the oxygen solubility. Equation (1) demonstrates that at the same P_{O_2}, the O_2 concentration increases with the oxygen solubility. The amount of oxygen, m_{O_2}, which is transported during the time interval, Δt, over the distance, Δl, into a tissue piece of an area, A, with a diffusion coefficient, D, is:

$$m_{O_2}/\Delta t = A \cdot D \cdot \alpha \, (\Delta P_{O_2}/\Delta l) \tag{3}$$

Equation (3) demonstrates clearly that with constant oxygen conductivity $(D \cdot \alpha)$, the spatial P_{O_2} difference, $\Delta P_{O_2}/\Delta l$, the local P_{O_2} gradient determines the magnitude of the diffusive transport. A large local O_2 consumption causes large O_2 fluxes, which produce large P_{O_2} gradients between the O_2-supplying capillary and O_2-consuming tissue. Thus, the local distribution of tissue P_{O_2} quantitatively reflects tissue oxygen supply.

[1]Max-Planck-Institut für Systemphysiologie, Rheinlanddamm 201, 4600 Dortmund 1, Federal Republic of Germany

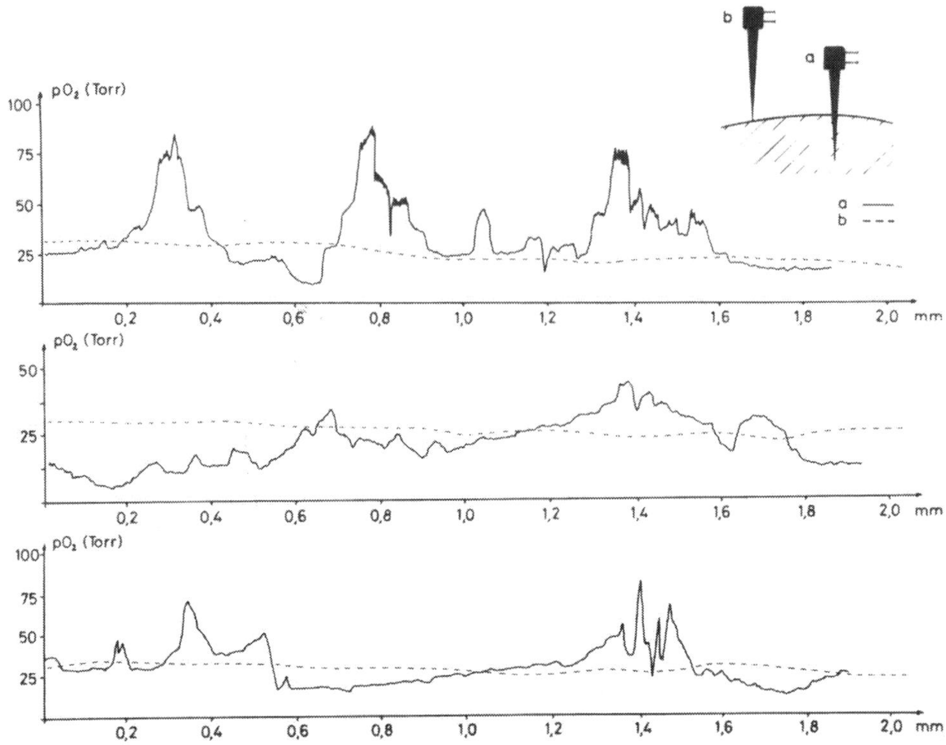

Fig. 1. P_{O_2} profiles within the cerebral cortex of the rat. With continuous speed of 150 μm/min, a membranized needle electrode (tip diameter 1–2 μm; *a*) was vertically inserted into the right hemisphere at three different sites of the exposed cortex. The other P_{O_2} electrode (*b*) measured the surface P_{O_2} during the experiment. Barbiturate anesthesia. After Baumgärtl and Lübbers [10]

In the steady state, oxygen supply by the capillary equals the tissue oxygen consumption, $\dot{V}_{O_2}$:

$$(C_{a,O_2} - C_{v,O_2}) \cdot \dot{B} = \dot{V}_{O_2} \tag{4}$$

$$C_{v,O_2} = C_{a,O_2} - (\dot{V}_{O_2}/\dot{B}) \tag{5}$$

where a signifies arterial, v venous, and $\dot{B}$ blood flow,

Equation (5) demonstrates that the venous O_2 concentration, C_{v,O_2}, depends on the blood flow, $\dot{B}$, in a hyperbolic way (circulatory hyperbola). Since capillary oxygen pressure and concentration are related to the O_2 dissociation curve, a similar dependence holds for the tissue P_{O_2}.

The existence of P_{O_2} gradients within the brain tissue between blood vessels was first recorded on the pial surface [3, 4]. Later, with the development of P_{O_2} microelectrodes of 1- to 5-μm-tip diameter by Silver [5], similar P_{O_2} profiles could also be measured within the brain tissue [6–9]. Figure 1 shows three P_{O_2} profiles of the cerebral cortex of the rat, which were obtained by puncturing perpendicularly the gray matter [10]. During the measuring period (ca. 15 min), the pial surface P_{O_2} remained constant (broken line in Fig. 1, $P_{O_2} = 32$ Torr), demonstrating a constant oxygen supply. Since the three-dimensional network of the brain capillaries lacks a preferential orientation [11], the tip of the puncturing electrode penetrated the tissue between different parts of the capillary network and consequently local tissue P_{O_2} varied. Sometimes, the tip of the electrode approached the arterial part of a vessel so that the tissue P_{O_2} came close to the arterial P_{O_2}, as in the upper panel of Fig. 1 at the three peak P_{O_2} values of 87, 86, and 76 Torr. Many tissue P_{O_2} values were below those of the venous P_{O_2}, which in Fig. 1 was close to the P_{O_2} of the broken line. In some experiments, the mean P_{O_2} of the gray matter was found to be independent of the depth of the puncture [9]; in other experiments, it decreased from the pial surface to deeper layers [12, 13]. The white matter had a lower mean tissue P_{O_2} [13].

For a correct interpretation of the spatial resolution of these P_{O_2} profiles, we have to take into account that the polarographic electrode influences the tissue P_{O_2} to be measured. The reason for this influence is that during the polarographic measurement, O_2 is reduced on the cathode surface. This oxygen diffuses from the tissue to the cathode, thereby changing the tissue P_{O_2}. To minimize this influence, electrodes with a small cathode surface, covered with a membrane, have to be used. Our needle electrode consisted of a Pt wire fused into a glass needle. The Pt cathode had a diameter of 0.5–1.0 μm. The Ag/AgCl reference electrode was sputtered on the shaft of the glass needle. The tip of the electrode had a small recess, which was filled and covered with a membrane, e.g., of polystyrene or collodium. The total outer diameter amounted to 1–2 μm. A rough estimate shows that in a homogeneous medium, 90% of the oxygen would come from a sphere the radius of which is about 3.15 times the diameter of the cathode, i.e., for our needle electrode a distance of about 1.6–3.15 μm. Since the mean capillary distance in the gray matter of the brain is about 60 μm, this analysis demonstrates that the used needle electrode was able to register P_{O_2} profiles between the capillaries with sufficient spatial resolution. It may be mentioned that this does not hold any more for an electrode with a 10-μm cathode, since in a homogeneous medium it would register the mean P_{O_2} of a tissue sphere with a diameter of 64 μm [10].

Normal Values of Tissue P_{O_2}

A good way to present the variability of P_{O_2} values in these profiles is to plot local P_{O_2} values as a P_{O_2} histogram [14]. Figure 2 shows the P_{O_2} histogram of the gray matter of the guinea pig brain measured by using recessed and membranized P_{O_2} needle electrodes with a tip diameter of 1–2 μm. On the abscissa, the P_{O_2} is plotted in classes of 5 Torr; on the ordinate, the percentage of the frequency of P_{O_2} values lying in the corresponding class is plotted. Only a few P_{O_2} values are larger than 70 Torr and come close to the arterial P_{O_2}. The skewed distribution is caused by the small O_2-binding capacity of the hemoglobin in the high P_{O_2} range, but additionally by the fact that O_2 diffuses into the tissue, not only along the capillary, but also along small arterioles and veins. The diffusive gas exchange along arterioles of 60–80 μm was demonstrated experimentally

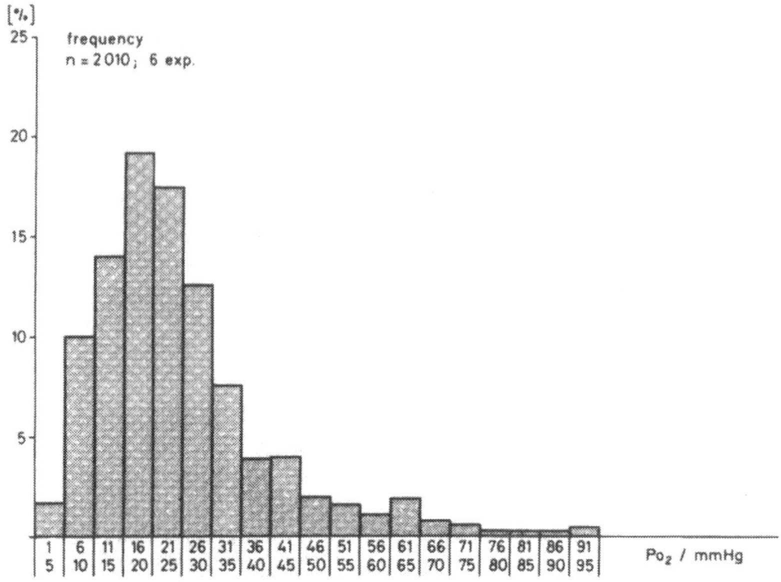

Fig. 2. P_{O_2} histogram of the blood-perfused guinea pig brain. Technique as in Fig. 1. Mean P_{O_2}, 23.3 Torr; median, 18 Torr. *n* number of measurements; six experiments, ten punctures. Barbiturate anesthesia

[15–17] and simulated by model calculations [18]. In P_{O_2} classes below 70 Torr, the ordinate increases gradually. This increase reflects partly the increasing O_2-binding capacity of hemoglobin. The maximun is in the range of 15–19 Torr. About 75% of all values are below the venous P_{O_2}. Similar histograms of the brain cortex are found in other species [5, 7, 9, 19].

To quantify the spatial variability of the local P_{O_2}, the P_{O_2} change over a distance of 10 μm was determined and is presented as a P_{O_2} gradient histogram. Figure 3 shows that in about one-third of all measurements, the P_{O_2} change over 10 μm was smaller than 1 Torr, and in about two-thirds of all cases smaller than 2 Torr.

Only 20 % of all gradients were larger than 10 Torr. The largest gradient of 24 Torr was only measured twice. This quantifies the impression of the P_{O_2} profiles in Fig. 1 that steep P_{O_2} gradients are not very frequent. Therefore, mean "local" P_{O_2} values, as for example measured by a 15-μm Pt electrode covered with a 12-μm cellophane and 12-μm Teflon membrane, still give a reasonable picture of the local P_{O_2} distribution of the brain. Since puncturing always causes trauma, in some cases it is preferable to use P_{O_2} surface electrodes. We used membrane-covered multiwire electrodes with eight Pt wires of a diameter of 15 μm, which were about 300–600 μm apart [20]. The comparison between P_{O_2} histograms measured by needle electrodes and P_{O_2} surface histograms measured by multi-wire P_{O_2} surface electrodes revealed that in the blood-perfused brain there is practically no difference in form, but the mean values of the P_{O_2} surface histogram may be shifted to somewhat higher values. In blood-free perfused prepara-

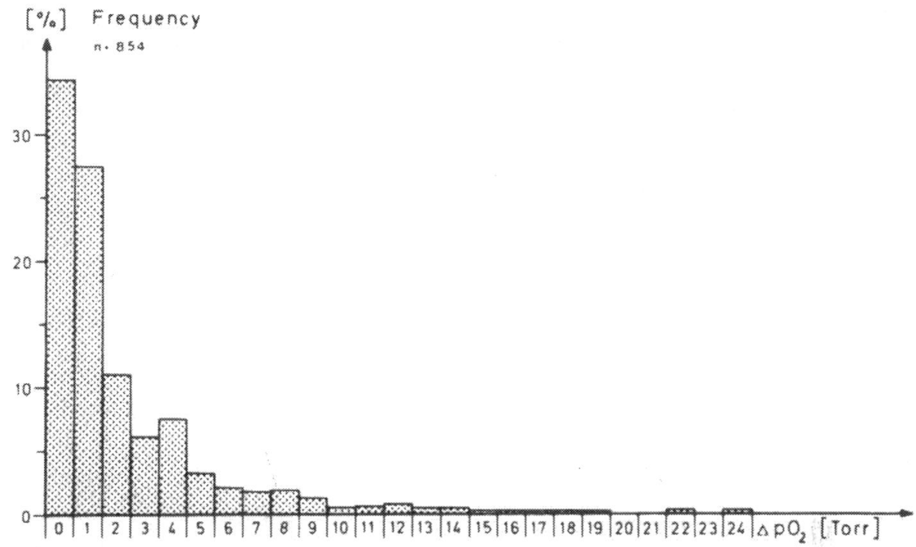

Fig. 3. Histogram of P_{O_2} gradients (over a distance of 10 μm) in the gray matter of the rat brain. Technique as in Fig. 1. In two-thirds of all measurements, the P_{O_2} gradients were smaller than 2 Torr. After Baumgärtl and Lübbers [10]

tions, however, large differences were observed [21].

Figure 4a demonstrates a surface P_{O_2} histogram of a hypoxic human brain [22]. In this P_{O_2} histogram, the number of low P_{O_2} values is increased. Low P_{O_2} values are also found with normal O_2 supply. Sometimes, tissue P_{O_2} values are practically zero, but single low P_{O_2} values cannot be taken as a sign of tissue hypoxia, since mitochondria have a critical P_{O_2} of about 0.1 Torr [23, 24], and in this low range P_{O_2} values cannot be correctly measured with polarographic P_{O_2} electrodes. However, the relative increase of the number of low P_{O_2} values causing a left shift of the P_{O_2} histogram (as seen in Fig. 4a) can be used as a reliable sign of tissue hypoxia. Figure 4b shows the normalization of the left-shifted P_{O_2} histogram after extirpation of an arteriovenous malformation of the cortex. This demonstrates in which way the P_{O_2} histogram can be used to evaluate the O_2 supply situation of a tissue. These findings show also that neither a single nor a mean tissue P_{O_2} value nor the venous P_{O_2} can be used to detect unequivocally tissue hypoxia.

Jöbsis and his group [25] concluded from measurements of the redox state of cytochrome aa_3 that relative hypoxia may exist in the brain with a normal physiological oxygen supply. They found that the redox state of cytochrome aa_3 was about 70% instead of the expected "normal" redox state of 90%–95%. However, such optical measurements in blood-perfused organs in vivo are very difficult. Since large perimitochondrial P_{O_2} gradients cannot be expected [26], there is no evidence for such a relative hypoxia from P_{O_2} measurements. This is in agreement with nuclear magnetic resonance (NMR) measurements of the energy state [27] and with measurements of the nicotinamide adenine dinucleotide NADH/NAD redox state [28] (see also Fig. 8a).

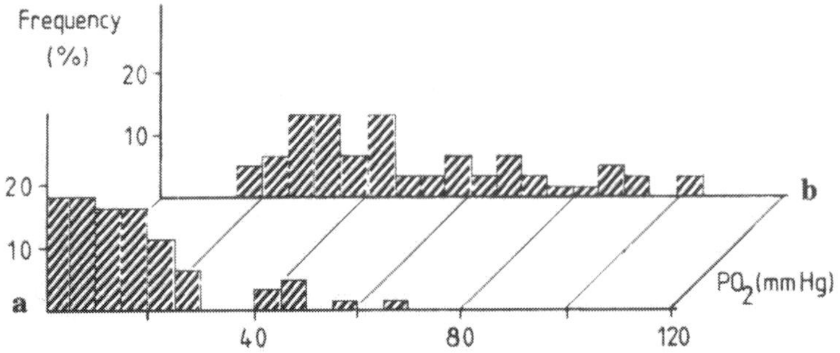

Fig. 4a, b. P_{O_2} histogram measured **a** before and **b** after extirpation of an arteriovenous malformation in adjacent cortex. The left-shifted hypoxic histogram (**a**) normalized after the operation (**b**). After Schultheiss et al. [22]

Tissue P_{O_2} and Blood Flow

As demonstrated in eq. (5), there is a hyperbolic dependence of the venous O_2 concentration on the flow. A similar relationship can be deduced for the tissue P_{O_2}, even if one takes into account the nonlinearity of the O_2 dissociation curve and the distribution of the P_{O_2} gradients within the tissue. Ivanow et al. [18] estimated that the normal flow velocity in the brain capillaries is so adapted that it lies in the mean range of the circulatory hyperbola, i.e., flow changes should be accompanied by distinct P_{O_2} changes. This, indeed, has often been observed, when the tissue P_{O_2} of the gray matter measured by 15-μm Pt surface electrodes was compared with heat clearance measurements [29]. With heat clearance, usually tissue volumes of several cubic millimeters are monitored. To obtain information about capillary circulation, we used a method with a higher spatial resolution, the pH_2/H_2 clearance method according to Lübbers and Stosseck [30–32]. When a bare palladinized pH_2 electrode of a diameter of 15 μm is used, the catchment volume includes about one to four capillaries. For a 100-μm pH_2 electrode, the number of capillaries increases to about 100. Figure 5a demonstrates that despite a constant regional flow, local microflow varies between 0 and 480 ml/(100 g·min), with a median of about 100 ml/(100 g·min) [33]. The four measuring sites are characterized by four different symbols. These measurements do not demonstrate the classic capillary recruitment with repeated stop and flow, but another kind of flow regulation—regulation by gradual variation of local microflow. Figure 5b compares pH_2/H_2 clearance measurements using pH_2 electrodes of three different diameters—100 μm, 50 μm, and 15 μm—which, as already mentioned, have considerably different catchment volumes. The 15-μm electrode shows the largest variability. It covers the microflow range between 0 and 590 ml/(100 g·min), with a mean value of 158 ± 123 ml/(100 g·min). The lowest class—0–49 ml/(100 g·min)—is the largest one. The mean value of the 50-μm electrode is 143 ± 60 ml/(100 g·min). The 100-μm electrode covers the microflow range between 30 and 300 ml/(100 g·min), with a mean value of 144 ± 55 ml/(100 g·min). There is still some argument about the validity of the pH_2/H_2 evaluation method [32], but in these experiments regional flow was measured simultaneously by Xe^{133} clearance. The regional flow in a tissue

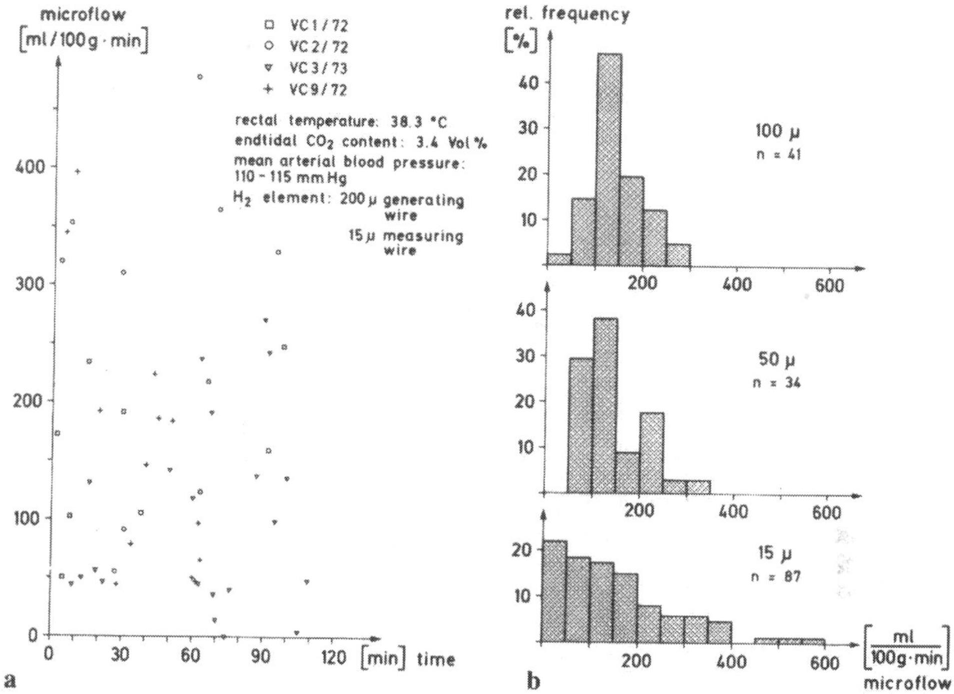

Fig. 5. a Temporal variations of microflow in the gray matter of the cat brain. Microflow (one to four capillaries) was measured at the same site for 2 h with a pH_2/H_2 surface electrode. The electrode was fixed on the gyrus suprasylvius of the cat cortex. barbiturate anesthesia. **b** Histogram of microflow measured with a 15-μm, 50-μm, and 100-μm pH_2 electrode. The histogram of the 15-μm pH_2 electrode shows the largest variability of microflow. During the experiments, regional flow was measured by Xe^{133} clearance and amounted to 107 ± 28 ml/(100 g·min). Barbiturate anesthesia

volume of about 1/2 cm^3 amounted to 107 ± 28 ml/(100 g·min) (n = 48). This demonstrates that the variability of the regional flow does not correctly reflect the simultaneous variability of the microflow. Since even with small P_{O_2} needle electrodes (tip diameter of 1–2 μm), we never observed such large variations of the local tissue P_{O_2}, we assume that in the gray matter each tissue site is supplied by several capillaries, so that the effect of flow variations in a single capillary is diminished by the contribution of the flow in the neighboring capillaries. These flow variations could be part of the total flow regulation in the capillary network; however, how this is brought about is unknown and needs further investigation. Nervous influence on the capillaries as well as signal processing by the endothelium have to be discussed. Glial cells may contribute to the local regulation. It may be mentioned that with autoradiographic methods, it was found that the density of the perfused capillary correlates well with local blood flow and metabolism, i.e., glucose utilization [34].

Regional flow often shows rhythmic variations—especially in nonanesthetized animals—which are independent of blood pressure waves or respiratory and metabolic rhythms [4, 35, 36]. Manil et al. [36] found that 70% of the frequency power spectrum of oscillations is in the range of 0.03–0.3 Hz (2–20/min; maximun, 6 and 15/min). Since frequency phase and amplitude vary spatially, local vascular oscillators must be present. The oscillations are sensitive to α-blocking agents; cooling decreases the frequency. The oscillations disappear in hypoxia, strong vasodilation, and vasoconstriction [35].

As far as blood pressure changes are accompanied by changes in local flow, tissue P_{O_2} changes correspondingly [29]. The intact brain shows excellent autoregulation of total and regional flow in the blood pressure range of about 50–160 mmHg. Consequently, the steady state values of tissue P_{O_2} remain quite constant despite large blood pressure changes, as shown for example in Fig. 6. In these experiments, no changes in extracellular K^+ and H^+ activities are observed [37]. However, at the level of the microcirculation, there is an inhomogeneous reaction of microflow: At some sites, the microflow may remain constant, whereas it simultaneously increases at other sites [38].

The special arterial supply of the brain allows considerable compensatory flow reactions. Temes et al. [39] successively occluded three of the large neck arteries of the dog and found that in the remaining arteries flow increased in such a way that tissue P_{O_2} remained practically unchanged. However, after clamping the middle cerebral artery (MCA), flow compensation by collaterals was mostly insufficient, so that tissue P_{O_2} decreased [e.g., 40]. The P_{O_2} histogram has also been used to study the effect of drugs in pathological situations [e.g., 41].

A compensatory flow increase is observed during isovolemic hemodilution [40, 42]. Figure 7 shows the behavior of the tissue P_{O_2} of the cat brain measured by a seven-wire Pt surface electrode. During isovolemic hemodilution from a hematocrit (Hct) of 45% to 25%, all seven P_{O_2} traces remained almost constant, as did end-tidal CO_2 and the electrocorticogram; only blood pressure increased somewhat at a Hct of 25%. A similar constancy of tissue P_{O_2} was also observed during isovolemic hemodilution after MCA clamp. These are remarkable regulatory reactions!

Tissue P_{O_2} and Changes in Arterial Blood Gases

From many experiments, it is known that arterial P_{O_2} may decrease to about 60 mmHg without affecting the brain blood flow [e.g., 43]. The reaction threshold for the blood flow increase is at a P_{a,O_2} of about 50 mmHg. Similarly, respiration of a hypoxic gas mixture with an F_{i,O_2} of about 0.12 reduces arterial and tissue P_{O_2}. That this P_{O_2} decrease is not followed by a reactive hyperoxia can probably be taken as a sign of a sufficient oxygen supply. The respiration of a gas mixture with an F_{i,O_2} of 0.08 produces a larger decrease of tissue P_{O_2} and is followed by a distinct reactive hyperoxia [44]. Figure 8 demonstrates the reaction of tissue P_{O_2} to mild and severe arterial hypoxia measured simultaneously at seven different sites [45]. In Fig. 8a, respiration of a 10% O_2 mixture decreases tissue P_{O_2} to different but fairly constant levels. During the subsequent air respiration, the initial P_{O_2} values are reached with only slight fluctuations. During respiration of a 2% O_2 gas mixture, however, all tissue P_{O_2} values approach zero. Then, in air respiration, a distinct reactive hyperoxia is seen in six traces with different time-

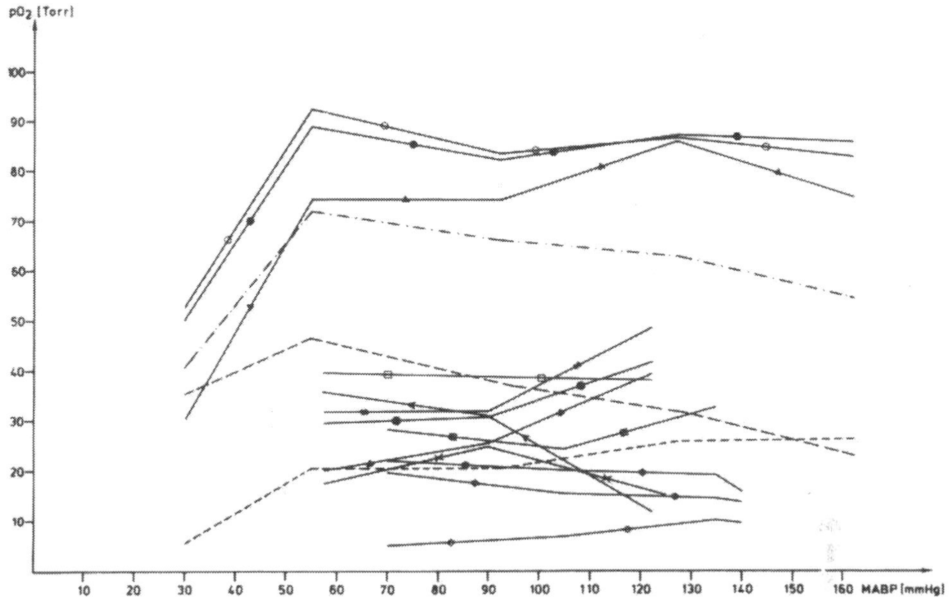

Fig. 6. Surface P_{O_2} of the cat brain during change in blood pressure. In the range of flow autoregulation, tissue P_{O_2} measured by a membrane-covered 15-μm Pt electrode remained almost constant. After Leniger-Follert [37]

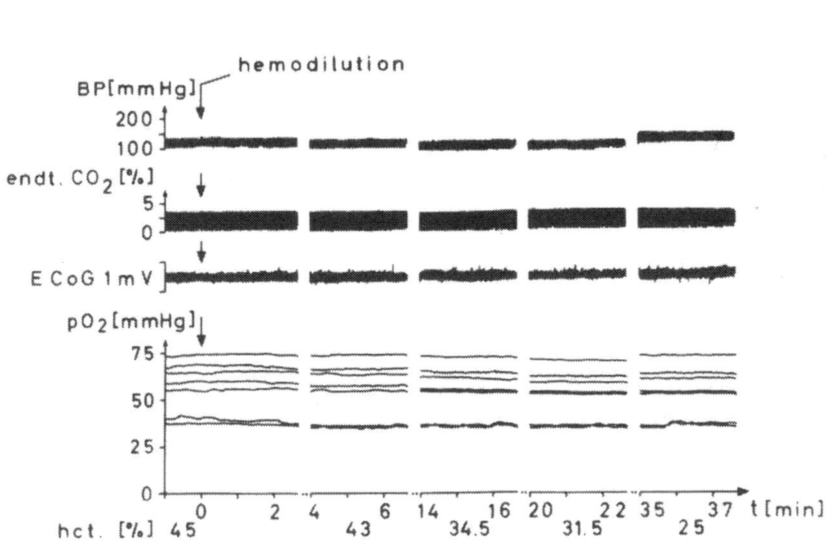

Fig. 7. Surface P_{O_2} of the cat brain during isovolemic hemodilution. P_{O_2} was measured by a multiwire membrane-covered P_{O_2} surface electrode (seven Pt wires of 15-μm diameter) without changing the measuring site. Hematocrit (*hct*) was changed stepwise by isovolemic hemodilution with 10% dextran 40 from 45% to 25%. *BP* blood pressure, *endt* CO_2 end-tidal CO_2, *ECoG* electrocorticogram. After Chan and Leniger-Follert [40]

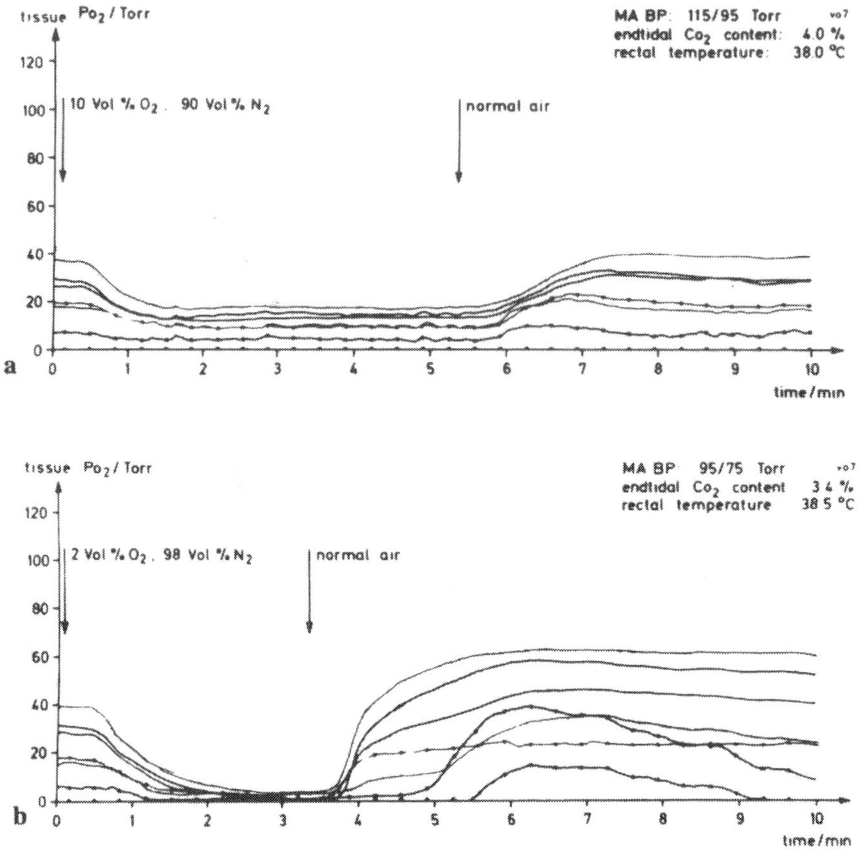

Fig. 8a, b. Local tissue P_{O_2} of the cat brain during mild and severe arterial hypoxia. Measuring technique as in Fig. 7. **a** Mild arterial hypoxia by respiring a gas mixture of 10% O_2 in N_2. **b** Severe arterial hypoxia by respiring a gas mixture of 2% O_2 in N_2. After Leniger-Follert et al. [45]

courses and different magnitudes; however, there is still one trace (in Fig. 8b the dotted line fourth from the bottom) which reaches its initial level without overshoot, demonstrating the heterogeneity of local reactions.

Simultaneous measurements of microflow with the pH_2/H_2 technique (100-μm diameter) reveal inhomogeneous flow reactions during hypoxia [46]. In Fig. 9, tissue P_{O_2}, microflow (pH_2 trace: increase of pH_2 means decrease of flow), and blood pressure are recorded simultaneously during respiration of a 5%O_2 gas mixture. It can be seen that there are three different types of flow reaction: (a) decrease of flow, (b) increase of flow, (c) flow passively follows the blood pressure. Despite these different local reactions of microflow, overall regional flow increased during hypoxia. These experiments demonstrate clearly that in the capillary range during hypoxia, there is a local redistribution of microflow. We think that in the brain tissue, capillaries or microareas exist with "luxury resting

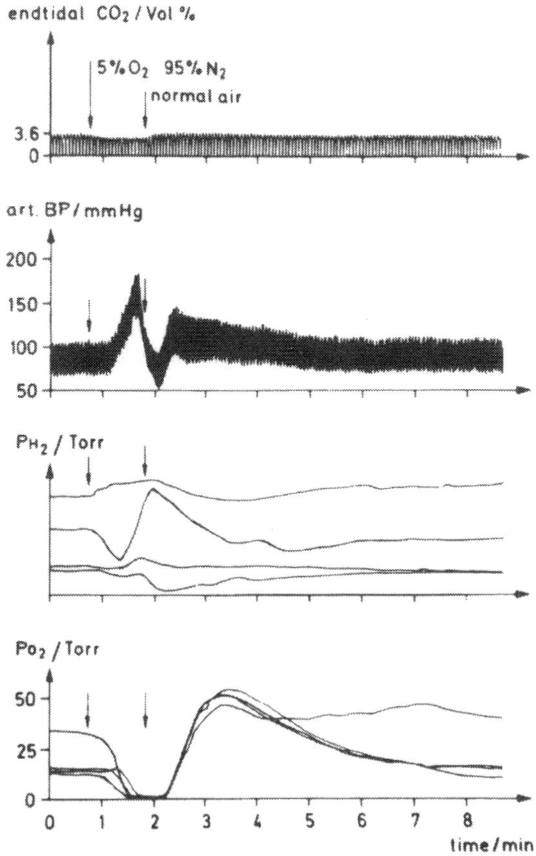

Fig. 9. Microflow, local tissue P_{O_2}, and blood pressure during severe arterial hypoxia. Local P_{O_2} was measured with a multiwire surface electrode (four Pt wires of 15-μm diameter), microflow by a pH_2/H_2 surface element (generating Pt wire, 200 μm; measuring wire, 100 μm). The electrode was in contact with the gyrus suprasylvius (exposed cat brain). Barbiturate anesthesia. After Lübbers and Leniger-Follert [46]

perfusion." This luxury perfusion of such "flow capillaries" allows blood to be diverted quickly to areas in which an increase of flow is needed without changing overall blood flow.

Respiration of gas mixtures with increased O_2 content increases the arterial P_{O_2}. This P_{a,O_2} increase is accompanied by a compensatory flow decrease so that only a moderate increase of tissue P_{O_2} results [35]. Burgess [47] observed that the compensatory vasoconstriction can be so large that in the awake rat, tissue P_{O_2} remains constant even when high pressure is applied causing a P_{O_2} of 5.4 bar. After anesthesia with barbiturate, this P_{O_2} constancy disappears. Vasoconstriction at high oxygen pressure could also be observed in isolated arteries, but there are regional differences in sensitivity [e.g., 48].

A more detailed analysis demonstrates that during hyperoxia the reactions of

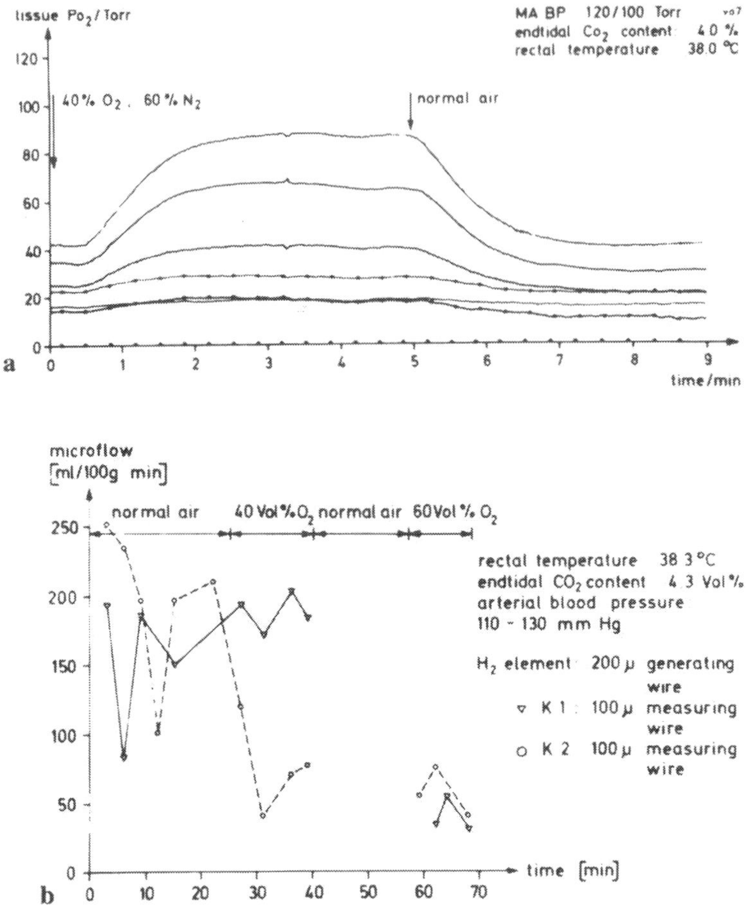

Fig. 10a, b. Local tissue P_{O_2} of the cat brain during arterial hyperoxia. Measuring technique as in Fig. 8. **a** During respiration of a 40% O_2 gas mixture, local P_{O_2} reacted differently at different sites. **b** Microflow measured simultaneously at two sites showed after respiration of a 40% O_2 gas mixture a decrease at one site and no change at the other, whereas after respiration of a 60% O_2 gas mixture microflow decreased at both sites. After Leniger-Follert et al. [45]

tissue P_{O_2} are heterogeneous. Figure 10 shows that, for example, at seven different sites about 350–600 μm apart, different P_{O_2} reactions occur after respiring a gas mixture with 40% oxygen in N_2. At some sites, tissue P_{O_2} increased and at other sites it remained almost constant. At one-third of all investigated sites, tissue P_{O_2} increased, whereas at the other two-thirds tissue P_{O_2} changed very little or remained constant. In a few cases, tissue P_{O_2} decreased or increased at first and then decreased. The local reaction pattern always remained constant. Simultaneous pH_2/H_2 microflow measurements showed that these different P_{O_2} reactions are caused by corresponding changes in microflow [45, 46]. In hyperoxia, flow compensation can occur in less than 1 s, since even with a quick and sensitive P_{O_2} electrode no change of tissue P_{O_2} was observable. This speaks in favor of an O_2 sensor reaction within the arterial vasculature. The compensatory flow reaction at high oxygen pressure is suppressed by anoxia, similar to the case in Fig. 9 with air respiration. It does also not occur in the hypoxic areas after MCA clamp [40]. Here, increase in arterial P_{O_2} always increased tissue P_{O_2}; this effect could probably be used therapeutically.

Entrei and Lund measured P_{O_2} histograms of the human brain and found that, as expected, at an F_{i,O_2} of 0.35 and 0.70 the P_{O_2} histogram was shifted to the right, but at 0.70% O_2 the P_{O_2} values were scattered over a larger P_{O_2} range [19]. This is the first sign of a disturbance of the microcirculation. At 100% O_2, the scattering of P_{O_2} values increased considerably, but now a relatively large number of low tissue P_{O_2} values are found so that, because of a maldistribution of the microcirculation, hypoxic hyperoxia occurred.

An increase of arterial P_{CO_2} increases total and regional flow as well as mean tissue P_{O_2} [45]. Under these conditions, microflow and local P_{O_2} react quite homogeneously with small or large increases. Grote et al. [49] demonstrated that hypocapnia produced a decrease of flow and a moderate left shift of the P_{O_2} histogram. In severe hypocapnia (P_{a,CO_2} = 12 Torr), however, the flow pattern (regional clearance by Kr^{85}) became nonhomogeneous and hypoxia developed, producing hypoxic hypocapnia.

Tissue P_{O_2} and Increased Neuronal Activity

Increase of neuronal activity is accompanied by an increase in the oxygen consumption of the brain and a corresponding increase of flow. Figure 11 shows that an increase of neuronal activity by electrical stimulation induces an increase of microflow (pH_2/H_2 clearance, 100-μm electrode), which is so large that local tissue P_{O_2} increases in spite of the increase of oxygen consumption [32]. Extracellular pH initially becomes alkaline because CO_2 is washed out by the large flow, but later H^+ ions and CO_2 reduce the pH. Similarly, an increase of tissue P_{O_2} is found after somatosensory stimulation [50]. This corresponds well with the reported relatively large flow increase [51]. There are some reports about a P_{O_2} decrease during activity [52], but with an intact circulation we have never observed such a P_{O_2} decrease as a repeatable reaction. It may be that different anesthesia is responsible for a different reactivity of the circulation. Also, during seizures, local tissue P_{O_2} increases [53]. The increase may vary, independent on the duration of the seizures [54]. It was found that with the onset of neuronal activity, the activity of extracellular potassium increased very quickly. Simultaneous measurements of microflow and K^+ activity demonstrated that local flow increases parallel with the increase of K^+ activity [55]. These results are in accordance with the assumption that the increase of K^+ activity triggers the flow increase so that changes in the neuronal membrane, which accompany the neuronal activity, are the first sign of the flow increase. Later, metabolic signals such as H^+ ions, CO_2, and adenosine may modulate this signal.

a b c

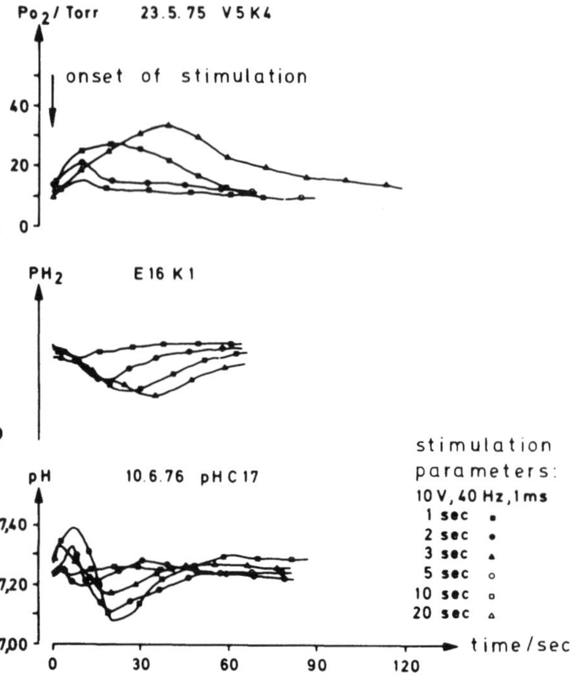

Fig. 11a–c. Local tissue P_{O_2}, microflow, and extracellular H^+ activity in the brain cortex of the cat during and after electrical stimulation. Time of stimulation was varied, whereas amplitude and frequency remained constant. With the onset of stimulation, **a** local tissue P_{O_2} and **b** microflow (pH_2) increased; **c** pH at first showed on alkalotic and then an acidotic change. pH_2/H_2 clearance: Decrease of pH_2 signifies increase of flow. After Lübbers and Leniger-Follert [46]

Conclusion

Oxygen is supplied to the brain tissue by diffusing out of the capillary blood into the tissue. Thereby, within the tissue, P_{O_2} gradients are produced, the steepness of which depends on the geometry of the tissue and the amount of oxygen transported. Along the capillary, P_{O_2} decreases from the arterial inflow to the venous outflow. This decrease depends on the O_2 consumption of the tissue, $\dot{V}_{O_2}$, the blood flow, $\dot{B}$, and the arterial O_2 capacity; it is further determined by the O_2 dissociation curve. Thus, within the tissue, a P_{O_2} field is formed which reflects tissue oxygen supply. The largest P_{O_2} values approach the arterial P_{O_2} level, the smallest ones are close to the critical mitochondrial P_{O_2} level. The lowest tissue P_{O_2} values are distinctly smaller than those of the venous P_{O_2}. Since the O_2 profiles show that large P_{O_2} gradients are rare, one can conclude that capillary geometry and flow are well adapted to the O_2 as well as to the metabolic needs. The P_{O_2} field can be quantitatively described by a P_{O_2} histogram. Experiments have shown that in many cases, surface P_{O_2} histograms can also be used to characterize the O_2 supply of the brain. In the lower P_{O_2} range, the shape of the

P_{O_2} histogram is much influenced by the O_2 capacity of the blood. Hypoxia is characterized by an increase of low P_{O_2} values (left-shifted P_{O_2} histogram). In hyperoxia, pathological situations can be detected by a larger "scattering" of P_{O_2} values (maldistribution).

Under normal conditions, the local tissue P_{O_2} value is quite constant. After a disturbance, it mostly reaches the initial P_{O_2} again, i.e., the tissue maintains the "set point" of its oxygen delivery constant. This set point, however, can be influenced, e.g., by drugs, anesthetics, but also by extracellular ions as well as by the sympathetic nervous system. All these substances and reactions affect the tissue P_{O_2} by their influence on the local circulation.

Simultaneous measurements of local microflow (flow in one to four capillaries) and local tissue P_{O_2} showed that the large variability of the capillary flow was not accompanied by similar changes in tissue P_{O_2}. We take this as a sign that each part of the tissue is always supplied by several capillaries. Probably, in the capillary network, flow is regulated in such a way that a decrease in one capillary may be accompanied by a corresponding increase in the other. There is no evidence for a "stop and flow" regulation (capillary recruitment), but for a regulation by large variations of the flow velocity. Since the surface P_{O_2} electrode and the pH_2/H_2 element can be made transparent, these measurements can be combined with microscopic observations.

Changes in the O_2 supply by adjustments of the arterial oxygen capacity (hematocrit) are compensated by increased flow so that oxygen delivery is maintained at constant local P_{O_2} values. A similar situation is observed during blood pressure changes: In the range of flow autoregulation, tissue P_{O_2} remains constant.

Increase of arterial P_{O_2} is accompanied by decrease of regional flow so that the tissue P_{O_2} increase is distinctly diminished. The very quick flow compensation would indicate an oxygen sensor in the arterial inflow. Severe hyperoxia can cause a maldistribution of microflow with local hypoxia. At a normal set point of the P_{O_2} histogram, small reductions of P_{a,O_2} seem to keep the oxygen delivery unchanged by increasing the O_2 extraction, which is accompanied by a decrease of tissue P_{O_2} but not followed by a reactive hyperemia after returning to normal P_{a,O_2}; there is no sign of tissue hypoxia. Larger arterial hypoxia shows a redistribution of microflow so that flow is reduced in the "high-flow capillaries" and increased in the adjacent area. This is a very local regulation, which does not necessarily affect regional flow. The different local reactions to the same stimulus are difficult to explain; in the brain, glial cells could be involved.

Neuronal activity increases tissue O_2 consumption and causes larger P_{O_2} gradients within the tissue, producing a decrease of a mean P_{O_2}. However, the increase of local flow, which is triggered by the increase of extracellular K^+ activity (i.e., signal from the neuronal membrane), increases oxygen delivery so that tissue P_{O_2} increases. Later, other substances such as pH, CO_2, and adenosine, i.e., metabolic signals may modulate the flow regulation.

The advantage of the P_{O_2} as well as the pH_2/H_2 microflow measurements, is that with these methods the reaction of the microcirculation can be continuously followed and that with regard to the spatial resolution, they are in the range of microscopic observation.

References

1. Opitz E, Palme F (1944) Darstellung und Höhenanpassung im Gebirge durch Sauerstoffmangel: III. Mitt. Graduierung der Höhenkrankheit durch das Elektroencephalogramm. Pflügers Arch 248: 330
2. Opitz E, Schneider M (1950) Über die Sauerstoffversorgung des Gehirns und den Mechanismus von Mangelwirkungen. In: Krayer O, Lehnartz E, v. Muralt A, Rein FH (eds) Ergebnisse der Physiologie, biologischen Chemie und experimentellen Pharmakologie, vol. 46. Springer, Berlin—Göttingen—Heidelberg, pp 126–261
3. Rémond A (1948) Aspects physiopathologiques de l'oxygène cortical. Revue Neurologique 80: 579–588
4. Davies PW, Bronk DW (1957) Oxygen tension in mammalian brain. Fed Proc 16: 689–692
5. Silver IA (1965) Some observations on the cerebral cortex with an ultramicro, membrane-covered, oxygen electrode. Med Electron Biol Engng 3: 377–387
6. Lübbers DW (1968) The oxygen pressure field of the brain and its significance for the normal and critical oxygen supply of the brain. In: Lübbers DW, Luft UC, Thews G, Witzleb E (eds) Oxygen transport in blood and tissue. Thieme, Stuttgart, pp 124–139
7. Whalen WJ, Ganfield R, Nair P (1970) Effects of breathing O_2 or $O_2 + CO_2$ and of the injection of neurohumors on the P_{O_2} of cat cerebral cortex. Stroke 1: 194–200
8. Metzger H (1973) Geometric considerations in modeling oxygen transport processes in tissue. Adv Exp Med Biol 37B: 761–772
9. Smith RH, Guilbeau EJ, Renau DD (1977) The oxygen tension field within a discrete volume of cerebral cortex. Microvasc Res 13: 233–240
10. Baumgärtl H, Lübbers DW (1983) Microcoaxial needle sensor for polarographic measurement of local O_2 pressure in the cellular range of living tissue. Its construction and properties. In Gnaiger E, Forstner H (eds) Polarographic oxygen sensors. Springer, Berlin—Heidelberg, pp 37–65
11. Bär T (1980) The vascular system of the cerebral cortex. In: Brodal A, v. Limborgh J, Ortmann R, Töndury G (eds) Advances in anatomy, embryology and cell biology, vol. 59. Springer, Berlin—Heidelberg—New York
12. Nair P, Whalen WJ, Buerk D (1975) P_{O_2} of cat cerebral cortex: Response to breathing N_2 and 100% O_2. Microvasc Res 9: 158–165
13. Metzger H, Heuber S, Steinacker A, Strüber J (1978) Staining of P_{O_2} measuring points demonstrated for the rat brain cortex. Adv Exp Med Biol 94: 49–55
14. Lübbers DW (1969) The meaning of the tissue oxygen distribution curve and its measurement by means of Pt electrodes. Progr Resp Res: 3: 112–123
15. Stosseck K (1970) Hydrogen exchange through the pial vessel wall and its meaning for the determination of the local cerebral blood flow. Pflügers Arch 320: 111–119
16. Duling BR, Kuschinsky W, Wahl M (1979) Measurements of the perivascular P_{O_2} and tissue P_{O_2} in the vicinity of the pial vessels of the cat. Pflügers Arch 383: 29–34
17. Ivanov KP, Derry AN, Vovenko EP, Samoilov MO, Semionov DG (1982) Direct measurements of oxygen tension at the surface of arterioles, capillaries and venules of the cerebral cortex. Pflügers Arch 393: 118–120
18. Ivanov, Kislayokov Yu Ya, Samoilov MO (1979) Microcirculation and transport of oxgyen to neurons of the brain. Microvasc Res 18: 434–441
19. Eintrei C, Lund N (1986) Effects of increases in the inspired oxgyen fraction on brain surface oxgyen pressure fields in pig and man. Acta Anaesthesiol Scand 30: 194–198
20. Kessler M, Lübbers DW (1966) Aufbau und Anwendungsmöglichkeit verschiedener P_{O_2}-Elektroden. Pflügers Arch 291: 82
21. Heinrich U, Hoffmann J, Baumgärtl H, Yu B, Lübbers DW (1985) Oxygen supply of the blood-free perfused guinea pig brain at three different temperatures. Adv Exp Med Biol 191: 77–84
22. Schultheiss R, Assad F, Leniger-Follert E, Pfeiffer G, Wassmann H, Wüllenweber R

(1985) Measurement of tissue P_{O_2} on the brain surface: Clinical application of the polarographic method. In: Hartmann A, Hoyer S (eds) Cerebral blood flow and metabolism measurement. Springer, Berlin-Heidelberg, pp 487–490
23. Oshino N, Sugano T, Oshino R, Chance B (1974) Mitochondrial function under hypoxic conditions: The steady states of cytochrome a,a_3 and their relation to mitochondrial energy states. Biochim Biophys Acta 368: 298–310
24. Lübbers DW (1981) Tissue oxgyen supply and critical oxygen pressure. Adv Physiol Sci 25: 3–11
25. Hempel FG, Jöbsis FF, LaManna JL, Rosenthal MR, Saltzman HA (1977) Oxidation of cerebral cytochrome aa_3 by oxygen plus carbon dioxide at hyperbaric pressures. J Appl Physiol 43: 873–879
26. Clark A Jr, Clark PAA (1985) Local oxygen gradients near isolated mitochondria. Biophys J 48: 931–938
27. Hilberman M, Subramanian VH, Haselgrove J, Cone JB, Egan JW, Gyulai L, Chance B (1984) In vivo time-resolved brain phosphorus nuclear magnetic resonance. J Cerebr Blood Flow Metab 4: 334–342
28. Dora E, Kovach AGB (1987) Role of hypoxia and acetylcholine in the regulation of cerebral blood flow. Adv Exp Med Biol 215: 237–248
29. Lübbers DW (1966) Methods of measuring oxygen tensions of blood and organ surfaces. In: Payne JP, Hill DW (eds) Oxygen measurements in blood and tissues. Churchill, London, pp 103–132
30. Lübbers DW, Stosseck K (1970) Quantitative Bestimmung der lokalen Durchblutung durch elektrochemisch im Gewebe erzeugten Wasserstoff. Naturwissenschaften 57: 311
31. Stosseck K, Lübbers DW (1970) Determination of microflow of the cerebral cortex by means of electrochemically generated hydrogen. In: Russel RWR (ed) Brain and blood flow. Pittman, London, pp 80–84
32. Leniger-Follert E Lübbers DW (1976) Behavior of microflow and local P_{O_2} of the brain cortex during and after direct electrical stimulation. Pflügers Arch 366: 39–44
33. Leniger-Follert E, Lübbers DW (1973) Mikrozirkulation und Sauerstofftransport im Gehirn. Verh Dtsch Ges Kreislaufforsch 39: 22–27
34. Klein B, Kuschinsky W, Schröck H, Vetterlein F (1986) Interdependency of local capillary density, blood flow, and metabolism in rat brains. Am J Physiol 251: H1333-H1340
35. Clark LC Jr, Misrahy G, Fox RP (1958) Chronically implanted polarographic electrodes. J Appl Physiol 13: 85–91
36. Manil J, Bourgain RH, v. Waeyenberge M, Colin F, Blockeel E, De Mey B, Coremans J, Paternoster R (1984) Properties of the spontaneous fluctuations in cortical oxygen pressure. Adv Exp Med Biol 169: 231–239
37. Leniger-Follert E (1985) Oxygen supply and microcirculation of the brain cortex. Adv Exp Med Biol 191: 3–19
38. Leniger-Follert E, Lübbers DW (1975) Interdependence of capillary flow and regional blood flow of the brain. In: Langfitt TW, McHenry LC Jr, Reivich M, Wollmann H (eds) Cerebral circulation and metabolism. Springer, New York, pp 46–48
39. Temes G, Lantos J, Török B (1985) Correlations between the quantity of cerebral flow, brain surface P_{O_2} and EEG in the dog. Res Exp Med 185: 121–129
40. Chan R, Leniger-Follert E (1983) Effect of isovolemic hemodilution on oxygen supply and electrocorticogram in cat brain during focal ischemia and in normal tissue. Int J Microcirc Clin Exp 2: 297–313
41. Wiernsperger N, Gygax P, Danzeisen M (1978) Cortical P_{O_2} distribution during oligemic hypotension and its pharmacological modifications. Ärzneim Forsch Drug Res 28(I): 768–770
42. Messmer K, Sunder-Plassmann L, Jesch F, Görnandt L, Sinagowitz E, Kessler (1973) Oxgyen supply to the tissues during limited normovolemic hemodilution. Res Exp Med 159: 152–166

43. Grote J, Schubert R (1982) Regulation of cerebral perfusion and P_{O_2} in normal and edematous brain tissue. In: Loeppky JA, Riedesel ML (eds) Oxygen transport to human tissues. Elsevier North Holland, Amsterdam pp 169–178
44. Metzger H, Erdmann W, Thews G (1971) Effect of short periods of hypoxia, hyperoxia, and hypercapnia on brain O_2 supply. J Appl Physiol 31: 751–759
45. Leniger-Follert E, Lübbers DW, Wrabetz W (1975) Regulation of local tissue P_{O_2} of the brain cortex at different arterial O_2 pressures. Pflügers Arch 359: 81–95
46. Lübbers DW, Leniger-Follert E (1978) Capillary flow in the brain cortex during changes in oxygen supply and state of activation. In: Cerebral vascular smooth muscle and its control. Ciba Foundation Symposium 56. Elsevier, Excerpta Medica, North Holland, Amsterdam, pp 21–47
47. Burgess DW (1975) The regulation of brain tissue oxygen tension under conditions of increased barometric pressures. In: Payne JP, Hill DW (eds) Oxygen measurements in biology and medicine. Butterworths, London, pp 217–230
48. Rubanyi G, Paul RJ (1985) Two distinct effects of oxgyen on vascular tone in isolated porcine coronary arteries. Circ Res 56: 1–10
49. Grote J, Zimmer K, Schubert R (1981) Effects of severe arterial hypocapnia on regional blood flow regulation, tissue P_{O_2} and metabolism in the brain cortex of cats. Pflügers Arch 391: 195–199
50. Leniger-Follert E, Hossmann K-A (1979) Simultaneous measurements of microflow and evoked potentials in the somatomotor cortex of the cat brain during specific sensory activation. Pflügers Arch 380: 85–89
51. Fox PT, Raichle ME (1986) Focal physiological uncoupling of cerebral blood flow and oxidative metabolism during somatosensory stimulation in human subjects. Proc Natl Acad Sci USA 83: 1140–1144
52. Metzger H (1978) The influence of electrical stimulation on cortex P_{O_2} level in the rat brain. Adv Exp Med Biol 94: 713–720
53. Leniger-Follert E (1984) Mechanisms of regulation of cerebral microflow during bicuculline-induced seizures in anaesthetized cats. J Cereb Blood Flow Metab 4: 150–165
54. Caspers H, Speckmann E-J (1972) Cerebral pO_2, pCO_2 and pH: Changes during convulsive activity and their significance for spontaneous arrest of seizures. Epilepsia 13: 699–725
55. Urbanics R, Leniger-Follert E, Lübbers DW (1978) Time course of changes of extracellular H^+ and K^+ activities during and after direct electrical stimulation of the brain cortex. Pflügers Arch 378: 47–53

Microvascular Permeability: Its Disturbance in Disease

LAURENCE H. SMAJE[1]

The main function of the microcirculation is exchange. In order to fulfill this role, material must be brought to the microvasculature by convection and then be transported across the permeable portions of the capillary wall to the tissues by a mixture of convection and diffusion.

The following equation describes the process of net *fluid* exchange in a modern form of Starling's principle:

$$J_v = L_pA\ ([P_c - P_t] - \sigma_d\ [\pi_c - \pi_t]) \tag{1}$$

Where J_v = fluid flux, L_p = filtration coefficient, A = area available for exchange, P = hydrostatic pressure, c = within capillary, t = in interstitium, σ_d = osmotic reflexion coefficient, and π = protein (colloid) osmotic pressure.

A glance at the equation reveals that an increased fluid flux could be the result of a change in the membrance coefficents (increased L_p, increased A, or decreased σ_d) or an increase in the net transmural force $[\Delta P - \Delta\sigma_d\pi]$. Failure of lymph drainage could also obviously lead to accumulation of tissue fluid.

Solute exchange occurs both by convection and diffusion:

$$J_s = P_sA\Delta C + Jv\ [1 - \sigma_f]\bar{c} \tag{2}$$

Where J_s = solute flux, P_s = permeability of microvascular wall, ΔC = solute concentration difference across the wall, $\bar{c}$ = mean solute concentration in the exchange channels in the membrane, and σ_f = solvent drag reflexion coefficient.

Equation 2 is an oversimplified version of the real situation and non-linear flux equations provide a better fit to experimental data. Equation 2 is useful, however, in that it is easy to see that the first term reflects diffusion, and the second convection. Small solutes like glucose and respiratory gases exchange almost exclusively by diffusion. As molecular size increases, P falls and, despite the increasing σ_d, the contribution of convection increases. Some claim that exchange of plasma proteins is mainly convective in nature [1].

Solute exchange can thus be altered not only by changes in capillary permeability as such, but also by changes in area, concentration gradients and convective forces. A comprehensive coverage of the changes in capillary per-

[1]Department of Physiology, Charing Cross and Westminster Medical School, University of London, London W6 8RF, England

meability in disease is thus impossible in the time available and I have decided to concentrate on three areas of clinical relevance that have been studied in my laboratory under the supervision of my colleague John Tooke. These are pre-menstrual oedema, fluid exchange in diabetes mellitus and essential hypertension. The thesis I wish to explore is that in each of these cases, many of the pathophysiological findings can be explained by a relative increase in capillary hydrostatic pressure gradient rather than any change in permeability as such.

Pre-menstrual Oedema

Ankle oedema is commonly associated with the pre-menstrual syndrome and although associations with fluctuations in female sex hormones or abnormalities in the renin-angiotensin-aldosterone system have been found, the exact mechanism involved remains obscure. The observation that oedema is precipitated by assumption of the upright posture and reduced by vasoconstrictor drugs suggests that undue pooling of blood in the dependent extremities may be responsible [2].

In normal non-pre-menstrual subjects, however, a marked reduction in foot blood flow is induced on standing or on lowering the limb below horizontal (Fig. 1). It is thought that this is the result of pre-capillary vasoconstriction in response to the increased hydrostatic pressure in the dependent vessels mediated largely by a sympathetic axon reflex [3]. In the dependent limb, the increased hydrostatic pressure would give rise to increased capillary filtration. An increased pre-capillary resistance, however, would limit the expected rise in capillary pressure. Furthermore, as filtration occurs from the extremely slow blood flow, oncotic pressure in the vessels rises, thereby limiting further fluid filtration [4]. A compromised vasoconstrictor response would thus tend to lead to postural oedema.

In view of the association of pre-menstrual oedema with posture and the evidence that vascular smooth muscle is affected by female sex hormones, Hassan and Tooke have studied the postural vasoconstrictor response at different stages of the menstrual cycle [2] and in women using oral contraceptive [5]. Details of the methods can be found in their papers but in brief, blood flow was measured both on the dorsum of the foot and the plantar surface of the big toe using a laser Doppler flowmeter and foot circumference was measured simultaneously with a mercury-in-rubber strain gauge. Measurements were made on subjects acclimatized in a temperature-controlled room firstly lying horizontal and then with the foot lowered 50 cm below the heart. In women with ovulatory cycles, postural changes in flow were measured during menstruation (days 1–2), during the follicular phase (days 12–15), and during the luteal phase (days 21–26) and hormone levels were measured at the same time. Women taking combined oral contraceptive pills (30 μg ethinyl oestradiol and 150 μg levonorgestrel) were studied on the last of 7 pill-free days (day 7) and the last day of pill ingestion (day 28). Three men were used as controls on two separate occasions at least 1 week apart. Postural flow changes are expressed as [(control flow − dependent flow) ÷ control flow] × 100.

Figure 2 shows that while there is a tendency for blood flow in the horizontal limb to increase during the cycle, this is not striking in either the dorsum of the foot or on the plantar surface of the big toe. Flows in the latter region are higher

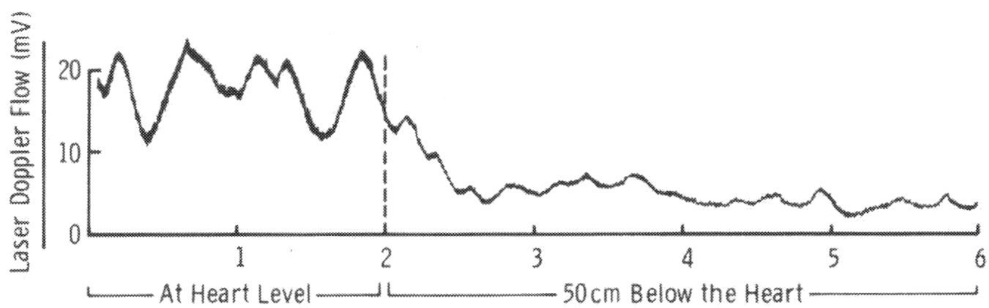

Fig. 1. Blood flow in the dorsum of the foot of a recumbent subject measured with a laser-Doppler flowmeter, firstly in the horizontal position and then with the foot lowered 50 cm below the heart. Mean flow is determined planimetrically from the 2-min period prior to the change in posture and during the 4th min in the dependent position. After Hassan (unpublished data)

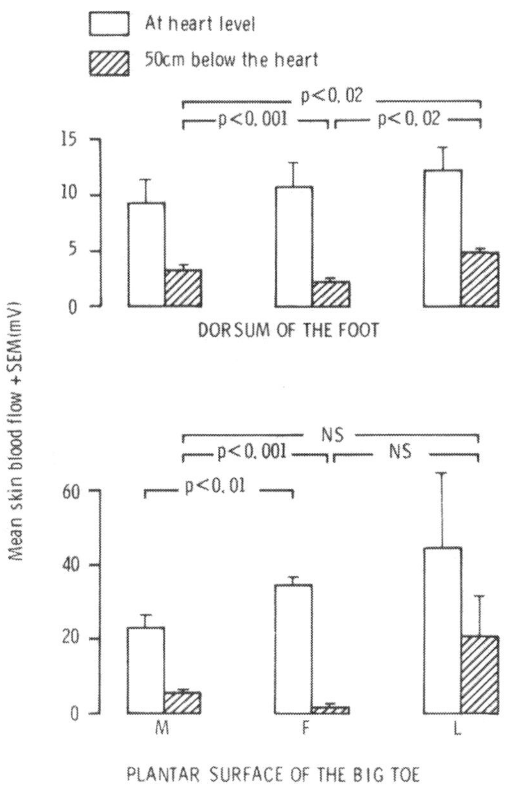

Fig. 2. Vasoconstrictor response to lowering the foot 50 cm below the heart at different stages in the normal menstrual cycle. *M* menstruation, *F* follicular phase, *L* luteal phase. After Hassan et al. [2]

because of the presence of arteriovenous (AV) anastomoses, which are not thought to be present on the skin of the dorsum. In all cases, lowering the limb 50 cm below the heart leads to a vasoconstriction, which is much less marked in the luteal phase. This is shown more clearly in Fig. 3, in which the postural responses are shown together with foot swelling rates. The two are reciprocally

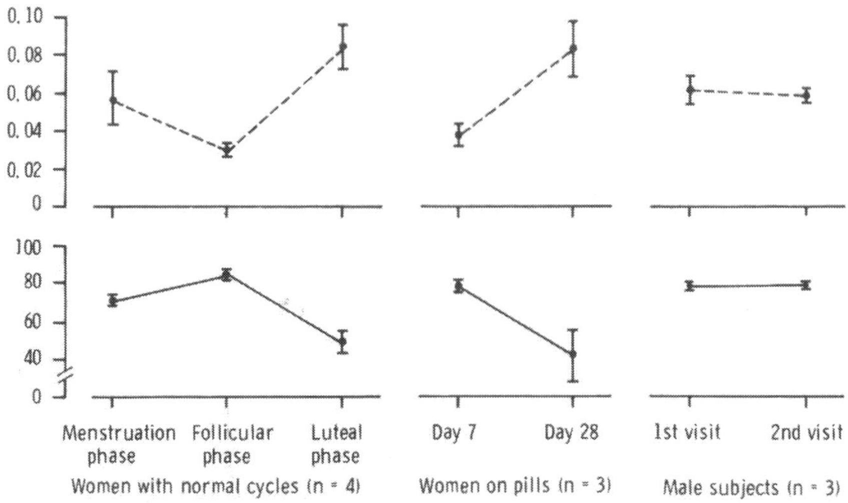

Fig. 3. Foot swelling rate in the dependent position and postural fall in blood flow (see text for details) under different hormonal conditions. Note that a lower number on the *flow scale* indicates a poorer vasoconstrictor response. Redrawn from Hassan et al. [2] and Hassan and Tooke [5]

related. As would be expected, the more effective the vasoconstriction, the lower the swelling rate. The relatively poor pre-menstrual vasoconstrictor response was also observed in women taking oral contraceptives and Fig. 3 summarizes these findings together with those in three male controls. It may be worth noting that there was a significant positive correlation between duration of pill use and skin blood flow measured in the dependent position and that in women with pre-menstrual oedema the total duration of pill use was significantly greater.

The reasons for the poor postural vasoconstrictor response in the pre-menstrual phase were not explored in this study, although typical hormonal changes were observed. It is not known which limb of the veni-arteriolar reflex is affected—the afferent signal, the neural response or the vascular smooth muscular contraction. It is clear, however, that capillary pressure and filtration are increased in the pre-menstrual phase of women with normal ovulatory cycles or on oral contraceptives and that their oedema can be correlated with this and no specific increase in vascular permeability as such need be postulated.

Diabetes Mellitus

Microangiopathy is a characteristic complication of diabetes and there would be widespread agreement that capillary permeability is increased in diabetic microangiopathy. Clinical findings include retinal exudates, proteinuria and neuropathic oedema; experimentally there is evidence for increased macromolecular permeability, capillary diffusing capacity and capillary filtration coefficient [6]. Before accepting that permeability per se is increased, it is necessary, as before, to examine whether increased transmural forces could be responsible.

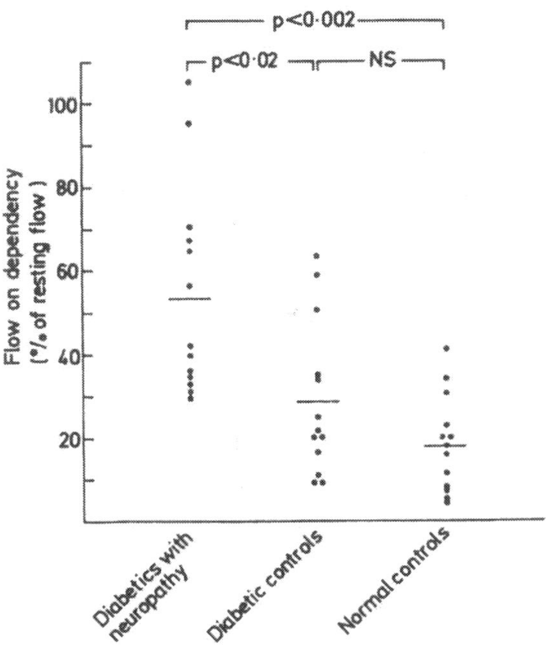

Fig. 4. Laser-Doppler flow on the plantar surface of the left big toe in response to lowering the foot 50 cm below the heart in diabetics with and without neuropathy and in age-matched controls. After Rayman et al. [7]

In diabetics Rayman et al. [7] found an impaired postural vasoconstrictor response, shown in Fig 4, associated with which is an increased foot swelling rate on dependency. The changes were significant only in diabetics with neuropathy although the mean vasoconstrictor response was also reduced in diabetic patients with no signs of sensory or autonomic neuropathy. Since postural vasoconstriction is probably a sympathetic axon reflex [3], an impairment probably reflects an early manifestation of autonomic neuropathy. The vasoconstrictor response may thus be a more sensitive indicator of autonomic disease than conventional tests.

In the present context, the important point to note is that as the veno-arteriolar reflex is less active than in normals, measurements of capillary filtration coefficient (CFC) may be affected. CFC is measured from the slope of the swelling rate at known pressures applied to a venous occlusion cuff [8]. Normally this procedure will induce a vasoconstrictor response and the value obtained will thus underestimate the true value. In diabetics, the veno-arteriolar reflex vasoconstriction is compromised, as shown above, and the relatively high CFC obtained may be explained without recourse to invoking permeability increase. The increase in diffusing capacity, which is also found in diabetes [9], cannot be so explained, however, as the measurements of diffusion capacity were made with a maximally vasodilated muscle bed.

The evidence for increased macromolecular permeability in human diabetic subjects is based on measurements of transcapillary escape rate (TER). In this technique, the plasma concentrations of radiolabelled protein are followed after bolus intravenous injection. Concentration falls as protein equilibrates with the extracellular space. The rate at which this occurs will depend on the factors in

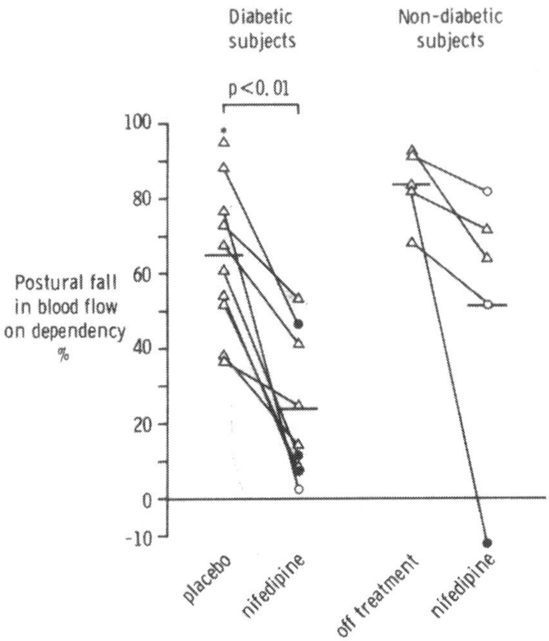

Fig. 5. Postural fall in skin flow on dependency in diabetic and non-diabetic hypertensives treated with nifedipine. Individual values shown. *Bars* show means of the group. After Williams, Rayman, and Tooke

Eq. 2 but in view of the heterogeneity of the bed involved, the fact that radiolabelled protein may not be treated exactly like native protein and that lymphatic return is ignored, interpretation is difficult and controversial.

Despite its theoretical drawbacks TER is widely used and probably does at least reflect the rate of transcapillary protein transport. Both TER and renal albumin excretion are increased in diabetes, particularly in poorly controlled diabetics. In young diabetics, improved control leads to restoration of the TER towards normal [6].

Poor diabetic control seems to lead to vasomotor instability [6] and it may be that the increased TER can be at least partly explained by increased capillary pressure in consequence of this.

A characteristic morphological change found in diabetic capillaries is basement membrane thickening [6]. The thickness of the basement membrane depends on transmural hydrostatic pressure [10]. At heart level, nail-fold capillary pressure does not seem to be altered much [11], but the compromised veno-arteriolar reflex will lead to increased capillary pressure in dependent limbs. Hypertension is commonly associated with diabetes and the calcium entry blocker nifedipine is commonly used to treat the hypertension. Unfortunately, this often leads to oedema. The effects of nifedipine have been investigated in diabetic and non-diabetic hypertensives by studying the postural vasoconstrictor response. Figure 5 shows that in both groups, the vasoconstrictor response is attenuated by nifedipine. This may come as no great surprise in view of its mode of action but it serves to emphasize that in diabetics with a compromised vasoconstrictor response, attenuating it still further by hypotensive agents may precipitate oedema and the dangerous sequelae that could follow.

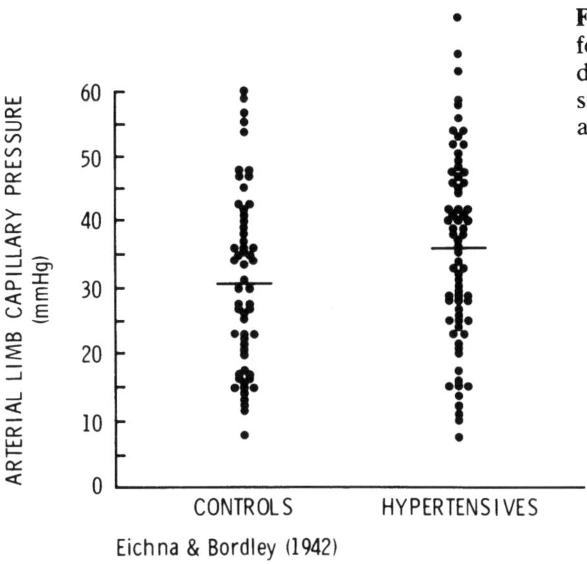

Fig. 6. Pressure in human nail-fold capillaries measured by direct micropuncture in hypertensives and controls. After Eichna and Bordley [12]

In summary, early in diabetes mellitus a sympathetic autonomic neuropathy appears to develop which leads to a reduced veno-arteriolar reflex. This will lead to increased capillary pressures, which will explain in part the increased basement membrane thickening, increased CFC and increased TER. At the same time there are also clear increases in microvascular permeability. Understanding of the changes observed requires dissection of the relative contribution of the changes in both capillary pressure and capillary membrane coefficients.

Essential Hypertension

The clinical significance of essential hypertension is reflected by the amount of research effort expended in investigating the disease both in man and experimental models. Curiously enough, however, the only study in which direct measurements of capillary pressure have been made is that by Eichna and Bordley [12]. They used direct micropuncture to measure capillary pressure in the nail-fold and, although the hypertensive group had a mean pressure greater than controls, it was claimed that this difference was insignificant (Fig. 6). The selection of both patients and controls was unsatisfactory by modern criteria, but nonetheless it has become the accepted view that capillary pressure is not raised in essential hypertension. Since cardiac output is also normal in the established disease, it is generally held that increased peripheral resistance is confined to the pre-capillary section of the microvasculature.

It is difficult to reconcile this view with a great deal of indirect evidence suggesting that capillary pressure is raised in essential hypertension. Plasma volume is reduced with a normal or expanded extra-cellular fluid volume. Macromolecular exchange (as meausred by TER) is also raised in proportion to mean arterial pressure (Fig. 7) [13]. More significantly perhaps, the increase in TER for albu-

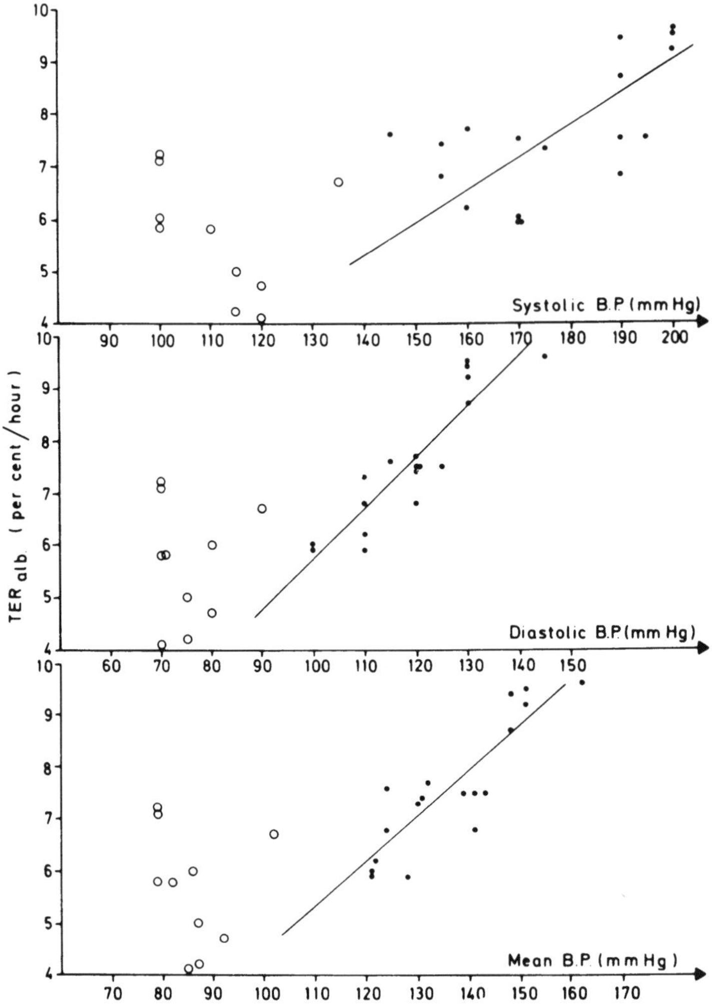

Fig. 7. Relation between transcapillary escape rate of albumin (TER alb) and systolic, diastolic and mean systemic arterial blood pressure ($P < 0.001$ in the hypertensive groups.) There was no correlation within the control group (*open circles*). After Parving and Gyntelberg [13]

min is proportionately the same as that for globulin (Fig. 8) [14], suggesting that the sieving properties of the vasculature are unchanged. This suggests that either the effective exchange area is increased or hydrostatic pressure is increased. The association between hypertension and increased venous tone, reduced venous compliance and by implication increased venular resistance, would also lead to an increased capillary pressure. Rarefaction of arterioles or capillaries, which has been reported in humans and animals, would also do so [15]. It was thus timely to re-examine capillary pressure in essential hypertension using direct measurement and this has been done by our group [15]. Pressure was measured

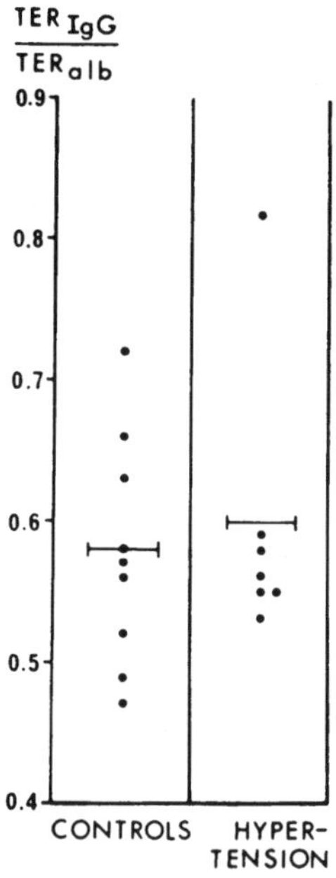

Fig. 8. Ratio of transcapillary escape rate of IgG and albumin in normo- and hypertensive subjects. *Solid lines* represent the mean values. After Parving et al. [14]

Table 1. Details of experimental groups

	Age (yrs)	Sex		Skin temp. (°C)	Blood pressure (mmHg)
		M	F		
Normotensive controls	46.2 ± 15.0	5	4	28.0 ± 3.0	124.6/76.6 ± 12.1/6.5
Subjects with hypertension	49.4 ± 13.1	5	4	28.7 ± 3.1	165.5/104.0 ± 24.7/10.0

All figures are expressed as means ± SD. The difference in blood pressure was the only finding to reach statistical significance ($P < 0.01$, Student's *t*-test). After Williams et al. [15]

using the Servonull technique in the apical loop of nail-fold capillaries in acclimatized subjects lying on a couch with their arms held at heart level. Newly diagnosed hypertensives screened for known causes of hypertension were matched with controls for age, sex, race and skin temperature at the time of study.

Table 1 summarizes details of the experimental groups and Fig. 9 the capillary pressure measurements. It is interesting to note that there also appears to be a relationship between mean arterial pressure and capillary pressure (Fig. 10). Even more gratifying was our observation that in two of the three patients who subsequently received treatment, both arterial and capillary pressures fell, while in the third, who failed to respond to treatment, both arterial and capillary pressure actually rose.

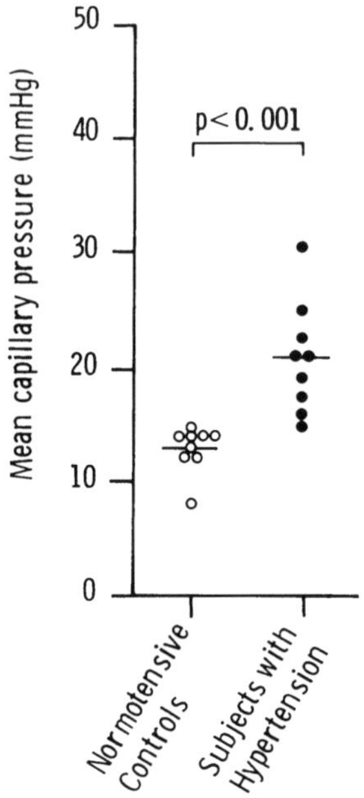

Fig. 9. Capillary pressure in the apex of nail-fold capillaries measured by direct micropuncture with the arm held horizontal at heart level. Newly diagnosed patients with essential hypertension were compared with matched controls. Two to five vessels were cannulated in each subject and each *point* represents the mean pressure in the cannulated vessels in that subject. After Williams et al. [15]

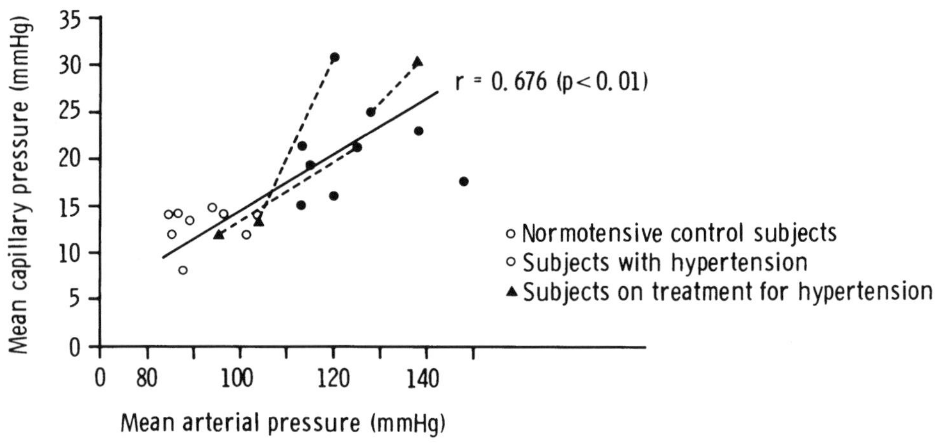

Fig. 10. Relation between capillary pressure (mean of all cannulations in each subject) and systemic arterial pressure (mean of all readings in each subject). Three of the patients were studied again after 2 weeks of anti-hypertensive treatment. After Williams et al. [15]

If pressure in the apical regions of nail-fold capillaries is representative of values elsewhere, then the present observations require a reappraisal of the orthodox view that essential hypertension is a consequence of an exclusive increase in pre-capillary resistance. Post-capillary resistance increases as well, leading to an increase in capillary hydrostatic pressure. Previous observations suggesting an increase in capillary pressure are consistent with the current observation, and new possibilities in relation to therapeutic interventions become apparent. Does capillary pressure follow changes in arterial pressure in all therapeutic regimes and, if not, is this of diagnostic or prognostic significance? On the basis of the present finding it is necessary to reconsider the appropriateness of those animal models of hypertension that do not lead to increases in capillary pressure.

Summary

Oedema associated with the pre-menstrual syndrome, diabetes and particularly in nifedipine-treated hypertensive diabetics can be largely explained without the need for invoking a specific increase in permeability. The failure of the veno-arteriolar reflex leads to increased capillary pressure and the increased capillary pressure leads to increased fluid and protein filtration. The increased CFC, TER and basement membrane thickening seen in diabetes can thus be partly explained.

In essential hypertension, contrary to classic views, capillary pressure is raised roughly in proportion to the mean arterial pressure. The increased TER in hypertension can thus also be largely explained.

Changes in permeability undoubtedly do occur in diabetes mellitus, but the main purpose of the present paper is to serve as a reminder that before permeability increase is invoked as an explanation for increased solute and water flux in disease states, increased capillary pressure in the dynamic situation must be excluded.

References

1. Lassen NA, Parving H-H, Rossing N (1974) Filtration as the main mechanism of overall transcapillary protein escape from the plasma. Microvasc Res 7: 1–4
2. Hassan A, Carter G, Tooke JE (1986) Postural vasoconstriction in the human foot during the menstrual cycle. J Physiol 382: 44P
3. Henriksen O, Sejrsen P (1976) Local reflex in microcirculation in human cutaneous tissue. Acta Physiol Scand 98: 227–231
4. Noddeland H, Aukland K, Nicolaysen G (1981) Plasma colloid osmotic pressure in venous blood from the human foot in orthostasis. Acta Physiol Scand 113: 447–454
5. Hassan AAK, Tooke JE (1988) Effect of combined oral contraceptive therapy on the postural vasoconstrictor response in the human foot. Postgrad Med J (in press)
6. Tooke JE (1987) The microcirculation in diabetes. Diabetic Medicine 4: 189–196
7. Rayman G, Hassan A, Tooke JE (1986) Blood flow in the skin of the foot related to posture in diabetes mellitus. Br Med J 292: 87–90
8. Michel CC, Moyses C (1987) The measurement of fluid filtration in human limbs. In: Tooke JE, Smaje LH (eds) Clinical investigation of the microcirculation. Martinus Nijhoff, Boston, pp 103–126
9. Trap-Jensen J, Alpert JC, Garcia del Rio H, Lassen NA (1967) Capillary diffusion capacity for sodium in skeletal muscle in long-term juvenile diabetes mellitus. Acta Med Scand [Suppl] 476: 135–146
10. Williamson JR, Vogler NJ, Kilo C (1969) Estimation of vascular basement membrane thickness. Diabetes 18: 567–578

11. Tooke JE (1980) A capillary pressure disturbance in young diabetics. Diabetes 29: 815–819
12. Eichna LW, Bordley J (1942) Capillary blood pressure in man. Direct measurements in the digits of normal and hypertensive subjects during vasoconstriction and vasodilatation. J Clin Invest 21: 711–729
13. Parving HH, Gyntelberg F (1973) Transcapillary escape rate of albumin and plasma volume in essential hypertension. Circ Res 32: 643–651
14. Parving HH, Jensen AE, Westrup M (1977) Increased transcapillary escape rate of albumin and IgG in essential hypertension. Scand J Clin Lab Invest 37: 223–227
15. Williams SA, Boolell M, MacGregor GA, Smaje LH, Wasserman S, Tooke JE (1988) Capillary hypertension in subjects with essential hypertension. (submitted)

Microcirculation Dysfunction in an Environment of Weightlessness

SYOTEN OKA[1]

Introduction

A cell-free marginal zone is formed in blood flow through microvessels as well as in small glass tubes. The cell-free zone is called the plasma zone, since it consists mainly of plasma. The plasma layer is several micrometers thick and vanishes when the flow ceases. The thickness depends not only on the flow velocity but also on the tube diameter and hematocrit. Because of the biconcave disk shape and the deformability of red blood cells, the fluid mechanical treatment of radial migration of red blood cells becomes difficult. The mechanism for the formation of plasma layer is not yet clear.

From a rheological point of view, the plasma layer plays an important role in reducing the flow resistance of blood in microvessels as well as in glass tubes. Since plasma viscosity is only one-third that of blood viscosity, the plasma layer behaves like lubricating oil. It can be shown that the effect of the plasma layer is particularly significant in smaller vessels.

It is an accepted belief that the plasma layer is not caused by gravity. Nevertheless, I maintain that gravity plays an important role in the formation of the plasma layer. Let us consider the Boycott phenomenon [1], i.e., the increased sedimentation rates of erythrocytes in inclined tubes (Fig. 1). This phenomenon is caused by settling of erythrocytes from the upper wall, which produces a plasma region; the plasma region should rise by natural convection and, similarly, the denser blood near the lower wall should flow downward. The upflow of plasma near the upper wall can actually be observed. The existence of the plasma region in inclined tubes is entirely due to gravity. The "accepted" opinion that the plasma layer is not caused by gravity is explained by the fact that the plasma layer is observed in both vertical and horizontal tubes.

Let us now consider the microvessels in human organs on earth. Since each portion of the microvessels is generally inclined to the vertical regardless of posture, a plasma region should also be produced, and this would greatly reduce the flow resistance of blood in microcirculation. This new idea has not yet been demonstrated because of the difficulty in obtaining actual proof.

[1] National Cardiovascular Center Research Institute, 7–1, Fujishirodai 5-chome, Suita, Osaka, 565 Japan

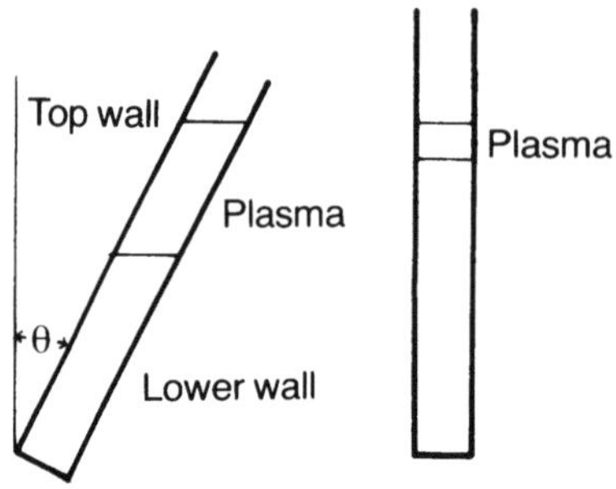

Fig. 1. Erythrocyte sedimentation rate in an inclined tube and a vertical tube

Let us next consider a material body within a spaceship revolving around the earth. As is well known, the earth's gravitation equals that of centrifugal force. Thus, the environment within such a spaceship is one of weightlessness or zero gravity. Of course, the centrifugal force is not completely equal to the gravitational force for various reasons; thus, the expression "environment of near-zero gravity" may be more accurate. From the above, it follows that the flow rate of the microcirculation during a spaceflight should be remarkably decreased as compared with that on the earth.

Theoretical Aspects

As was mentioned above, the plasma region should be produced only on the upper wall of each portion of the microvessels in an organ. It is rather difficult, however, to analyze such an asymmetric blood flow in inclined microvessels. Since we are dealing with the blood flow in extremely complicated microvessels of organs as a whole, a statistical approach is indicated, and so a simplified model of a number of microvessels surrounded by a plasma layer of uniform thickness δ may be adopted (Fig. 2). For simplicity, let us assume that the blood flow in such a model is laminar, steady, and Newtonian and that δ is very small compared with the inner radius R of the vessel. Then, the flow rate Q is given by:

$$Q = \frac{\pi R^4}{8\eta} \frac{\Delta p}{L} \left\{ 1 + \frac{4\delta}{R} \left(\frac{\eta}{\eta_p} - 1 \right) \right\} \tag{1}$$

where $\Delta p/L$ is the pressure gradient and η and η_p are, respectively, the viscosities of blood and plasma. The first term is the well known Poiseuille flow, and the second term represents the effect of the plasma layer. Obviously, the second term is negligible for larger blood vessels, while it plays an important role in the microcirculation.

Let us consider a straight portion of a microvessel with an angle of tilt θ from vertical (Fig. 3). The acceleration of gravity effective in producing a plasma region at the upper wall is given by the component $g\sin\theta$ perpendicular to the axis of the tube, where g is the acceleration of gravity; $g = 9.80$ m/s^2 on earth. Even in the blood flow through a vertical tube $\theta = 0$, a plasma region can be observed. Therefore, the "uniform" thickness δ of the plasma layer in a tube of radius R may statistically be written as the sum of two terms δ_0 and δ_g, where δ_0

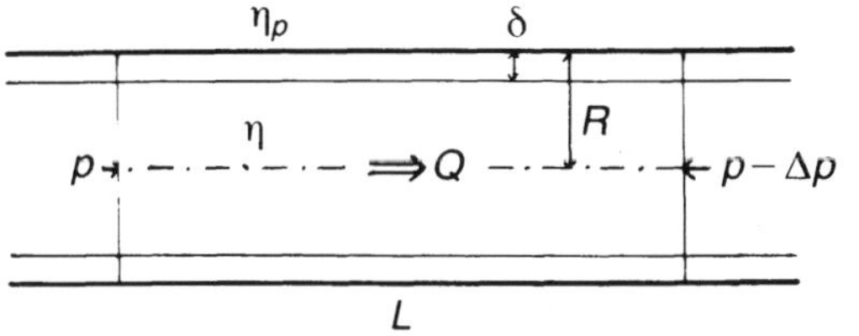

Fig. 2. Model of a microvessel surrounded by a plasma layer of uniform thickness δ

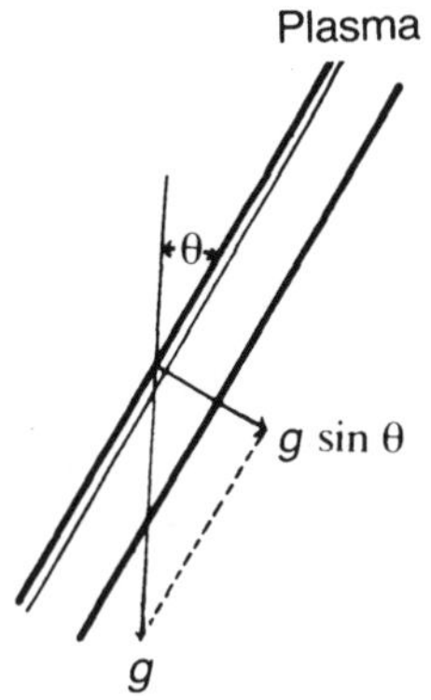

Fig. 3. Continuous production of a plasma region in an inclined microvessel by gravity

is independent of g, while δ_g is proportional to g:

$$\delta = \delta_0 + \delta_g \tag{2}$$

δ_0 is equal to the thickness of the plasma layer in blood flow through a vertical tube.

Consequently, Eq. (1) is written as:

$$Q_E = \frac{\pi R^4}{8\eta}\frac{\Delta p}{L}\left\{1 + \frac{4(\delta_o + \delta_g)}{R}\left(\frac{\eta}{\eta_p} - 1\right)\right\} \tag{3}$$

on earth. If we assume that the pressure gradient $\Delta p/L$ and the blood viscosity η remain the same in space as on earth, the flow rate in an environment of zero gravity will become:

$$Q_S = \frac{\pi R^4}{8\eta}\frac{\Delta p}{L}\left\{1 + \frac{4\delta_o}{R}\left(\frac{\eta}{\eta_p} - 1\right)\right\} \tag{4}$$

the term δ_g disappears here. Obviously, the flow rate Q_S in space is less than the corresponding flow rate Q_E on earth in accordance with our expectation.

Let us denote the reduction rate of the blood flow by:

$$\alpha = \frac{Q_E - Q_S}{Q_E} \tag{5}$$

Substitution of Eqs. (3) and (4) gives:

$$\alpha = \frac{4(\eta/\eta_p - 1)\delta_g/R}{1 + 4(\eta/\eta_p - 1)(\delta_2 + \delta_g)/R} \tag{6}$$

Table 1. Reduction rate α for several values of δ_0/D

δ_0/D (%)	1.0	1.5	2.0	2.5	3.0	3.5	4.0
α (%)	12	16	20	22	25	27	28

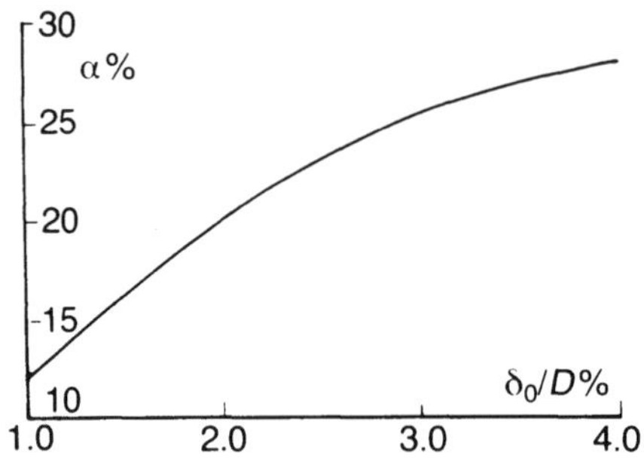

Fig. 4. Plot of α against δ_o/D

If we take the usual viscosity values of $\eta_p = 1.33$ cP and $\eta = 4.04$ cP, then Eq. (6) becomes simplified to:

$$\alpha = \frac{16.3\delta_g/D}{1 + 16.3(\delta_0 + \delta_g)/D} \tag{7}$$

where D = 2R is the inner diameter of the vessel. Note that the observed values of δ_0/D are usually within the range of 4%–2%, the values being larger for smaller vessels [2].

It is regrettable that the value of δ_g is entirely unknown at present. If we assume simply:

$$\delta_g = \delta_0 \tag{8}$$

for the present, then the reduction rate α can be calculated for various values of δ_0/D within the range of 1.0%-4.0% (Table 1). It is noteworthy that the corresponding values of α are found up to 12%–28%. The reduction rate α is also plotted against δ_0/D in Fig. 4. δ_g is probably much larger than δ_0 in consideration of the vigorous upflow of plasma in inclined tubes.

Conclusion

The flow rate of the human microcirculation in any organ will be remarkably reduced during spaceflight compared with the flow rate on earth. The reduction rate is greater in smaller microvessels than in larger ones. This theoretical study on microcirculatory dysfunction in an environment of weightlessness strongly emphasizes the beneficial role of gravity, which has not yet been observed in the microcirculation of man and animals on earth.

The increase in the flow resistance of the microcirculation in spaceflight results, of course, in decreased flow resistance in the systemic circulation.

A decrease in the flow rate of blood is one of the various symptoms experienced by astronauts in space [3], in agreement with the conclusion of the present simplified theoretical study.

Discussion

Several assumptions are made in this simplified theoretical approach. The assumptions that blood flow is laminar, steady, and Newtonian may be generally valid in the microcirculation. It is assumed that the pressure gradient in space remains the same as on earth. Sandler [4] reports that human blood pressure shows no marked change in spaceflight. It is assumed that blood viscosity during spaceflight remains the same as on earth. Dintenfass [5] reports that erythrocytes retain their normal shape in space; they do form aggregates, but such aggregates are smaller than the corresponding aggregates obtained on earth. Since the aggregation of erythrocytes is closely related to blood viscosity, the measurement of blood viscosity in spaceflight is very much desired.

The Fahraeus effect shows that the blood viscosity depends on hematocrit in the microvessels. Therefore, the blood viscosity 4.04 cP in Eq. (6) should be replaced by smaller values depending upon the tissue.

This study has been limited to the blood flow within a microvessel without permeability. Apelblat et al. [6] studied the microvessel-tissue fluid exchange based on Krogh's model. The tissues region was treated as an isotropic porous medium to which Darcy's law is applicable.

In water, the body weight is almost equal to the surface force buoyancy. I believe that these conditions are not the same as true weightlessness or zero gravity. Although the body weight is equal to buoyancy, gravity still acts on the erythrocytes to form a plasma region in the microvessels, such that no appreciable change occurs in the microcirculation in swimming.

A number of investigations have been presented on cardiovascular disorders during spaceflight, such as the weightlessness-induced headward fluid shift, decrease in heart size and fall in cardiac output usually associated with a fall in stroke volume and decrease in heart rate [4]. The effects of the headward fluid shift and other disorders on the flow rate of blood in microcirculation need to be investigated in future studies.

References

1. Boycott AE (1920) Sedimentation of blood corpuscles. Nature 104: 532
2. Charm SE, Kurland GS (1974) Blood flow and microcirculation. Wiley, New York, p 73
3. Nicogossian A, Buchanan P (1984) Life sciences considerations for long duration manned space missions. John F Kennedy Space Center
4. Sandler H (1986) Zero-G fluid mechanics in animal and man. In: Lantz SA, King AI (eds) Advances in Bioengineering. Am Soc Mech Eng, New York, p 80
5. Dintenfass L (1985) Mystery of red cell aggregation under zero gravity. Med J Australia 143: 281–283
6. Apelblat A, Katzir-Katchalsky A, Silberberg A (1974) A mathematical analysis of capillary-tissue fluid exchange. Biorheology 11: 1

Chapter 2
Multiple Organ Failure

How Hyperoxemia May Lead to Ischemia in Multiple Organs and Possibly to Organ Failure

NIELS LUND[1]

The causes and effects of hypoxemia have been the subjects of innumerable investigations. It is intuitively understood, and has been scientifically shown, that in most instances hypoxemia is harmful to human beings. However, the negative effects of normobaric hyperoxemia are less well known to the clinician.

Oxygen Transport in Organs

The first organ which is reached by oxygen is the lung. Historically, right-to-left intrapulmonary shunt has been measured while administering an FiO_2 of 1.0, i.e., 100% oxygen, the hypothesis being that an FiO_2 of 1.0 should eliminate the shunting effect of inequalities of ventilation and perfusion [1]. This hypothesis was questioned by several groups in the mid-1970s and the early 1980s. Douglas and co-workers [2] showed that venous admixture increased when FiO_2 was above 0.6, Shapiro et al, [3] found an increase in intrapulmonary shunting at an FiO_2 of 1.0. Finally, Oliven et al. [4] reported an increase in pulmonary venous admixture as FiO_2 was increased from 0.21 to 0.4. It is, thus, fairly well established that high inspired fractions of oxygen influence arterial blood oxygenation adversely.

However, it is easy to reach high arterial oxygen levels on a short-term basis until the long-term pulmonary toxic effects of oxygen come into play and, among other effects, create a gas diffusion barrier. Thus, what happens downstream when arterial blood with high oxygen pressures reaches the tissues? High oxygen levels in this context are defined as a p_aO_2 above 130 mmHg. Many methods have been used to assess tissue oxygenation. Several groups have used the multipoint surface oxygen electrode first described by Kessler and Lübbers in 1966 (Fig. 1) [5].

If we begin with the pump, i.e., the heart, studies done by Walfridsson [7] on pig hearts (Fig. 2) show that an arterial pO_2 above 140 mmHg leads to abnormal

[1]Department of Anesthesiology, University of Rochester, School of Medicine and Dentistry, Rochester, NY 14642, USA

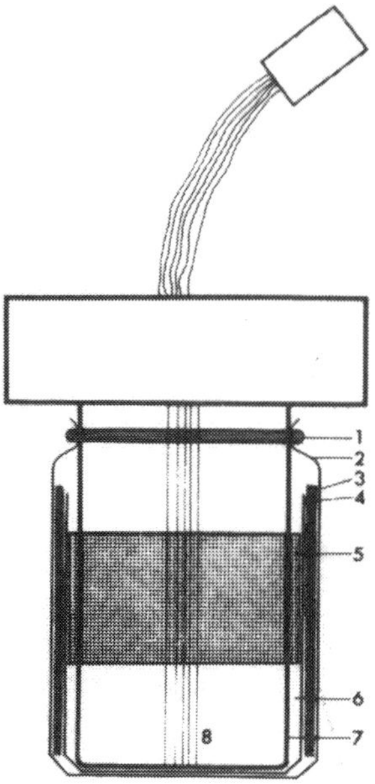

Fig. 1. Oxygen surface electrode of Kessler and Lübbers [5]. *1* Rubber ring, *2* Teflon membrane, *3* plastic ring, *4* cellophane membrane, *5* Ag/AgCl anode, *6* 0.2 *M* KCl, *7* glass nucleus, *8* platinum wires. Reproduced with kind permission of Acta Anaesthesiologica Scandinavica [6]

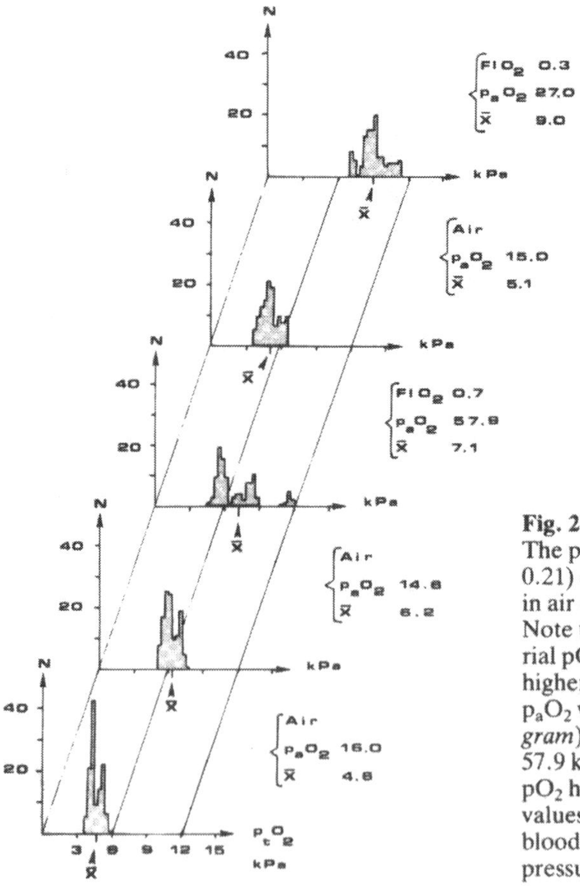

Fig. 2. Histograms from pig heart. The pig was breathing either air (FiO_2 0.21) or increased fractions of oxygen in air (FiO_2 0.3 and 0.7, respectively). Note that during air breathing an arterial pO_2 (p_aO_2) below 15 kPa led to a higher mean tissue pO_2 ($\bar{x}$) than when p_aO_2 was 16.0 kPa (*lowermost histogram*). When FiO_2 was 0.7, p_aO_2 was 57.9 kPa; the corresponding tissue pO_2 histogram shows a scattering of values (indicating maldistribution of blood flow). *N* number of oxygen pressure values, p_tO_2 tissue pO_2

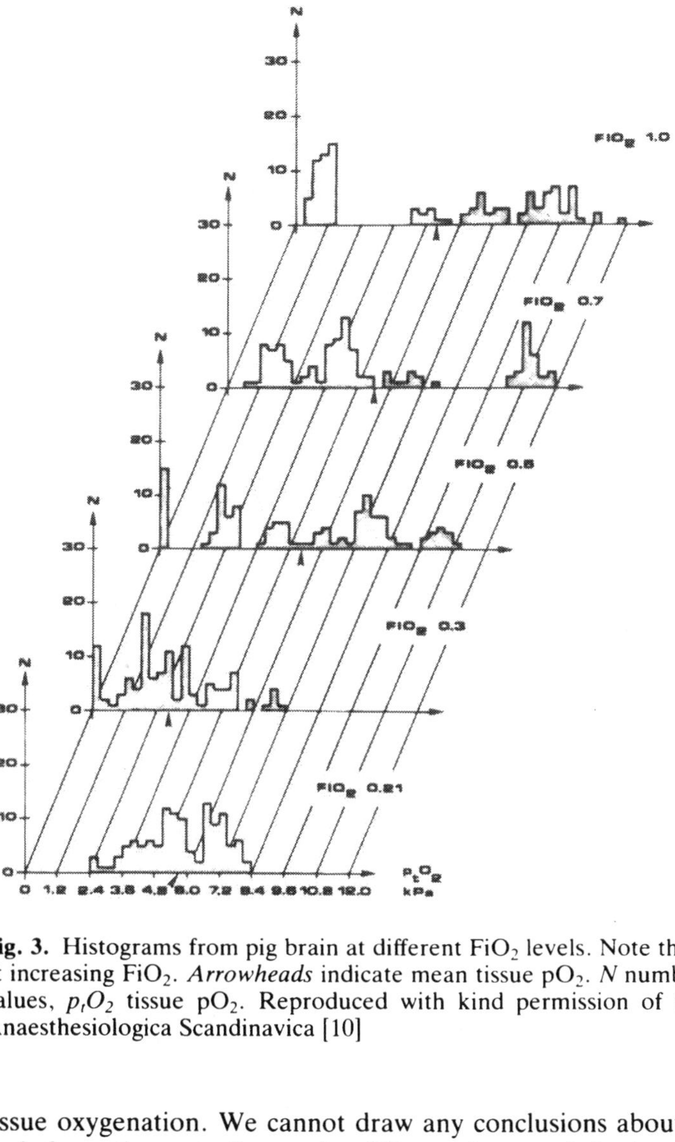

Fig. 3. Histograms from pig brain at different FiO_2 levels. Note the increasing scattering at increasing FiO_2. *Arrowheads* indicate mean tissue pO_2. *N* number of oxygen pressure values, p_tO_2 tissue pO_2. Reproduced with kind permission of the authors and Acta Anaesthesiologica Scandinavica [10]

tissue oxygenation. We cannot draw any conclusions about the whole heart as such from these studies as the different layers of the heart are supplied with microvessels and oxygen in different ways. Interestingly, Bourdeau-Martini and co-workers in 1974 [8] described a decrease in myocardial capillary density when p_aO_2 was increased from 120 to 300 mmHg. Above 300 mmHg, the capillary density again increased.

Another important part of the body is the brain. Eintrei [9] and Eintrei and Lund [10] studied the effects of high arterial oxygen levels both in pigs (Fig. 3) and humans during neurosurgery. The conclusion drawn from these studies was that an arterial oxygen level above 115 mmHg will lead to a maldistribution of brain oxygenation with an increase in the number of areas with low oxygen levels.

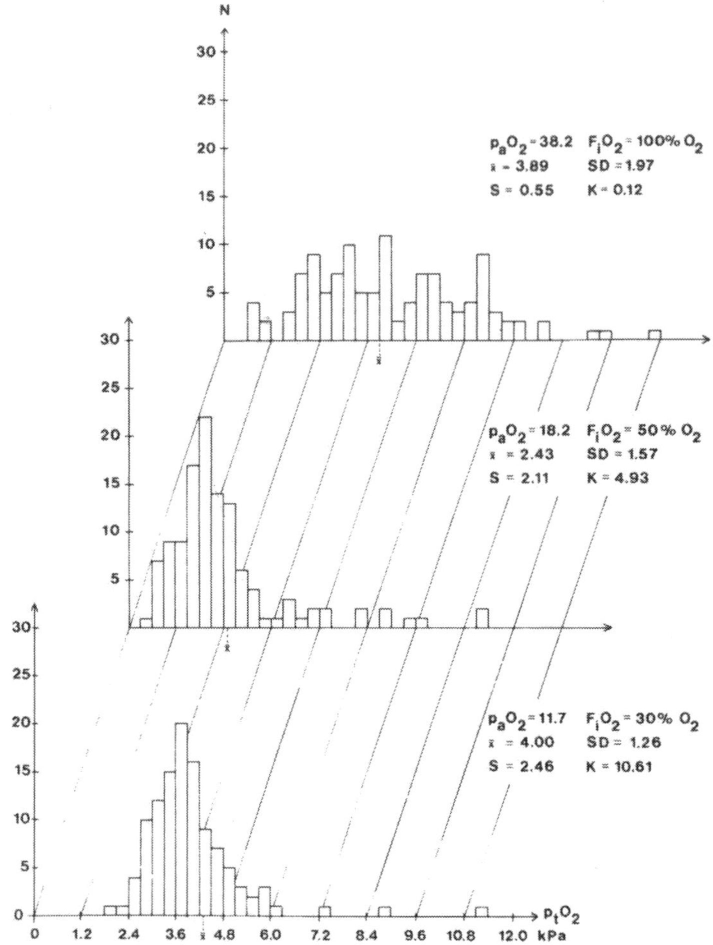

Fig. 4. Histograms from the brachioradial muscle in a ventilated, critically ill patient registered at different arterial oxygen pressures. The *lower histogram* is normal. The *middle histogram* shows a lower mean value and the beginning of scattering of tissue pO_2 values. The *upper histogram* is abnormal. *N* number of oxygen pressure values, p_tO_2 tissue pO_2, FiO_2 inspired oxygen concentration, $\bar{x}$ mean, *SD* standard deviation, *S* skewness, *K* kurtosis. Reproduced with kind permission of the authors and Acta Anaesthesiologica Scandinavica [12]

A less important part of the body, at least in terms of survival, is the skeletal muscle. However, skeletal muscle constitutes a large proportion of the body and it is important in situations when the blood volume is redistributed. Studies by Lund [11] and Lund et al. [12] have indicated that skeletal muscle (Fig. 4) is not different from any other tissue with respect to the effects of high arterial oxygen levels. In parallel with the findings by Bourdeau-Martini et al. in the myocardium, Lindbom and co-workers in 1980 [13] published data on the capillary density in skeletal muscle. When ambient pO_2 was elevated progressively from

5 to 100 mmHg, capillary density fell from 269/mm² to 6/mm². When the muscle was exposed to atmospheric oxygen tension (i.e., above 150 mmHg) there were no perfused capillaries at all.

Other organs than those mentioned above have been studied in different animals, and they show parallel results, i.e., high arterial oxygen levels affect capillary blood flow and tissue oxygenation.

Blood Flow Maldistribution

What causes maldistribution of the blood flow? Many factors have been investigated, mostly by Duling and co-workers. Duling and Jackson [14] showed that oxygen-induced constriction of arterioles was not mediated by nerves or oxygen effects on the surrounding parenchyma, but that oxygen acts locally on a component of the arteriolar wall or blood. In 1982, Proctor and Duling [15] concluded

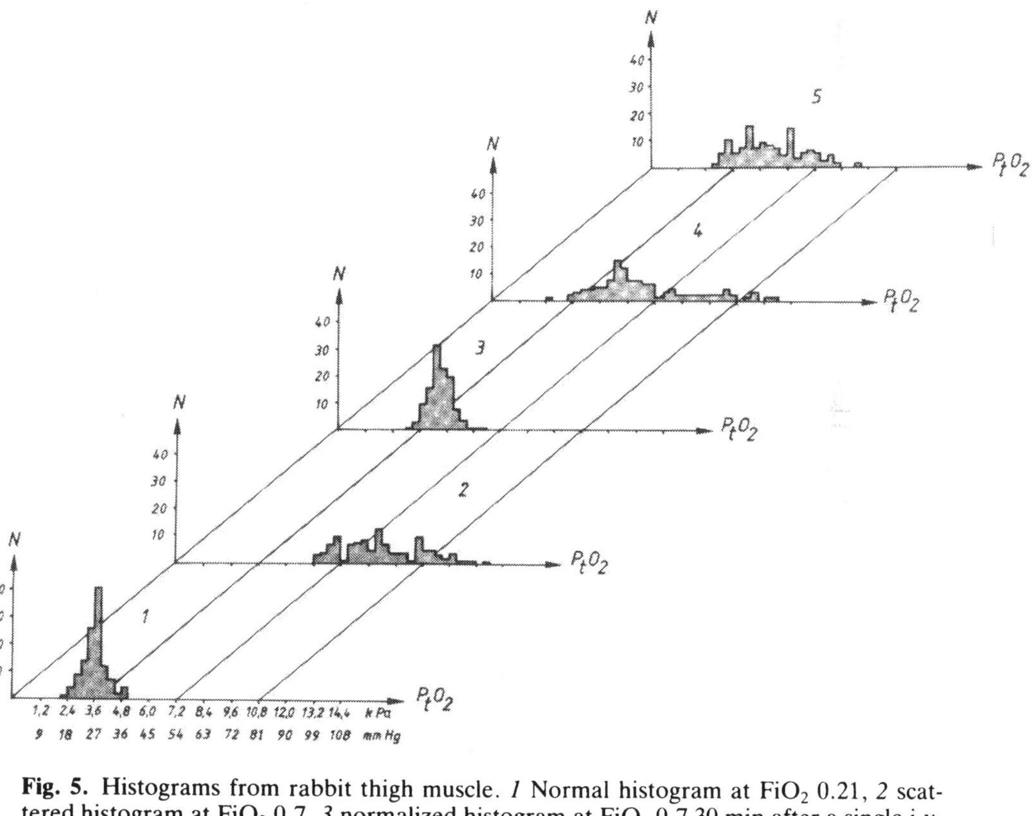

Fig. 5. Histograms from rabbit thigh muscle. *1* Normal histogram at FiO_2 0.21, *2* scattered histogram at FiO_2 0.7, *3* normalized histogram at FiO_2 0.7 30 min after a single i.v. injection of ketanserin 0.07 mg × kg bw^{-1}, *4* scattered histogram at FiO_2 0.7 90 min after the single i.v. injection of ketanserin 0.07 mg × kg bw^{-1}, *5* scattered histogram at FiO_2 0.7 after an additional single i.v. dose of ketanserin 0.035 mg × kg bw^{-1}. *N* number of oxygen pressure values, p_tO_2 tissue pO_2. Reproduced with kind permission of the authors and Critical Care Medicine [18]

that the release of superoxide radicals into the extracellular space was not involved in local microvascular control of muscle blood flow. Very recently, Jackson has shown that prostaglandins are not involved either [16]. Kessler et al. [17] have suggested that "signal oxidases" may be involved in the regulation of capillary flow distribution. In 1986, Thorborg et al. [18] found indications that ketanserin, a serotonin-S_2 receptor antagonist, counteracts the microcirculatory effects of hyperoxemia (Fig. 5).

Conclusion

A great deal is known about the distribution of blood flow in different microvascular beds. We have some knowledge about what regulates the distribution of blood flow. It is known from the work of many authors that most, if not all, organs in the body respond negatively to high arterial oxygen levels, i.e., tissue pO_2 decreases in large tissue areas. We know very little about the long-term effects of oxygen on different organs. In all probability oxygen in itself cannot kill a person acutely, but the long-term effects of high arterial oxygen pressures are clearly negative.

Developments in drugs may allow us to treat patients with high levels of oxygen without closing the microcirculation. However, it is not known whether in this way even more harm may be caused, e.g., through the increased production of free oxygen radicals.

I do not think that hyperoxemia alone can cause extensive organ damage on a short-term basis, but adding excessively high oxygen levels to other injury factors is definitely not helpful. Also, when hemoglobin is fully saturated, little is gained by increasing the inspired fraction of oxygen.

Acknowledgments. Several of the studies were supported by grants from the Swedish Medical Research Council (02042, 05956), the County Council of Östergötland, Sweden (15/82, 96/82, 98/82, 14/83, 16/84, 085/84, 088/84, 092/84), the Swedish Society of Medical Sciences (346), the Tore Nilson Foundation (83/94, 84/20, 85/5) and the Faculty of Medicine, Linköping University, Sweden.

References

1. Berggren S (1942) The oxygen deficit of arterial blood caused by nonventilating parts of the lung. Acta Physiol Scand [Suppl] 11: 1–92
2. Douglas ME, Downs JB, Dannemiller FJ, Hodgess MR, Munson ES (1976) Change in pulmonary venous admixture with varying inspired oxygen. Anesth Analg 55: 688–95
3. Shapiro BA, Cane RD, Harrison RA, Steiner MC (1980) Changes in intrapulmonary shunting with administration of 100 percent oxygen. Chest 77: 138–141
4. Oliven A, Abinader E, Bursztein S (1980) influence of varying inspired oxygen tensions on the pulmonary venous admixture (shunt) of mechanically ventilated patients. Crit Care Med 8: 99–101
5. Kessler M, Lübbers DW (1966) Aufbau und Anwendungsmöglichkeit verschiedener PO_2-Elektroden. Pflügers Arch ges Physiol 291: R82

6. Lund N (1978) Methods for measuring tissue oxygen tension. Acta anaesth scand suppl 70: 183–5
7. Walfridsson H (1985) Myocardial oxygen pressure of the border zone. Linköping University Medical Dissertations No 199
8. Bourdeau-Martini J, Odoroff C, Honig CR (1974) Dual effect of oxygen on magnitude and uniformity of coronary intercapillary distance. Am J Physiol 226: 800–10
9. Eintrei C (1985) Blood flow and oxygen pressure in cerebral cortex. An experimental and clinical study. Linköping University Medical Dissertations No 210
10. Eintrei C, Lund N (1986) Effects of increases in the inspired oxygen fraction on brain surface oxygen pressure fields in pig and man. Acta Anaesthesiol Scand 30: 194–198, 599
11. Lund N (1979) Studies on skeletal muscle surface oxygen pressure fields. Linköping University Medical Dissertations No 71
12. Lund N, Jorfeldt J, Lewis DH, Ödman S (1980) Skeletal muscle oxygen pressure fields in artificially ventilated critically ill patients. Acta anaesth scand 24: 347–53
13. Lindbom L, Tuma RF, Arfors K-E (1980) Influence of oxygen on perfused capillary density and capillary red cell velocity in rabbit skeletal muscle. Microvasc Res 19: 197–208
14. Jackson WF, Duling BR (1983) The oxygen sensitivity of hamster cheek pouch arterioles. In vitro and in situ studies. Circ Res 53: 515–25
15. Proctor KG, Duling BR (1982) Oxygen-derived free radicals and local control of striated muscle blood flow. Microvasc Res 24: 77–86
16. Jackson WF (1986) Prostaglandins do not mediate arteriolar oxygen reactivity. Am J Physiol 250: H1102–8
17. Kessler M, Höper J, Harrison DK, Skolasinska K, Klövekorn WP, Sebening F, Volkholz HJ, Beier I, Kernbach C, Rettig V, Richter H (1984) Tissue O_2 supply under normal and pathological conditions. In: Lübbers DW, Acker H, Leniger-Follert E, Goldstick TK (eds) Oxygen transport to tissue: V. Plenum Press, New York and London, pp 69–80
18. Thorborg P, Sjöberg F, Lund N (1986) Serotonin—a regulator of tissue oxygenation? Crit Care Med 14: 395

Multiple Organ Failure in Low Cardiac Output Syndrome After Cardiac Surgery

Keiji Kumon[1], Kazuhiko Tanaka[1], Takahiko Hirata[1], Yoshitsugu Kitoh[2], and Tsuyoshi Fujita[2]

Major advances in the care of critically ill patients have resulted in fewer deaths. However, multiple organ failure (MOF) remains a principal cause of fatality. Low cardiac output syndrome after cardiac surgery (LOS) is defined as the imbalance of oxygen demand and supply in tissues as the result of impaired cardiac function [1]. Insufficient oxygen delivery due to LOS produces MOF [2]. Here, we present an analysis of MOF in LOS patients after open heart surgery as well as continous measuring of mixed venous oxygen saturation ($S\bar{v}O_2$) for estimating oxygen metabolism in LOS upon MOF.

Subjects

From 1977 to 1986, a total of 4179 patients after open heart surgery were treated postoperatively at the ICU of the National Cardiovascular Center. LOS was defined as a decrease of cardiac index to less than 2.2 l/min/m^2, necessitating the administration of large doses of inotropic agents with or without an assist circulation. Under this definition, LOS developed in 884 patients (21.2%).

Organ Failures in LOS Patients

The criteria for organ failure used in this study are listed in Table 1. We found some organ failure caused by LOS in 553 patients (62.6%) of the LOS patients.

The incidence of impaired organs in LOS patients and the clinical results are listed in Table 2. Respiratory failure and acute renal failure were the most common complications in LOS patients. The most common course of MOF in LOS was the following: LOS initially triggered respiratory failure and/or acute renal failure. Difficult controlling these complications subsequently resulted in MOF, which was aggravated by various complicated activators, such as infection, shock disseminated intravascular coagulation (DIC), malnutrition [2].

Intensive Care Unit[1], Cardiovascular Surgery[2], National Cardiovascular Center, 7-1, Fujishirodai 5-chome, Suita, Osaka, 565 Japan

Table 1. Criteria for organ failures

Condition	
Respiratory failure	Respiratory index ($A\text{-}aDo_2/Pao_2$) > 1.5 or necessitated prolonged mechanical ventilation
Acute renal failure	Serum creatinine > 2.0 mg/dl or necessitated dialysis
Hepatic failure	Serum bilirubin > 3.0 mg/dl
Disseminated intravascular coagulation	FDP > 20 μg/ml and platelet count < $7.0 \times 10^4/mm^3$ or rapid fall
Central nervous system failure	Altered levels of consciousness and/or seizures
Gastrointestinal bleeding	Necessitated transfusion

FDP fibrin or fibrinogen degradation product, *$A\text{-}aDo_2$* alveolar-arterial oxygen tension difference

Clinical Results

The clinical results of LOS patients associated with some organ failure were extremely poor; the mortality of patients with respiratory failure was 38.7% and that of other organ failures exceeded 50%, as indicated in Table 2. Figure 1 also shows the clinical results after open heart surgery. The overall mortality was 5.5%, and it was 0.9% in patients free from LOS. The mortality of LOS patients without associated organ failure was 5.2%, remaining in a lower range. However, in the LOS patients with complicated organ failure, the mortality elevated inevitably as the number of failed organs increased. Therefore, it can be said that organ failure has played a vital role in the clinical results of patients after open heart surgery.

Clinical Aspects on Major Organ Failure in LOS

Respiratory Failure

We found three types of respiratory failure in LOS patients: lung edema or congestion due to increased pulmonary capillary pressure in left ventricular failure, an increase of the ventilation-perfusion ratio caused by right ventricular failure or pulmonary hypertension, and acute respiratory distress syndrome due to pulmonary endothelial damage associated with open heart surgery [2].

Acute Renal Failure

Acute renal failure in LOS develops according to the following process. First, a reduction of renal blood flow leads to oliguria or anuria. Then, reduced oxygen supply allows ischemic damage of the parenchyma and dysfunction of the

Table 2. Incidence of impaired organs in LOS patients and the clinical results

Impaired organ	Incidence (%)	Mortality (%)
Respiratory failure	48.8	38.7
Acute renal failure	30.9	55.3
Hepatic failure	22.3	50.3
DIC	17.3	59.5
Gastrointestinal bleeding	11.0	64.9
CNS failure	16.4	62.1

LOS low output syndrome, *DIC* Disseminated intravascular coagulation, *CNS* Central nervous system

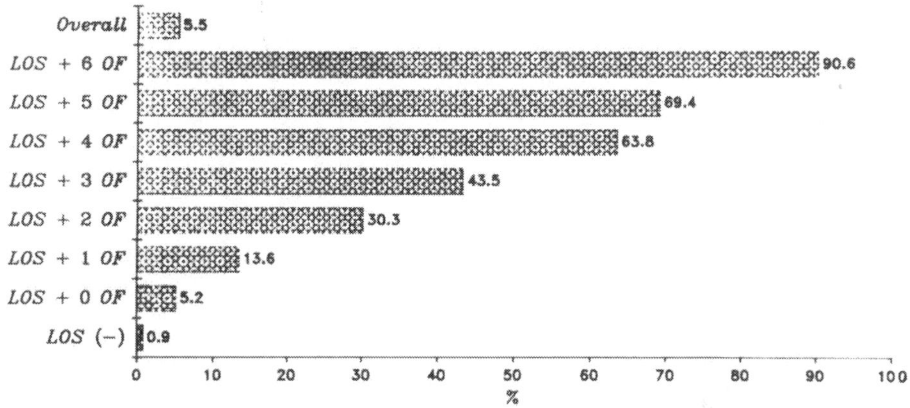

Fig. 1. Clinical results of open heart surgery. *LOS* low output syndrome, *OF* organ failure

mitochondria. This leads to cell swelling due to Na-K pump failure in the cell membrane. Swollen cells compress the intercellular renal capillaries, facilitating the ischemia and finally leading to acute tubular necrosis [2, 3].

Hepatic Failure

Hepatic failure due to LOS is classified clinically into two types—the ischemic and intrahepatic cholestatic types. The ischemic type is caused by low perfusion to liver tissue, leading to centrilobular necrosis. We found increases in the serum levels of hepatic enzymes in this type. The second type is initially caused by congestion of the liver due to right ventricular failure. The laboratory findings consist of elevation of direct bilirubin without concomitant increases of enzymes. This type of hepatic failure is also triggered and/or aggravated by the cell swelling after ischemia, infection, and drug intoxication [2].

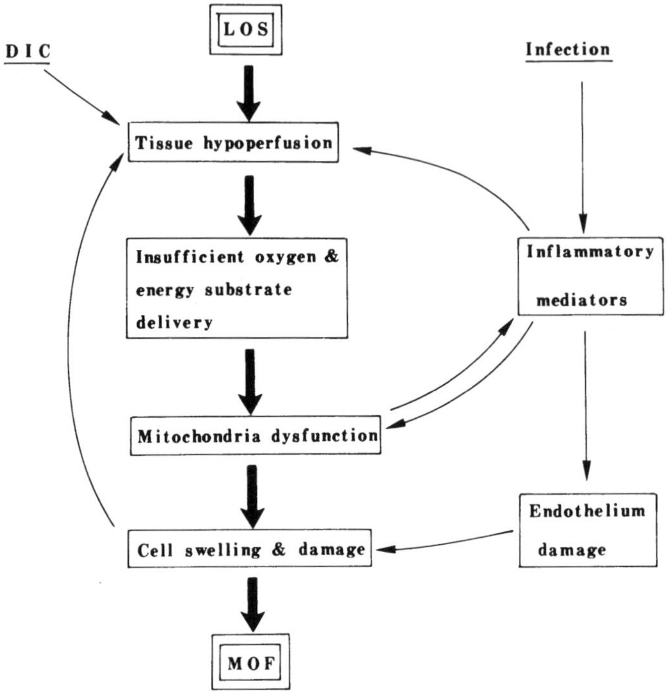

Fig. 2. Schematized hypothesis on the main mechanism responsible for cell damages due to low cardiac output syndrome (*LOS*). *DIC* disseminated intravascular coagulation, *MOF* multiple organ failure

Mechanism of Cell Damage Due to LOS

Figure 2 schematizes our hypothesis on the main mechanism responsible for cell damage due to LOS. First, insufficient oxygen and energy substrate delivery produce initial cell damage [3]. Then, swollen cells induced by the initial damage cause compressive obstruction of the capillaries, promoting the ischemia. Moreover, this cell damage is facilitated by various inflammatory mediators, such as the complement system, vasoactive substances, arachidonic cascade, lysozome enzyme, interleukin 1, toxic radical [4]. Finally, these lead to irreversible cell damage and result in MOF [2].

Continuous Measurement of $S\bar{v}o_2$ in LOS upon MOF

The development of initial cell damage depends on both the severity and duration of insufficient oxygen delivery in LOS. For estimating the oxygen metabolism, we measured continuously $S\bar{v}o_2$ by fiberoptic reflection oximetry in patients after cardiac surgery [5, 6].

Figure 3 shows the changes in $S\bar{v}o_2$ early after operation for acquired valvular diseases. The $S\bar{v}o_2$ levels of uneventful cases were stable at around 75% during

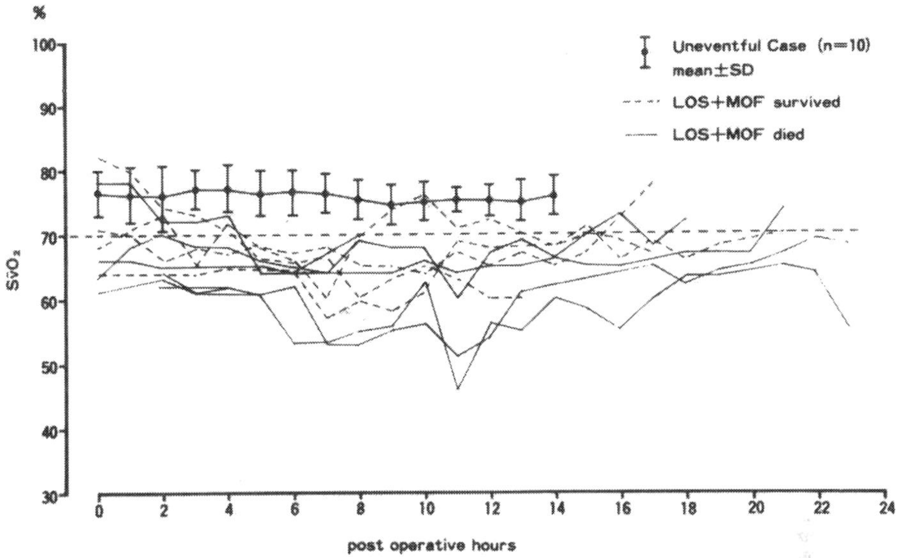

Fig. 3. Changes in mixed venous oxygen saturation ($S\bar{v}o_2$) after open heart surgery. The *closed circles* ± SD indicate ten uneventful cases. The *broken lines* indicate patients who survived the development of MOF due to LOS. *Solid lines* indicate patients who died due to MOF caused by LOS

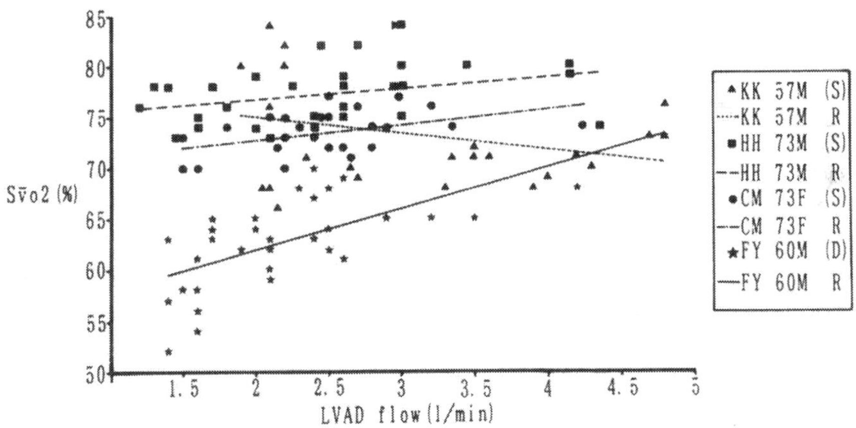

Fig. 4. Changes in $S\bar{v}o_2$ during weaning from left ventricular assist device (*LVAD*). *S* survived, *D* died, *R* regression line

the study periods. In contrast, in each case, the $S\bar{v}o_2$ of MOF patients decreased to less than 70% for several hours during the study periods, reflecting the insufficient oxygen delivery in LOS.

We also measured $S\bar{v}o_2$ continuously in patients who required circulatory support by left ventricular assist device (LVAD). Figure 4 shows the changes in

$S\bar{v}o_2$ in four patients during the weaning from LVAD. The $S\bar{v}o_2$ of a patient who died due to MOF developed after LVAD removal decreased associated with a reduction of the blood flow previously supported by LVAD. In contrast, the $S\bar{v}o_2$ of the other three patients who were successfully weaned from LVAD and survived was maintained at relatively high levels independent of the reduction of the supported blood flow, indicating sufficient oxygen delivery.

From these findings, continuously measuring $S\bar{v}o_2$ and keeping $S\bar{v}o_2$ above 70% is recommended to prevent the complicated organ failures due to LOS.

Summary

The insufficient oxygen delivery in LOS triggers MOF, which can be aggravated by secondary ischemia at the microcirculation level and by inflammatory mediators. The organ failure due to LOS plays a vital role in the clinical results of open heart surgery.

For estimating initial insufficient oxygen delivery in LOS, continuous measuring of $S\bar{v}o_2$ is useful. Keeping $S\bar{v}o_2$ above 70% is recommended to prevent the initial organ damage in LOS.

References

1. Dietzman RH, Ersek RA, Lillehei CW, Castaneda CW, Lillehei RC (1969) Low output syndrome. Recognition and treatment. J Thorac Cardiovasc Surg 57: 138
2. Kumon K, Tanaka K, Hirata T, Naito Y, Fujita T (1986) Organ failures due to low cardiac output syndrome following open heart surgery. Jpn Circ J 50: 329–335
3. Chaudry IH, Clemens MG, Baue AE (1981) Alterations in cell with ischemia and shock and their correction. Arch Surg 116: 1309
4. Keller GA, West MA, Cerra FB, Simmons RL (1985) Macrophage-mediated modulation of hepatic function in multiple-system failure. J Surg Res 39: 555–563
5. Schmidt CR, Frank LP, Forsythe SB, Estafanous FG (1984) Continuous $S\bar{v}o_2$ measurement and oxygen transport patterns in cardiac surgery patients. Crit Care Med 12: 523–527
6. Kuwabara M, Kumon K, Hirata T, Tanaka K, Kawazoe K, Kitoh Y, Nakajima N, Fujita T (1986) Usefulness of continous measuring of mixed venous oxygen saturation ($S\bar{v}o_2$) in cardiac surgery. Jpn J Thorac Surg 39: 686–689

Deteriorating Defense Mechanism for Bacterial Infection and High Incidence of Endotoxemia in Surgical Patients Developing MOF

Masaru Ishiyama, Chiyuki Watanabe, Takashi Ichikura, Kojiro Kuroiwa, Satoru Inoue, Takeyuki Hiramatsu, and Yasuhiko Morioka[1]

Introduction

Multiple organ failure (MOF), a clinical concept first reported by Tilney et al. [1], is a critical state in which the function of vital organs or physiological systems progressively or sequentially deteriorates during hemodialysis for patients with acute renal failure following surgery for a ruptured abdominal aneurysm. Baue [2], Eiseman et al. [3], Fry et al. [4], and others describe similar pathophysiological sequelae which appear in various critically ill patients, including subjects who have undergone gastrointestinal surgery. These authors coincidentally emphasize that most MOF cases are accompanied by severe bacterial infection and that the mortality of MOF is extremely high.

We experienced 55 MOF cases in 2501 patients who underwent various abdominal surgical procedures over the past 6 years. The major cause of MOF was postoperative infection such as intra-abdominal or intrathoracic abscess, cholangitis, and pneumonia. On the other hand, nonseptic causes included hepatic failure following hepatectomy or esophageal transection, massive hemorrhage, and so on. Most of these latter cases of MOF indicated certain septic signs such as fever, leukocytosis, or endotoxemia. Endotoxin in the bloodstream, as one of the lethal factors, was positive in over 90% of the patients to whom the Limulus test was applied, regardless of whether they were septic or nonseptic [5].

It is thus apparent that the bacterial factor is most contributory in establishing the clinical features of MOF, although there may be many other contributing factors. Furthermore, an immunocompromised state may be present which directly brings about bacterial infection.

Effective elucidation of the conditions leading to intractable sepsis and MOF was accomplished by a retrospective analysis of postoperative patients including the 55 MOF cases mentioned above. The plasma opsonic index (OI) was employed as a parameter of immunodefense activity. The OI assaying technique was first proposed by Hirsch and Strauss and modified by Alexander et al. [6]

[1]First Department of Surgery, Faculty of Medicine, University of Tokyo, 3-1, Hongo 7-chome, Bunkyo-ku, Tokyo, 113 Japan

Method

Clinical Analysis of 55 MOF Cases

The contributing factors which lead to MOF arising in surgical patients were assessed by performing surgical procedures on MOF patients, followed by an investigation of the preoperative risk factors of these patients.

Evaluation of Immunological Defense Mechanism in Surgical Patients

Measurement of Plasma OI . The OI measurement technique employed was that of a modified method of Alexander et al. [6].

Patients' samples. Five milliliters of each patient's blood were taken by venipuncture, using 0.5 ml sodium citrate. After centrifugation, the supernatant was dialyzed using seamless cellulose tubing (Union Carbide Corp., Danbury, CT, USA) to eliminate any antibiotics present and was passed through a 0.22-μm millipore filter (Millipore Corporation, Bedord, MA, USA) to ensure the removal of bacteria from the plasma. Plasma free of both antibiotics and bacteria was stored at −80°C for subsequent OI assay.

Pooled normal human plasma. The plasma of several healthy volunteers was treated in exactly the same way as the plasma of MOF patients and was pooled as a control sample at −80°C.

Normal human neutrophil preparation. The blood obtained from a healthy volunteer was mixed with about a half volume of Dextran T-70 and left to stand at room temperature for 45 min. After the supernatant was washed twice with isotonic saline, the neutrophil preparation was prepared at a concentration of 10^7/ml.

Bacteria. *Escherichia coli* 075 (10^7/ml) was prepared.

Hank's balanced salt solution. The actual procedure used to determine the plasma OI is schematized in Fig. 1. Briefly, 0.1 ml *E. coli* 075 in saline and 0.04 ml of each patient sample were mixed with 0.36 ml Hank's balanced salt solution in two separate sterile glass tubes. Then, 0.1 ml neutrophil preparation was added to one of the tubes. The same procedure was carried out for the control samples. After the sets of four glass tubes were incubated for 3 h at 37°C with shaking, the bacteria were counted on agar culture media.

As the final step, the OI was calculated by the formula given in Fig. 1, with the OI indicating the opsonic activity percentage of pooled normal human plasma.

Plasma OI as Indicator of Defense Activity. The clinical evaluation of the OI involved a correlation between the preoperative value of the OI and incidence of postoperative infection, a correlation between the OI and the nutritional index, and a comparison of the changing patterns in the day to day OI values in patients

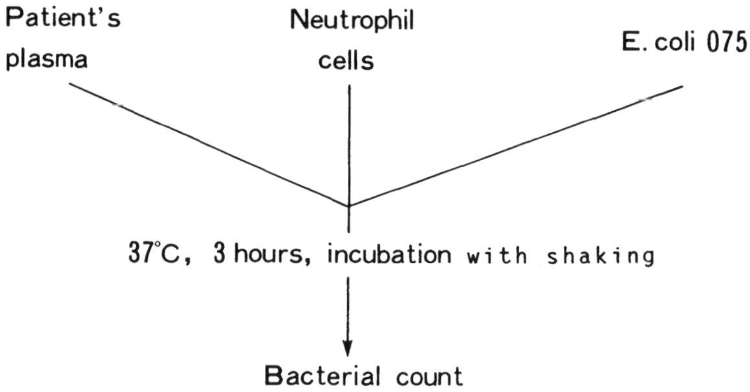

$$OI = \frac{\log P(-) - \log P(+)}{\log C(-) - \log C(+)}$$

Fig. 1. Opsonic index (OI). *P*(−), bacterial counts after incubation with patient's plasma; *P*(+), bacterial counts after incubation with patient's plasma and W.B.C.; *C*(−), bacterial counts after incubation with pooled plasma; *C*(+), bacterial counts after incubation with pooled plsams and W.B.C.

postoperation. The OI values on the day before operation and on postoperative days 2, 4, 6, and 8 for the patients who had undergone various types of abdominal surgery were determined and compared.

Results

The surgical procedures performed in the 55 MOF cases are listed in Table 1. As shown in this table, the majority of MOF patients (33 cases, 60%) underwent fairly extensive procedures, e.g., pancreatoduodenectomy, hepatectomy, subtotal esophagectomy, while 22 patients underwent rather minimal procedures, such as subtotal gastrectomy and partial intestinal resection. This suggests that large stress as a result of the surgical procedure may be a contributing factor in postoperative morbidity. Another important factor is the patient's condition. The MOF cases studied presented various surgical risks, as shown in Table 2; the major factors were aging, liver dysfunction, and emaciation due to advanced malignacy.

As is clear in Table 3, in the cases where the preoperative OI values were low (<0.8), the morbidity for postoperative infection was significantly higher than in the high-OI (≥ 0.8) cases. Therefore, the risk of postoperative infection may be indicated by the preoperative OI value.

Figure 2 indicates a significant correlation between OI and serum albumin titers. There were also similar correlations between the OI values and other nutritional indices, i.e., the serum c3 level, CH50, and rapid turnover proteins. This suggests that nutritional debasement is one of the major causes of a low opsonic activity level.

Table 1. MOF and surgical procedure

Surgical procedure	No. of cases
Right lobectomy of liver and pancreatoduodenectomy	2
Hepatectomy	7
Subtotal esophagectomy	8
Total gastrectomy	8
Esophageal transection	4
Abdominal aneurysmectomy	4
Other	22
Total	55

Table 2. Risk factors in the background of MOF cases

Risk factor	No. of cases
Aging (over 70 years old)	18
Emergency	11
Liver cirrhosis	11
Obstructive jaundice	7
Diabetes mellitus	6
Advanced cancer	2
Leukemia	1
Chronic renal failure	1
Adrenal insufficiency	1

Table 3. Preoperative value of opsonic index and morbidity of postoperative infection

Preoperative opsonic index	Postoperatively infected cases	
	No.	Percent
≥ 0.8 ($n = 67$)	16	24
< 0.8 ($n = 57$)	36*	63

*$P < 0.001$

The serial daily values of OI in patients who had undergone subtotal gastrectomy characteristically lowered just after the operation and recovered within 3 or 4 postoperative days. On the other hand, the group of patients who had undergone more extensive surgical procedures showed a more profound lowering of the OI value immediately after the operation and a low OI value which tended to be prolonged (Fig. 3, asterisk; statistically significant).

Figure 4 demonstrates the characteristic change in the postoperative daily OI values in elderly patients. The upper curve is the daily mean value of the postoperative OI change in the younger (≤ 59 years) patients who underwent subtotal gastrectomy, while the lower curve represents the elder (≥ 70 years) patients undergoing the same procedure. The postoperative lowering of the OI

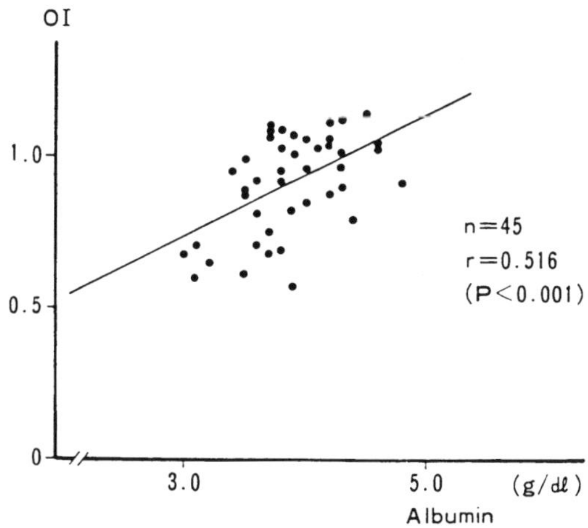

Fig. 2. Albumin and OI (preoperative)

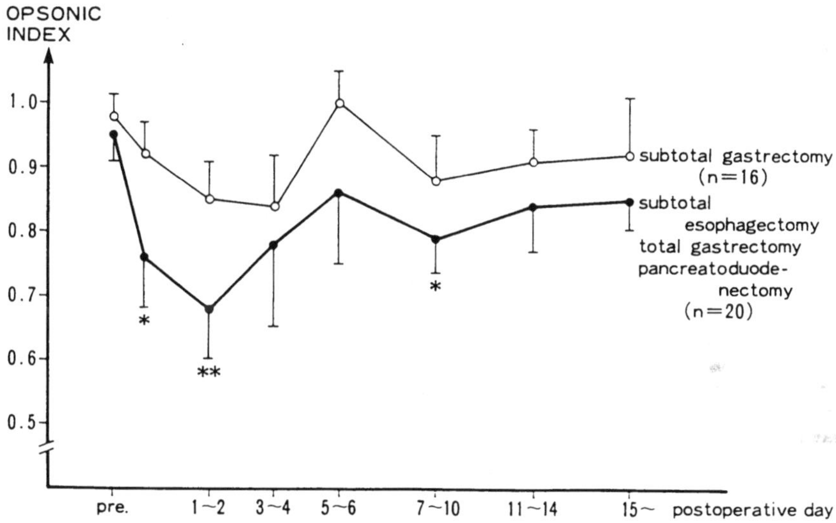

Fig. 3. Postoperative change in OI

values in the older group is clearly larger than in the younger group. It is assumed that in older patients, the same surgical procedure may produce greater damage, and that the postoperative period of older patients may produce a compromised state for bacterial incursion.

In these cases associated with liver cirrhosis, the postoperative debasement of OI values was more remarkable, as is clear in Fig. 5. This may be because the synthesis of opsonic proteins is considerably lowered in these patients.

The effect of a postoperatively administered high-calorie elemental diet on OI is shown in Fig. 6. The postoperative daily OI values of patients who had undergone subtotal esophagectomy or total gastrectomy were very low as shown by the broken line in Fig. 6. The patients received less than 500 kcal/day glucose

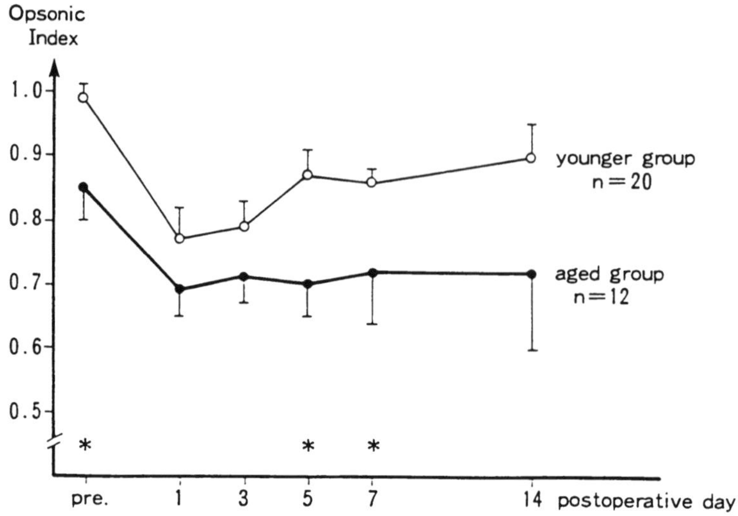

Fig. 4. Postoperative change in OI for younger and aged groups

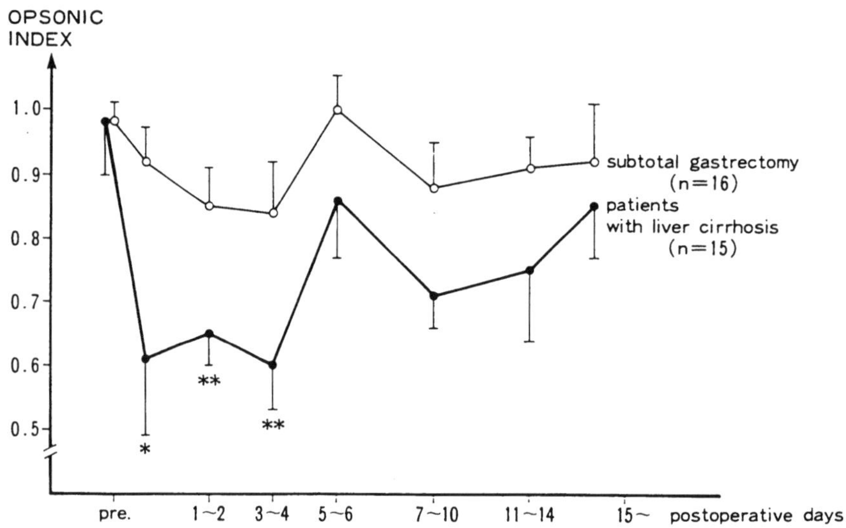

Fig. 5. Postoperative OI change in patients with liver cirrhosis

solution for around 5 postoperative days; even later oral intake proved insufficient. On the other hand, the patients who had undergone the same procedures and were given more than 30 kcal/day/kg body weight of elemental diet through a jejunal catheter from the 4th or 5th postoperative day for 7 days showed markedly improved OI values postoperatively, as shown by the solid line in Fig. 6.

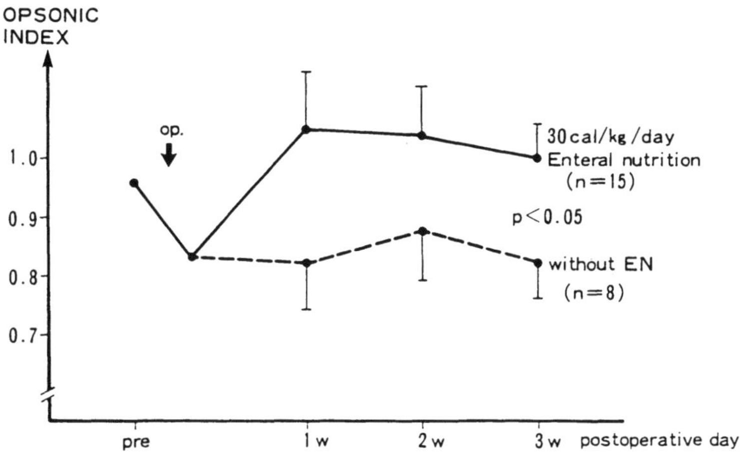

Fig. 6. Effect of enteral nutrition on OI

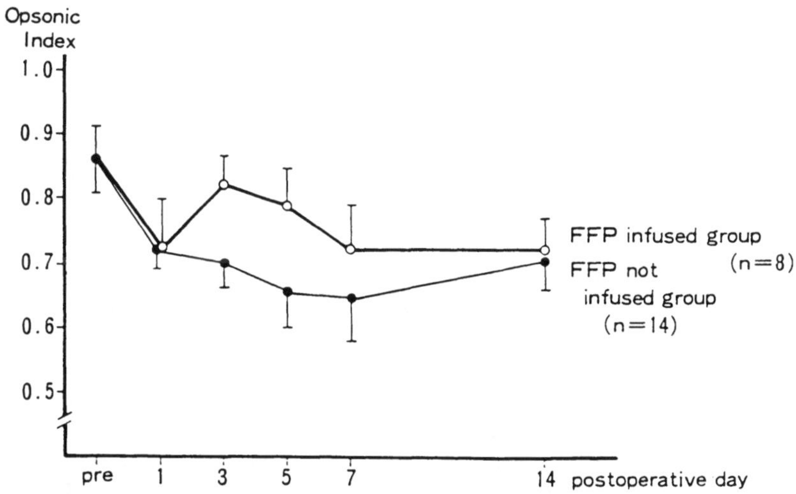

Fig. 7. Postoperative change in opsonic index (elderly patients)

Another more rapidly effective therapy for the low opsonic state is the administration of human fresh frozen plasma (FFP), which contains sufficient opsonic proteins. In the elderly, the postoperative OI values were very low and low titers tended to be prolonged, as is clear from the lower curve of Figs. 4 and 7. However, the changing pattern of OI values in the older patients who were infused with more than 240 ml/day FFP for the first 5 postoperative days was very similar to that of the younger group as is evident from in the upper curve of Fig. 7.

In the liver cirrhosis group indicated in Fig. 8, a sufficient effect of FFP administration on the postoperative OI values was obtained by more than 800 ml FFP/day.

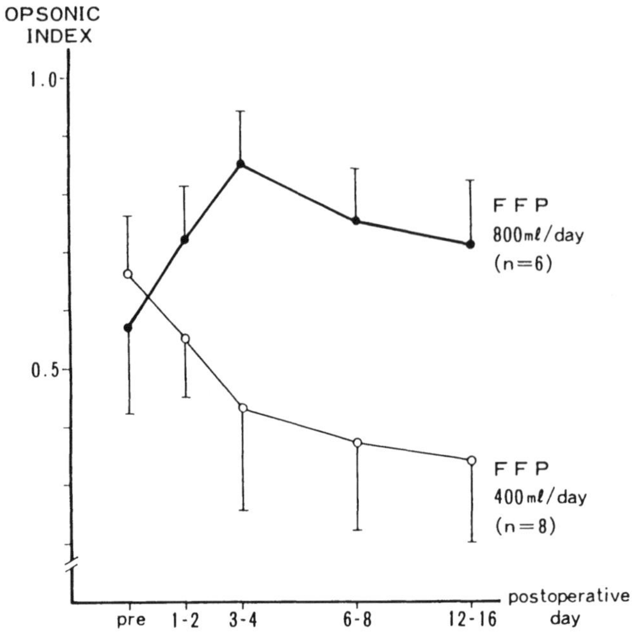

Fig. 8. OI change after hepatectomy

Discussion

Plasma OI is a clinically reliable parameter for ascertaining the sensitive state for bacterial infection. According to the papers by Alexander et al. [6, 7], the OI value may be dabased when the patient incurs major physical injury, i.e., trauma, surgical procedure, thermal burn, sepsis, and also may be debased by severe malnutrition or lowered protein synthesis. Consumption and reduced production of opsonic proteins may debase the plasma opsonic activity.

Opsonic activity determined by the present technique mainly depends on the plasma complement activity. However, the plasma C3 level or the value of CH50 is not a parameter of opsonic activity. This is because when the C3 or CH5O level is very low, the OI is also low, although many samples show a low level of OI even though the C3 level or CH5O value are within normal levels.

In vitro, in plasma inactivated by 56°C 30-min heating or cobra venom factor, the opsonic activity is restored by adding a very small amount of the C3-rich fraction extracted from normal human plasma using polyethyleneglycol.

Additionally, the C3-rich fraction demonstrated therapeutic effects on experimental animal peritonitis. It contains five times as much C3, properdin, and factor B as does normal plasma.

The OI of inactivated plasma mixed with the C3-rich fraction is higher than the OI of the C3-rich fraction itself. Therefore, components of the alternative pathway of complement activation must be essential for maintaining plasma opsonic activity, although other components in the plasma may also contribute.

MOF cases generally exhibit various previous physical injuries and risk factors. These contribute to deterioration of the defense activity against bacteria. Bacterial infection or bacterial toxins thus appear to contribute to establishing the clinical features of MOF.

MOF is, in a sense, a critical state that allows bacterial entry through reduced defense mechanisms, which may be caused by major injuries and risk factors. Thus, two methods would seem to be effective in MOF prophylaxis or therapy: pre- or postoperative nutritional supplies via intravenous or enteral routes and the administration of a sufficient volume of human FFP in certain cases, such as those which severe infection, elderly patients, or the presence of liver dysfunction requiring the immediate effects of opsonin [8].

Occasionally, the volume of FFP may be overloaded. In such a case, we can expect the C3-rich fraction to be useful whereby a very small amount is capable of restoring the opsonic activity of the enfeebled plasma. Further investigation into the appropriate fraction, however, is necessary.

References

1. Tilney LN, Bailey GL, Morgan AP (1973) Sequential system failure after rupture of abdominal aortic aneurysms. Ann Surg 178: 117–122
2. Baue AE (1975) Multiple progressive or sequential system failure. Arch Surg 110: 779–781
3. Eisemman B, Beart R, Norton L (1977) Multiple organ failure. Surg Gynecol Obstet 144: 323–326
4. Fry OF, Pearlstein L, Fulton RL, Polk HC Jr (1980) Multiple system organ failure, the role of uncontrolled infection. Arch Surg 115: 136–140
5. Ishiyama M, Watanabe C, Tamakuma S (1984) Clinical aspects of endotoxemia. In: Homma JY, Westphal O et al. (eds) Bacterial endotoxin. Verlag Chemie, Weinheim, pp 307–313
6. Alexander JW, McClellan MA, Ogle CK, Ogle JD (1976) Consumptive opsoninopathy: possible pathogenesis in lethal and opportunistic infection. Ann Surg 184: 672–678
7. Alexander JW, Ogle CK, Stinnett JD, MACMillan BG (1978) A sequential, progressive analysis of immunologic abnormalities and infection following severe thermal injury. Ann Surg 188: 809–815
8. Watanabe C, Stinnett JD, Alexander JW (1982) Evaluation of serum replacement therapy for bacterial infection in complement-depleted guinea pigs. J Clin Surg 1: 27–31

Prediction and Diagnosis of Low Cardiac Output Syndrome After Open-Heart Surgery: An Echocardiographic Study

SHINTARO BEPPU, HIROSHI SAKAKIBARA, NORIO TANAKA, KUNIO MIYATAKE, SEIKI NAGATA, YUNG-DAE PARK, FUMIO OMORI, SHIRO IZUMI, MASAKAZU YAMAGISHI, KAZUHIKO TANAKA, KEIJI KUMON, and YASUHARU NIMURA[1]

Introduction

Although there are various causes of multiple organ failure (MOF), low cardiac output syndrome (LOS) is the major cause after open-heart surgery. The hemodynamic situation is unstable, and LOS frequently occurs soon after cardiac surgery. Therefore, it would be helpful if LOS could be predicted beforehand. Once LOS occurs, early diagnosis of its cause is indispensable to adequate treatment. We examined the above two points using echocardiography.

Subjects and Methods

The general subjects of this study were 298 adult patients who underwent open-heart surgery from May 1986 to February 1987. Of these patients, 88 suffered from LOS. In studying the prediction of LOS from preoperative cardiac function, 91 of the above patients were selected. As indices of cardiac function, left ventricular end-diastolic and end-systolic diameters and the fractional shortening were assessed by echocardiography less than 1 month before cardiac surgery. Of the 298 patients, 42 underwent echocardiographic examination soon after surgery; there were 27 LOS patients among them. Both left ventricular diameter and regional wall motion abnormality and abnormality of the extracardiac space were examined.

The echocardiograph used was a Toshiba SSH-11A, SSH-60A, or SSH-65A with a 2.5- or 3.75-MHz transducer. After open-heart surgery, transesophageal echocardiography was performed in 31 patients whose conventional echocardiograms, from the precordial approach, did not yield good image quality. The transesophageal transducer used was a commercially available Toshiba EPB-37SR. The transducer is installed on the tip of the gastrofiberscope. The cross section of the echocardiographic image is perpendicular to the longitudinal axis of the fiberscope. The frequency of ultrasound is 3.75 MHz, and the visual angle 90°. The tip of the fiberscope can be bent to fit the inner wall of the esophagus by

[1]National Cardiovascular Center Research Institute and Hospital, 7–1, Fujishirodai 5-chome, Suita, Osaka, 565 Japan

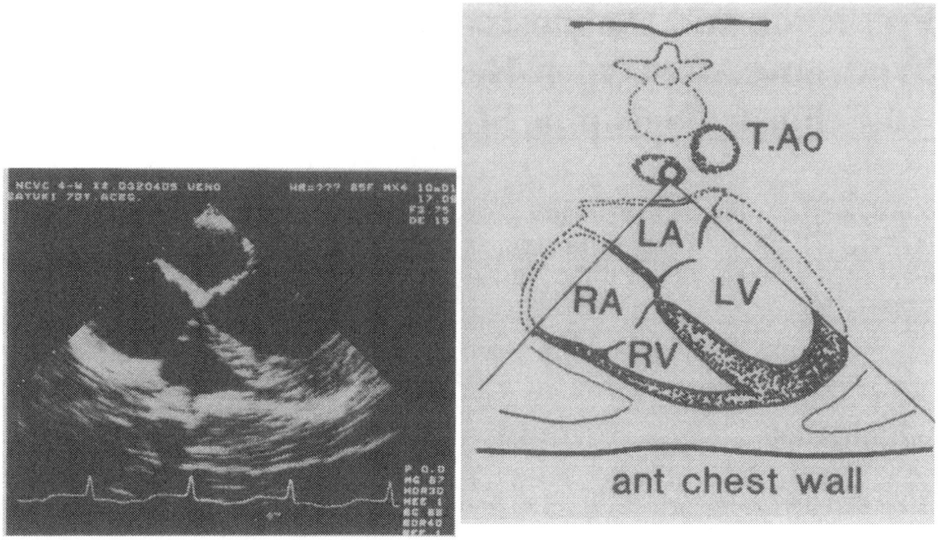

Fig. 1. A transesophageal echocardiogram showing the four-chamber view. The *top* of the echocardiogram corresponds to the position of the esophagus. *LA* left atrium, *LV* left ventricle, *RV* right atrium, *T.Ao* thoratic aorta

manually manipulating the rotary knob. The heart is observed from behind by this means (Fig. 1).

After open-heart surgery, cardiac function is influenced by perioperative complications such as myocardial ischemia, myocardial infarction, ventricular tachycardia, and ventricular fibrillation. To elucidate the significance of perioperative problems in the occurrence of LOS, the influences of anoxic cardiac arrest time and perioperative myocardial infarction were also examined.

Results

Perioperative Problems

Anoxic cardiac arrest time was significant to the occurrence of LOS (Fig. 2). While LOS occurred in only 24% of the patients with an arrest time of less than 2 h, 42% of the patients with an arrest time of over 2 h suffered from LOS ($P < 0.05$). The complication of perioperative myocardial infarction was also significant with regard to LOS. While 74% of the patients with perioperative myocardial infarction had LOS, it occurred in only 25% of the patients without such infarction ($P < 0.01$).

Prediction of LOS

The left ventricular end-diastolic and end-systolic diameters and systolic percentage of fractional shortening (FS) in each group are shown in Fig. 3. The

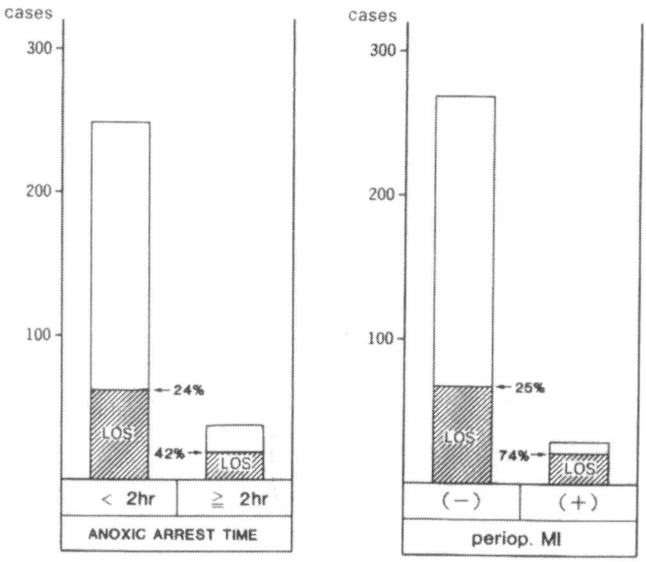

Fig. 2. Adverse effect of prolonged cardiac anoxic arrest time and perioperative myocardial infarction vis-à-vis the occurrence of LOS after surgery

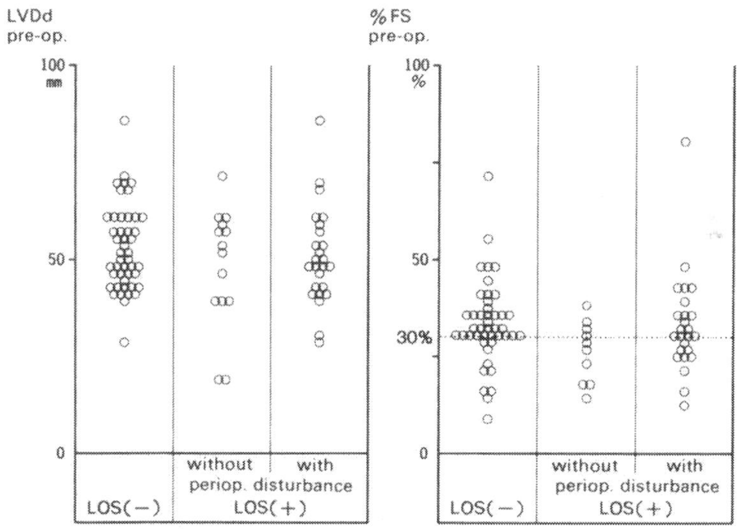

Fig. 3. Left ventricular end-diastolic diameter (*LVDd*) and percentage of fractional shortening (*%FS*) before surgery in patients with and without LOS after surgery. The patients with LOS are grouped by the complications at perioperative disturbances

variables do not differ among the groups. However, excluding the patients with perioperative complications, 30% seems to be the critical value for prediction of LOS after surgery. LOS occurred in only 10% of the patients with over 30%, in contrast to almost 40% of the patients with FS below 30% ($P<0.05$).

a 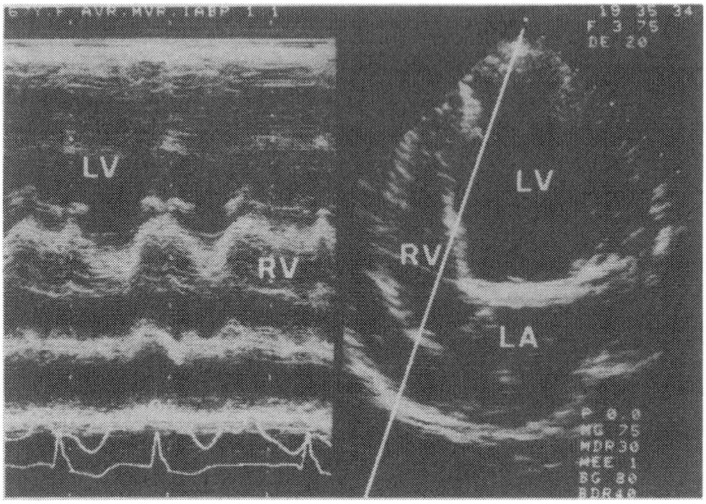 b

Fig. 4a, b. The apical four-chamber view of an LOS patient. The interventricular septum shows systolic dyskinetic motion, as indicated by the M-mode echocardiogram in **a**. The beam direction for the M-mode is indicated by the *line* in **b**

Echocardiographic Features of LOS Patients

Reduced wall motion of the left ventricle was diagnosed in 18 of 27 LOS patients by echocardiography. However, electrocardiography did not show any evidence of myocardial infarction in two of the patients with newly developed left ventricular wall motion abnormalities. In one patient who underwent aortic and mitral valve replacement and suffered LOS after surgery, for example, electrocardiograms did not show obvious ST-T wave abnormalities, indicating myocardial infarction despite serum creatine phosphokinase elevation to over 3000 units. On the other hand, echocardiography demonstrated the abnormal motion of the ventricular septum (Fig. 4). The area of abnormal motion was greatly responsible for the LOS in this patient.

In 2 of 27 LOS patients, cardiac tamponade due to pericardial effusion was diagnosed by echocardiography as the cause of the LOS. Echocardiography demonstrated the characteristic motion of the right atrial and right ventricular wall motion. In another 7 of the 27 LOS patients, conventional echocardiography did not show the deterioration of the left ventricular wall motion or pathological accumulation of effusion surrounding the heart. However, transesophageal echocardiography disclosed the accumulation of blood coagula in front of the right atrial wall inside the pericardial space (Fig. 5). In these patients, the end-diastolic dimension was relatively small, though FS was not low (Fig. 6). It was thought that the accumulated blood coagula interfered with adequate distension of the heart. It is noteworthy that there was no specific motion of the right atrial or right ventricular wall, indicating cardiac tamponade with fluid accumulation. The blood coagula were removed by reopening the chest wall in two patients,

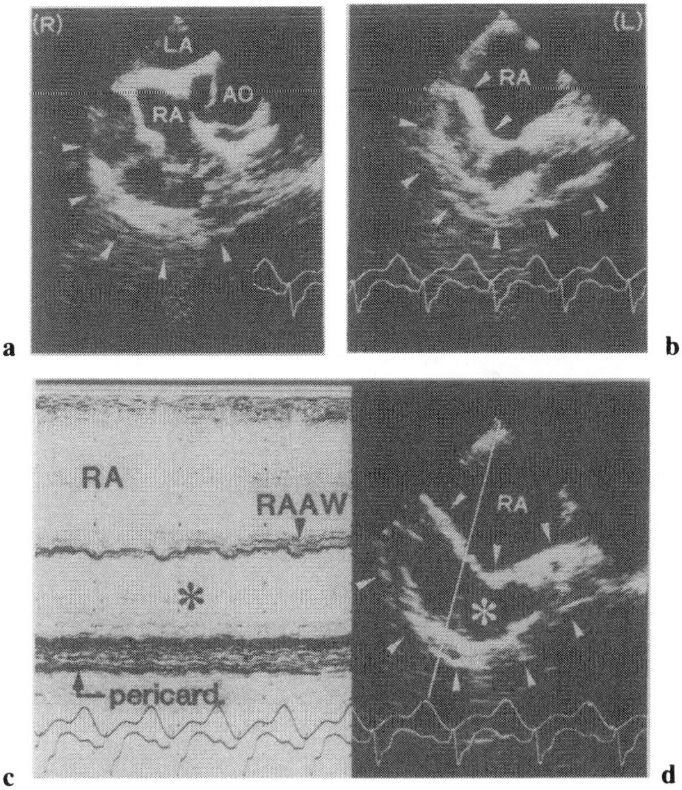

Fig. 5a–d. Transesophageal echocardiograms in a patient with LOS, whose conventional echocardiography from the anterior chest wall shows no obvious abnormalities. **a** The level of the upper part of the heart; **b** the base; **c** near the center of the heart. Localized accumulation of coagula (*arrowheads*) in the pericardial space is shown in front of the right atrial wall. **d** M-mode echocardiogram recorded via the beam direction indicated by the *white line* on the two-dimensional echocardiogram in **c**. The right atrial anterior wall hardly moves

and the LOS state was relieved. In the other five patients, blood coagula were not removed and LOS was prolonged but gradually relieved.

Discussion

Prediction of LOS

None of the echocardiographic parameters was predictive as an index of LOS, though low cardiac function as assessed by FS tends to precede LOS after cardiac surgery. Perioperative complications are more significant than cardiac function before surgery vis-à-vis LOS occurrence. Prolonged cardiac anoxic arrest

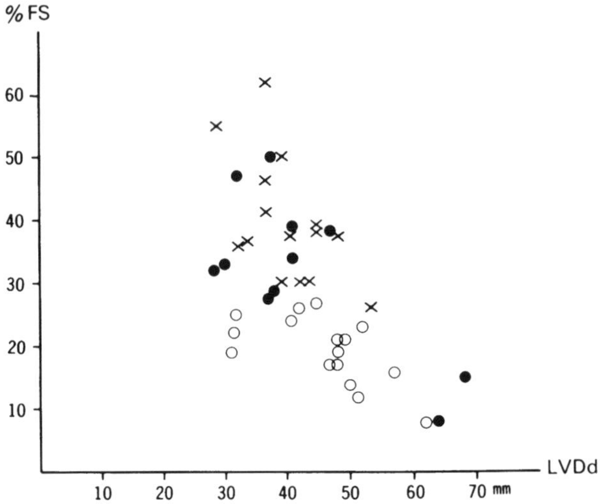

Fig. 6. Echocardiographic indices of left ventricular function in patients with and without LOS after surgery. The patients without LOS (×) are located at the *upper left*. The patients with LOS (o) at *lower right* indicate that LOS patients generally have a relatively large ventricular cavity with poor contraction. The patients with cardiac tamponade (●) show that the percentage of fractional shortening is not low but the end-diastolic dimension is relatively small, indicating that the left ventricle cannot distend adequately

time is a precursor of LOS. It seems that cardioplegia does not always protect the heart muscle from anoxia for many hours. It is likely that perioperative myocardial infarction deteriorates ventricular systolic function. The problem is that perioperative myocardial infarction cannot always be diagnosed accurately by electrocardiography, though echocardiography is useful in monitoring the wall motion of the heart and in estimating cardiac function in such cases.

Use of Echocardiography

Immediate after open-heart surgery, conventional echocardiography from the precordial approach is not always possible, because the ordinary position of the transducer may be near the surgical wound in the chest wall, and the air trapped in the thorax cavity, as a result of the open chest procedure, interferes with ultrasound penetration. In such cases, transesophageal echocardiography is useful for monitoring the heart. The advantage of this method is that the image quality is superior because there are no obstructions to the ultrasound passage. Moreover, it has the advantage of clearly demonstrating the right side of the heart. In general, the right side of the heart is invisible to conventional echocardiography; i.e., abnormalities of the right side of the heart cannot be diagnosed without transesophageal echocardiographic examination.

Specific Cause of LOS

Deterioration of left ventricular systolic function is the general cause of LOS, i.e., the ordinary LOS patient has a relatively large ventricular cavity with poor contraction. Patients with cardiac tamponade, however, are unusual; the left ventricular cavity is small and systolic function is preserved despite LOS. This means that the left ventricle cannot distend adequately.

Cardiac tamponade by the accumulation of pericardial effusion is a well-known cause of impaired distension of the heart. However, the significance of the coagula tamponade after cardiac surgery has not been clarified. The following are characteristic features of coagula tamponade. Blood coagula are usually localized in front of the right atrium and ventricle, which may be due to a midline incision and incomplete check of bleeding. Some patients with accumulation of blood coagula suffer from LOS as a result of impaired distension of the heart. Although the accumulation of blood fluid or coagula in a wide area of the pericardial space can be detected even by conventional echocardiography from the anterior chest wall, the localized accumulation of blood coagula in front of the right atrium can only be detected by esophageal echocardiography.

In summary, patients with low cardiac function before surgery tend to have LOS. However, in most patients, LOS results from complications in the perioperative phase, such as prolonged anoxic arrest time and myocardial infarction. Usually, LOS occurs as a result of ventricular contraction failure. However, among patients with LOS, impaired distension of the heart is the cause of LOS. In such cases, inotropic agents do not relieve the abnormal hemodynamics. It is important to diagnose the cause of LOS accurately for adequate treatment. Echocardiography, especially transesophageal, is useful in differentiating between two types of LOS.

The Effect of Multiple Organ Failure on the Regulation of the Circulation with Special Reference to the Microcirculation

DAVID H. LEWIS[1]

Introduction

The evolution of shock research in the latter half of this century has been one of investigating more and more complex experimental models as the mechanisms behind the less complex clinical situations become better understood. Such an understanding has usually led quite quickly to clinical application of the newly gained information. Thus, pure hemorrhagic shock models gave way to models of combined traumatic-hemorrhagic shock, and these have in turn given way to models of sepsis-endotoxin shock. It is also true that the clinical situations are never as "pure" as the experimental models, so that while trauma and sepsis can be separated in the laboratory they are often combined in the clinic. Failure to recover from these pathological conditions in a relatively rapid time frame leads to organ failure and at the end of the line is the specter multiple organ failure.

It is the purpose of this communication to discuss briefly a few of the disorders of microcirculatory regulation that are felt to be of importance in the progression of the pathophysiology of shock and may well play a role in the evolution of multiple organ failure. There are many important aspects of this problem, but in the space provided the points that will be discussed include only sympathoadrenal control at the microcirculatory level and the role of vascular endothelium in microcirculatory control.

Sympathoadrenal Control of Microcirculation

The major microvascular and metabolic effects of activation of the sympathoadrenal system in response to a serious threat to the organism are as follows:

- Increase in peripheral vascular resistance due mainly to precapillary arteriolar vasoconstriction. This has also the effect of maintaining a normal blood viscosity in the microcirculation.
- Decrease in capacitance due mainly to vasoconstriction of veins and venules
- Decrease in mean net capillary hydrostatic pressure, resulting in a net influx of extravascular fluid into the circulation

[1]Clinical Research Center, Faculty of Health Sciences, University Hospital, S-581 85 Linköping, Sweden

Table 1. Relationship between myocardial blood flow and myocardial blood volume. After Fukuyama et al. [7]

Myocardial blood flow ($ml \times min^{-1} \times g\ tissue^{-1}$)	Myocardial blood volume ($ml \times g\ tissue^{-1} \times 10^{-3}$)
> 1.5	25
1.5–1.2	33
1.2–0.9	42
0.9–0.6	58
0.6–0.3	88
< 0.3	130

- Increase in the size of the capillary bed available for exchange due to an opening up of "precapillary sphincters"
- Increase in extracellular osmolality transferring fluid from the intracellular compartment to the extracellular space. This is due to the combination of hyperglycemia (release of glucose from the liver) and insulin resistance.

This demonstrates what happens in the series-coupled microvascular elements in a typical bed. The sense of the response is similar in the various parallel-coupled beds, i.e., the different organs, but is obviously expressed to different degrees for each element. The sum total of the response involves activation of both alpha (vasoconstriction) and beta (vasodilatation and metabolic response) receptors and is dependent, among other things, upon receptor and nerve fiber density [1] and cotransmitter activation [2]. Note that all of these responses are compensatory in nature. They work toward enabling the organism to survive the insult. In their absence, survival is not possible [3]. It has been suggested that the sympathetics are important in the maintenance of a normal, low microvascular blood viscosity and that this is accomplished in part by vasoconstriction [4], since vessel size is a major determinant of microvascular hematocrit [5]. This is thought to be the explanation for the beneficial effect of normovolemic hemodilution in prolonged, low-flow states [6] as well as the inverse relationship between microvascular blood flow and microvascular blood volume in organ failure [7]. Table 2, taken from the data of Fukuyama and co-workers [7], shows that as blood flow in the myocardium decreases from the normal level there is an increasing level of blood volume in the segment involved. These data are in agreement with the observations of Engler and co-workers [8] that a polymorphonuclear leukocyte causing obstruction to blood flow in a myocardial capillary (see below) has a "tail" of impacted, concentrated red blood cells behind it.

The effect of shock and impending organ failure is to impair the ability of the sympathoadrenal system to exert its normal control function on the microcirculation. As the shock progresses and as organ failure appears, the degree of dysregulation increases. This occurs to varying degrees in all of the parallel-coupled beds and affects all levels of the series-coupled vessels. The exact mechanism remains to be elucidated, but it appears not to be due to failure of nerve transmission or failure of transmitter release. The presence of transmitter inhibitors has been described [9], and much work has gone into finding the one, single mediator responsible for the failure of the sympathoadrenal responsiveness. Certainly, one of the most fascinating aspects of the disorder of the regulatory phenomenon in shock is the apparent paradox of the role of the sympathoadrenal system. It is necessary for survival at the onset of the pathophysiological condition but appears to be a lethal factor late in the process. At what point does this reversal occur? Can one single point in time or one single location in the organism be recognized as *the* causative factor? What is the factor (or factors) responsible? It is not simply that the regulatory mechanisms become less effective. It is rather that in the attempt to maintain regulation, the regulatory apparatus acts in a decompensatory fashion. The final answer to this riddle will no doubt come when we understand the nature of the regulatory mechanisms at the cellular and molecular level. It is clear, however, that a fundamental understanding here will enable us to manipulate these regulatory phenomena in such a way as to abrogate their decompensatory action and restore their effectiveness. This may well be accomplished by bypassing the normally utilized receptor mechanisms, most probably with specific pharmacological agents or even the organism's own naturally occurring, but as yet poorly understood, "mediators." This type of manipulation is one approach to combating the effect of the "toxins" that are the unavoidable accompaniment of the septic state and multiple organ failure. This could provide life-saving therapy, when simple removal of the septic focus does not reverse the pathophysiology.

Role of Vascular Endothelium

As our understanding of the many and varied functions of the vascular endothelium increases, it is becoming more and more evident that this cell plays a central role in the pathophysiology of shock and multiple organ failure. Some of this cell's important functions are given below.

Permeability barrier. The essential role of the endothelium as a barrier between the intravascular and extravascular compartments has long been recognized. We are learning continually about the molecular mechanisms involved in the site and manner of transport of substances of varied molecular size and charge. The importance of the immediate postcapillary venules in conveying protein to the interstitium has been established. The question of active contractility of endothelial cells as a mechanism for altering permeability is still open to question, but it would appear that permeability as such is not constant. Changes in permeability, both increase and decrease, may well be used in normal situations and are of paramount importance in multiple organ failure.

Metabolism. It is now recognized that the endothelial cell is highly active in the handling of blood-borne substances. This is seen most clearly in the lung because of the large volume of endothelial cells in this organ but is true for all organs. Removal of "unwanted" circulating agents is one of the functions of the endothelium, and impairment of this function is seen in organ failure. For example, in our studies of the handling of substances during their first passage through the lung, the transfer of lidocaine from the blood to the lung was altered in patients with respiratory distress [10]. In like manner, naturally occurring substances as well as drugs normally handled by vascular endothelium will display altered pharmacokinetics in multiple organ failure. The endothelium is also responsible for the production of many substances, and with impaired metabolism this function too will be interfered with. Thus, in the presence of an impaired pulmonary handling of substances coming to it, toxic factors normally removed from the venous return will reach the systemic circulation. Similarly, substances normally released from the lung into the systemic circulation will be lacking.

Vascular tone. The observation that certain substances produce vasodilatation by releasing a relaxant factor from the endothelium that acts on the vascular smooth muscle [11] has increased greatly our knowledge of vascular control, even if the final answer has not yet been found. What is unfortunate at the present time is that the concept of an endothelium-derived relaxant factor leads to uncertainty about events in the pathological state. With our previous understanding of the origin of vasomotion, it was taken for granted that a substance either did what it was supposed to do or for one reason or another failed to do what it was supposed to do. What we are faced with now, however, is entirely different. A given substance, and this includes many of the mediators released in shock and circulating during multiple organ failure, will cause vasodilatation *if* the endothelium is intact and capable of producing an endotheium-derived relaxant factor. However, if the endothelium is absent or if it is incapable of producing an endothelium-derived relaxant factor, then this same substance will now cause vasoconstriction. The original descriptions of this occurrence were made on large vessels, but the endothelium in the microcirculation does display the same phenomenon [12]. In addition, as workers at the Mayo Clinic have observed, there are also endothelium-derived constricting substances [13]. Therefore, the question as to what the state of responsiveness of the microvasculature is in any pathological situation resides not only with the function of the vascular smooth muscle but also with the function of the endothelium as well. This complicates the picture greatly and makes it impossible at the present time to predict in any given situation where the failure lies. It does, however, hold future promise in providing another point at which new therapeutic regimens can be applied.

Leukocytes. It has become clear in recent years that polymorphonuclear leukocytes accumulate not only in inflamed tissue but also in ischemic and injured tissue [14]. This is due to activation of these cells, causing them to obstruct capillaries and carpet the walls of postcapillary venules. Our observations on the effects of ischemia on skeletal muscle capillaries would suggest that changes in the endothelial cell membrane may also play a role in this phenomenon. The resultant swelling of some of the capillary endothelial cells reduces the capillary lumen and can well provide a mechanical hindrance to the passage of these large, stiff cells [15]. The trapping of polymorphonuclear leukocytes in the microcirculation not only reduces the size of the capillary bed available for flow but it also increases resistance to flow at the level of the postcapillary venules. This latter phenomenon can be responsible in part for a net outward flux of fluid from the intravascular compartment. In addition, the presence of activated polymorphonuclear leukocytes provides a highly concentrated and localized source of oxygen-free radicals and a host of destructive enzymes. All of these factors can clearly play a role in the production of organ failure.

Concluding Remarks

In the normal situation, the microcirculation is regulated both by centrally originating and locally derived control mechanisms. The central control is exercised in large part via the sympathoadrenal system, whose action at the outset of a threatening situation is compensatory in nature and necessary for the survival of the organism. This response changes as the disease state progresses, becoming at some point decompensatory. The mechanism responsible for this turnabout is poorly understood. One factor may well be the presence of inhibitors at the level of synaptic transmission. Loss of regulation at the microcirculatory level leads to changes in vasomotion, changes in the net balance of fluid transfer, and a pathological distribution of flow in the capillary bed. The effect on the vascular endothelial cells in the shock situation compounds the situation and may be a causing factor. Without normally functioning endothelium in the microcirculation there will also be alterations in the status of vasomotion, permeability of the vascular barrier, and distribution of blood flow within the capillary bed. Increased understanding of the molecular basis for these pathological changes will lead to new therapies in multiple organ failure.

Acknowledgments. The original results reported in this communication were supported in part by grants-in-aid from the Swedish Medical Research Council (project nr. 02042), the Swedish National Defence Research Institute (project nr. D60), the County Council of Östergötland, and Linköping University.

References

1. Burnstock G, Griffith SG, Sneddon P (1984) Autonomic nerves in the precapillary vessel wall. J Cardiovasc Pharmacol 6: S344–S353
2. Lundberg JM, Fried G, Pernow J, Theodorsson-Norheim E (1986) Corelease of neuropeptide Y and catecholamines upon adrenal activation in the cat. Acta Physiol Scand 126: 231–238
3. McKechnie K, Dean HG, Furman BL, Parratt JR (1985) Plasma catecholamines during endotoxin infusion in conscious unrestrained rats: Effects of adrenal demedullation and/or guanethedine treatment Circ Shock 17: 85–94
4. Lewis DH (1987) Do the sympathetics play a role in the maintenance of microvascular hematocrit? Fed Proc 46: 1532
5. Lipowsky HH, Usami S, Chien S (1980) In vivo measurement of "apparent viscosity" and microvessel hematocrit in the mesentery of the cat Microvasc Res 19: 297–319
6. Lewis DH, Schmid-Schönbein H (1981) Rheology and vasomotion: A validation of hemodilution as a rational therapeutic manuever. In: Schmid-Schönbein H, Messmer K, Rieger H (eds) Hemodilution and flow improvement. Bibliohca Haemat nr. 47. Karger, Basel, pp 122–126
7. Fukuyama T, Sobel BE, Roberts R (1984) Microvascular deterioration: implications for reperfusion. Cardiovasc Res 18: 310–320
8. Engler RL, Schmid-Schönbein GV, Pavelec RS (1983) Leukocyte capillary plugging in myocardial ischemia and reperfusion in the dog. Am J Pathol 111: 96–111

9. Bond RF, Bond CH, Peissner LC, Manning ES (1981) Prostaglandin modulation of adrenergic vascular control during hemorrhagic shock. Am J Physiol 241: H85–H90
10. Jorfeldt L, Lewis DH, Löfström JB, Post C (1983) Lung uptake of lidocaine in man as influenced by anesthesia, mepivicaine infusion or lung insufficiency. Acta Anesthesiol Scand 27: 5–9
11. Furchgott RF, Zawadski JV (1980) The obligatory role of endothelial cells in the relaxation of arterial smooth muscle by acetylcholine. Nature 288: 373–376
12. Rosenblum WI, Nelson GH, Povlishock JT (1987) Laser-induced endothelial damage inhibits endothelium-dependent relaxation in the cerebral microcirculation of the mouse. Circ Res 60: 169–176
13. Shepherd JT, Vanhoutte PM (1985) Spasm of the coronary arteries: Causes and consequences (the scientists' viewpoint). Mayo Clin Proc 60: 33–46
14. Lewis DH, Gidlöf A, Behm KE, Bengtsson M-B, Menschik A (1987) White cells in shock ischemia. In: Schlag G, Redl H (eds) First Vienna shock forum: A. Pathophysiological role of mediators and mediator inhibitors in shock. Liss, New York, pp 63–74
15. Gidlöf A, Lewis DH, Hammersen F (1988) The effect of prolonged total ischemia on the ultrastructure of human skeletal muscle capillaries. A morphometric analysis. Int J Microcirc: Clin Exp 7: 67–86

Hemorheological and Coagulofibrinolytic Aspects in Multiple Organ Failure After Open Heart Surgery

NOBUKO TSUSHIMA[1] and TSUYOSHI FUJITA[2]

Introduction

The purpose of this study was to elucidate the pathophysiological mechanism of multiple organ failure (MOF) after open heart surgery through analyses of hemorheology by blood viscosity and its related factors, the index of hemorheological oxygen delivery according to the method of Chien [1], and coagulofibrinolytic factors before, during, and after operation. Diagnosis of MOF was made according to the clinical criteria at our hospital [2].

Methods and Materials

Thirty-eight patients with valvular disease who underwent open heart surgery (20 male, 18 female) aged between 20 and 70 years (average 52.5 ± 12.2 years) were studied. Diagnosis of MOF was made retrospectively 1 month after open heart surgery.

Eleven patients with MOF (four male, seven female) aged between 39 and 70 years (average 50.0 ± 12.4 years) and 27 patients with good convalescence after surgery (non-MOF; 16 male, 11 female) aged between 20 and 68 years (56.6 ± 11.2 years) were compared. Thirty-six healthy volunteers (33 male, 3 female) aged between 19 and 48 years (average 30.3 ± 3.5 years) were used as normal controls (Table 1). Blood specimens from the cubital vein were mainly used with the exception of arterial blood on the 1st postoperative day.

Examinations of hematological, chemical, hemorheological, and coagulofibrinolytic factors were performed four times: (a) preoperatively, (b) 1st postoperative day, (c) 1 week, and (d) 2 weeks after operation. Additional examinations were performed in cases of MOF.

Analyses

We tested hematological indices by THMS, H-6000 (Technicon, USA), and serum cholesterol, triglyceride, albumin, globulin, and total protein by standard

Department of Internal Medicine[1], Department of Surgery[2], National Cardiovascular Center Hospital, 7–1, Fujishirodai 5-chome, Suita, Osaka, 565 Japan

Table 1. Patients undergoing valvular operation

Valve	n	Age (years)[a]	Non-MOF	MOF
M	10	51.0 ± 13.4	8	2
A	12	52.1 ± 14.3	10	2
M + A	4	50.0 ± 12.1	2	2
M + T	8	55.9 ± 9.1	5	3
M + A + T	4	55.8 ± 13.3	2	2
Total	38	52.5 ± 12.2	27	11

M mitral valve operation, *A* aortic valve operation, *T* tricuspid valve operation, *non-MOF* cases whose postoperative convalescence was good, *MOF* cases with postoperative multiple organ failure (three organs and system failure)
[a] Means ± SD

biochemical methods. Plasma fibrinogen (Fbg) was tested by the thrombin method, and antithrombin III (AT-III), plasminogen (PLG), and α_2 plasmin inhibitor (α_2-PI) by the chromogenic substrate (Daiichikagaku, Japan) method (COBAS-FARA, USA). We tested α_1-antitrypsin (α_1-AT) and α_2-macroglobulin (α_2-M) by the SRID (Hechst, Federal Public of Germany) method, (COBAS-FARA, USA), FDP by the LPIA (Teikokuzoki, Japan) method, (COBAS-FARA, USA), fibrinopeptide A (FPA) and fibririnopeptide B (FPB) by the RIA-PEG (IMCO, Sweden) method, FDP-D dimer (FDP-D.D) by the ELISA (AGEN, Australia) method, and tissue plasminogen activator (tPA) by the ELISA (American Diagnostica, USA) method.

The viscosity of whole blood and plasma at the shear rates of 94.5 and 0.376 s^{-1} were measured by Low Shear-30 (CONTRAVES, England).

The hemorheological index of oxygen delivery was calculated from hematocrit (Ht) divided by blood viscosity (ηB) [Ht/ηB] [1].

Statistics

Student's *t*-test or Welch's *t*-test was used for intergroup dfferences. The method of paired comparison was adopted to assess the differences between preoperative and postoperative day 1 and week 1 and 2 values for the above-mentioned factors. If *P* values were less than 0.05, the statistical difference was held to be significant. All results are described as means ± SE with the exception of age, which is given as means ± SD.

Results

The following description is limited to the results showing a $P < 0.1$ statistical difference or trend of change between MOF and non-MOF.

Preoperative Factors

These are summarized in Table 2.

Table 2. Preoperative factors

	Non-MOF	MOF	Difference
Age (years)	56.6 ± 11.2	50.4 ± 12.4	NS
Ht (%)	40.4 ± 0.9	34.8 ± 1.6	**
PLT (× 10³/mm³)	192.1 ± 12.2	153.0 ± 15.0	†
Neutro (%)	53.2 ± 1.9	60.4 ± 2.5	**
T-chol (mg/dl)	193.0 ± 6.7	166.2 ± 10.3	**
Trig (mg/dl)	162.3 ± 18.1	87.8 ± 8.4	***
Fbg (mg/dl)	300.3 ± 11.1	350.2 ± 21.3	**
FDP (μg/ml)	13.8 ± 0.5	15.3 ± 0.8	†
α_1AT (mg/dl)	243.9 ± 9.5	282.2 ± 10.1	***
Viscosity (mPa.s)	5.1 ± 1.5	4.6 ± 1.6	**

NS not significant, *Ht* hematocrit, *PLT* platelets, *Neutro* neutrophils, *T-chol* total cholesterol, *Trig* triglyceride, *Fbg* fibrinogen, *FDP* fibrin degradation product, $\alpha_1 AT$ α_1 antitrypsin, †$P<0.1$, **$P<0.01$, ***$P<0.001$

Blood cell factors. The Ht in MOF of at 34.8% ± 1.6% was significantly lower than that in non-MOF at 40.4% ± 0.9% ($P<0.01$). Platelets in MOF at 153.0 ± 15.0 × 10³/mm³ showed a decrease compared with those in non-MOF at 192.1 + 12.2 × 10³/mm³. Neutrophils in MOF were significantly higher than in non-MOF.

Serum and plasma factors. Both total cholesterol and triglycerides in MOF were significantly lower than in non-MOF ($P<0.01$ and $P<0.001$, respectively).

Fbg, FDP-D.D, and α_1AT in MOF were significantly higher than in non-MOF ($P<0.01$, $P<0.1$, and $P<0.001$, respectively).

Whole blood viscosity. In MOF, whole blood viscosity at 4.6 ± 1.5 mPa.s was significantly lower than in non-MOF at 5.1 ± 0.7 mPa.s ($P<0.01$). Whole blood viscosity in normal controls at 5.07 ± 0.08 mPa.s was significantly higher than in both MOF and non-MOF ($P<0.01$).

Factors During Operation

The amount of blood transfusion, anesthesia, and operation time in MOF were significantly greater than in non-MOF ($P<0.01$, $P<0.001$, and $P<0.001$, respectively; Table 3). Anoxic arrest time and extracorporeal circulation (ECC) time in MOF tended to be longer than in non-MOF.

Pre- and Postoperative Changes in Whole Blood Viscosity

Whole blood viscosity at the shear rate of 94.5 s^{-1} in MOF was elevated significantly after surgery and subsequently stayed at this higher level, whereas in non-MOF whole blood viscosity decreased significantly after surgery, thereafter fluctuating but staying at the lower level (Fig. 1). Whole blood viscosity at the shear rate of 0.376 s^{-1} showed almost the same change as that of 94.5 s^{-1} postoperatively.

Table 3. Factors during operation

	Non-MOF	MOF	Difference
Blood transfusion (ml)	1214.8 ± 404.3	2772.0 ± 537.0	***
Anoxic arrest time (min)	89.3 ± 4.8	105.6 ± 8.1	†
ECC time (min)	148.1 ± 8.4	231.1 ± 42.4	†
Anesthesia time (min)	390.0 ± 19.2	565.0 ± 42.0	***
Operation time (min)	332.3 ± 17.9	516.4 ± 46.4	***

Figures are means ± SE
ECC extracorporeal circulation
†$P<0.1$, **$P<0.01$, ***$P<0.001$

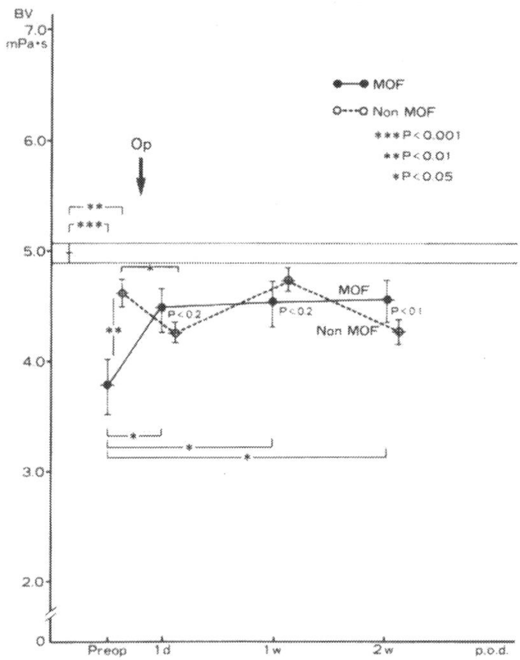

Fig. 1. Whole blood viscosity at the shear rate of 94.5 s^{-1} with the change in time pre- and postoperatively in MOF and nonMOF groups. Whole blood viscosity was increased significantly after operation and subsequently stayed at a higher value in the MOF group; in the non-MOF group, it decreased significantly after operation and subsequently fluctuated moderately. *Gray zone* represents the control value of whole blood viscosity as means ± SE

Pre- and Postoperative Change in Index of Oxygen Delivery (Ht/ηB)

The index of oxygen delivery in normal controls was 8.7% ± 0.1%/mPa.s (Fig. 2); in MOF this was 8.7% ± 0.2%/mPa.s and in non-MOF 8.8% ± 0.1% preoperatively, with no significant difference between these values and those of normal controls.

The index in non-MOF decreased gradually until 2 weeks after surgery, show-

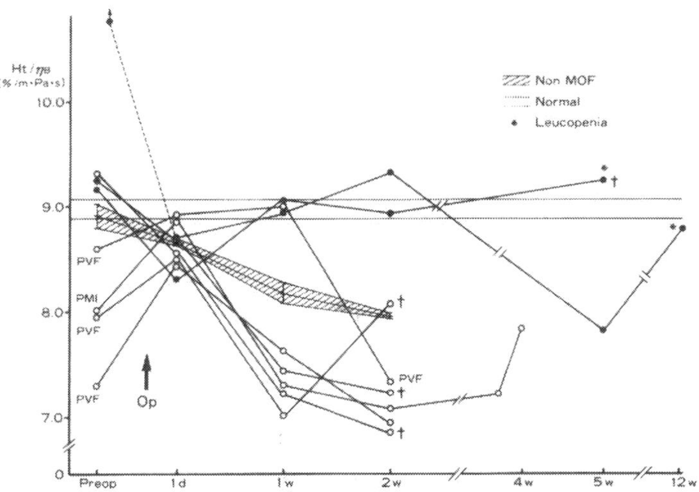

Fig. 2. Index of oxygen delivery (Ht/η_B) with the pre- and postoperative change in time. Hemorheological index of oxygen delivery was calculated hematocrit (*Ht*) divided by blood viscosity (η_B) in MOF and non-MOF groups. Index of oxygen delivery is demonstrated as *gray zone* in normal and as *hatched shading* in non-MOF. Oxygen delivery even in the non-MOF group descends gradually up to 2 weeks after operation; that in the MOF group diverges extremely preoperatively, reaching a similar value at the 1st day and attaining a lower level than that of non-MOF except in the cases with leukopenia at 1 and 2 weeks after operation. *PVF* prosthetic valve failure, *PMI* perioperative myocardial infarction

ing a significant decrease compared with the preoperative value. From the index in MOF, two postoperative groups of patients were seen lower and higher values than in non-MOF after 2 weeks. Cases with a higher index in MOF showed leukopenia.

Postoperative Change in Fibrinolysis

FDP in non-MOF revealed no abnormal increase after surgery; in MOF, however, it demonstrated a significant increase 1 week after surgery, subsequently tending to decrease with no significant increase on the 1st postoperative day. On the other hand, FDP-D.D in non-MOF revealed a gradual increase for up to 2 weeks after surgery; in MOF, however, the greatest increase was evident 1 week after surgery, subsequently tending to decrease with a significant increase on the 1st postoperative day.

FPB_β showed no significant change in non-MOF, showing a significant increase from the 1st day to 2 weeks after surgery in MOF (Fig. 3).

Discussion

Significantly lower blood viscosity in MOF before operation could be mainly explained by a decrease in the preoperative lower level of Ht in MOF because

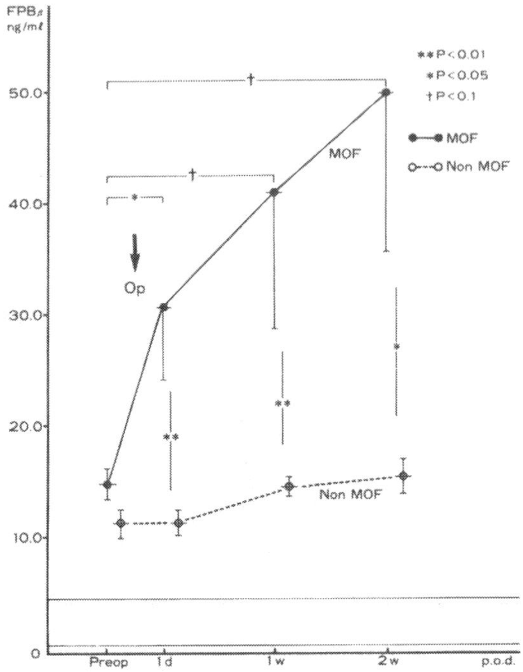

Fig. 3. FPBβ_{15-42} with the change in time pre- and postoperatively in the MOF and non-MOF groups. Both groups showed higher values than the control group (*gray zone*, means ± SE). In MOF group, FPBβ_{15-42} elevated significantly after operation, increasing for up to 2 weeks after operation; in non-MOF group, it stayed at almost the same level with the time-course of the operation

preoperative serum and plasma factors influencing blood viscosity such as total cholesterol triglycerides, Fbg, FDP, and α_1AT were higher in MOF than in non-MOF. A long-established preoperative hemorheological condition, as reflected in the low blood viscosity level, is maintained by a balanced interplay between the total blood flow, oxygen content of the blood, and the metabolic activity of each organ under the poor hemodynamic conditions of valvular disease.

The following have been widely accepted as preoperative factors affecting postoperative MOF in valvular disease: pulmonary hypertension, giant left atrium, and myocardial hypertrophy [3]. These changes represent the ultimate deterioration in the hemodynamics due to valvular disease, including myocardial damage, and may lead to an imbalance between the distribution of total blood flow, oxygen content of the blood, oxygen delivery, and the metabolic activity of each organ.

An increase in blood viscosity after open heart surgery was reported by Balas et al. [4] and a decrease in blood viscosity by isovolumetric hemodilution has been recommended by Messmer [5] from the viewpoint of oxygen transport and tissue perfusion, resulting in improvement in blood fluidity. In the present study, the blood viscosity after operation revealed a significant increase in MOF and significant decrease in non-MOF. A large surgical invasion even resulted in normalized valvular function by perhaps causing an imbalance in the established relation between blood distribution, oxygen content of blood, oxygen delivery, and metabolic activity of an organ.

Longer anoxic arrect, extracorporeal circulation, anesthesia, and operation time together with a larger amount of blood transfusion were significant factors in MOF (Table 2). Whenever the hemodynamics and metabolic activity of an organ are affected by larger surgical invasions during operation, blood fluidity (hemorheological factors), which is normally of limited significance in the tissues and circulation, might become a crucial factor for tissue supply, including the myocardium, by virtue of its effect upon flow within the microcirculation.

The hemorheological index of oxygen delivery in MOF decreased to lower values than in non-MOF with the exception of cases with leukopenia, which showed normal values at 2 weeks after operation. A lower index of oxygen delivery could explain the cricial condition of MOF. The fact that cases with leukopenia showed a normal index of oxygen delivery may suggest the detrimental effect of leukocytes in oxygen delivery.

FPA, which is an index of thrombin activity, was elevated in both non-MOF and MOF pre- and postoperatively as compared with normal controls. FDP in MOF was elevated significantly at 1 week after operation, while in non-MOF it stayed at less than 20 μg/ml for 2 weeks after operation. FPB_{β} in MOF, which is a marker of plasmin digestion of fibrinogen and an index used in the diagnosis or investigation of disseminated intravascular coagulation (DIC), was significantly higher than in non-MOF (Fig. 3).

A hypercoagulable and hyperfibrinoloytic state together with pre- and postoperative abnormalities of platelet function in valvular disease, especially, in MOF, could be a pathophysiological mechanism of MOF [6, 7].

Summary

Eleven cases of MOF and 27 cases of non-MOF after valvular surgery were studied. The blood viscosity of MOF was significantly lower than in non-MOF before surgery. The blood viscosity of MOF increased significantly, while that of non-MOF decreased significantly after surgery. The hemorheological index of oxygen delivery in MOF reached a lower level than in non-MOF after surgery. Fibrinopeptide $B_{\beta_{15-42}}$ increased significantly from the 1st day to 2 weeks after surgery in MOF.

Acknowledgments. The authors gratefully acknowledge the assistance of Dr. T. Omae and are indebted to Drs. Keiji Kumon, Kazuhiko Tanaka, Tadashi Kato, Kohei Kawazoe, and Yoshitsugu Kito for their collaboration.

References

1. Chien S (1981) Hemorheology in diseases: Pathophysiological significance and therapeutic implications. Clin Hemorheol 1: 419–442

2. Kumon K, Tanaka K, Hirota T, Naito Y, Fujita T (1986) Organ failures due to low cardiac output syndrome following open heart surgery. Jpn Circ J 50: 329–335
3. Yutani C, Imakita M, Ueda H, Tanaka K, Kawazoe K, Fujita T (1984) Histopathological study of multiple organ failure following cardiac valve replacement. Prog Cardiovasc Dis Res 5: 184–202
4. Balas P, Bastonnis E, Stamatoponlos C, Lianou M (1974) The influence of surgical trauma in blood viscosity. Angiology 25: 249–255
5. Messmer K (1981) Stabilization of the circulation by hemodilution in elective and cardiac surgery. In: Effros RM, Schmid-Schoenbein H, Ditzel J (eds) Microcirculation. Academic, New York, pp 299–313
6. Mohr R, Golan M, Martinowitz U, Rosner E, Goor DA, Romot B (1986) Effect of cardiac operation on platelets. J Thorac Cardiovasc Surg 92: 434–441
7. Bagge L, Lilienberg G, Nystrom SO, Tyden H (1986) Coagulation, fibrinolysis and bleeding after open-heart surgery. Scand J Thorac Cardiovasc Surg 20: 151–160

Organ Failure and Disseminated Intravascular Coagulation

Robert M. Hardaway[1]

Disseminated intravascular coagulation (DIC) involves the formation of fibrin from fibrinogen. This results in two important effects: (a) The onset of a clotting defect due primarily to the using up of clotting factors faster than they can be manufactured. (b) The precipitation of fibrin fibers primarily on the most available surface, that of red cells (Fig. 1). This results in the formation of red cell conglomerates, which occlude the microcirculation. It is this second effect which is our present concern.

DIC concerns the microcirculation most because: (a) the microcirculation is most easily occluded being extremely small in diameter, especially the capillaries; (b) the blood flow is slowest since the microcirculation has the largest total diameter of the circulatory system; (c) it greatly affects cellular nutrition because the capillaries are the sites of delivery of nutrition to the cells and pick up of cell metabolites.

Cells cannot survive a total cutoff of capillary perfusion for more than a very

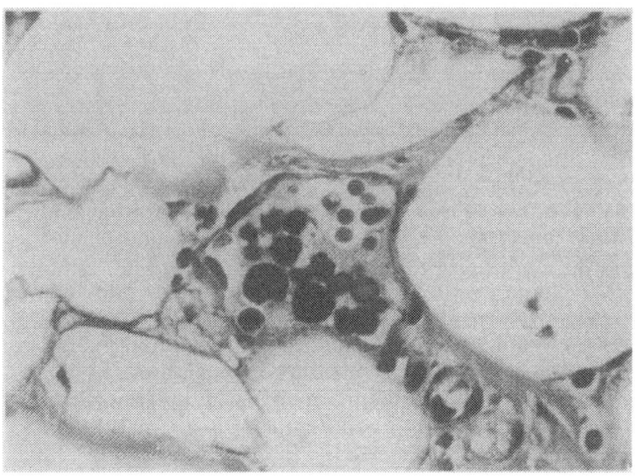

Fig. 1. Lung of patient dying of septic shock. Note the fibrin-coated red cells in the pulmonary vessel

[1]Department of Surgery, Texas Tech University School of Medicine, El Paso, Texas, USA

short time. The exact time may vary from a few minutes for nerve cells to a few hours for some other less active cells. The absence of removal of cell metabolites, particularly lactic acid, is probably the first factor responsible for destroying the cells, even sooner than the absence of oxygen delivery. When capillary flow slows or stops and oxygen is delivered in inadequate amounts, the cell converts from aerobic to anaerobic metabolism (Fig. 2). The end product of anaerobic metabolism is lactic acid, rather than CO_2 and water produced by aerobic metabolism. As long as some capillary flow is maintained, this lactic acid is picked up and carried away. However, if capillary flow stops completely, even for a short time, lactic acid rapidly accummulates in and around the cell. The pH of the cell and surrounding extracellular fluid rapidly falls to very low levels below pH 7 or even below pH 6. This happens even though the pH of the circulating blood may remain normal (Fig. 3). Cellular enzymes cannot function in this low pH. The sodium pump fails. Sodium and water pass into the cell and

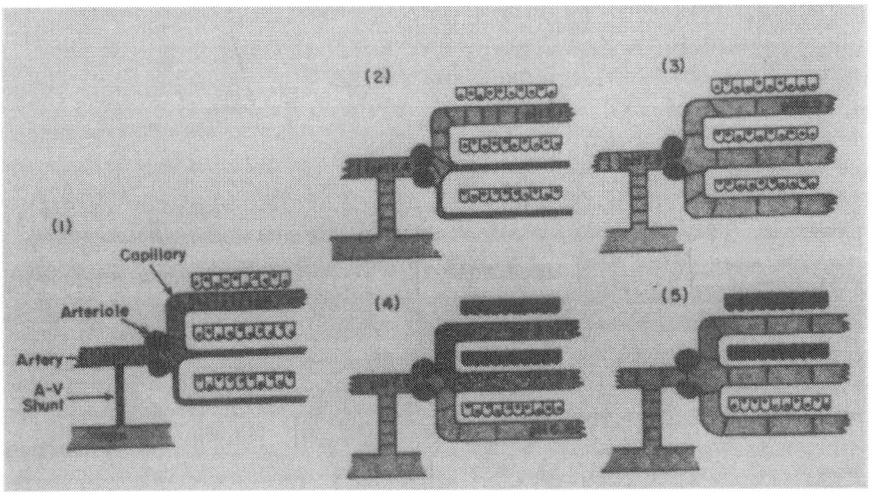

Fig. 2. A small artery ending in an arteriole with sphincter-like action. The arteriole feeds three capillaries, each feeding a group of cells. *1* Normal condition: Arterioles are fairly widely opened. Only one capillary is being perfused, while the others rest. Capillaries open in rotation on demand of the cells adjacent to them. Constant perfusion is not necessary. Blood flow through the capillary is rapid. pH drop across the capillary is minimal. *2* Phase I, shock, vasoconstriction. This is due to cathecholamines after hemorrhage and trauma. The arteriole constricts, letting less blood through. There is hypotension in the artery, capillary flow is showed. *3* Phase II, shock, capillary dilation (expansion of vascular space). All capillaries are open on demand of their cells. Blood flow through all capillaries is extremely slow, pH drop across the capillary is marked. *4* Phase III, shock, disseminated intravascular coagulation, late shock. Hemolysis has aided the slow flowing acid blood in two of the capillaries to clot, stopping perfusion completely in these capillaries. The cells nourished by these capillaries are dying. Blood flow through the remaining capillary is sluggish. The circulating blood is incoagulable. *5* Phase IV, irreversible shock. The arteriole has opened somewhat after replacement of blood volume. Capillary clots have been lysed by endogenous fibrinolysin, restoring the circulation. However, the cells supplied by the formerly clotted capillaries are not dead. This produces areas of focal necrosis and if sufficiently widespread causes tissue and organ failure

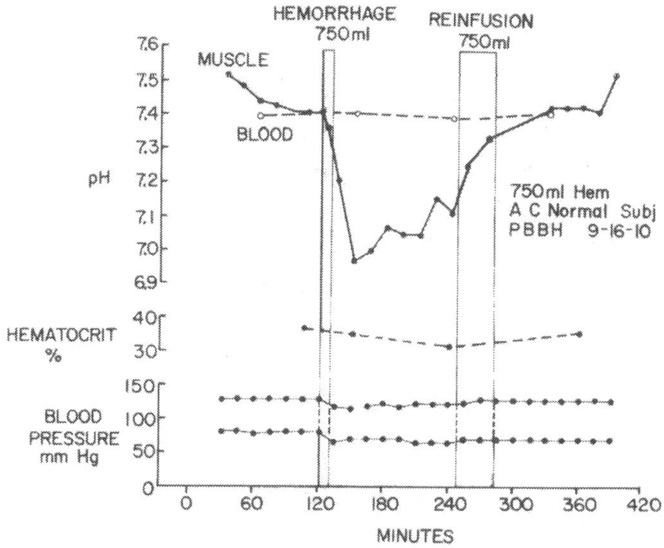

Fig. 3. Mild hemorrhage causes no change in arterial pH but a marked fall in tissue pH

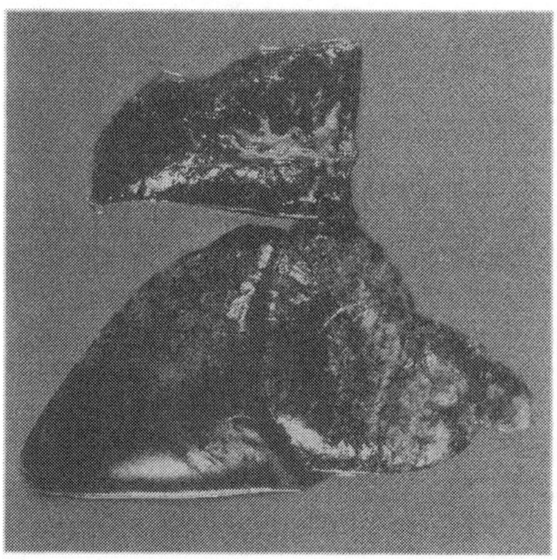

Fig. 4. Lung of dog subjected to hemorrhagic shock

potassium passes out of the cell. The cell swells up and dies. If capillary perfusion is not quickly restored, areas of cellular necrosis rapidly spread. If this happens beyond a certain extent, organ failure results. This is particularly important in vital organs such as the liver, kidney, and heart. In the lungs, swelling of the endothelium opens up large holes in the capillary walls allowing not only liquid components of the blood to flow out of the capillary but cellular components as well (Fig. 4). This creates the picture of "shock lung" or adult respiratory distress syndrome (ARDS).

The body attempts to restore capillary perfusion in two ways. Profibrinolysin or plasmin is activated at the same time that DIC is taking place. This soon lyses

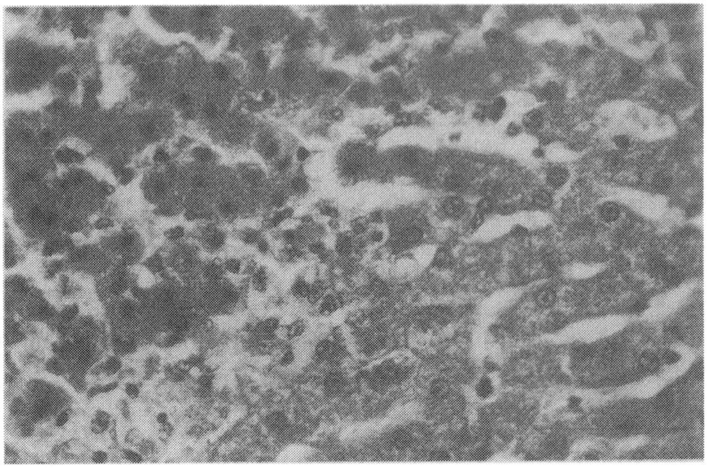

Fig. 5. Liver of dog subjected to hemorrhagic shock. Note the area of necrosis *above* and normal liver cells *below*

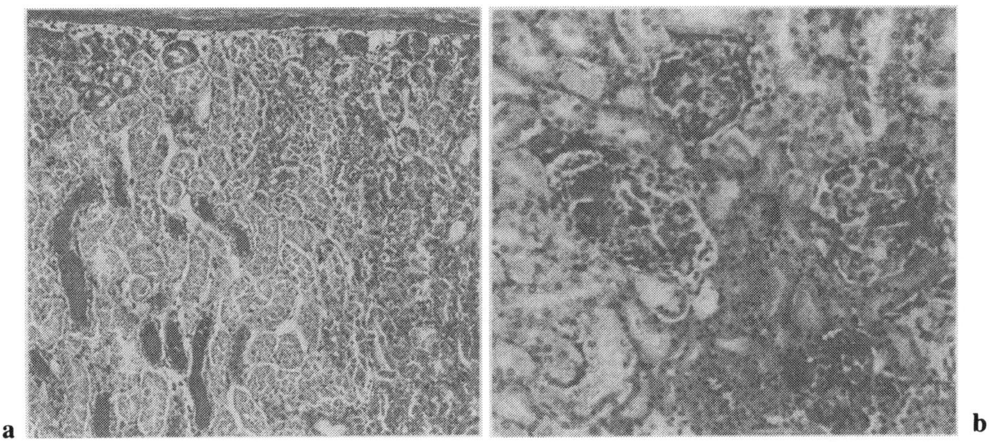

Fig. 6. a Kidney of dog subjected to hemorrhagic shock. Note the areas of necrosis (*left*) and normal tissue (*right*). **b** Kidney of dog subjected to hemorrahgic shock. Note the area of necrosis and fibrin thrombi

the clots in the capillaries and circulation may be restored (Fig. 2). If this takes place in time, cell necrosis will be halted. However, the fibrinolysin may exacerbate the clotting defect already present due to the consumption coagulopathy which has been going on. Also, the body attempts to restore blood flow by pulling in extracellular fluid to improve the blood volume and by speeding up the heart, increasing cardiac output in an attempt to force out the clots. This may be effective particularly if intravenous fluids are given, with the arterioles being opened by vasodilating drugs if necessary.

If epsilon amino caproic acid (EACA) is given, perhaps in an attempt to con-

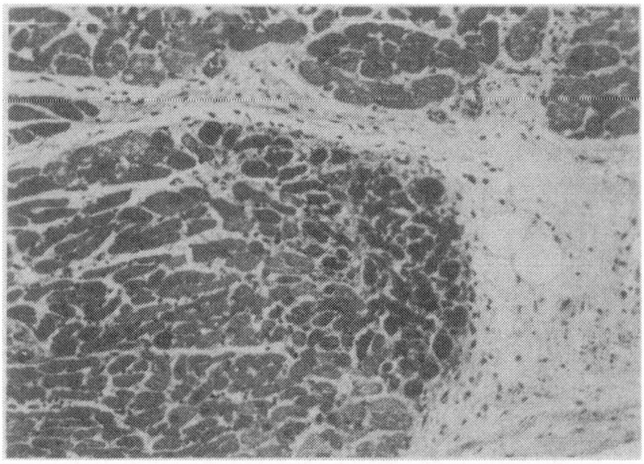

Fig. 7. Heart of patient dying of septic shock. Note the small area of necrosis

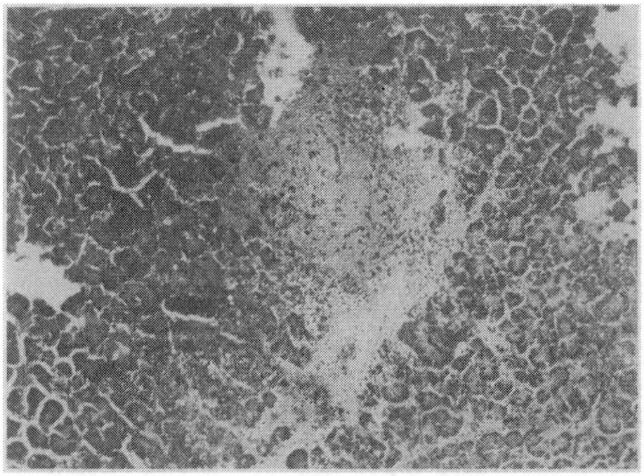

Fig. 8. Pancreas of dog subjected to hemorrhagic shock. Note the focal area of necrosis

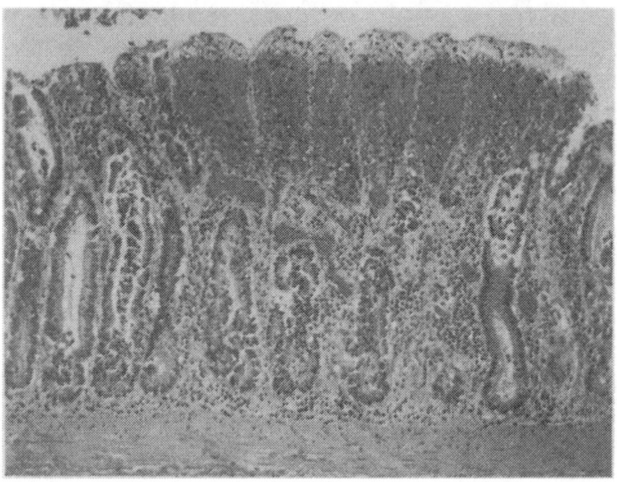

Fig. 9. Gut of dog subjected to hemorrhagic shock. Note the superficial area of necrosis

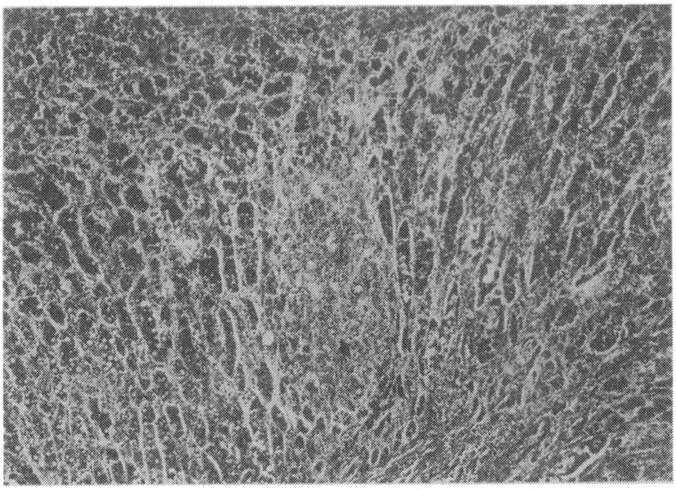

Fig. 10. Adrenal gland of dog subjected to hemorrhagic shock. Note the small area of necrosis

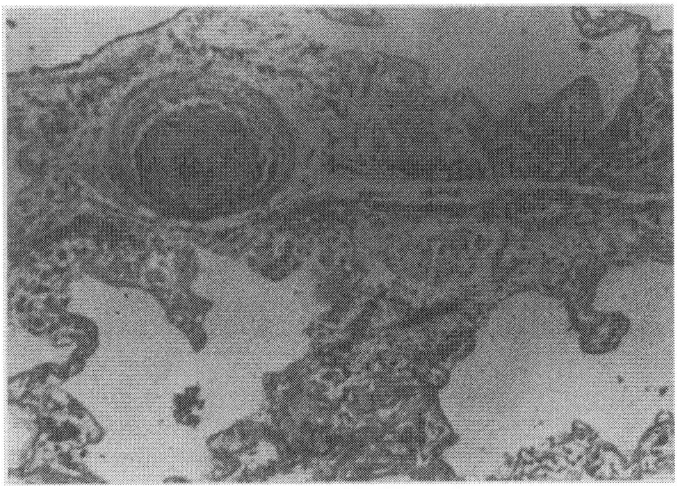

Fig. 11. Lung of patient dying of shock. Note edema of alveolar walls, fibrinous exudate lining some alveoli, and intravascular thrombus

trol fibrinolytic bleeding, fibrinolysis is halted, capillary clots remain, and extensive tissue necrosis results. It is in this case that the true extent of capillary clotting may be seen at autopsy. Otherwise, the capillary clots are usually lysed by the time of autopsy and are not seen in tissue sections.

Examples of tissue necrosis resulting in organ failure are often seen in the liver (Fig. 5), kidney (Fig. 6), heart (Fig. 7), pancreas (Fig. 8), gut (Fig. 9), adrenal (Fig. 10), and lung (Fig. 11).

Tissue enzymes liberated by dying cells offer laboratory evidence of this cell death (Figs. 12–14).

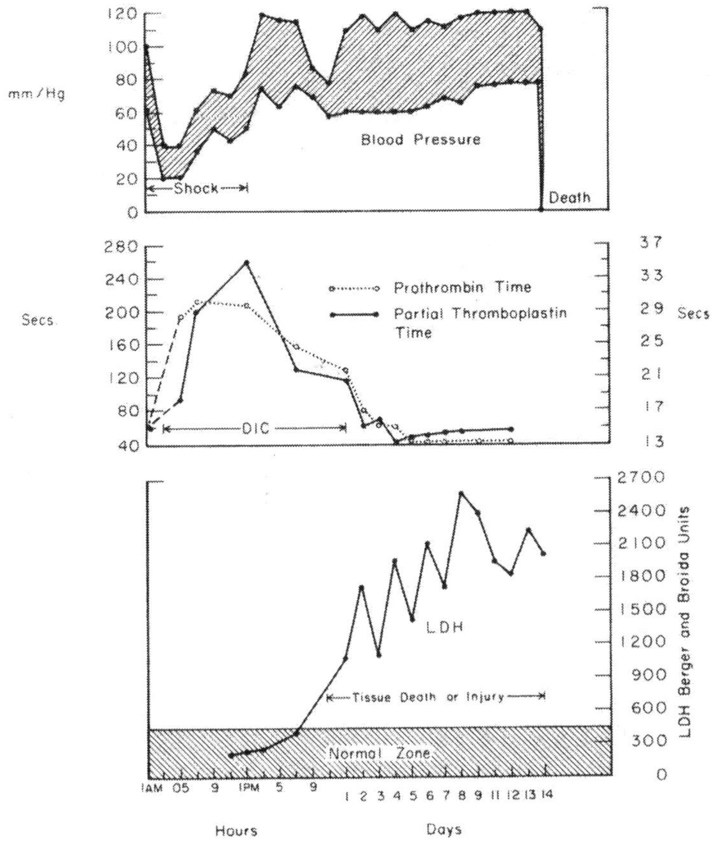

Fig. 12. Patient who died in septic shock. Note the episode of DIC followed by increasing lactate dehydrogenase (*LDH*) and death

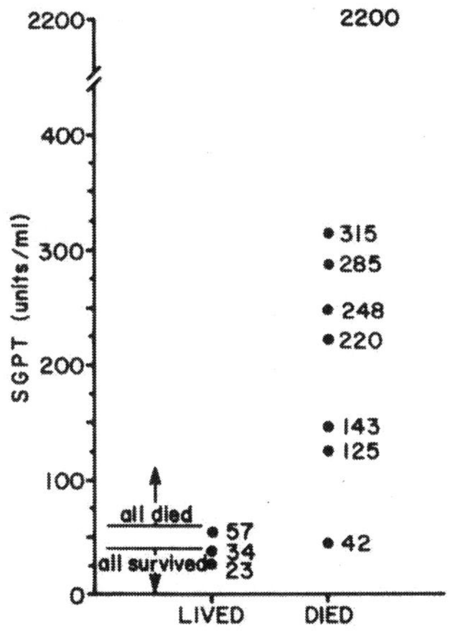

Fig. 13. Patients in severe shock. Note that above 100 units/ml serum glutamic-pyruric transaminase (*SGPT*) all the patients died; less than 60 units/ml SGPT all survived

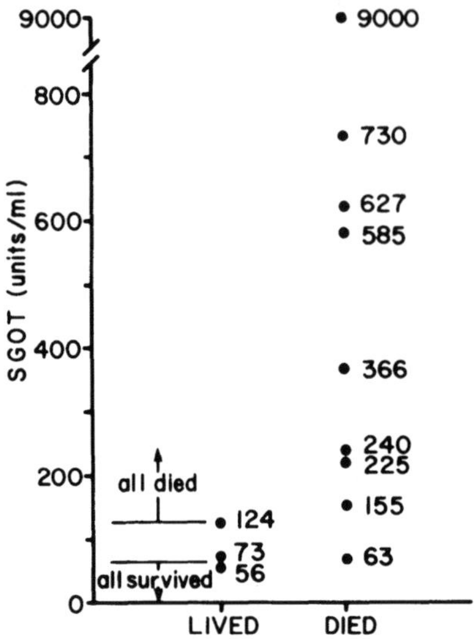

Fig. 14. Patients in severe shock. Note that above 150 units/ml serum glutamic-oxaloacetic transaminase (*SGOT*) all the patients died; less than 60 units/ml SGoT all survived

Microrheological Aspects: Their Crucial Role in Multiple Organ Failure

Leopold Dintenfass[1]

Introduction

Sequential breakdown in a number of crucial organs, such as the heart, kidneys, lungs, liver or brain, may take place over a span of seconds or many weeks. The crucial parameter in such a breakdown will be blood rheology, or more exactly, hyperviscosity of blood. Blood hyperviscosity can be due to elevation of any one of the blood viscosity factors: elevation of plasma viscosity, elevation of packed cell volume (Haematocrit), elevation of the degree of aggregation of red cells (and especially the presence of large compact clumps of red cells), increase in the internal viscosity and rigidity of red cells, increase in the number and rigidity of the white cells, and presence of platelet aggregates. Blood hyperviscosity may be accompanied by an increase of the viscosity of whole blood, but it may be present in spite of normal or even decreased viscosity of whole blood when one of the viscosity factors is abnormally increased. The crucial role of blood hyperviscosity is especially apparent in the microcirculation. The effect of increased rigidity of blood cells or aggregates or clumps of blood cells, or the presence of microthrombi, microemboli or other products of blood coagulation is amplified by the "inversion phenomenon" in the microcapillary flow [1, 2].

A slowdown of blood flow, occlusion, and/or rheological intermittent spasm-like conditions leads to deprivation of the tissue of oxygen, prevents outflow of metabolites, affects heat transfer, interferes with communication by chemical messengers, results in hypoxia and anoxia, initiates blood coagulation, etc., creating a vicious circle and inducing the syndromes of blood hyperviscosity, in effect, hyperviscosaemia. [3].

The interaction between hyperviscosity and coagulation cascades is not restricted to an increase of aggregation of red cells with increased fibrinogen level and/or fibrin formation; hyperviscosity per se affects biochemical reactions and synthesis of lipids, etc.

Our bodies are based on mechanochemical-electrical processes; such processes are particularly evident in the red cell membrane.

Failure of a crucial organ or organs is influenced by genetic and environmental

[1]Department of Medicine, University of Sydney, NSW 2006, and Clinical Haemorheology Department, Rachel Forster Hospital, Redfern, NSW 2016, Australia

factors, especially stress. Even with such a simple genetic marker as ABO blood groups, there is a significant difference in viscosity function for the A, O, and B groups. Stress, depression, anxiety, etc. influence significantly the levels of blood viscosity factors; pain and psychosomatic pain are related to abnormal blood rheology and, through it, to abnormal chemical reactions and electrical phenomena. Again, a vicious circle is evident.

Notwithstanding the complexity of factors and events in multiple organ failure, the crucial parameters can be recognized, and these include the rigid red cell and rigid clumps of blood cells on the one hand and the amplification mechanism for disturbances in the microcirculation, namely, the inversion phenomenon.

Red Cell

Blood is a very complex fluid. While at near-zero flow velocities the viscosity of whole blood may be 100 to 10000-fold higher than that of water, at high flow velocities it may be only twice that of water. But under certain circumstances, an increased pressure may lead to an apparent increase in the viscosity of blood. Generally, however, the most remarkable aspect of blood is that it remains fluid at nearly 100% concentrations of red cells. In contrast to blood, suspensions of rigid particles already exhibit the consistency of concrete at concentrations of about 65%.

This remarkable property of blood corresponds to that of an ideal emulsion (which does not exist in actuality), i.e., a suspension of fluid drops in which the interfacial layer (membrane) does not prevent the drops or cells from remaining fluid.

Determinations of the fluidity/rigidity or deformation of red cells have been carried out recently; including the use of a variety of filtration methods. The rigidity of red cells can also be estimated from the viscosity of blood measured at relatively high shear rates (above 180 s^{-1}) when the red cell aggregates are presumed to break down and disperse.

Dintenfass suggested an equation for blood viscosity [4, 5]:

$$\eta_r = (1 - TkC)^{-2.5}$$

in which η_r is the relative viscosity of blood, i.e., viscosity of blood defined at high shear rates divided by the viscosity of plasma, however as in many rotational viscometers plasma exhibits flow instability, it is safer to define plasma viscosity in a capillary viscometer; T is Taylor's adapted factor by which the volume of red cells is effectively decreased due to internal circulation within the red cells, this T is calculated from the viscosity equation; k is a coefficient related to plasma trapping (entrainment) and also can be obtained from this equation as part of the Tk factor; and C is the volume concentration of red cells.

The numerical value of Taylor's factor is:

$$T = (p + 0.4)/(p + 1)$$

in which p is the ratio of the apparent internal viscosity of the fluid drop to the viscosity of plasma.

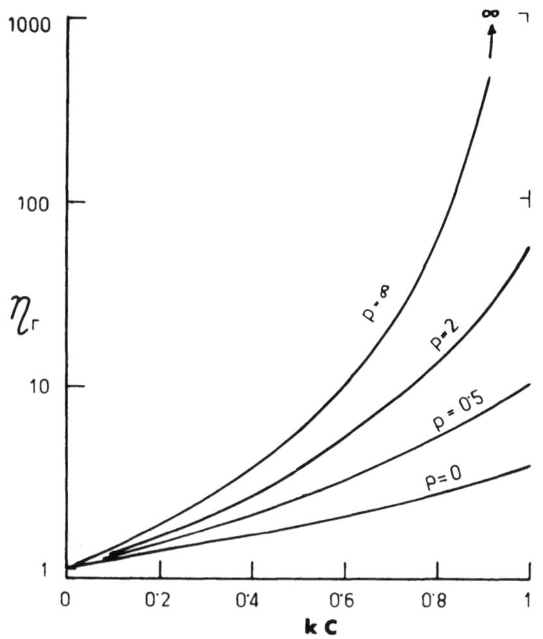

Fig. 1. Relative viscosity of blood as a function of concentration of red cell (C) and the *ratio* of the internal viscosity of red cells and the viscosity of plasma ($p = \eta_i/\eta_{pl}$); the curves are drawn from Dintenfass' blood viscosity equation. Note that the lowest values of p correspond to disorders such as Waldenström's macroglobulinaemia, in which plasma viscosity is very high. Normal values are about p = 2; when rigidity of the red cells increases, p climbs towards infinity. Coeffcient k and T are related by an empirical equation [2]: K = {0.0066/(1/T = 0.99)} + 1.01

To calculate the rigidity of the red cell Tk, we can use the following transformed equation:

$$TkC = (\eta_r^{0.4} - 1)/\eta_r^{0.4}$$

Note that the relative viscosity is dimensionless and that C is a volume fraction; one can obtain the relative viscosity taken to exponent 0.4 using either a logarithmic slide rule or a proper calculator. The T value cannot be smaller than 0.4 or larger than 1.0; however, Tk can show any value between 0.4 and 1.67—the latter for rigid particles or rigid cells. Normal Tk values are up to 0.95, and values of Tk above 1.0 are abnormal.

The effect of rigidity of the red cells on the relative viscosity of blood at different kC values and at shear rates at which the cells are disaggregated, is illustrated in Fig. 1. When p is zero and the equivalent T is 0.4, the contribution of red cells to blood viscosity is very small; when p is infinity and T is 1, there is a pronounced increase of blood viscosity with an increase of concentration of cells (or particles). Note that kC includes packing factor, which in rigid particles is about 1.6. For details see Dintenfass [2, 3, 6].

A more complete equation for blood viscosity, at any shear rate, is given as:

$$\eta_r = (1 - \alpha_D k_D T_D C)^{-2.5}$$

in which the subscript D indicates the influence of shear rates, while the term α reflects the state of aggregation of red cells and, thus, the concurrent increase in the free volume of the disperse phase. (An analysis of the experimental data based on this equation is given in Dintenfass [1])

Rigid Aggregates of Red Cells

It has been presumed for a long time that the aggregation of red cells is of little importance in the microcirculation. This concept was based on findings made in normal subjects and pregnant women, showing aggregates of red cells to be basically rouleaux or a network based on rouleaux. It is unlikely that rouleaux present a risk factor in the circulation, as they break down easily. In extreme cases, networks formed by rouleaux can lead to high blood viscosity at low shear rates and even to a high yield point (although this is a function of time). However, there may be a spectrum of aggregates ranging from rouleaux to compact clumps, and the latter may show a resistance to breakdown and present a problem in the microcirculation. Such complex and compact clumps have been observed by Knisely et al. in their in vivo antemortem studies [7] and were reported later by Talstad [8] and Dintenfass [1]. In his more recent studies, Dintenfass described compact aggregates in patients with heart disease, various forms of cancer, diabetes, etc. [9]. These studies were carried out using the parallel-plate slit-capillary viscometer (a space-rated version of which was employed on the space shuttle "Discovery" in 1985 [10]. Our studies showed that single compact aggregates of red cells may contain 50 000 or more red cells under conditions of stasis.

The degree of red cell aggregation (size of aggregates and kinetics) depends on the flow velocity (shear rate) and intrinsic properties of blood. When the flow rate is constant, the size and morphology of aggregates depends on the plasma proteins, toxins, antigens, etc.

Inversion Phenomenon

The flow through the microcirculation depends on two additional factors: (a) the Fahraeus-Lindqvist phenomenon, whereby an apparent decrease of blood viscosity occurs as the caliber of the capillary (or small blood vessel) decreases, and (b) on the inversion phenomenon of Dintenfass [2, 3], in which a sudden and dramatic increase in the apparent viscosity of blood (and a sudden and dramatic increase in the resistance to flow) takes place at a critical vessel radius (Fig. 2). This critical radius can be as small as 2 μm or as large as 10, 20, or 100 μm, depending on the rheology of the blood cells and on the presence of rigid red cells, rigid white cells, rigid platelet aggregates, or rigid red cell aggregates. Thus, we have a mechanism by which even a slight elevation in the rigidity of blood cells can be amplified through the inversion phenomenon, affect the resistance to flow in the tissues, and influence the apparent value of localized blood viscosity.

The inversion phenomenon represents a microrheological system of special

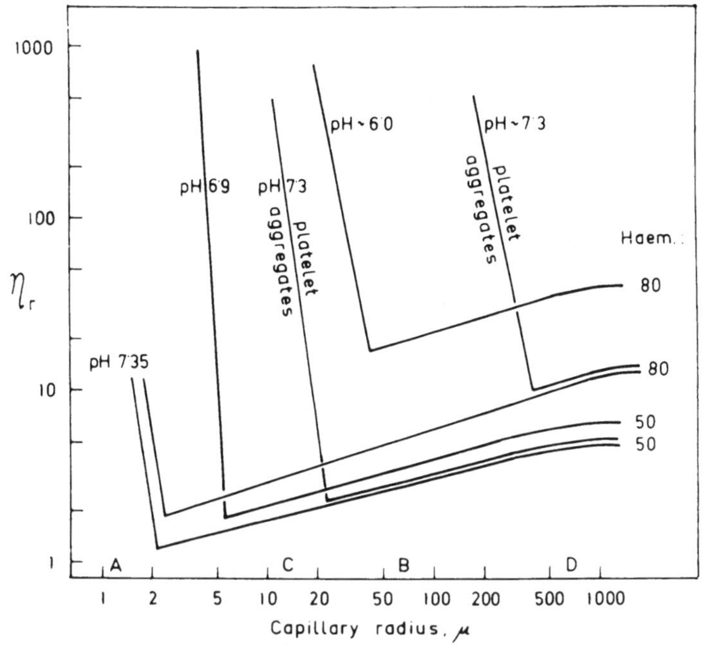

Fig. 2. Inversion phenomenon. The relative viscosity of blood decreases when the capillary (or blood vessel) bore decreases, in accordance with the Fahraeus-Lindqvist phenomenon. However, at a certain critical bore, there is a sudden increase in the apparent viscosity, which is largely independent of haematocrit. The inversion depends on the rheology of blood cells and, in particular, on the rigidity of red cells, presence of platelet aggregates, presence of rigid compact clumps of red cells, ect. Red cells can be affected by pH and tonicity, or type of haemoglobin

relevance to the microcirculation. As this phenomenon can be intermittent or spasm-like, it can provide a counterpart to the arterial spasm, which is of specific importance in the coronary circulation [3, 11].

It should be noted that haematocrit per se is of minor importance. As platelet aggregates play a pronounced role in the inversion phenomenon, a short review of the relevant coagulation mechanism will be given.

Dynamic Coagulation and Thrombus Formation, Suspension Coagula

Platelet aggregates, microthrombi, and microemboli may lead to crucial occlusions amplified by the inversion phenomenon. As the role of flow velocity and shear rates, morphology and durability of thrombi in the formation time is not fully appreciated, a short description is needed.

Platelet aggregation can be enhanced by the shear rate, and platelet aggregates may be a by-product of coagulation in addition to being produced by deterioration and degradation of the original thrombi. Fibrinogen products may also be partly a direct result of coagulation under specific high shear rates or a by-product of deteriorating thrombi [12, 13]. The "casting" shear rate determines the final properties of clots and artificial thrombi (in any particular type of donor or disease). Starting from a nearly zero shear rate to high shear rates, we can observe the formation of red thrombi, red-white thrombi, white thrombi, and suspension coagula (i.e., suspensions of platelet aggregates, and fibrin-platelet aggregates). In parallel, the clotting times vary from many minutes at zero shear rate, through a few minutes at mediums shear rates, to a few seconds at shear rates above 400 s^{-1}. There is a simultaneous change in the morphology, from red cells enmeshed in a fibrin network, through masses of platelets, to individual particles of platelets and fibrin.

Viscosity, morphology, and formation times of clots, red thrombi, white thrombi, and suspension coagula are all dependent on the microrheological processes affected by velocity gradient (shear rate): if the latter is progressively increased, the systems change in the following manner: (a) through the progressive orientation of the fibrin network and, in extreme cases, through the formation of globular fibrin particles (shearing forces may lead to stretching and bending of macromolecules and, through directional shearing stresses, may affect polymerization; (b) through the progressive disaggregation of red cell aggregates followed by a progressive escape of red cells from the fibrin network (note that the aggregation of red cells in the blood of patients with thrombosis is related to the consistency of their red thrombi); (c) through the progressive aggregation of platelets, the degree of aggregation, and the rate of aggregation depending on the casting shear rates and on the intrinsic adhesiveness of platelets peculiar to the individual subject; (d) through the influx of mechanical energy, which might affect the chemical or mechanical integrity of blood cells, with a possible release of additional coagulation factors; and (e) through a facilitated diffusion and collision frequency of the coagulation factors and co-factors.

The mode of coagulation at stasis or very slow flow of blood will proceed through the stages of rapid aggregation of red cells, hypoxia or anoxia-induced degeneration of the red cell membrane, and formation of fibrin networks. At the other extreme, very high shear rates, such as in the stenotic regions, will lead to rapid formation of platelet aggregates and/or fibrin particles; such stenotic regions shoot microemboli into the distal circulation. Disintegrating thrombi (disintegration is much more rapid in abnormal blood, such as in renal failure, hypertension or atherosclerosis, and diabetes) also release microthrombi into the circulation. All modes of coagulation can lead to the formation of microemboli, which will affect the distal circulation, such effects being amplified by the inversion phenomenon.

Mechanism of Rheological Damage

Increase of blood viscosity factors may lead to capillary stasis, thrombosis, localized infection, or gangrene in the heart muscle, kidneys, brain, liver, etc., or in an arterial wall. Two schemas are presented: one leading to infarction and thrombosis (Fig. 3), and the other leading to cancer metastases (Fig. 4). I believe that similar rheological mechanisms play a role in both types of event.

A series of primary causes, including metabolic, genetic, viral, psychological, can induce the formation of abnormal blood viscosity factors, which then have

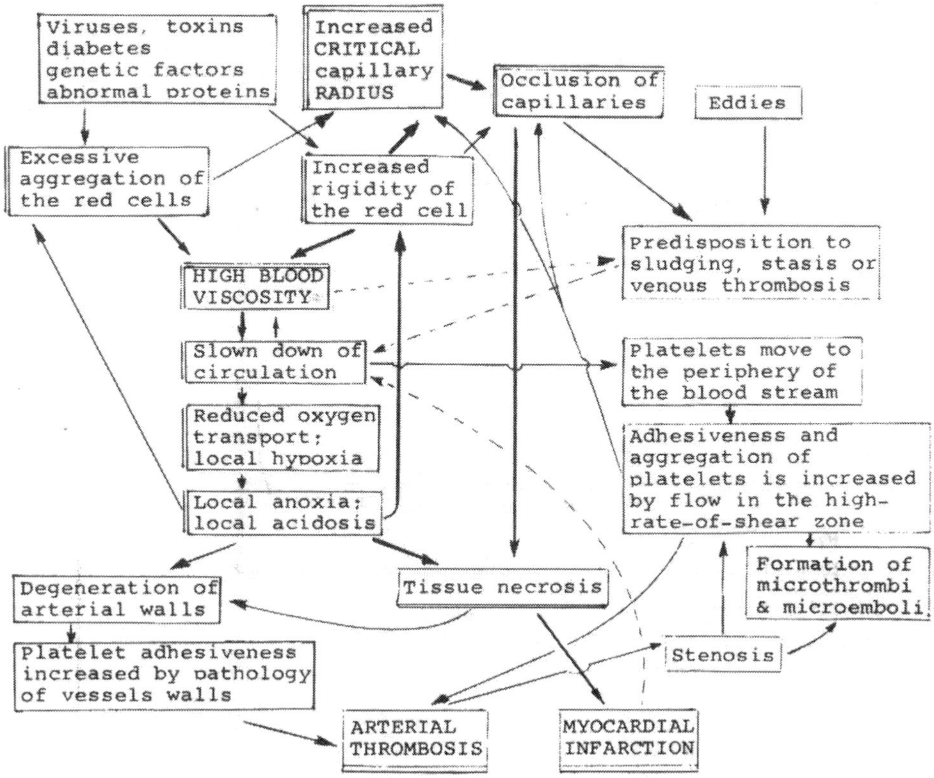

Fig. 3. The pattern of changes leading to thrombosis or infarction in the of microrheology of blood. Blood viscosity increase (or increase in blood viscosity factors) can be originally induced by infection, toxins, abnormal proteins, metabolic disorders, cancer, etc. and can lead to a slowing down of the flow with a range of haemodynamic changes as illustrated. Vicious circles can be formed which enhance the abnormality of individual blood viscosity factors. Copyright owner is L Dintenfass

immediate effects in the microcirculation and subsequent macroeffects, such as myocardial infarction, cerebrovascular incident, gangrene (Fig. 5). A series of vicious circles may appear which reinforces the original trend to enhance the macroeffect.

The timing of such events could be precipitated by a number of factors, including stress and diet, which might lead to a temporary increase in one of the blood viscosity factors (e.g., rigidity of red cells, aggregation of red cells, haemoconcentration, activity of white cells, platelet aggregation).

Thresholds for different organs and tissue (in respect of an increase or rather degree of increase, or degree of abnormality of blood viscosity factors) within each individual may differ depending on genetic factors and the response to environmental stress (including infections, weather, diet, interpersonal relationships, physical activity, mental activity, life philosophy). All the listed factors influence blood viscosity or blood subphases and affect tissue perfusion. Drugs, cigarette smoking, and alcohol consumption influence the aggregation of red

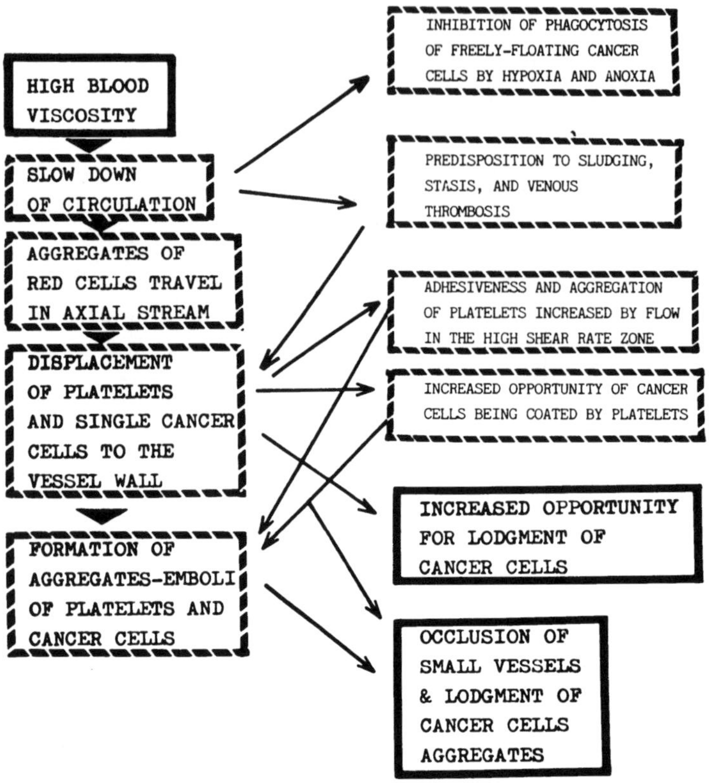

Fig. 4. Hypothesis for rheologically enhanced metastases. It is suggested that an increase of aggregation of red cells leads to displacement of freely floating cancer cells towards the vessel wall with the subsequent formation of cancer cell-platelet aggregates, which might show increased capacity for sticking to the vessel wall or occluding a small vessel

cells as well as other viscosity and clotting factors.

Studies in a range of diseases showed few patients with normal blood viscosity factors; very few normal subjects showed any abnormal viscosity factors. Blood viscosity factors and functions have been investigated in the following disorders in the Biorheology and Haemorheology Department, Kanematsu Memorial Institute, Sydney Hospital and Department of Medicine, University of Sydney (1963–1984): ischaemic heart disease, myocardial infarction, renal failure, cadaveric renal transplants, diabetes (maturity and juvenile onset), retinopathy (diabetic and hypertensive), peripheral arterial disease, hypertension, malignant melanoma, Waldenström's macroglobulinaemia, acute leukaemia, chronic leukaemia, haemophilia, polycythaemia, deep vein thrombosis, depressive anxiety, psychosomatic pain, and cancer [3]. Where abnormal viscosity factors were present, such an increase in the factors was a precursor to subsequently observed disorders including cerebral incidents, arterial occlusion, myocardial infarction. Even in athletes, the determination of blood viscosity factors appeared to be a better indicator of future health pattern than biochemical or clinical tests.

It was possible to establish correlations between the blood viscosity factors

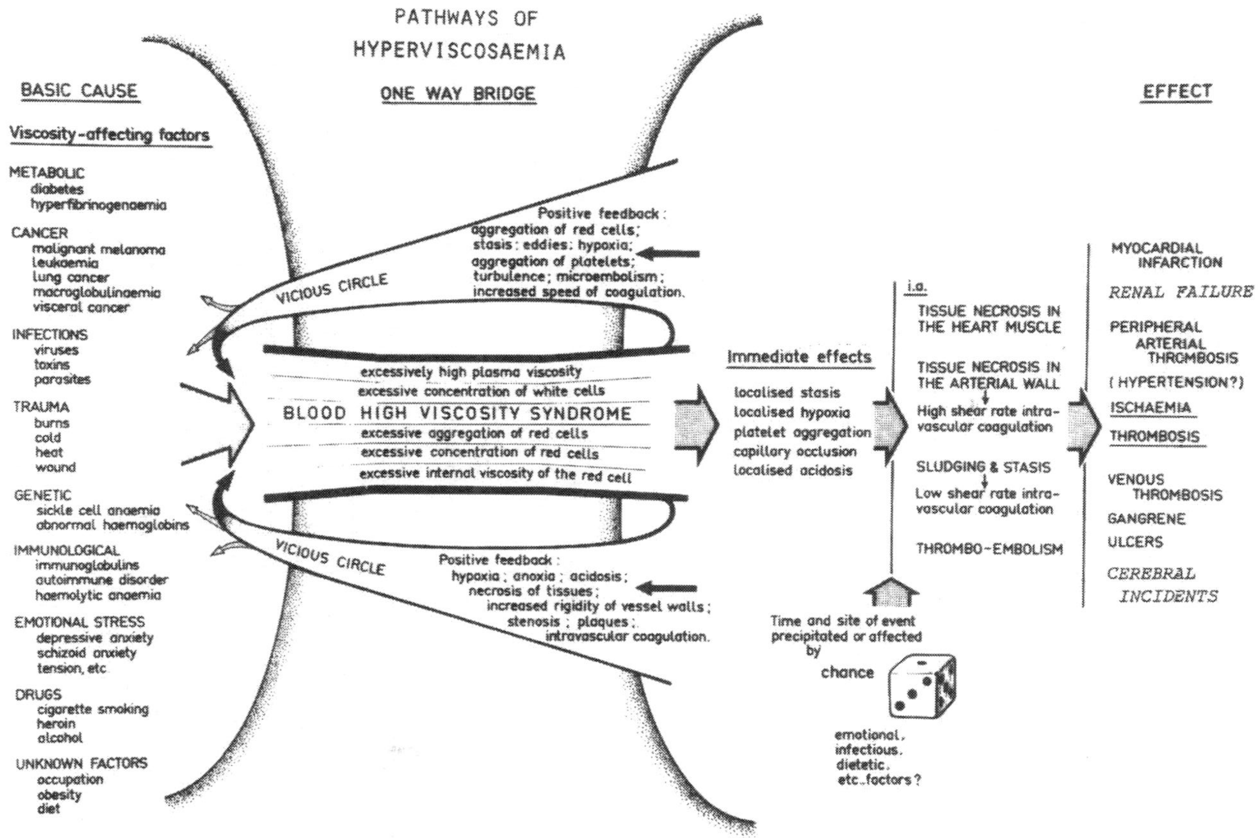

Fig. 5. A large series of original causes, from infections and drugs to cancer and metabolic discorders, leads to increase of blood viscosity factors, and through microeffects in the microcirculation (including stasis and occlusion) induce hypoxia and tissue demage, with the final result being infarction, thrombosis, and failure of particular organs. Many vicious circles lead to reinforcement of the pathological condition and subsequent increase in intensity of disease. Precipitation of catastrophic events could be promoted or initiated by dehydration, fever, cigarette smoking, psychological stress, etc. Copyright owner is L Dintenfass

and arterial blood pressure, ST-segment depression, SGOT (aspartate transaminase) or SGBT, and other enzymes indicating destruction of the tissue, parathyroid hormone, blood sugar level, and paraproteins [3].

It was also possible from such parameters as submaximal work output to consider patients and normals as a continuum, i.e., there was a continuous increase in blood viscosity factors from the healthiest subjects towards the those with the most severe disease [14].

Even survival time has been established as a function of a number of blood viscosity factors in malignant melanoma patients (although the sample, even if statistically significant, is still rather small) [3]. In further discussion of the role of hyperviscosity in multiple organ failure, it should be stressed that death from a heart attack does take place in subjects with intact and healthy coronary arteries and, after exclusion of an arterial spasm, one can blame a localized increase in the viscosity of whole blood, the presence of rigid clumps of red cells and/or white cells and/or platelets, or rigid red cells or rigid white cells in the case of the smallest blood vessels.

It is of particular interest to note that in aging patients, at least three pathological conditions can be observed simultaneously, and Thompson found in 1986 that in nearly 600 patients aged over 70 years, eight diseases were present simultaneously: obesity, hypertension, type 2 diabetes, atherosclerosis, cancer, endogeneous depression, autoimmune depression, and immunosuppression [15].

As shown by Dintenfass [2, 3] hyperviscosity is present in diabetes, cancer, depression, and hypertension. Hypertension and cancer are both characterized by increased rigidity of red cells and increased thrombus formation [3]. A clinical link between hypertension and cancer was described by Dyer et al. [16]. The correlations between hyperviscosity and anxiety and depression was made by Dintenfass and Zador [17], while others described an impairment of immunological functions as a result of depression and psychological stress [18].

If oxygenation of the blood is not critically diminished, any decrease of oxgyen consumption is due to inadequate microcirculation. In shock patients, inadequate tissue perfusion is always followed by a decrease in the total oxygen uptake, although superficially haemodynamics appear to be adequate [19]. The status the microcirculation is the decisive factor in the development and course of shock. Neuhof [19] stated in particular that: (a) the microcirculation may be impaired in many ways and the pattern and degree of disorder may differ from organ to organ and even within the same organ; and (b) a microlocal capillary perfusion and/or metabolism cannot be representative of the true situation of the organ or of the status of the total microcirculation.

Neuhof particularly stressed that it is impossible to interpret the status of microcirculation from haemodynamics, especially in septic shock. In hyperdynamic septic shock, capillary gas exchange is impaired and the total oxygen uptake is highly reduced despite augmented cardiac output.

In cardiogenic shock, occlusion of the coronary arteries by rigid red cells, red cell aggregates, microthrombi, microemboli, transient aggregates of blood cells, temporary localized haemoconcentration, and thus a localized increase in the blood viscosity will affect the myocardium and survival. Cardiogenic shock is often characterized by severe lactic acidaemia, which leads to increase rigidity and aggregation of red cells and, in turn, is amplified by these rheological phenomena.

Any increase in rheological factors, especially sudden increases, will affect primarily the mucosa and submucosa of the stomach, then the kidneys, adrenals, muscle, etc.

Endotoxins can induce stagnant anoxia of the viscera. Toxins increase aggregation of red cells, cause increase of blood viscosity, and lead to stagnantion and stasis, with a further increase in blood viscosity factors and predisposition to intravascular coagulation, the latter being a source of microemboli. The production of catecholamines can be increased by endotoxin stimulation.

Thus, we can say that although cardiorespiratory patterns may move differently in different types of shock, the common denominator of shock is abnormality of blood flow in the microcirculation. Thus, the main parameter should be the rheology of blood and various contributions of the blood subphases to blood viscosity and blood flow or stasis. Different subphases of blood and different patterns of viscosity factors may exhibit a similar low-flow or no-flow condition; but the pattern of viscosity factors may be characteristic of specific shock Furthermore, Shoemaker [20] stated that the onset of shock can be present in a patient prior to recognition; it should indeed be possible to recognize the presence of shock or the presence of a risk stage by study of the blood viscosity factors. On the other hand, Shoemaker claims that a method of estimating the distribution of systemic blood flow and oxygen transport could be used to assess the perfusion defect of acute peripheral circulatory failure.

In this review of the mechanism of rheological damage, so far mainly mechanical types of damage have been considered. However, it appears lately from different types of studies [21–23] that increased viscosity itself also affects the biochemical reactions within the cell membrane and other cells. Thus, the haemolysis of red cells may be affected by plasma viscosity; the synthesis of lipids may be affected by the viscosity of plasma or interstitial fluid.

This would seem to return to the mechanochemical (teinochemical) principle suggested by Kuhn [24]: namely, that there is a reciprocal effect between a mechanical (or hydrodynamic) system and the chemical reactions within such a system. Thus, the external stresses may lead to appreciable changes in ionization or chemical activity [1]. Perhaps such stresses may ever be transformed into a different pattern of adsorption or cell interaction; vice versa, chemical changes within the cell (or clot) might influence mechanical performance (or retraction). As this area has not been adequately explored, it is simply noted here that another dimension might be opening.

Thus, the time interval between sequential and progressive failure of different organs may be affected by haemorheological factors, genetic and environmental factors, psychological factors, unknown interactions between the chemistry and mechanics of blood cells and blood vessels, which, in their turn, may also be affected by genetic and environmental factors

Conclusions

The common factor to all these diseases and disorders is blood hyperviscosity, which also includes rheologically active products of coagulation.

Our bodies are to a high degree self-repairing mechanisms. However, for self-repair to function properly, the flow of blood must be unimpaired. Many causes lead to an increase of blood viscosity factors and to occlusions in the microcirculation. However, many of these causes could be counteracted by rheological intervention: bleeding, haemodilution, and anti-aggregation drugs, and drugs affecting the fluidity/rigidity of the red cells or white cells.

One of the self-controlling mechanisms is suggested to be blood viscosity autoregulation via viscosity receptors [3, 25–28]. Viscoreceptors, which are believed to sense the rigidity of red cells and viscosity of whole blood, may fail when a sudden excessive increase in blood viscosity factors does take place. Perhaps a decrease of such factors, imposed externally, may bring the autoregulation into proper function again.

The potential scope to fight multiple organ failure is by control of blood rheology.

Acknowledgments. Support from the CSIRO Endowment Fund and from the Sir Zelman Cowen University Fund is hereby acknowledged.

References

1. Dintenfass L (1971) Blood microrheology, viscosity factors in blood flow, ischaemia and thrombosis. Butterworths, London
2. Dintenfass L (1976) Rheology of blood in diagnostic and preventive medicine. Butterworths, London
3. Dintenfass L (1985) Blood viscosity, hyperviscosity and hyperviscosaemia. MTP Press and Kluwer, Lancaster
4. Dintenfass L (1968) Internal viscosity of the red cell and a blood viscosity equation. Nature 219: 956–958
5. Dintenfass L (1969) The internal viscosity of the red cell and the structure of the red cell membrane. Considerations of the liquid crystalline structure of the red cell interior and membrane from rheological data. Mol Cryst 8: 101–139
6. Dintenfass L (1977) Theoretical aspects and clinical applications of the blood viscosity equation containing a term for the internal viscosity of the red cell. Blood Cells 3: 367–374
7. Knisely MH, Warner L, Harding F (1960) Ante-mortem settling. Microscopic observations and analyses of the settling of agglutinated blood-cell masses to the lower sides of vessels during life: a contribution to the biophysics of disease. Angiology 11: 535–550
8. Talstad I (1971) The morphology of erythrocyte sedimentation rate (ESR). Acta Med Scand 190: 7–10
9. Dintenfass L (1985) Red cell aggregation in cardiovascular diseases and crucial role of inversion phenomenon. Angiology 36: 315–326
10. Dintenfass L, Jedrzejczyk H, Willard A (1982) Photographic, stereological and statistical methods in evaluation of aggregation of red cells in disease: I. Kinetics of aggregation. Biorheology 19: 567–577
11. Maseri A, L'Abbate A, Baroldi G (1978) Coronary artery spasm as a possible cause of myocardial infarction: a conclusion derived from study of preinfarction angina. N Engl J Med 299: 271–272
12. Dintenfass L (1967) Dynamics of blood coagulation. Introducing a new coagulation factor "velocity gradient." Haematologia 1: 387–400
13. Dintenfass L, Stewart JH (1968) Formation, consistency and degradation of artificial

thrombi in severe renal failure. Effect of ABO blood groups. Thromb Diath Haemorrh 20: 267–284
14. Dintenfass L, Lake B (1977) Blood viscosity factors in evaluation of submaximal work output and cardiac activity in man. Angiology 28: 788–798
15. Thompson K (1986) Not the James Mackenzie lecture—a concept of disease to educate the new type of doctor: discussion paper. J Roy Soc Med 79: 729–783
16. Dyer AR, Stamler J, Berkson DM, Lindbert HA, Stevens E (1975) High blood pressure: a risk factor for cancer mortality? Lancet 1: 1051–1056
17. Dintenfass L, Zador I (1977) Hemorheology, chronic anxiety and psychosomatic pain: an apparent link. Lex et Scientia 13: 154–162
18. Bartrop RW, Luckhurst E, Lazarus L, Kiloh LG, Penny R (1977) Depressed lymphocyte function after bereavement. Lancet 1: 834–836
19. Neuhof H (1982) Clinical problems in shock: microcirculation and peripheral gas exchange. Clinical Hemorheology 2: 691–703
20. Shoemaker WC (1979) Pathophysiology and therapy of shock states: use of hemodynamic and oxygen transport variables to predict survival and to guide therapy. In: The organ in shock. Upjohn, Kalamazoo, pp 75–87
21. Yedgar S, Eilam O, Shafrir E (1985) Regulation of plasma lipid levels by plasma viscosity in nephrotic rats. Am J Physiol 248: E10–E14
22. Yedgar, S., Weinstein DB, Patschi W, Schonfeld G, Casanada FE, Steinberg D (1982) Viscosity of culture medium as a regulator of synthesis and secretion of very low density lipoproteins by cultural hepatocytes. J Biol Chem 257: 2188–2192
23. Hovav E, Halle C, Yedgar S (1987) Viscous macromolecules inhibit erythrocyte hemolysis induced by snake venom phospholipase A_2. Biorheology (in press)
24. Kuhn W (1960) Prinzip der Erzeugung mechanischer Energie durch makromolekulare Systeme. Makromolek Chemie 35: 200–220
25. Dintenfass L (1976) Malfunction of viscosity-receptors (viscoreceptors) as the cause of hypertension. Am Heart J 92: 260–263
26. Dintenfass L (1977) Hypothesis of viscoreceptors: malfunction of viscoreceptors and viscosity-controllers in hypertension and polycythaemia. Bibliot Anat 16: 478–480 (9th European Conference on Microcirculation, Antwerp 1976)
27. Dintenfass L (1980) Autoregulation of blood viscosity in health and disease. Vascular Surgery 14: 227–237
28. Dintenfass L (1981) Hyperviscosity in hypertension. Pergamon, Sydney

Histopathological Study of Multiple Organ Failure Following Open Heart Surgery

Chikao Yutani, Masami Imakita, and Hatsue Ishibashi-Ueda[1]

Introduction

Although the recent development of intensive care unit (ICU) has made it possible to reduce the mortality due to failure of one vital organ, it is reported that multiple organ failure (MOF), defined as serious and sequential disturbances in more than two organs [1], is associated with most postoperative deaths.

According to Roberts [2], organ failure following open-heart surgery can usually be ascribed to low cardiac output syndrome (LOS), the cause of which is still unknown.

The aim of this study is to elucidate the pathological sequences of MOF from morphological analyses of patients who died of MOF after cardiac valve replacement (VR) and aortocoronary bypass graft surgery (ACBG).

Materials and Methods

During the period from June 1977 to June 1986, approximately 1200 patients were autopsied at the Division of Pathology, National Cardiovascular Center (NCVC). Of the 1200 autopsied cases, 91 were submitted for MOF study, diagnosis of which was made according to the clinical criteria.

The 91 cases were composed of 63 cases of VR and 28 cases of ACBG. We divided them into five groups according to the time from operation to death, namely less than 1 week, less than 1 month, less than 2 months, less than 1 year, and more than 1 year.

In the clinical data, we compared extracorporeal circulation (ECC) time, anoxic arrest time, the volume of blood transfusion, and so on; diagnosis of LOS was made according to the criteria of ICU at NCVC.

The hearts, lungs, liver, and other organs were histopathologically examined, particularly with respect to contraction band necrosis as evidence of myocardial damage [3–5], the Heath-Edwards classification [6] for pulmonary hypertension, and hemorrhagic centrilobular necrosis as a sign of ischemic hepatic change [7].

[1]Division of Pathology, National Cardiovascular Center, 7–1, Fujishirodai 5-chome, Suita, Osaka, 565 Japan

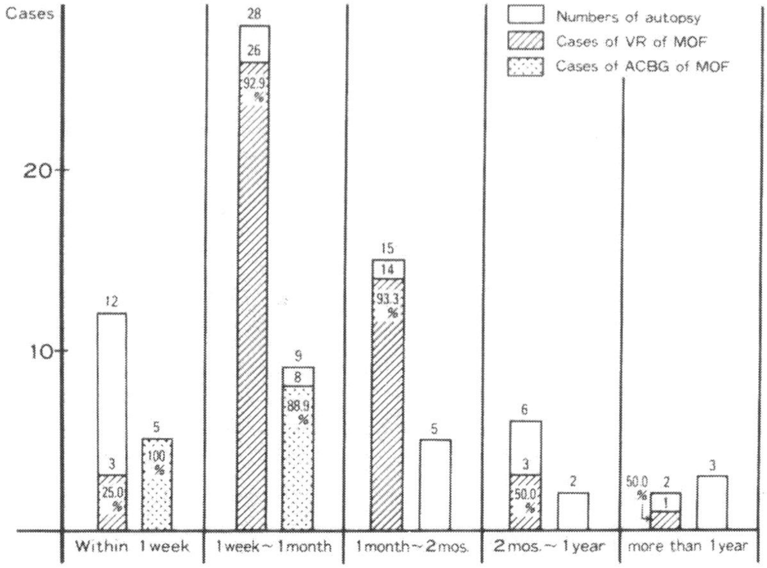

Fig. 1. Frequency of multiple organ failure (*MOF*) in cases following cardiac valve replacement (*VR*) and aortocoronary bypass surgery (*ACBG*)

Multiple formalin-fixed tissue blocks were taken for histological examination and sections were routinely stained with hematoxylin and eosin. Masson trichrome, Heidenhain's iron hematoxylin, and elastica van Gieson's stains were also used in some cases.

Results

Frequency of MOF

MOF occurred in 74.6% and 46.4% of autopsy cases with VR and ACBG, respectively. In the cases of VR, the peak of incidence of MOF was between 1 week and 2 months; most MOF cases in ACBG occurred within 1 month (Fig. 1).

MOF After VR

The longer the extracorporeal circulation (ECC) time and anoxic arrest time the patients received in the course of operation, the more easily they fell into MOF (Fig. 2).

The following morphological aspects of the heart were examined: weight, giant left atrium [8], thrombus formation, and myocardial necrosis. The peak of incidence of each factor was between 1 week and 2 months, which nearly correlated to heart weight (Fig. 3)

Myocardial necrosis was in particular considered to be very important because

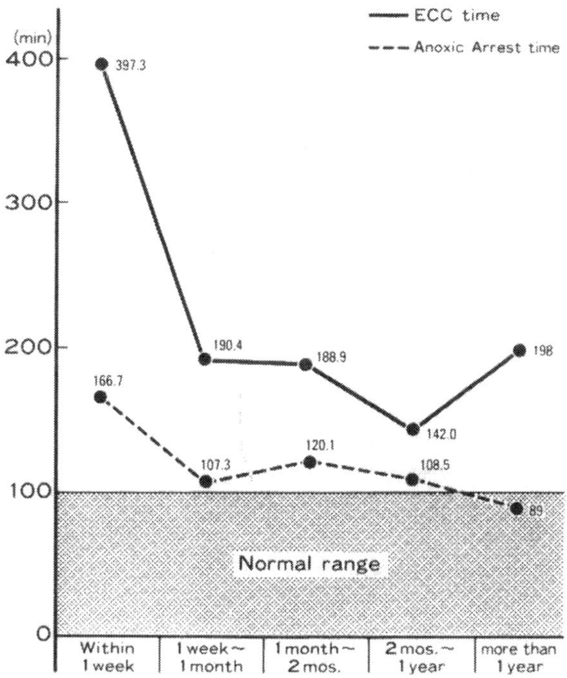

Fig. 2. Extracorporeal circulation time (*ECC*) and anoxic arrest in cases of MOF following VR

this lesion may lead to LOS; we, therefore, paid close attention to myocardial contraction band necrosis, hemorrhage, and their distribution (Fig. 4). Contraction band necrosis was most frequently found within 1 week and was associated with a high incidence of myocardial hemorrhage.

Jaundice is a reliable indicator in the clinical diagnosis of MOF. Sepsis, cardiac sclerosis, hemorrhagic centrilobular necrosis, cholangitis, volume of blood transfusion, and ECC time were investigated as contributing factors for jaundice (Fig. 5). Cardiac sclerosis ($P < 0.05$), cholangitis ($P < 0.005$), and the volume of blood transfusion ($P < 0.05$) were significantly related to jaundice.

With respect to the histological findings of the lungs, pneumonia, chronic changes, i.e., organizing edema (exudate), and septic thickening were most frequently observed between 1 week and 2 months after VR, which was similar to the frequency of cardiac and hepatic changes. The grade of pulmonary hypertension ranged between Heath-Edwards grades I and II

MOF After ACBG

In cases of MOF after ACBG 13 of 28 patients died with 1 month (Table 1). Hemorrhagic myocardial infarcts [9] were seen in 7 of 13 patients; hemorrhagic centrilobular necrosis of the liver occurred in 10 of 13 patients.

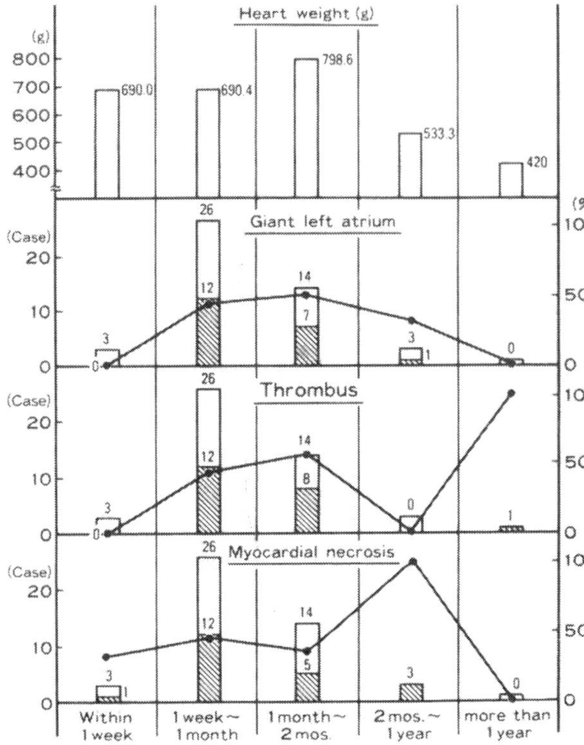

Fig. 3. Cardiac pathology in cases of MOF following VR

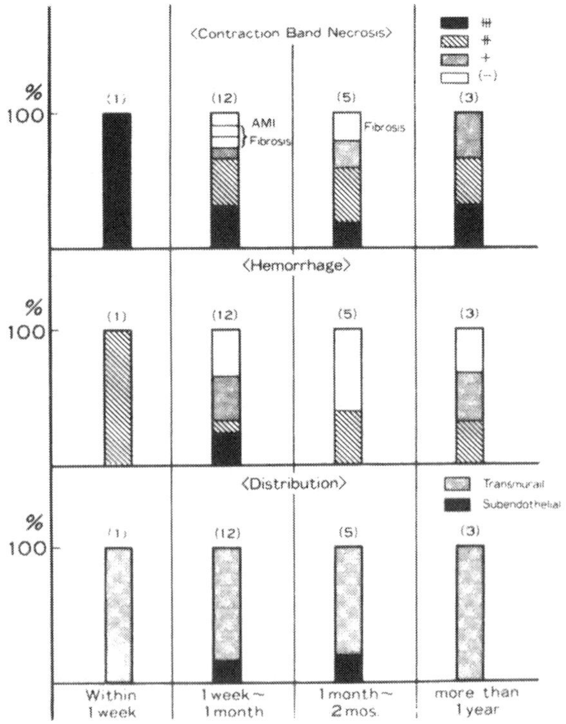

Fig. 4. Myocardial findings in cases of MOF following VR

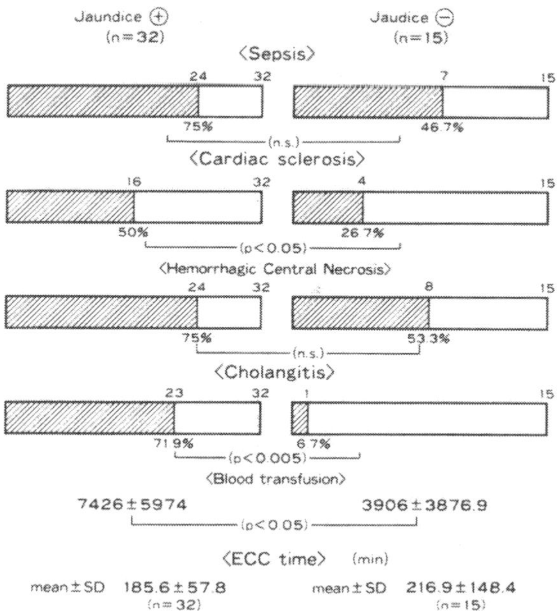

Fig. 5. Jaundice in cases of MOF following VR

Discussion

According to Schoen et al. [10], the causes of death after cardiac valve replacement may be divided into three categories: (a) those related to underlying cardiac vascular conditions and the surgery to correct them, (b) those related to complications of the prosthesis, and (c) those unrelated to the heart, blood vessels, or prosthesis. As seen in our study, early deaths are preponderantly due to the poor condition of the heart with valvular disease or complications of the operative procedure, including ECC, cardioplegia, and so forth.

Myocardial necrosis, which may be responsible for LOS as could be recognized in our study, is an important and not infrequent myocardial complication of cardiac operations that occasionally compromises survival [11].

The etiology of myocardial necrosis cannot be ascertained from the morphological data presented. The current theory is that transient anoxia and reperfusion play a major role. Nevertheless, the results of this study are consistent with those of previously reported autopsy series after cardiac valve replacement [10].

As to the etiology of myocardial contraction band necrosis, some of the ways in which such an injury can be produced—internal electric shock, potassium deficiency, stress, catecholamines, corticoid, and reperfusion—occurred in cases of temporary occlusion of a coronary artery and cardiopulmonary bypass [4]. It should be considered that the etiology of myocardial contraction band necrosis as well as postoperative jaundice [12] may be multifactorial.

In the cases of MOF after VR, judging from the histopathological findings, LOS preoperatively took place as a result of many causes, as described above, and was followed by infection which may have induced pneumonia, cholangitis, pancreatitis, and, finally, a septic state, leading to shock and death (Fig. 6).

Table 1. Pathology of multiple organ failure in patients following aortocoronary bypass surgery

	Age (years)	Sex (M:F)	Sepsis	DIC[a]	LVAD[b]	Weight (g)			
						Heart	Lungs	Liver	Kidneys
Within 1 week ($n = 5$)	64.4	4:1	0	1	0	468.3	865. 0	1440.0	326.7
1 week–1 month ($n = 8$)	62.9	7:1	6	1	1	556.7	1181 .3	1656.3	378.6

Table 1. (*continued*)

	Heart		Lungs			Liver			Kidneys ATN[e]	Cholesterol emboli
	OMI	Hemorrhagic MI	Pneumonia	ARDS[c]	Hemorrhage	Jaundice	HCN[d]	Cholangitis		
Within 1 week ($n = 5$)	4	3	1	0	0	2	5	0	5	3
1 week–1 month ($n = 8$)	6	4	3	1	2	5	5	1	4	0

[a] Disseminated intravascular coagulation
[b] Left ventricular assist device
[c] Adult respiratory distress syndrome
[d] Hemorrhagic centrilobular necrosis
[e] Acute tubular necrosis
OMI old myocardial infarct, *MI* myocardial infarct

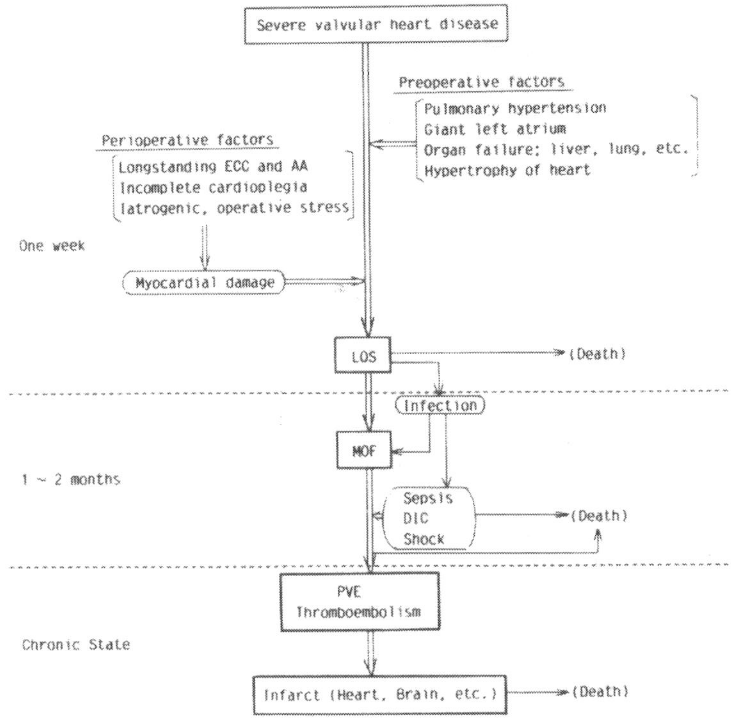

Fig. 6. Pathological sequence of MOF after cardiac valve replacement. *ECC* extracorporeal circulation, *AA* anoxic arrest, *LOS* low output syndrome, *MOF* multiple organ failure, *PVE* prosthesis valve endocarditis

Summary

The development of the intensive care unit (ICU) has made it possible to reduce the mortality in major surgery and save many patients. However, some patients die despite the ICU; the leading cause of death in ICUs is reported to be due to multiple organ failure (MOF).

We reviewed the records of 91 patients who died of MOF after cardiac valve replacement (VR) and aortocoronary bypass graft surgery (ACBG) and who underwent autopsy at the National Cardiovascular Center from 1977 through 1986. The frequency of MOF in VR was 74.0%, ACBG 46.4%, and the peak of numbers in MOF cases was within 7–2 months. A common finding in this particular series was myocardial necrosis, which may be responsible for low cardiac output syndrome (LOS) in or after operation. On the other hand, jaundice was the most reliable hallmark in making a diagnosis of MOF in the clinical course, which may be due to acute cholangitis in VR patients and hemorrhagic centrilobular necrosis in ACBG patients

It is also concluded that chronic changes, e.g., cardiac cirrhosis, pulmonary hypertension, may be an important factor in LOS as a prediposing factor of MOF.

References

1. Eiseman B, Beart R, Norton L (1977) Multiple organ failure. Surg Gynecol Obstet 144: 323
2. Roberts WC (1973) Pathologic anatomy of cardiac valve replacement: a study of 224 necropsy patients. Progress in Cardiovascular Diseases 15: 539–587
3. Morales AR, Fine G, Taber RE (1967) Cardiac surgery and myocardial necrosis. Arch Pathol 83: 71–79
4. Reichenbach DD, Benditt EP (1968) Myofibrillar degeneration: A response of the myocardial cell to injury. Arch Pathol 85: 189–199
5. Gotlieb A, Masse S, Allard J, Huang S (1977) Concentric hemorrhagic necrosis of the myocardium, A morphological and clinical study. Human Pathol 8: 27–37
6. Wagenvoort C, Wagenvoort N (1977) Pulmonary hypertension in cardiac left to right shunts. Pathology of pulmonary hypertension. Wiley, New York, pp 56–94
7. Arcidi JM, Moore GW, Hutchins GM (1981) Hepatic morphology in cardiac dysfunction, A clinicopathologic study of 1000 subjects at autopsy. Am J Pathol 104: 159–166
8. Kawazoe K, Beppu S, Takahara Y, Nakajima N, Tanaka K, Ichihashi K, Fujita T, Manabe H (1983) Surgical treatment of giant left atrium combined with mitral valvular disease. J Thorac Cardiovasc Surg 85: 885–892
9. Geft IL, Fishbein MC, Hashida J, Ninomiya K, Nishizawa K, Haendchen R, Venkatesh N, Y-Rit J, Yano J, Ganz W (1984) Effects of late coronary artery reperfusion after myocardial necrosis is complete. Am Heart J 107: 623–629
10. Schoen FJ, Titus JL, Lawrie GM (1983) Autopsy-determined causes of death after cardiac valve replacement. JAMA 249: 899–902
11. Kirklin JW, Corti VR, Blackstone EH (1979) Prevention of myocardial damage during cardiac operation. N Engl J Med 301: 135–141
12. Sherlock DS (1981) Disease of the liver and biliary system, 6th edn. Blackwell, Oxford, pp 188–189

Multiple Organ Failure: Clinical Implications to Macro- and Microcirculation

KONRAD MESSMER[1], UWE KREIMEIER[1], and FRITHJOF HAMMERSEN[2]

As result of improved primary resuscitation, a smaller number of all patients suffering from trauma, multiple injuries, and shock succumb within the first critical hours, except those with lethal injury to the vital organ. However, even though these patients present with stable hemodynamic conditions for days or weeks after the injury, dysfunction of one or several of their organs becomes apparent and these patients eventually die from late complications of the primary insult, in sepsis and multiple organ failure (MOF) [6, 37]. Baker [4] has demonstrated that age, severity of the injury, shock with arterial pressures below 80 mmHg, and, most importantly, the duration of shock are the crucial factors in the development of MOF. MOF can be the end-stage of shock in both low-flow and high-flow states. As a common denominator of all forms of shock appears the maldistribution of cardiac output, with critical reduction of nutritional blood flow in the vital organs and initiation of shock-specific microcirculatory disturbances [28, 36].

Hypotheses for Development of MOF

During recent years, four major hypotheses have been forwarded to explain the pathogenesis of multiple organ system failure after trauma and/or shock: (a) In patients with severe injury and/or after major surgery, activation of the sympathetic nervous system leads to the sympathoadrenergic reaction and consequently to a redistribution of cardiac output to the various organs. Since the splanchnic organs are rich in α-adrenergic receptors, vasoconstriction is most pronounced in this region, particularly in the vascular bed of the superior mesenteric artery. Consequently, blood supply to the intestine is reduced, whereby the integrity of the mucosal barrier is compromised so that microorganisms can enter the systemic circulation provoking bacteremia, endotoxinemia, and eventually sepsis and septic shock [9]. (b) Bacteria invade the lungs, liver, and kidneys;

[1] Department of Experimental Surgery, University of Heidelberg, Im Neuenheimer Feld 347, 6900 Heidelberg 1, Federal Republic of Germany
[2] Department of Anatomy, Technical University of Munich, Biedersteiner str. 29, 8000 Munich, Federal Republic of Germany

within these tissues, they activate macrophages and monocytes to release cytokines, including interleukin-1 (IL-1) and TNF small peptides known to affect the function of most organs and tissues [14]. (c) Multiple organ failure is considered to be the result of a general activation of the immune systems [31]. (d) MOF is promoted by shock-specific impairment of the microcirculation, focal ischemia, and local reperfusion injury [28, 29]. The latter triggers the adherence of leukocytes to the endothelial surface, the release of oxygen free radicals, and the generation of mediators which in turn activate the cascade systems, i.e., the arachidonic acid pathway, complement, and the coagulation system [15, 27].

The last hypothesis implies that primary resuscitation, despite normalizing the macrohemodynamic parameters does not restore microcirculatory function. Therefore, regional or focal ischemia may persist and the function of the given organs might deteriorate as a result of these ischemic lesions and even more so by local reperfusion injury.

In fact, the damage of tissues and organs remote from the site of injury is enhanced by reperfusion and reoxygenation after temporary ischemia. One of the causes of this phenomenon is the generation of oxygen free radicals, which induce lipid peroxidation and thereby have the potential to initiate irreversible denaturation of cellular proteins [18, 27, 32]. Of particular importance is the interaction between polymorphonuclear granulocytes (PMN) and the endothelial cells in the microvasculature, first characterized by sticking of marginated leukocytes, which later migrate into the tissue [19]. This reaction is triggered by the complement factor C5a activated by the tissue damage, inflammation, and particularly by endotoxin. C5a in turn stimulates PMN to adhere to the endothelial wall, with subsequent leukostasis and plugging of capillaries and postcapillary venules [2, 33, 34]. As a consequence, the tissue supplied by these microvessels becomes ischemic and damaged.

Shock-Specific Impairment of Microcirculation

Within the vascular bed, the α-receptor-mediated constriction elicited by shock and trauma affects predominantly the precapillary arterioles, but also the postcapillary venules. Constriction of the precapillary resistance vessels results in reduction of the driving pressures, local flow velocities, and the number of perfused capillaries. At the same time, the spontaneous arteriolar vasomotion is suppressed. Loss of arteriolar vasomotion alters the dynamics of the microcirculation dramatically with a special impact on the distribution of microvascular blood flow, fluidity of blood within the microvascular segments, and transcapillary fluid exchange [20]. The microvascular perfusion becomes static and heterogeneous, and the relationship between microvascular flow and the capillary surface area available for exchange of nutrients and metabolites (permeability surface area product) is critically reduced [1]. Since capillary perfusion dissociates into tissue compartments with stagnant flow and complete stasis adjacent to tissue compartments perfused by plasma, the tissue nutrition is compromised and the drainage of cellular metabolites becomes insufficient. Hypoperfusion, hypoxia, and reduction of transcapillary exchange surface cause local accumulation of acid metabolites from anaerobic cell metabolism. The local acidosis alters the responsiveness of the microvascular segments to endogeneous catecholamines in the sense that the precapillary resistance vessels dilate, while the postcapillary venules remain constricted. Since the outflow from the postcapillaries is already severely compromised by the excessive deterioration of blood fluidity (red cell aggregation at low-flow velocity), the net result of the altered microvascular reactivity—shock-specific vasomotion—is forcible shifts of ions, fluid, and macromolecules into the interstitium with further impairment of the flow conditions and flow properties of the blood within these microvessels [28]. By this mechanism, hypoperfusion is aggravated and a viscious circle is established at the level of the microcirculation. The microvessels being occluded for rheological reasons (red cell aggregation) and/or by leukocyte plugging [3] might hinder reperfusion during primary resuscitation; therefore, focal ischemia can persist despite normalization of cardiac output, arterial pressure, and global organ blood flow.

Hyperdynamic Endotoxinemia

As already mentioned, bacteremia, endotoxinemia, and sepsis often precede the development of MOF. It is today well recognized that the initial phase of sepsis and septic shock is characterized by a high-flow state, termed the hyperdynamic circulatory state, which was first described by Waisbren [38]. Only at a later time does the hyperdynamic circulatory state turn into hypodynamic septic shock. The diagnosis of incipient septic shock should no longer rely on the result of bacterial cultures but on the evidence of bacterial endotoxin in the systemic circulation: With the modern assays available [10, 16], endotoxin (lipopolysaccharides) can be detected in peripheral blood long before blood cultures provide positive results. The presence of measurable amounts of endotoxin in the systemic circulation indicates that the clearance capacity of the reticuloendothelial system (RES) has been exhausted and that the endotoxin has started an array of reactions, including the pyrogen reaction, stimulation of the humoral immune response, activation of the coagulation and complement system, and tissue release reactions [29]. Among the latter, the activation of monocytes and macrophages with the release of interleukin-1 and TNF appears to be of particular importance concerning the development of MOF. When endotoxin enters the circulation, it damages the endothelial cell surface and thereby favors the formation of wall-adhering aggregates of platelets and leukocytes. In addition to its effect on the endothelial wall, endotoxin stimulates the generation and release of various compounds which are vasoactive in nature and potentially increase microvascular permeability. One should, therefore, expect severe microvascular disturbances secondary to the exposure to endotoxin during the hyperdynamic phase of septic shock, i.e., when cardiac output is high and total organ blood flow appears normal.

Microcirculatory Failure in Hyperdynamic Endotoxinemia

Our group has recently analyzed the blood flow distribution during acute endotoxinemia. The experimental data were obtained from pigs receiving a con-

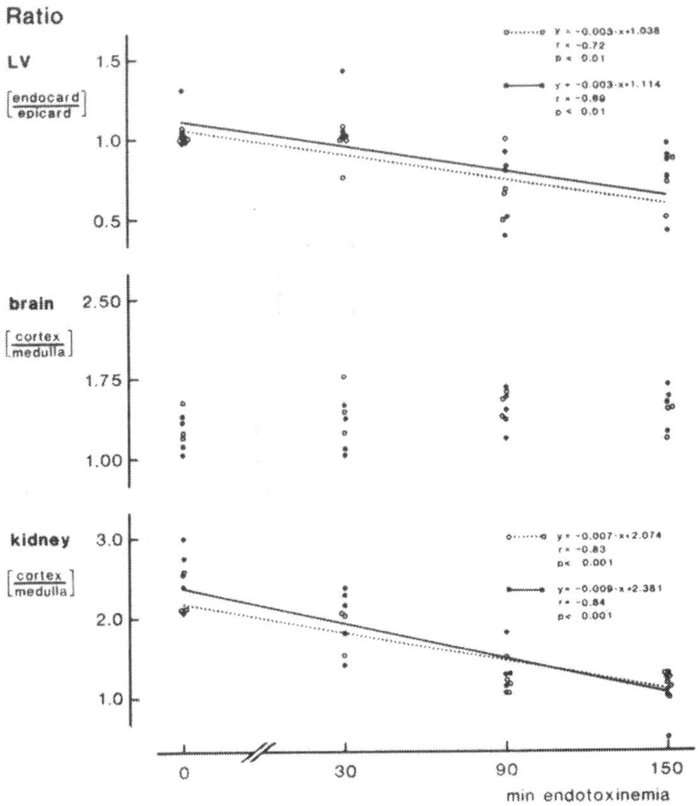

Fig. 1. Hyperdynamic endotoxinemia in the pig: Changes in intraorgan blood flow distribution dependent upon the time of endotoxinemia induced by two different doses of *Salmonella abortus equi* endotoxin (○····○ total dose 3.8 μg/kg b.w., ●—● 13 μg/kg b.w.). It should be noted that the fall of the endo-/epicardial flow ratio in left ventricle (*LV*) and of the cortex/medulla ratio in the kidney occurs in parallel, independent of the total dose of endotoxin administered. After Messmer et al. [29]

tinuous infusion of *Salmonella abortus equi* endotoxin. The analyses included central hemodynamics, lung function, gas exchange, regional organ blood flow (using radioactive-labeled microspheres; 15 μm in diameter), and the concentration of endotoxin in the plasma [23].

The infusion of small doses of endotoxin into the vena cava inferior resulted in hyperdynamic endotoxinemia with high cardiac output and low peripheral resistance. Blood flow to the right ventricle, kidney, cerebral cortex, and skeletal muscle remained in the control range, whereas a temporary fall and recovery of blood flow was observed in the left ventricle, gastric mucosa, small intestine, and pancreas. The only organ presenting a significant and progressive reduction in blood flow was the spleen [23].

Despite only minor changes in global organ blood flow, hyperdynamic endotoxinemia initiated a redistribution of intraorgan blood flow in the heart and

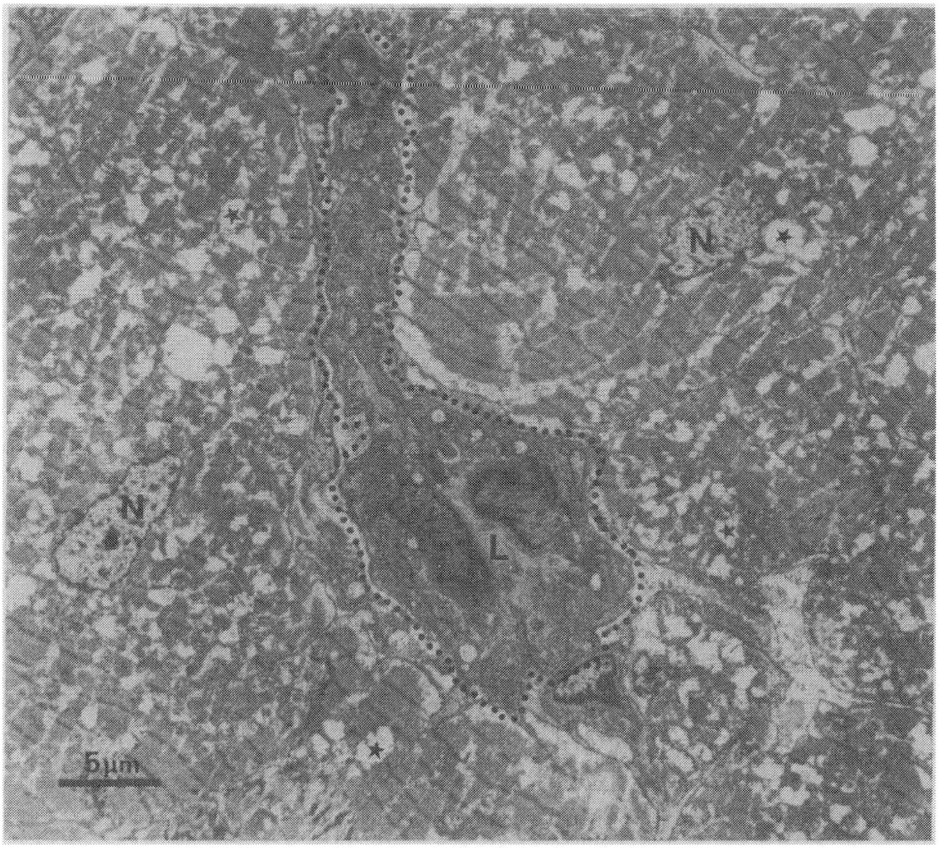

Fig. 2. Hyperdynamic endotoxinemia in the pig: Electron micrograph of midmyocardium showing severe damage to the cardiomyocytes exemplified by the swollen mitochondria, which appear as structureless empty vacuoles (*asterisk*). *Outlined by black dots* is a completely occluded capillary. *N* myocardical nucleus, *L* capillary lumen. × 4000

kidneys. These changes are depicted in Fig. 1, where the endocardial/epicardial flow ratio (left ventricle) and the cortex/medulla flow ratio (kidney) are presented according to the duration of endotoxinemia. Figure 1 reveals a decrease in the endo-/epicardial and the cortex/medulla flow ratio, indicating redistribution of microcirculatory flow in the heart and kidney with underperfusion of the endocardium and renal cortex, respectively. Furthermore, Fig. 1 shows that the redistribution of microvascular flow in the heart and kidney occurs very early, because the different doses (3.8 μg/kg or 13 μg/kg b.w. endotoxin) given during the 150-min observation period yielded similar changes in blood flow ratios. These findings indicate that microvascular perfusion is severely compromised though global blood flow to these organs remained normal. The measurements by means of the microspheres were corroborated by our electron-microscopic findings. The micrographs in Figs. 2 and 3 were derived from the midmyocar-

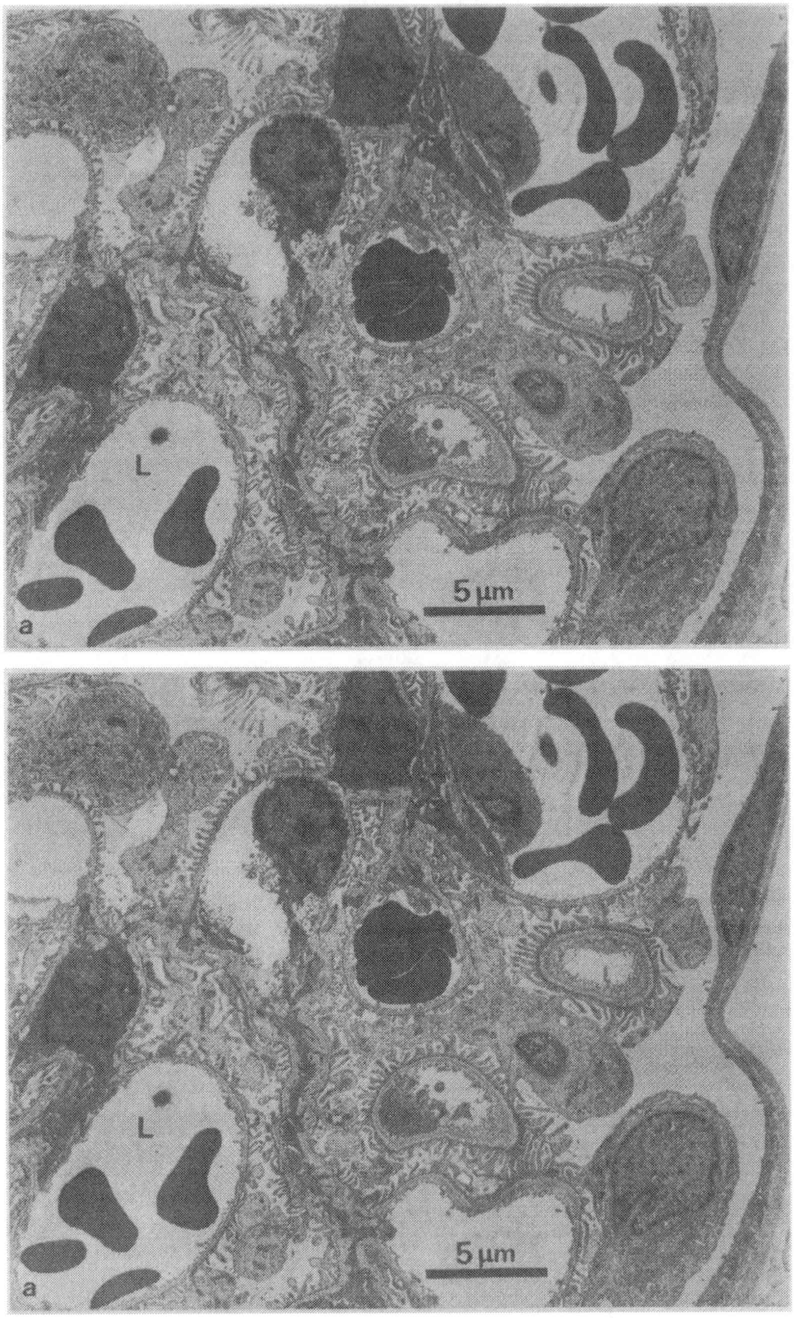

Fig. 3a, b. Hyperdynamic endotoxinemia in the pig: Electron micrographs taken at the same magnification from renal glomeruli of **a** control and **b** experimental animals. Following endotoxin infusion for 80 min, the capillary lumina (*L*) appear dilated and they contain membrane-bound blisters (*asterisks*), varying in size and contents. These structures develop either as vacuoles or blebs within the endothelial cytoplasm, to which they remain connected by delicated stalks (*arrow*) until they are finally pinched off into the lumen. In contrast, the podocytes appear completely normal. × 4500 dium and kidney of a pig with hyperdynamic endotoxinemia; both organs were perfusion fixated in situ with the animal still alive. It should be noted that the section from the midmyocardium (Fig. 2), the total flow of which was still in the normal range, reveals severe damage to the cardiomyocytes and one capillary is completely occluded by endothelial cell swelling and entrapped blood cells, therefore rendering ischemic the myocardial cells downstream from the occlusion. Severe structural alterations were also observed in the capillaries of the kidneys (Fig. 3), which might explain the redistribution of renal blood flow demonstrated by the microspheres measurements.

These new data suggest that focal ischemia is present from the very beginning of endotoxinemia and persists while the disease progresses into sepsis and septic shock, a fact emphasizing in particular the pivotal role of endotoxin in the development of MOF.

Cellular and Humoral Reactions

As already mentioned, tissue damage and endotoxin are potent stimuli to elicit cellular and humoral reactions through the activation of macrophages and monocytes. These cells release cytokines, among them interleukin-1 (IL-1) and tumor necrosis factor (TNF; cachectin). Through interaction with a membrane receptor, IL-1 activates phospholipase A_2 and consequently the arachidonic cascade with the end-products prostaglandins and leukotrienes [14, 17]. Depending upon the amount and ratio of eicosanoids produced [5, 7] and upon the tissue content of monocytes and macrophages, localized constriction, dilatation, blockade of microvascular segments by leukocytes, and increased microvascular permeability are encountered. IL-1 and TNF represent probably the most important mediators impairing organ function after tissue damage, inflammation, and exposure to endotoxin, because both cytokines do not exclusively affect the neutrophils, but concomitantly affect the brain, liver, bone marrow, skeletal muscle, pancreas, and bone joints [14, 39]. Fever, anorexia, uptake of amino-acids by the liver with the release of acute-phase proteins, release of neutrophils from the bone marrow, proteolysis and release of amino-acids from skeletal muscle, insulin release, and activation of fibroblasts with collagen proliferation are all events mediated by IL-1 and are typical for septic patients [39]. The proteolysis factor, demonstrated by Clowes et al. [11] and Loda et al. [24] during infection and septicemia, represents a small molecular fragment of IL-1. Since both cytokines interfere with the function of most the organs, they appear as significant pathogenetic factors contributing to the development of MOF (Fig. 4).

Therapeutic Implications

Persisting microcirculatory failure, focal ischemia, and local reperfusion injury have been cited as factors initiating MOF after primary resuscitation from trauma and shock and also in the initial hypercirculatory state of septic patients. This notion calls for a redirection of the presently used therapeutic means so as to prevent and abolish the microcirculatory defects and, in addition, to cope with the endotoxin liberated from the bacteria.

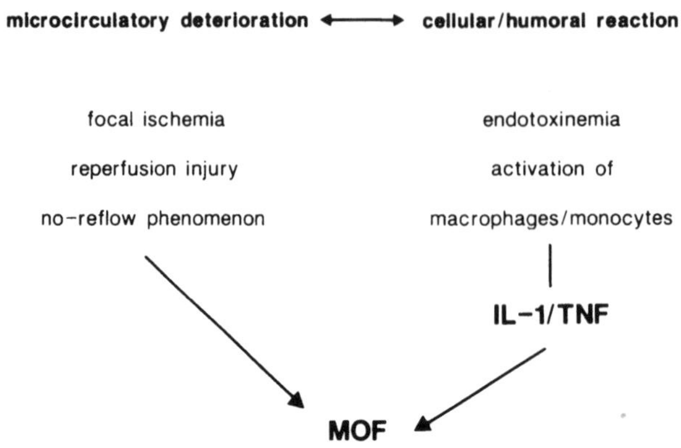

Fig. 4. Pathways into multiple organ failure (*MOF*), propagated by both microcirculatory failure and the cellular and humoral reactions elicited by endotoxin

It has to be realized that primary resuscitation as performed today by the infusion of isooncotic colloid or isotonic crystalloid solutions does not efficiently restore normal microcirculatory flow nor does this volume therapy safely prevent focal microcirculatory defects and tissue lesions. In contrast to these conventional fluids, a strongly hyperosmolar saline solution appears advantageous, because it allows the period the patient is in shock to be reduced and restores the macrohemodynamic parameters, but most importantly it restores the nutritional perfusion of the vital organs.

Hypertonic salt solutions were found to be exceedingly efficient in the treatment of severe hemorrhagic hypotension and refractory hypovolemic shock in animals and man [13, 21, 22, 25, 26, 30]. Intravenous infusion of small volumes (4 ml/kg b.w.) of hyperosmolar solutions (7.2% – 7.5% saline) provoke an instantaneous rise in cardiac output above normal with the release of systemic vasoconstriction. The findings from our most recent studies [22] addressing the effects of hypertonic solution on nutritional blood flow indicate that small-volume resuscitation with hypertonic saline and even more so with hypertonic/hyperoncotic saline/dextran reestablishes both the cardiac output and nutritional blood flow to brain, heart and adrenals within minutes. The new concept of small-volume resuscitation with hyperosmolar/hyperoncotic solutions is presently being explored by various laboratories all over the world. While animal experiments have already demonstrated that these solutions are a safe means of reestablishing normal microcirculatory perfusion, it will be difficult, if not impossible, to prove that with initial restoration of microcirculatory flow and prevention of focal ischemia with its sequelae, a safe prophylaxis from MOF can efficiently be achieved [22].

The second new means of preventing the development of MOF consists of eliminating endotoxin from the systemic circulation. This concept requires first of all that endotoxin be detected in the blood and body fluids at a very early time and, secondly, that techniques are developed to eliminate endotoxin from or inactivate endotoxin within the organism. Inactivation of endotoxin by antibodies, elimination by plasmapheresis, immunoabsorption, and adsorption of

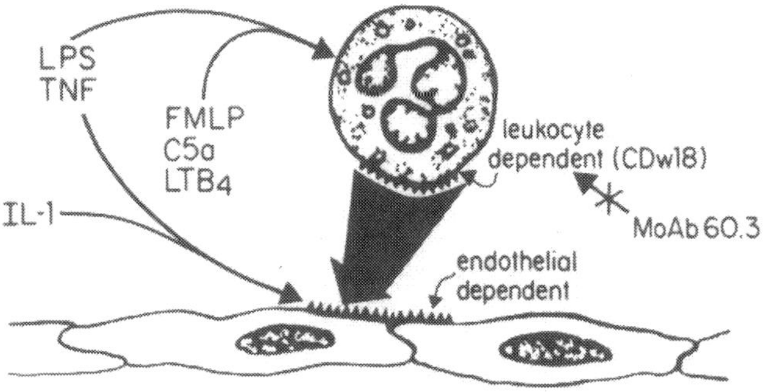

Fig. 5. Leukocyte-endothelium interaction is promoted by two mechanisms: leukocyte dependent and endothelium dependent. Chemotactic factors initiate adherence through the leukocyte-dependent mechanism, which involves the adhesive membrane complex CDw18 and can be blocked by MoAb 60.3. Interleukin-1 (*IL-1*) promotes leukocyte adherence through an endothelium-dependent mechanism. Endotoxin (*LPS*) and tumor necrosis factor (*TNF*) promote leukocyte adherence by both pathways. After Arfors et al. [2]

endotoxin with polymyxin B are modalities presently under investigation [8, 12, 29].

Finally, the PMN should become the target of new therapeutic strategies to prevent temporarily their interaction with the endothelium of the microvessels (Fig. 5). Recent results suggest that this goal might be achieved by means of monoclonal antibodies directed against the leukocyte membrane complex, responsbile for the sticking of the cell to the endothelium [2] or by drugs affecting postischemic PMN-endothelium interaction [35].

References

1. Appelgren KL (1972) Perfusion and diffusion in shock. Acta Physiol Scand Suppl 378: 1
2. Arfors KE, Lundberg C, Lindbom L, Lundberg K, Harlan M (1987) A monoclonal antibody to the membrane glycoprotein complex CDw18 (LFA) inhibits PMN accumulation and plasma leakage in vivo. Prog Appl Microcirc 11: 270
3. Bagge U, Braide M (1985) Microcirculatory effects of white blood cells in shock. Prog Appl Microcirc 7: 43
4. Baker CC (1986) Epidemiology of trauma: the civilian perspective. Ann Emerg Med 15: 1389
5. Ball HA, Cook JA, Wise WC, Halushka PV (1986) Role of thromboxane, prostaglandins and leukotrienes in endotoxic and septic shock. Intensive Care Med 12: 116
6. Baue AE, Chaudry IH (1980) Prevention of multiple systems failure. Surg Clin N Amer 60: 1167
7. Bevilacqua MP, Pober JS, Wheeler ME, Contran RS, Gimbrone MA Jr (1985) Interleukin 1 acts on cultured human vascular endothelium to increase the adhesion of polymorphonuclear leukocytes, monocytes, and related leukocyte cell lines. J Clin Invest 76: 2003
8. Brock-Utne JG (1984) A breakthrough in the therapy of septic shock? South African Med J 65: 149

9. Carrico CJ, Meakins JL, Marshall JC, Fry D, Maier RV (1986) Multiple-organ-failure syndrome. Arch Surg 121: 196
10. Ten Cate JW, Büller HR, Sturk A, Levin J (eds) (1985) Bacterial endotoxins. Structure, biomedical significance, and detection with the limulus amebocyte lysate test. Liss, New York.
11. Clowes CHA Jr, George BC, Villee CA Jr, Saracis CA (1983) Muscle proteolysis induced by a circulating peptide in patients with sepsis or trauma. N Engl J Med 308: 545
12. Cohen J, Aslam M, Pusey CD, Ryan CJ (1987) Protection from endotoxemia: A rat model of plasmapheresis and specific adsorption with polymyxin B. J Infect Dis 155: 690
13. De Felippe J, Timoner J, Velasco IT, Lopes OU, Rocha-e-Silva M (1980) Treatment of refractory hypovolaemic shock by 7.5% sodium chloride injections. Lancet II: 1002
14. Dinarello CA (1984) Interleukin I. Rev Infect Dis 6: 51
15. Fleck A, Colley CM, Myers MA (1985) Liver export proteins and trauma. Brit Med Bull 41: 264
16. Fink PC, Grunert JH (1984) Endotoxinemia in intensive care patients: A longitudinal study with the Limulus Amebocyte Lysate Test. Klin Wschr 62: 986
17. Goldblum SE, Cohen DA, Gillespie MN, McClain CJ (1987) Interleukin-1-induced granuloytopenia and pulmonary leukostasis in rabbits. J Appl Physiol 62: 122
18. Granger DN, Dale A, Höllwarth M (1986) Role of oxygen radicals in ischemic bowel disorders. Pediatr Surg Int 1: 15
19. Hammersen F, Hammersen E (1987) The ultrastructure of endothelial gap formation and leukocyte emigration. Prog Appl Microcirc 12: 1
20. Intaglietta M (1986) The static versus the dynamic state of the microvasculature. In: Schmid-Schönbein GW, Woo SLY, Zweifach, BW (eds) Frontiers in biomechanics. Springer, New York, p 314
21. Kramer GC, Perron PR, Lindsey DC, HO HS, Gunther RA, Boyle WA, Holcroft JW (1986) Small-volume resuscitation with hypertonic saline dextran solution. Surgery 100: 239
22. Kreimeier U, Messmer K (1987) New perspectives in resuscitation and prevention of multiple organ system failure. In: Baethmann A, Messmer K (eds) Surgical research: Recent concepts and results. Springer, Berlin Heidelberg New York Tokyo p 39
23. Kreimeier U, Yang Zh, Messmer K (1987) The role of fluid replacement in acute endotoxin shock. In: Kox W, Bihari D (eds) Septic shock and the adult respiratory distress syndrome. Springer, Berlin Heidelberg New York Tokyo, p 179
24. Loda M, Clowes GHA Jr., Dinarello CA, Georges BC, Lane B, Richardson W (1984) Induction of hepatic protein synthesis by a peptide in blood plasma of patients with sepsis and trauma. Surgery 96: 204
25. Maningas PA, DeGuzman LR, Tillman FJ, Hinson CS, Priegnitz KJ, Volk KA, Bellamy RF (1986) Small-volume infusion of 7.5% NaCl in 6% dextran 70 for the treatment of severe hemorrhagic shock in swine. Ann Emerg Med 15: 1131
26. Mazzoni MC, Arfors KE, Intaglietta M (1987) Compartmental analysis of fluid shift between blood endothelium and interstitium during treatment of hypotensive hemorrhage with hypertonic solutions. In: Tsuchiya M, Asano M, Mishima Y, Oda M (eds) Microcirculation—An update, vol 1. Excerpta Medica, Amsterdam, p 289
27. McCord JM, Fridovich I (1978) The biology and pathology of oxygen radicals. Ann Int Med 89: 122
28. Messmer K (1983) Traumatic shock in polytrauma: circulatory parameters, biochemistry, and resuscitation. World J Surg 7: 26
29. Messmer K, Kreimeier U, Hammersen F (1988) Changes in the microcirculation in sepsis and septic shock. In: Reinhart K, Eyrich K (eds) Sepsis—An interdisciplinary Challenge. Springer, Berlin Heidelberg New York Tokyo
30. Nakayama S, Sibley L, Gunther RA, Holcroft JW, Kramer GC (1984) Small-volume

resuscitation with hypertonic saline (2.400 mosm/liter) during hemorrhagic shock. Circ Shock 13: 149
31. Nuytinck JKS, Goris RJA, Redl H, Schlag G, van Munster PJJ (1986) Posttraumatic complications and inflammatory mediators. Arch Surg 121: 886
32. Parks DA, Bulkley GB, Granger DN (1983) Role of oxygen free radicals in shock, ischemia and organ preservation. Surgery 94: 428
33. Redl H, Schlag G, Hammerschmidt DE (1984) Quantitative assessment of leukostasis in experimental hypovolemic-traumatic shock. Acta Chir Scand 150: 113
34. Sack FU, Funk W, Hammersen F, Messmer K (1987) Microvascular injury of skeletal muscle and skin after different periods of pressure induced ischemia. Prog Appl Microcirc 12: 282
35. Sack FU, Zeintl H, Menger MD, Hammersen F, Messmer K (1988) In-vivo quantification of postischemic PMN-endothelium-interaction in skeletal muscle and the influence of Bufedil. Circ Shock 24: 202
36. Thijs LG, Groeneveld ABJ (1987) The circulatory defect of septic shock. In: Vincent JL, Thijs LG (eds) Septic shock. Springer, Berlin Heidelberg New York Tokyo p 161
37. Trunkey DD (1983) Trauma. Sci Amer 149: 20
38. Waisbren BA (1964) Gram-negative shock and endotoxin shock (editorial). Am J Med 36: 819
39. Yurt RW (1984) Intermediary metabolism including mediator activation. In: Shires GT (ed) Shock and related Problems. Churchill Livingston, Edinburgh, p 111

Chapter 3
Gastroenterological Disorders

Structural Alterations of Mucosal Microvascular System in Human Chronic Gastritis

Yasunari Tsuchihashi[1], Toshio Tani[1], Kyohei Maruyama[1], Shozo Yorioka[1], Katsuhiro Okada[2], Hiromasa Sudo[2], Tsukasa Ashihara[1], Setsuya Fujita[1], and Keiichi Kawai[2]

Chronic gastritis is an important pathological condition of the gastric mucosa because the disease is thought to develop a predisposition to other gastric diseases [1], including, most seriously, gastric carcinomas [2, 3]. Although a large amount of information concerning glandular epithelial changes of the stomach in chronic gastritis has accumulated [4], our knowledge of vascular stromal changes in the diseased condition is surprisingly limited. Since glandular epithelial components and their surrounding vascular stroma have been shown to be structurally and functionally closely related to each other in the normal gastric mucosa [5], it is clearly important to study vascular stromal changes in chronic gastritis where diverse alterations of structures and cellular differentiations of the gastric glands are observed [4].

Since the study of Arnold [6], the anatomy of the vascular system of the stomach has been extensively studied using microdissections and dye-injection. Recently, soft X-ray microangiography [7] and scanning electron microscopy on resin molds of blood vessels [8] have been introduced to investigate the gastric vascular architecture, but these modern techniques have added very little information to the results of the classic studies of Mall [9].

It is worth mentioning here that in the studies mentioned above, little attention was paid to dynamic alterations of the mucosal vascular structure of stomachs more or less affected by chronic gastritis. More recently, Tabata used microangiographic techniques to study the structural alterations of the mucosal vascular system in chronic gastritis [10]. He succeeded to some extent in outlining the basic alterations of the vascular architecture; however, detailed structural relations between each remodeled, altered gland and changes in its surrounding vascular stroma were not determined, owing chiefly to the potential difficulties in adequate filling of all the microvessels with a contrast medium and the insufficient resolutional powers of the method. Tabata described dilatation of the superficial mucosal vessels in superficial gastritis, elongation and increase in the number of foveolar vessels in both hypertrophic and atrophic hyperplastic gastritis, and shortening and sparseness of the mucosal vessels in atrophic gastritis.

Department of Pathology[1] and Department of Preventive Medicine[2], Kyoto Prefectural University of Medicine, Kawaramachi Hirokoji, Kamigyo-ku, Kyoto, 602 Japan

To make possible detailed comparative histological studies between the structure of altered gastric glands and their surrounding vascular stroma in human chronic gastritis, we developed a method of local organ perfusion with India ink gelatin [11, 12]. The principle and practice of the method are virtually the same as those we used in experimental animals [5]. To avoid artificial dilatation or insufficient filling of mucosal microvessels, special care was taken to keep the perfusion pressures of both the arterial and venous sides within the physiological range. Surgically resected human stomachs bearing tumors received the perfusion, and the background mucosal areas affected by chronic gastritis were histologically examined using thick-sectioned microvascular preparations with a nuclear fast red stain; the adjacent thin sections were stained with hematoxylin-eosin or special mucin stains.

In the following, we describe our results on the characteristics of mucosal microvascular structures in chronic gastritis according to the currently used morphological classification of the diseased condition, i.e., chronic superficial gastritis, chronic atrophic gastritis, and gastric atrophy [13]. Since the changes are best appreciated in comparison with the normal condition, we describe first the structural characteristics of the vascular system of the nearly normal stomach. Presentation of images of a completely normal stomach was not possible with our material since the mucosae of tumor-bearing stomachs are generally quite diffusely affected by chronic gastritis [2].

Vascular Structure of Normal or Nearly Normal Gastric Mucosae

The normal or nearly normal gastric mucosa has a dense microvascular network with a remarkable structural regularity, being uniform horizontally and transitional vertically to the mucosal surface (Figs. 1, 2). According to the differences in density and the patterns of the mucosal microvessels, three distinct vascular zones that are horizontal to the mucosal surface can be distinguished in both the fundic and pyloric mucosae. The first is the proximal vascular zone of comparatively high vascularity (zone I), which spatially corresponds to the glandular portion of the gastric glands. The second is the middle vascular zone of decreasing vascularity (zone II), which spatially corresponds to the lower tubular portion of the gastric glands. The third is the distal vascular zone of increasing vascularity (zone III), which spatially corresponds to the upper tubular or superficial foveolae of the gastric glands. In the fundic mucosa, ascending mucosal capillaries arising from the muscularis mucosae form extensively anastomosing networks, which surround the glandular portion of each gastric gland, thus constituting the first vascular zone (zone I; Fig. 1). The density of the capillaries is much higher at the mucosal level, which corresponds to the upper half of the glandular portion of a gland, where the parietal cells are predominantly distributed, than at the lower half, where mainly the chief cells are distributed. This difference in vascular density merits subdivision of the first vascular zone into two parts—the lower half (zone Ia) and upper half (zone Ib). Specialization of zone Ib is considered to afford stromal support to the active secretory function of parietal cells and this is thought to require a large amount of fluid movement from the capillaries to the lumina of glands [14]. At the mucosal level, being

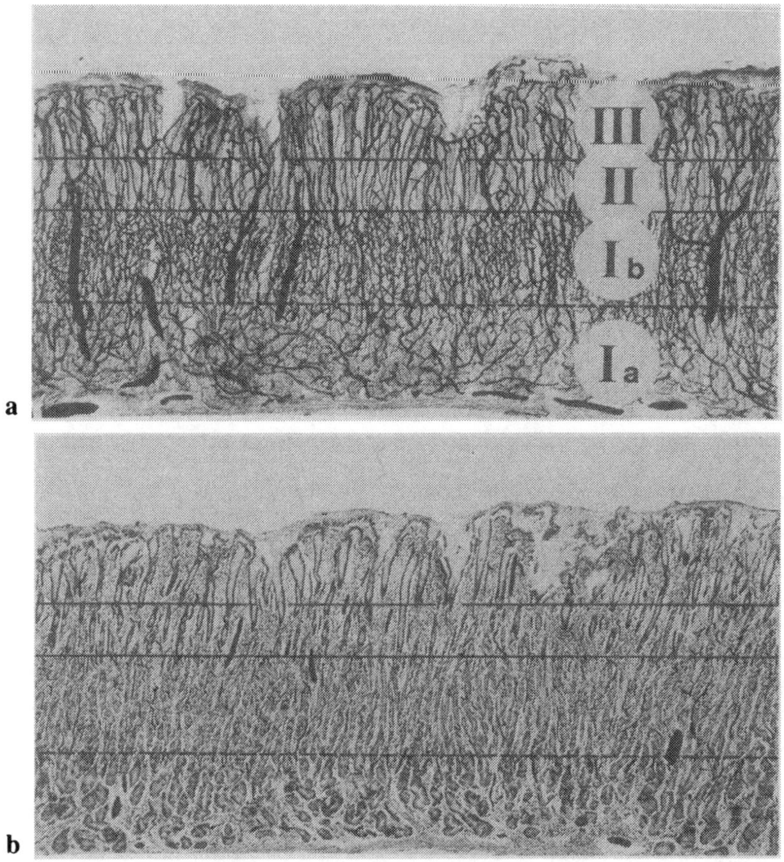

Fig. 1a, b. A microvascular preparation of nearly normal fundic mucosa stained with **a** nuclear fast red and **b** its adjacent thin section stained with H and E. Ascending mucosal capillaries form a dense anastomosing networks around each gastric gland. According to the density and patterns of the ascending mucosal capillaries, three vascular zones horizontal to the mucosal surface are identified—*I*, *II* and *III*. Zone *I* can be further divided into two parts—*Ia* and *Ib*. Zone *Ib* shows the highest density and corresponds to the mucosal level of an extensive parietal cell distribution

transitional from the glandular to the tubular portion of a gland, the ascending mucosal capillaries decrease quite suddenly in number and the vascular zone II is formed. This zone corresponds to the mucosal level, where the generative cells are present. Toward the mucosal surface, the ascending mucosal capillaries gradually increase in number and, apparently, in diameter. The capillaries merge into surface venular meshes. The uppermost part of the ascending mucosal capillaries together with the surface venular meshes constitute the third vascular zone (zone III). The surface venular meshes coalesce to form collecting venules, which run straight or oblique back toward the muscularis mucosa, with or without a few mutual junctions, and finally merge into the submucosal venous plexus.

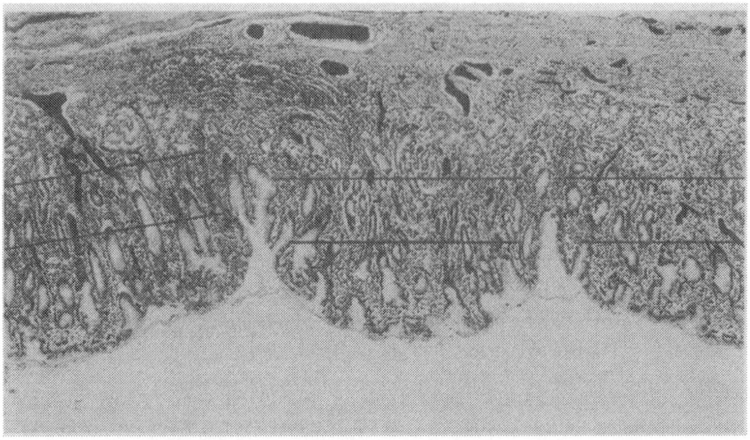

a

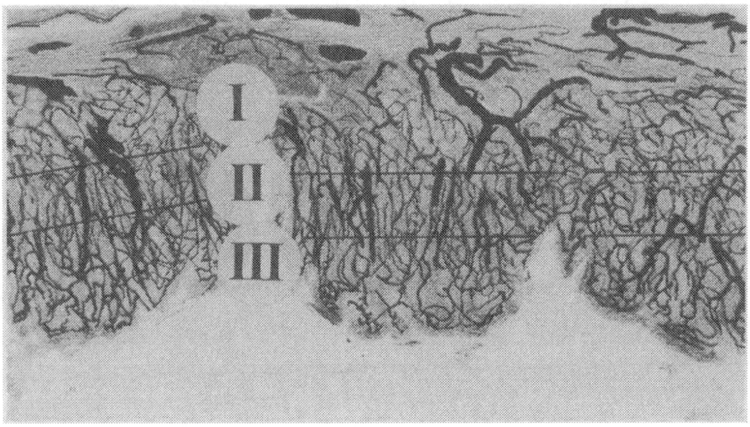

b

Fig. 2a, b. A microvascular preparation of relatively normal pyloric mucosa stained with **a** nuclear fast red and **b** its adjacent thin section stained with H and E. Three vascular zones can be identified as in the fundic mucosa. However, the vascular density is uniformly high in zone *I* and subdivision of this zone into two parts is not present. The proportion of zone *I* to zones *II* and *III* is lower in the pyloric than in fundic mucosae

In the pyloric mucosa, the microvascular structures are different to those in the fundic mucosa in several aspects (Fig. 2). The ascending mucosal capillaries form mutually anastomosing networks surrounding the glandular portion of each pyloric gland and constitute the first vascular zone (zone I) as in the fundic mucosa. Their density, however, is quite uniformly high and the subdivision of zone I into two parts is not present here. At the mucosal level, being transitional from the glandular to the tubular portion of a gland, the vascular density decreases and the vascular zone II is formed as in the fundic mucosa. Toward the mucosal surface, the vascular structures corresponding to the superficial mucosa, zone III, are expanded in accordance with the extension of foveolae in the pyloric mucosa. Collecting venules tend to run more obliquely and to have more mutual junctions within the mucosa than those of the fundic mucosa.

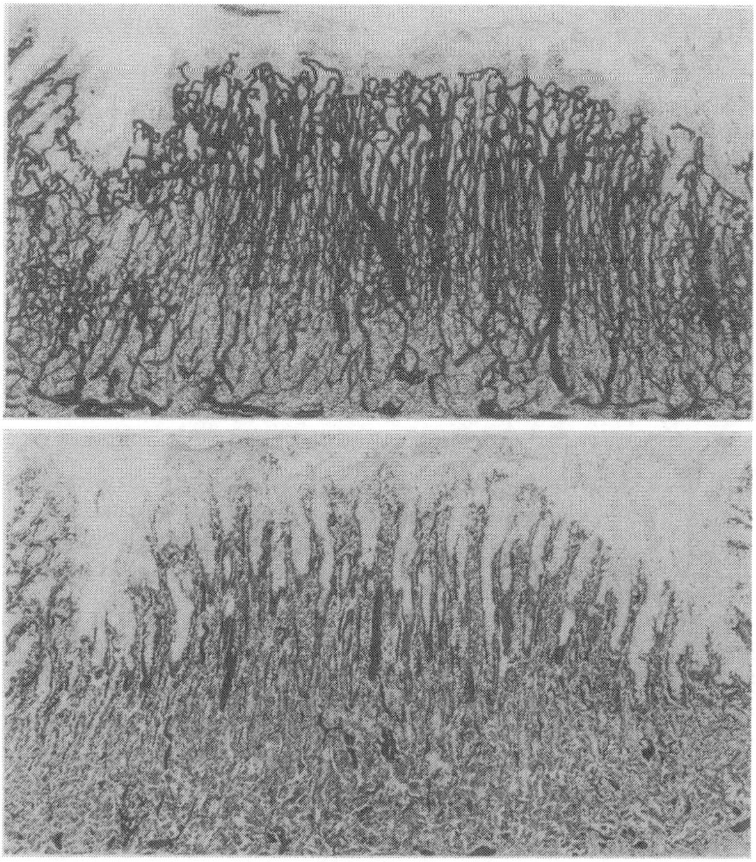

a

b

Fig. 3a, b. A microvascular preparation of the fundic mucosa affected by chronic superficial gastritis stained with **a** nuclear fast red and **b** its adjacent thin section stained with H and E. There is an expansion of zone *II* and *III* although zone *I* is relatively unchanged

Chronic Superficial Gastritis

In chronic superficial gastritis, the second and third vascular zones are expanded in contrast to a slight shortening of the first vascular zone (Fig. 3). These changes occur in accordance with elongation of the tubular portion and slight shortening of the glandular portion of the gastric glands. The third vascular zone often shows an increase in vascular density. Thick tortuous microvessels are seen just beneath the hyperplastic foveolar epithelium. The border between the second and third vascular zones becomes somewhat indistinct due to an increase in the diameters of most capillaries in these two zones. In the first vascular zone, particularly in its lower half (Ia), the vascular density appears slightly decreased. However, the high vascular density at the upper half of the first vascular zone (Ib) is well preserved and the distinction between zones Ia and Ib is still clear. These vascular structures are seen in accordance with the preservation of parietal cells and chief cells in chronic superficial gastritis.

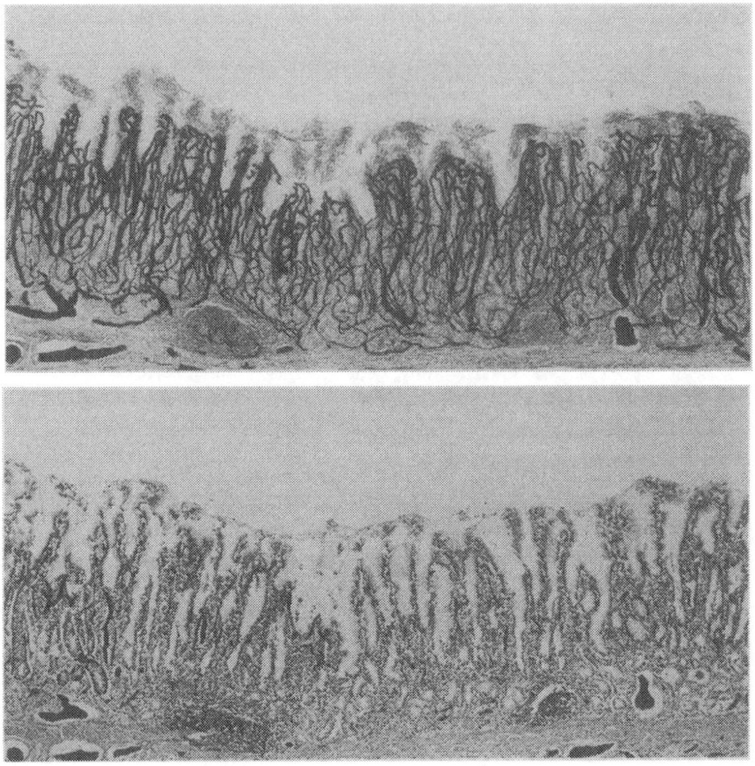

a

b

Fig. 4a, b. A microvascular preparation of the fundic mucosa affected by chronic atrophic gastritis stained with **a** nuclear fast red and **b** its adjacent thin section stained with H and E. There is a progressive shrinkage and rarefaction of the vascular system in zone *I*. These changes accompany a loss of parietal and chief cells and the appearance of mucous cells in the glands (pseudopyloric metaplasia). Zones *II* and *III* are irregularly expanded and the distinction between them is not clear. Intestinal metaplasia is occasionally developed where the mucosa has a somewhat villous surface and a dense subepithelial capillary network similar to the vascular structure of small intestinal villi develops

Chronic Atrophic Gastritis

In chronic atrophic gastritis, the first vascular zone is markedly shortened in contrast to the elongation of the second and the third vascular zones (Fig. 4). These changes are seen in accordance with the progressive atrophy of the glandular portion, elongation of the tubular portion, and hyperplasia of the foveolar epithelium of the gastric glands. The vascular density of the first vascular zone is focally or diffusely decreased. In the upper half of the first vascular zone, i.e., zone Ib, where the vascular density was originally particularly high and parietal cells were originally predominently distributed, the vascular density progressively decreases. As a result, the vascular density of zone I of the fundic mucosa is quite uniformly low and appear less dense than that of the the normal pyloric mucosa. The distinction between zones Ia and Ib is now virtually lost. These changes in the vascular pattern are seen in spatial accordance with such epithelial changes as a progressive loss of parietal cells and the appearance of pseudopyloric metaplasia in the atrophic glandular portion of the gastric glands. The basic patterns of the second and third vascular zones are similar to those seen in chronic superficial gastritis, but the vascular density is often irregularly decreased where the glandular density is decreased. Collecting venules tend to run more obliquely and have more mutual junctions than in normal mucosae. In the areas of intestinal metaplasia, the first vascular zone virtually disappears and the second and third vascular zones are markedly distended. In the focal areas of metaplastic intestinalized mucosa with a villous surface, the third vascular zone consists of a densely anastomosing subepithelial capillary network that resembles the vascular patterns of the small intestinal villi.

Gastric Atrophy

In gastric atrophy mucosa is thin, usually has quite a smooth surface, and contains sparsely distributed metaplastic intestinalized glands. The vascular density of all three vascular zones is markedly decreased and the first vascular zone virtually disappears (Fig. 5). Sparsely distributed ascending mucosal capillaries form a structure that resembles the vascular structure of colonic mucosa.

Changes in Mucosal Microvascular Structure and Significance in Gastric Disease

It was found that in the progression of chronic gastritis, a progressive decrease in the vascular density occurs at the mucosal level of the glandular portion of the gastric glands (zone I). This means that chronic gastritis causes a progressive deprivation of vascular stromal support to the secretory gastric functions and leads to a progressive loss of parietal and chief cells in the fundic mucosa. Mucous neck cells intercalated amongst the parietal cells appear more resistant to the rarefaction of vascular stroma than parietal cells. They are persistent and proliferate in situ [15] to form a pseudopyloric metaplasia. Achlorhydria or hypochlorhydria in chronic gastritis could be partly explained by a decreased vascular stromal support in zone I as well as by a decrease or loss of parietal cells. The rarefaction of vascular stroma in zone I may also cause impairment of the secretory function of the pyloric or pseudopyloric glands, leading to decreased mucosal defense [13] and a predisposition to peptic ulcer diseases. In the areas of pseudopyloric metaplasia, the rarefaction of the vascular stroma is generally more marked than in the pyloric mucosa proper, possibly forming a locus minoris resistentiae. This could partly explain the tendency for gastric ulcers to be found in the transitional zone, where extensive pseudopyloric metaplasia occurs. In chronic atrophic gastritis, the vascular zones II and III are expanded and the border between them becomes somewhat indistinct. These changes are found to correspond spatially to elongation of the foveolae and to an expanded distribution of the generative cells [16]. The changes would cause in-

a

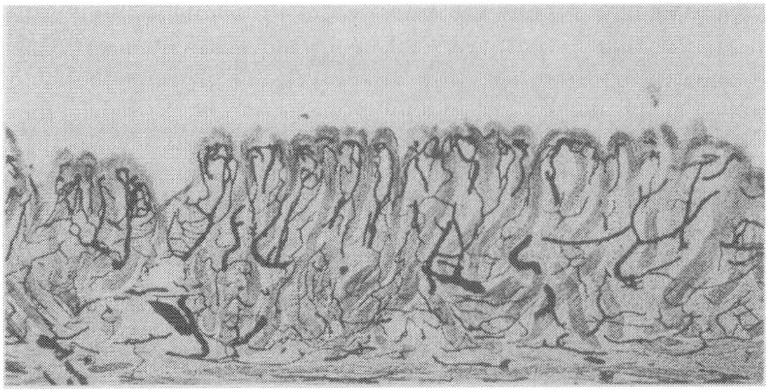

b

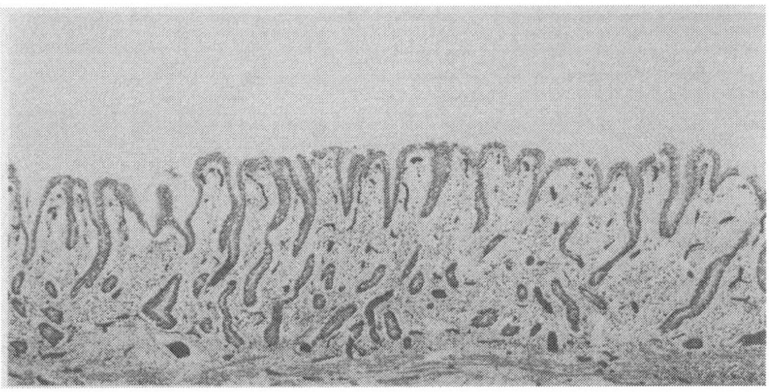

Fig. 5a, b. A microvascular preparation of the corpus mucosa showing gastric atrophy stained with **a** nuclear fast red and **b** its adjacent thin section stained with H and E. Vascular density is markedly decreased in every level of the mucosa. Zone *I* virtually disappears. The rarefied zones *II* and *III* show a vascular structure similar to that of the normal colon. The mucosa is markedly atrophic and has quite a smooth surface. Sparsely distributed intestinal type glands are seen

creased accessibility of various extrinsic factors in the gastric luminal contents to the generative cells, including carcinogen target cells. Since most of the carcinogenic influences come from the gastric lumen, these changes could constitute a predisposition to gastric carcinomas.

Conclusion

In chronic gastritis, profound structural changes of the mucosal microvascular structures occur. They involve a progressive shrinkage and rarefaction of the vascular stroma in zone I and extension of zones II and III. These changes are coupled with pseudopyloric and intestinal metaplasias and the development of a predisposition to peptic ulcer disease. The changes in zones II and III are coupled with extension of the foveolae and expanded distribution of the generative cells, which may eventually constitute a predisposition to gastric carcinomas.

Consideration of these basic alterations of the mucosal microvascular structures is essential for any physiological and pathological research into the gastric microcirculation.

Acknowledgments. The authors are grateful to Drs. S. Takahashi, T. Usui, and H. Sakabe and other members of staff of the Department of Surgery, Kuramaguchi Hospital, Kyoto, Japan for their kind help in our research. This work was supported in part by a Grant-in-Aid from the Ministry of Education, Science and Culture, Japan.

References

1. Gear MWL, Truelove SC, Whitehead R (1971) Gastric ulcer and gastritis. Gut 12: 639–645
2. Imai T, Kubo T, Watanabe H (1971) Chronic gastritis in Japanese with reference to high incidence of gastric carcinoma. J Natl Cancer Inst 47: 179–195
3. Sipponen P, Kekki M, Siurala M (1983) Atrophic chronic gastritis and intestinal metaplasia in gastric cacinoma. Cancer 52: 1062–1068
4. Morson BC (1978) The stomach. In: Symmers WSC (ed) Systemic pathology, 2nd edn. Churchill, Edinburgh, pp 1010–1052
5. Tsuchihashi, Y (1983) Studies on structure and function of the mucosal microvascular system of the gastrointestinal tract with special references to their relations to epithelial functions. J Kyoto Pref Univ Med 92: 59–81
6. Arnold (1847) Handbuch der Anatomie des Menschen, Vol II, Part I. Herder, Freiburg, pp 74–78
7. McAlister WH, Margulis AR, Heinbecker P, Spjut H (1962) Arteriography and microangiography of gastric and colonic lesions. Radiology 79: 769–782
8. Murakami T (1971) Application of the scanning electron microscope to the study of the fine distribution of the blood vessels. Arch Histol Jpn 32: 445–454
9. Mall F (1896) The vessels and walls of the dog's stomach. Johns Hopkins Hosp. Rep. 1: 1–36
10. Tabata T (1976) A microangiographic study on the vascular structures of chronic gastritis. Gastroenterol Endoscopy 18: 527–541
11. Tsuchihashi Y, Ashihara T, Fujita S (1984) Microvascular structures of the metaplastic human gastric mucosa. In: Seno S, Okada Y (eds) International cell biology. Academic, Japan, p 425
12. Fujita S, Sugihara H, Ito R, Tsuchihashi Y (1984) Biology of cancer cell-stroma interaction in carcinogenesis and cancer progression. Jpn J Cancer Chemother 11: 644–661
13. Robbins SL, Cotran RS, Kumar V (1984) Pathologic basis of disease, 3rd edn. Saunders, Philadelphia, pp 809–820
14. Guyton AC (1981) Textbook of medical physiology, 6th edn. Saunders, Philadelphia, pp 801–815
15. Yorioka S, Maruyama K, Kodama T, Takino T, Tsuchihashi Y (1986) Studies on experimental gastric mucosal atrophy: cell kinetic studies of mucosal lesions in rats induced by a single per os administration of acetic acid. In: Tsuchiya M (ed) Cytoprotection and cytobiology, 3rd edn. Excerpta Medica, Tokyo, pp 286–294
16. Tsuchihashi Y, Yorioka S, Tani T, Maruyama K, Ashihara T, Fujita S (1984) Studies on the stromal changes of the atrophic gastric mucosa with a special reference to the genesis of cancers, IX. Generative cell zone and vascular stroma in atrohic human gastric mucosa. Jpn J Cancer Res Gann (proc.) 43: 357

Chemical Mediators in Ethanol-Induced Increased Jejunal Microvascular Permeability

IVAN T. BECK, P.K. DINDA, DESMOND J. LEDDIN, MONICA RAY, IGOR PROKOPIW, and APRIL BOYD[1]

Introduction

The intraluminal ethanol concentration in the jejunum of man varies between 2% and 9% w/v [1] in the course of moderate drinking. This concentration is 15–100 times higher than that which occurs in the blood (0.08%–0.15%) during mild inebriation. Ethanol is transferred across the epithelial layer of the jejunum by simple diffusion [2]. The capillaries and postcapillary venules of the jejunal villus lie in close proximity to the epithelium. They are separated from the lumen only by a sheet of epithelial cells, the basal lamina of the villous core, and a very thin and loose connective tissue layer. Because of this, ethanol can reach the microvessels in high concentrations and could initiate microvascular damage.

We have, indeed, demonstrated in the past that 6% w/v intraluminal ethanol increased arterial blood flow [3–5] and caused capillary congestion [4] and mucosal hemoconcentration [5]. There was also increased capillary permeability due to a temporary retraction of endothelial cells and opening of interendothelial gap junctions in the jejunal mucosa [6]. These events were accompanied by an increase in plasma protein loss into the lumen [5]. An increase in capillary pressure, capillary surface area, and intraluminal protein loss was also demonstrated by Kvietys et al. [7].

All the above-described events are reminiscent of the early phase of inflammation. Furthermore, the electron-microscopic changes of the microvessels during ethanol infusion [6] resemble those reported to occur in other organs during the early phase of inflammation, or the infusion of histamine and other mediators [8–11]. In view of this, we initiated a series of studies to assess whether mediators of the early (vascular) phase of inflammation are involved in the ethanol-induced microvascular damage.

[1]The Gastrointestinal Diseases Research Unit, Department of Medicine and Department of Physiology, Queen's University, Hotel Dieu Hospital, Kingston, Ontario, K7L 5G2, Canada

General Methods

Experiments were carried out using either rabbits or dogs. All animals were anesthetized with sodium pentobarbital. Intraluminal plasma protein loss (in rabbits) or plasma albumin loss (in dogs) was taken as a measure of the microvascular damage. Intraluminal protein (albumin) loss was determined by measuring the clearance of intravenously injected ^{51}Cr- or ^{125}I-labeled autologous or bovine serum albumin into the lumen of the jejunum [5]. In all experiments (irrespective whether they were carried out on rabbits or dogs), two adjacent segments of the upper jejunum (just distal to the ligament of Treitz) were prepared. One of these (control segment) was perfused with Krebs-Ringer bicarbonate solution containing 10 m*M* glucose (KRBSG) and the other (ethanol-perfused segment) with KRBSG containing 6% w/v ethanol (KRBSGE). The perfusion lasted for 90 min, and the intraluminal protein or albumin loss was assessed in the effluent collected sequentially from each segment during 10-min periods over the 90-min perfusion.

Experiments and Results

The time-course of protein loss by the two segments (control and ethanol perfused) in normal anesthetized rabbits and dogs is shown in Fig. 1. In all our experiments, protein (albumin) loss in the control segment of normal animals of both species was low and remained stable throughout the 90-min perfusion period. In contrast, not only was the protein loss higher in the ethanol-perfused segments, but in both species the amount lost varied considerably among the 10-min collection periods. In rabbits, protein loss increased for up to 30–40 min and then declined in spite of continued ethanol perfusion. In dogs, the albumin

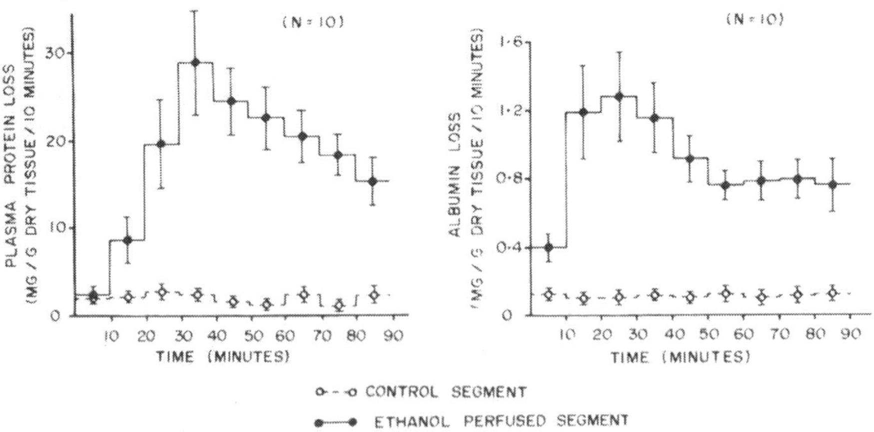

Fig. 1. Time-course of ethanol-induced intraluminal protein loss in control groups. Note that the ethanol-induced increase in protein loss peaked at 30–40 min in rabbits (*left panel*), but at 20–30 min in dogs (*right*). Values are given as means ± SEM

loss peaked at between 20 and 30 min. However, except for differences in the timing of the peak and the magnitude of the protein loss (rabbits lost more than dogs), the shape of the curves depicting the time-related changes were similar in the two species.

Involvement of Histamine in Ethanol-Induced Microvascular Damage

Two series of experiments were carried out. In the first series, two groups of rabbits were used. One group was "untreated" and received intravenous saline only; the other group—"histamine $H_1 + H_2$ receptor blocked"—received cimetidine (40 mg/kg as an i.v. bolus followed by 3.5 mg/kg/h i.v. infusion) plus promethazine (1.5 mg/kg i.v. bolus followed by 2.5 mg/kg/h i.v. infusion). We established that these doses of promethazine and cimetidine fully suppressed the dermal wheal-flare reaction and pentagastrin-stimulated acid secretion.

The results of the cumulative 90-min protein loss are shown in the left panel of Fig. 2. We found that the combination of $H_1 + H_2$ receptor blockade significantly depressed the ethanol-induced intraluminal protein loss. This finding is in keeping with the hypothesis that histamine plays a role in ethanol-induced microvascular damage. Three questions, however, remained unanswered in this study: (a) Are the effects of cimetidine and promethazine due to their antihistamine effects or to some other nonspecific pharmacological effect? (b) Are the results reproducible in other species? (c) Which of the histamine receptors (H_1 or H_2) plays a role in the ethanol-induced microvascular effects? To answer these questions, we repeated the above-described experiments with the following modifications: *Firstly*, a different set of histamine-receptor antagonists was

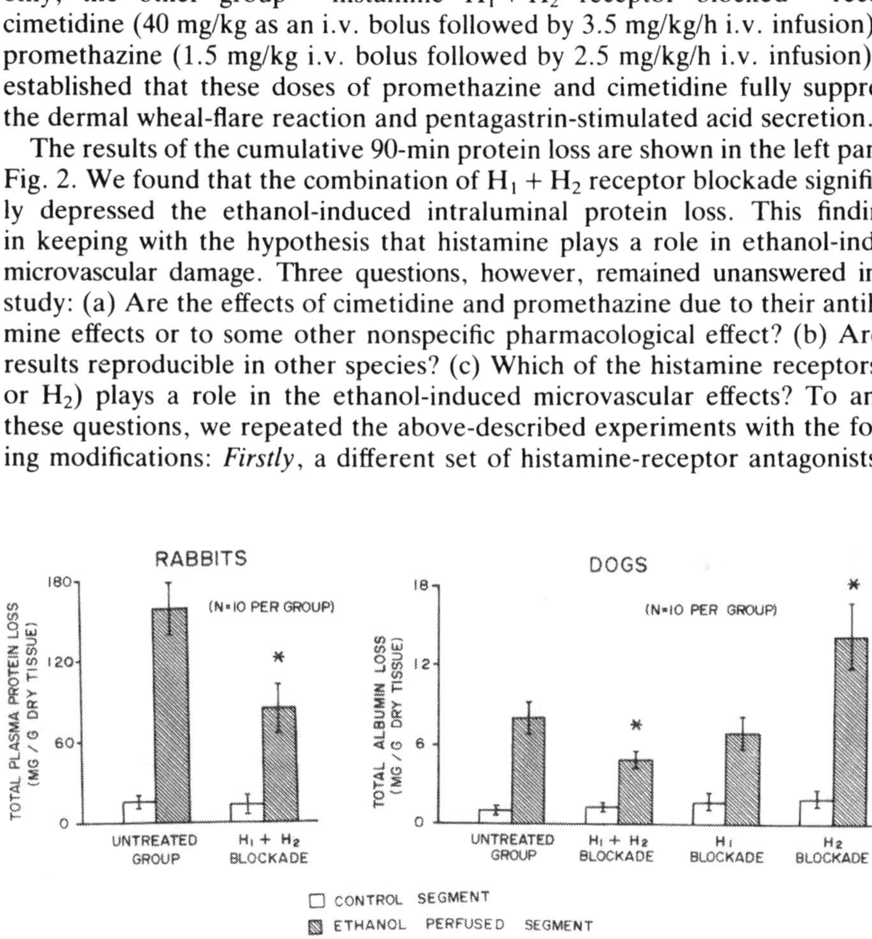

Fig. 2. Effect of histamine receptor antagonists on the ethanol-induced cumulative protein loss over the 90-min perfusion period. Combined $H_1 + H_2$ blockade in the rabbit (cimetidine and promethazine) and in the dog (ranitidine and chlorpheniramine) significantly reduced the protein loss induced by ethanol as compared with the untreated controls. In the dog, H_1 blockade (chlorpheniramine) alone was without significant effect and H_2 blockade (ranitidine) significantly increased ethanol-induced albumin loss. Values are given as means ± SEM. *Asterisks* denote that the value is significantly lower than the ethanol-perfused segments of the untreated group

used—chlorpheniramine (17 mg/kg infused over 90 min) for H_1, and ranitidine (12 mg/kg infused over 90 min) for H_2 blockade. *Secondly*, the experiments were carried out on dogs rather than rabbits. *Thirdly*, four groups were studied: untreated (no histamine blockade), H_1 plus H_2 receptor blocked (a combination of chlorpheniramine plus ranitidine), H_1 blocked (chlorpheniramine only), and H_2 blocked (ranitidine only). Again, in each animal the control jejunal segment was perfused with KRBSG, and the experimental segment with KRBSGE.

As shown on the right of Fig. 2, combined H_1 plus H_2 blockade significantly ($P < 0.05$) decreased the ethanol-induced albumin loss. H_1 blockade alone diminished albumin loss, but this was not statistically significant. Interestingly, H_2 blockade alone increased ablumin loss, both in the control- and the ethanol-perfused segments. In view of the significant decrease in albumin loss with the combination of ranitidine and chlorpheniramine, one can conclude that the inhibition of protein loss in rabbits by combined cimetidine and promethazine treatment was related to the specific antihistamine effects of these drugs. Furthermore, the involvement of histamine in the ethanol-induced miscrovascular damage is not species dependent, and neither H_1 nor H_2 blackade alone protects against the ethanol-induced microvascular injury. Blockade of H_2 receptors alone appears to accentuate the ethanol-induced injury. The elucidation of the cause of this merits further investigation.

Involvement of Arachidonic Acid Metabolites in Ethanol-Induced Microvascular Damage

Since complete blockade of H_1 plus H_2 receptors caused only 50% protection against the ethanol-induced increased protein loss, we postulated that other mediators, including the products of arachidonic acid metabolism, may also be involved in the process. The principal enzymes involved in the catabolism of arachidonic acid are cyclooxygenase and 5-lipoxygenase. The products of cyclooxygenase are the endoperoxidases (prostacyclins, prostaglandins, and the thromboxanes), while the products of 5-lipoxygenase are the derivatives of 5HPETE (leukotrienes B_4, C_4, D_4, and E_4) [12]. Similar to histamine, the leukotrienes (LT) have been reported (especially C_4, D_4, and E_4) to increase the permeability of capillaries and postcapillary venules. In contrast, prostaglandin E_2 is known to protect against microvascular injury caused by various noxious agents in the stomach [13].

Effect of inhibition of 5-lipoxygenase activity. In this study, we investigated whether the products of 5-lipoxygenase were involved in the jejunal microvascular injury induced by intraluminal ethanol. The experimental setup was similar to that of our $H_1 + H_2$ studies in the rabbit. A group of rabbits was given a selective inhibitor of 5-lipoxygenase (4-bromo-2, 7-dimethoxy-3H-phenothiazine-3-one — L-651, 392–Merck Frosst Canada Inc.) [14]. The drug was administered orally in two doses of 10 mg/kg, given 24 and 2 h prior to the experiment (treated group). A second group was "untreated." In each animal of both groups, one jejunal segment served as the control segment and an adjacent one as the ethanol-perfused segment. In the untreated group, leukotriene B_4

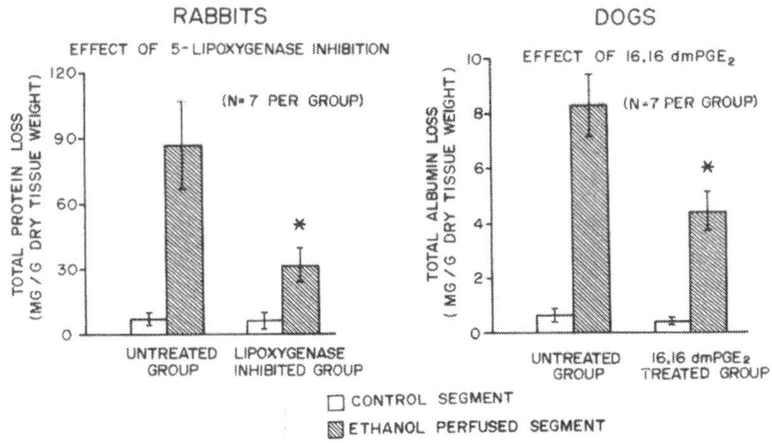

Fig. 3. *Left panel* shows the effect of 5-lipoxygenase inhibition (L-651, 392) on the ethanol-induced protein loss in the rabbit. *Right panel* depicts the effect of 16, 16 dmPGE$_2$ treatment in the dog on the ethanol-induced albumin loss. Both *panels* show cumulative loss over the 90-min perfusion period. The protein loss by the ethanol-perfused segments of the groups treated with these agents was significantly lower than that by the comparable segments of the untreated group; this is indicated by the *asterisks*

(LTB_4) generation (which was taken as the measure of 5-lipoxygenase activity) by the ethanol-treated segment was 265% higher ($P < 0.005$) than that by the control segment. Thus, ethanol stimulates 5-lipoxygenase activity. In the L-651, 392-treated group, LTB_4 generation decreased both in the control and ethanol-perfused segments by 78% ($P < 0.05$) and 35% (not significant), respectively as compared with the control segment of the untreated group. As can be seen on the left panel of Fig. 3, the protein loss in the ethanol-perfused segment was 13 times greater ($P < 0.01$) than in the control segment of the untreated group, but the increase was only five fold ($P < 0.05$) in the treated group. The difference in the ethanol-induced increase in protein loss between the two groups was significant ($P < 0.05$). Thus, ethanol perfusion increased 5-lipoxygenase activity and a selective inhibitor of this enzyme attenuated the microvascular injury (protein loss) caused by ethanol. These findings suggest that products of 5-lipoxygenase (LTs) are involved in the ethanol-induced microvascular injury.

The activity of 5-lipoxygenase can be measured by determining the generation of any of its products by the tissue. We have utilized LTB_4 for this purpose. The fact that we used LTB_4 as an index of the enzyme activity does not necessarily indicate that it is this LT which is involved in the ethanol-induced microvascular damage. As a matter of fact, LTB_4 has little effect on the microvasculature, and it is LTC_4 and LTD_4 which have been shown to increase vascular permeability [12]. Preliminary experiments in our laboratory have shown that a selective inhibitor of LTD_4 receptors (L-649, 923; Merck Frosst Canada) also inhibits the ethanol-induced protein loss. In view of this, further studies are needed to determine which LTs are the main contributors to the ethanol-induced protein loss.

Effect of 16, 16-dimethyl prostaglandin E_2(dmPGE$_2$). In this study, we investigated whether 16, 16-dmPGE$_2$ attenuates the ethanol-induced plasma albumin loss. The experimental setup was similar to that of the experiments described above. Two groups of dogs ($n = 7$ each) were used. One group was untreated; the other (dmPGE$_2$ treated) group received intravenously dmPGE$_2$ at a dose of 0.1 μg/kg as a bolus, followed by a steady infusion of 0.05 μg/kg/h throughout the experiment. A control jejunal segment was perfused with KRBSG and the ethanol-perfused segment with KRBSGE. As shown on the right of Fig. 3, the increase in cumulative albumin loss by the ethanol-perfused segment (over the control) was significantly less (by 45%) in the dmPGE$_2$-treated than in the untreated group ($P < 0.05$). Thus, this synthetic PGE$_2$ provided partial protection against the ethanol-induced jejunal microvascular damage. Even though an analogue was used in our experiments, it is tempting to suggest that local release of prostaglandin E_2 would also result in protection against the ethanol-induced microvascular injury.

Discussion

Both in the rabbit and the dog, the intraluminal protein (albumin) loss increased steadily until a peak was reached. After this, in spite of continuous perfusion (Fig. 1), it progressively declined, indicating an attenuation of the microvascular changes. This biphasic response to ethanol is reminiscent of the finding by Fox et al. [15] that superfusion of the cat and rat mesentery with histamine causes a large transient increase followed by a smaller sustained increase in vascular permeability. Furthermore, it has been reported that histamine infusion causes only a transient opening of the gap junctions; these junctions are widest at 5- to 10-min infusion and close after 15–30 min despite continuous histamine infusion [11]. These findings are similar to our previous report that continuous perfusion of the jeunal lumen with ethanol causes only transient retraction of endothelial cells (and consequently an opening of the interendoethelial gap junctions) of the microvessels of the villus tip [6]. Based on these reports on histamine and our finding that the microvascular effects of ethanol are attenuated by combined $H_1 + H_2$ blockade, it is tempting to postulate that the biphasic effect of ethanol on protein loss is related to a similar transient effect of histamine. At present, there is no explanation as to why the effect of histamine is biphasic, but it is possible that the histamine-induced endothelial cell damage leads to liberation of cyclooxygenase products (e.g., PGE$_2$), which tend to close the gap junctions opened by histamine. This is consistent with our finding that a prostaglandin analogue attenuates the microvascular effect of ethanol. Therefore, it is likely that the mild tissue injury induced by 6% w/v ethanol causes degranulation of mast cells and the release of injurious agents (e.g., histamine and leukotrienes). This in turn (similar to what has been reported as "adaptive cytoprotection" in the stomach [13]) results in the liberation of "cytoprotective" prostaglandins (PGE$_2$). It is then possible that low concentrations of this prostanoid cause the endothelial cells to relax and bring about closure of the gap junctions. Figures 4 and 5 depict the main features of this hypothesis. Clearly, this is an oversim-

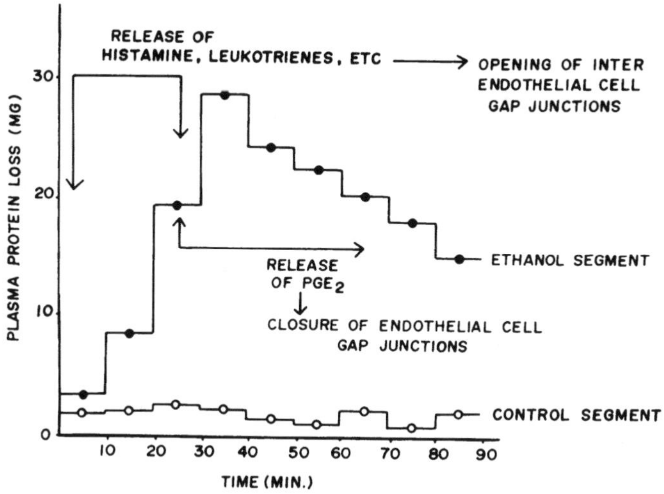

Fig. 4. Hypothesis for the biochemical mechanisms involved in the ethanol-induced opening and closure of gap junctions

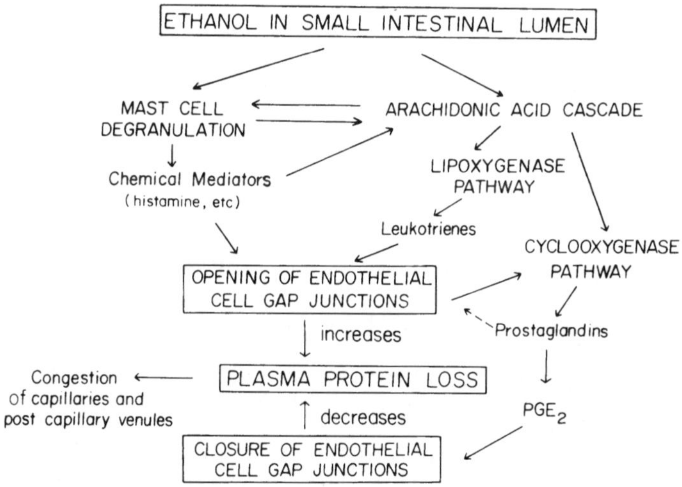

Fig. 5. Hypothesis for the mechanism of rise and decline of ethanol-induced protein loss (microvascular changes)

plification of the situation, since (except for the mast cell degranulation) the figures show only those events for which some experimental evidence has already been obtained in our laboratory. The actual events are probably much more complex, and further work is necessary to elucidate the roles of other mediators (e.g., other prostaglandins, thromboxanes, platelet-activating factor, kinins, free oxygen radicals) in the ethanol-induced microvascular damage.

Acknowledgment. This work was supported by grant MT. 4257 from the Medical Research council of Canada.

References

1. Millan MS, Dinda PK, Buell MG (1980) Villous damage induced by suction biopsy and by acute ethanol intake in the normal human small intestine. Dig Dis Sci 25: 513–25
2. Beck IT. (1977) Effects de l'alcool sur l'intestin grele. La Vie Med. Can Fr 6: 1049–1064
3. Buell MG, Beck IT (1983) Effect of ethanol on jejunal regional blood flow in the rabbit. Gastroenterology 84: 81–89
4. Buell MG, Dinda PK, Beck IT (1983) Effect of ethanol on morphology and total, capillary, and shunted blood flow of different anatomical layers of dog jejunum. Dig Dis Sci 28: 1005–1017
5. Buell MG, Beck IT (1984) Ethanol-induced mucosal microvascular stasis and enhanced plasma protein loss in the dog jejunum. Gastroenterology 86: 413–320
6. Beck IT, Buell MG, Morris GP (1986) Ethanol-induced vascular permeability changes in the jejunal mucosa of the dog. Gastroenterology 90: 1137–1145
7. Kvietys PR, Paterson WG, Russell JM, Barrowman JA, Granger DN, (1984) The role of the microcirculation in ethanol-induced mucosal injury in the dog. Gastroenterology 87: 562–571
8. Ham KN, Hurley JV (1965) Acute inflammation. An electron microscope study of turpentine-induced pleurisy in the rat. J Pathol Bacteriol 90: 365–377
9. Majno B, Palade GE, (1961) Studies in inflammation: I. The effect of histamine and serotonin on vascular permeability: an electron microscopic study. J Biophys Biochem Cytol 11: 571–605
10. Majno G, Gilmore V, Levanthal M (1967) On the mechanism of vascular leakage caused by histamine-type mediators. A microscopic study in vivo. Circ Res 21: 833–847
11. Casley-Smith JR (1980) The response of the microcirculation to inflammation: In: Weissman G (ed) The cell biology of inflammation. Handbook of inflammation, vol. 2. Elsevier, Amsterdam, pp 53–82
12. Vane J, Botting R (1987) Inflammation and the mechanism of action of anti-inflammatory drugs. FASEB J 1: 89–96
13. Robert A, Nezamis JE, Lancaster C, Davis JP, Field SO, Hanchar AJ (1983) Mild irritants prevent gastric necrosis through "adaptive cytoprotection" mediated by prostaglandins. Am J Physiol 245: G113–121
14. Guindon Y, Girard Y, Maycock A, Ford-Hutchinson AW, Atkinson PC, Belanger JG, Dallob A, DeSouse D, Dougherty H, Egan R, Goldbery MM, Ham E, Fortin R, Hamel P, Lau CK, Leblanc Y, McFarlane CS, Piechuta H, Therien M, Yoakim C, Rokach J (1987) L-651, 392: A novel, potent and selective 5-lipoxygenase inhibitor. In: Samuelsson B, Paoletti R, Ramwell PW (eds) Advances in prostaglandin, thromboxane, and leukotriene research. Raven, New York, 17: 554–557
15. Fox J, Galey F, Wayland H (1980) Action of histamine on the mesenteric microvasculature. Microvasc Res 19: 108–126

Gastric Microvascular Effects of the Pro-ulcerogenic Mediator PAF-Acether

BRENDAN J.R. WHITTLE[1], JUAN V. ESPLUGUES[1], and PAUL H. GUTH[2]

Introduction

Platelet-activating factor (PAF)-acether is an endogenous phospholipid that can be formed and released by a variety of cell types, including platelets, neutrophils, basophils, macrophages, monocytes and endothelial cells [1]. Its immediate precursor, lyso-PAF, is released from membrane-bound phospholipids by the action of phospholipase A_2, the enzyme which also releases arachidonic acid. Lyso-PAF, which has little or no intrinsic biological activity, is metabolized into PAF-acether by the action of acetyl CoA transferase and is subsequently broken down back to lyso-PAF by the action of the enzyme acyl hydrolase (Fig. 1). PAF-acether is a low-molecular-weight phospholipid characterized by an ether linkage at the 1' position (usually with a fatty acid chain of 16 or 18 carbons) and an acetyl group at the 2' position of a phosphatidylcholine giving the structure of 1-0-alkyl-2-0-acetyl-sn-glyceryl-3-phosphocholine (Fig. 2).

The release of PAF-acether has been implicated in the pathophysiology of several disease processes, including asthma, anaphylaxis or allergy and as a mediator of inflammation [1]. Furthermore, PAF-acether induces a range pathophysiological events that resemble shock states [2]. These actions include increased vascular permeability, haemoconcentration, hypotension and circulatory collapse, neutrophil aggregation and lysosomal enzyme release. PAF-acether is also the most potent endogenous pro-ulcerogenic mediator so far described [3], and thus its release during endotoxin or septic shock may contribute to the associated gastro-intestinal damage [4, 5]. Since changes in the microcirculation can underlie the pathogenesis of gastric damage, the effects of PAF-acether on the gastric mucosal microvasculature, using both histological techniques and blood flow measurements, were conducted.

[1]Department of Mediator Pharmacology, Wellcome Research Laboratories, Langley Court, Beckenham, Kent, BR3 3BS, England
[2]Center for Ulcer Research and Education, V.A. Wadsworth Hospital Center, Los Angeles, CA 90073, USA

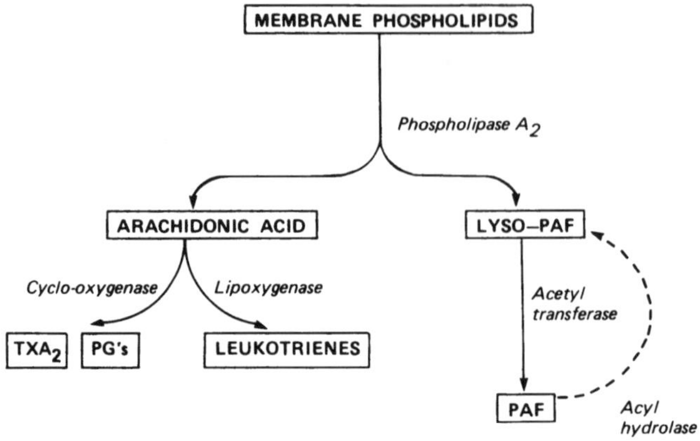

Fig. 1. Biosynthesis of PAF-acether from membrane phospholipids following stimulation of phospholipase A_2

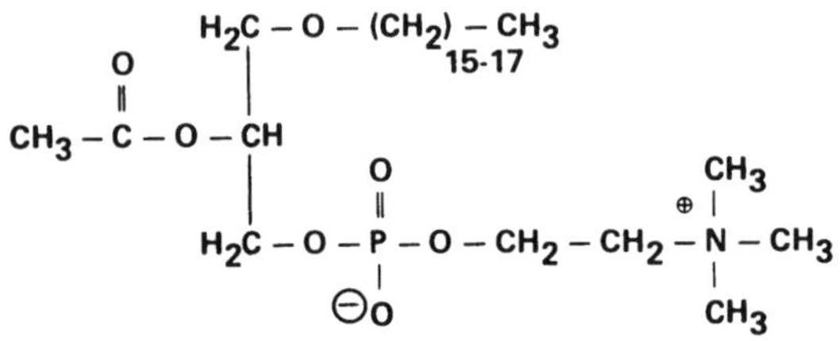

Fig. 2. Chemical structure of PAF-acether

Effects of Intravenously Administered PAF-Acether

Intravenous infusion of PAF-acether in low doses induced extensive damage to the rat gastric mucosa. This mucosal damage was macroscopically characterized as extensive hyperaemia and vasocongestion, with areas of haemorrhagic damage [3]. On histological evaluation, microvascular engorgement and congestion was the predominant feature, with extravasation of red blood cells being apparent as well as epithelial and glandular destruction; focal areas of necrosis extended throughout the mucosal tissues [6]. In addition to the congestion of the mucosal and submucosal microvasculature with red blood cells, the presence of white-cell aggregates within these vessels was observed, particularly at the base of the mucosal glands and submucosal vessels [6].

Effects of Close-Arterial Administration of PAF

To investigate the actions of local administration of PAF-acether on the integrity of the rat gastric mucosa and to evaluate its effects on the microvasculature using histological criteria, we utilized a technique for the close-arterial infusion of such mediators through the left gastric artery [7].

Male rats, deprived of food, but not water, for 18 h prior to study, were anaesthetized with sodium pentobarbitone and the stomach was exposed by a mid-line incision. The left gastric artery was freed from connective tissue under a stereomicroscope, and cannulated with a modified short 23-g Teflon cannula. Patency of the cannula was assured by observing the back-flow of blood. PAF-acether or the vehicle—0.25% bovine serum albumin (BSA) in saline—was infused into the left gastric artery for 10 min at a rate of 12.5 $\mu l\ min^{-1}$.

Twenty minutes after terminating the local intra-arterial infusion, the stomachs were removed and opened along the greater curvature. The stomach were pinned out, mucosal side up, to a wax block, immersed in neutral-buffered formalin and then photographed on colour transparency film. The extent of macroscopically visible damage was determined from these projected transparencies in a randomized manner via computerized planimetry using an Apple IIe system.

Two samples of the corpus and one sample of the antrum, existed from standardized regions, were processed by routine techniques prior to embedding paraffin. Sections (4 μm) were stained with haematoxylin and eosin and examined in a randomized coded manner under a light microscope. The 1-cm length of each section was divided into five or six fields, and each field further divided into four equal subsections. Each subsection was assessed for epithelial cell damage (type 1 damage, a score of 1 being assigned); glandular disruption, vasocongestion or oedema in the upper mucosa (type 2 damage, a score of 2); haemorrhagic damage in the mid- to lower mucosa (type 3 damage, a score of 3) and deep necrosis or ulceration (type 4 damage; a score of 4). Each subsection was evaluated on a cumulative basis, the maximum score for each subsection being 10, and the total maximum score for each field being 40. The overall mean value of the scores for each of the five or six fields was taken as the histological index for that section.

Local intra-arterial infusion (12.5 $\mu l\ min^{-1}$) of the vehicle (0.25% BSA is saline) for periods of 30–80 min caused no damage to the mucosal tissue, as assessed macroscopically or histologically (Fig. 3). Thus, there was sufficient collateral blood flow in the mucosa, derived from the submucosal vascular network and gastric muscle supplied by the gastro-epiploic and hepatic branches of the coeliac artery, to maintain mucosal integrity. This was further demonstrated by the substantial back-flow of blood from the left gastric artery observed after cannulation.

Local intra-arterial infusion of PAF-acether (5–50 ng $kg^{-1}\ min^{-1}$) for 10 min resulted in a dose-dependent increase in macroscopically assessed damage to the gastric mucosa, with 10 ng $kg^{-1}\ min^{-1}$ PAF-acether being the threshold dose for significant damage as compared with control. With the highest dose of PAF-acether studied (50 ng $kg^{-1}\ min^{-1}$), this damage affected 26.6% ± 5% of the surface of the mucosa. The appearance of this damage was comparable with that described following intravenous infusion and was characterized by extensive hyperaemia and haemorrhage, being located in the corpus region.

Histological examination following close-arterial infusion of PAF-acether indicated congestion in the mucosal and submucosal microvasculature throughout the antral and corpus regions, which was accompanied by extensive damage to the surface epithelium, dilatation of the gastric glands and subepithelial oedema where the epithelium had remained intact. The threshold dose for a significant increase in the overall histological index in the corpus mucosa with PAF-acether

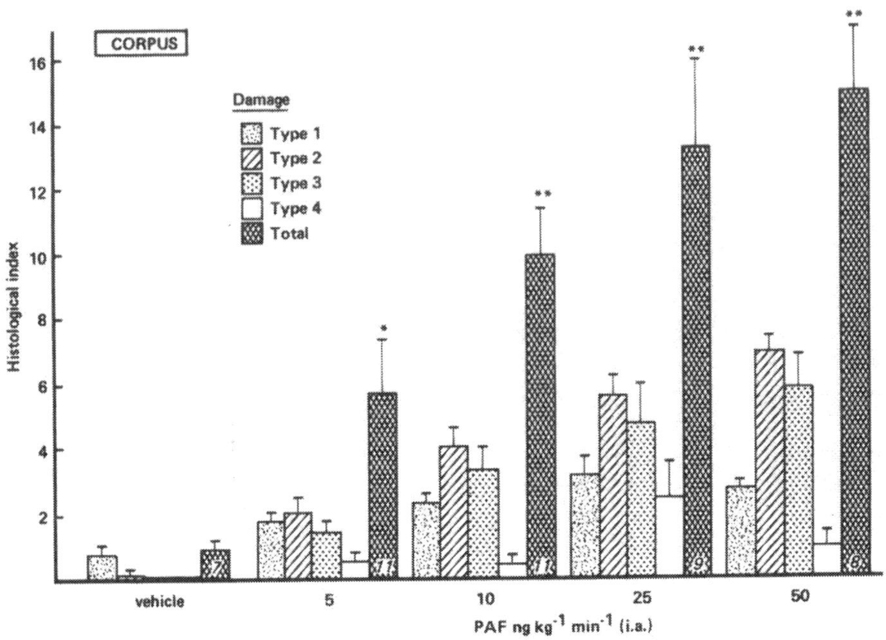

Fig. 3. Histological evaluation of the effects of local intra-arterial infusion of PAF-acether (5–50 ng kg^{-1} min^{-1}) on gastric corpus mucosa of the rat in vivo. The *data* are shown in terms of the histological score for various types of damage (types 1–4) and total histological index in the gastric corpus mucosa. *Results* are means ± SE mean of (*n*) values. For clarity, significant differences from vehicle control is given for total histological index only, where $*P<0.05$, $**P<0.01$

was 5 ng kg^{-1} min^{-1} (Fig. 3). At this dose, there was a significant increase ($P<0.05$) in the individual scores for epithelial cell disruption (type 1 damage), vasocongestion, glandular disruption, and haemorrhagic damage in the upper and mid-regions of the mucosa (type 2 and 3 damage). With the highest doses of PAF-acether, there were also areas of necrosis in the mucosa (type 4 damage), complete disruption of the glandular structure and, in some cases, deep ulceration and partial disappearance of the mucosa.

Although no damage to the antral mucosa was detected on macroscopic inspection, a significant increase in the histological index for the antral area was observed with PAF-acether (5–50 ng kg^{-1} min^{-1}), as shown in Fig. 4. This damage was characterized by the same histological features as observed in the corpus, with pronounced vasocongestion being observed in the microvasculature.

The threshold doses of PAF-acether for induction of macroscopic or histological damage in both antral and corpus regions following close-arterial infusion produced minimal systemic hypotension, with the fall in blood pressure (BP) being less than 20 mmHg. Furthermore, intravenous infusion of PAF-acether (25 ng kg^{-1} min^{-1}) produced a comparable fall in BP as the same dose infused locally, yet it induced minimal damage to the gastric mucosa as assessed

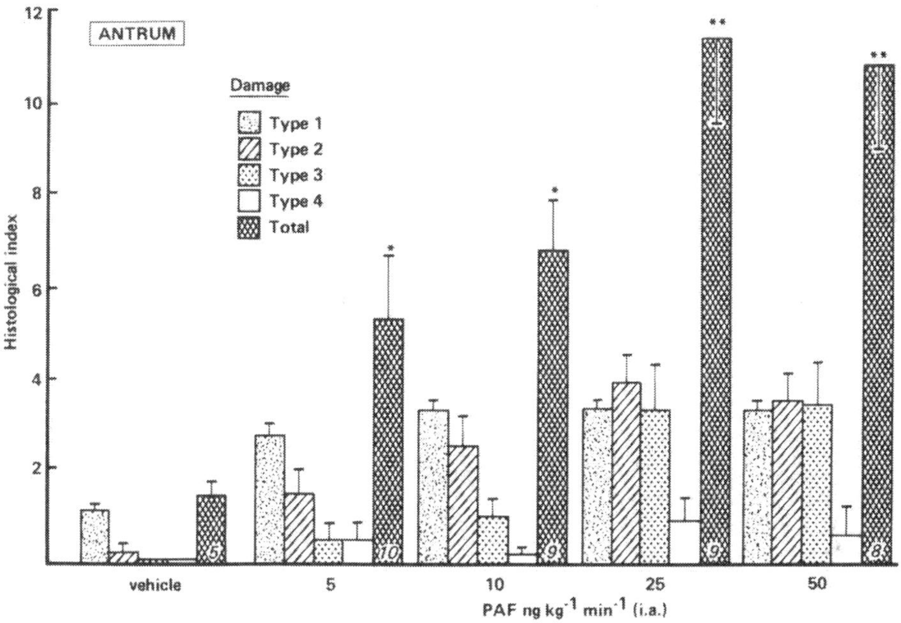

Fig. 4. Histological evaluation of the effects of local intra-arterial infusion of PAF-acether (5–50 ng kg^{-1} min^{-1}) on gastric antral mucosa of the rat in vivo. The *data* are presented as in Fig. 3

both by macroscopical and histological observation. These findings indicate that although systemic hypotension may contribute to the gastric damage induced by high doses of PAF-acether, especially when administered by the intravenous route, PAF-acether can induce extensive disruption of the mucosal tissue and microvasculature by more direct mechanisms.

The predominant histological feature of congestion and engorgement of the mucosal microvessels following both local and intravenous administration of PAF-acether suggested that vascular stasis may be an important mechanism underlying the mucosal damage. Such stasis could have been brought about by direct vasoconstrictor effects on the submucosal arterioles and venules resulting in a reduction in mucosal blood flow, or by other microvascular changes. To investigate such possibilities, the effects of PAF-acether on blood flow in the rat gastric mucosa were determined.

Actions of PAF-Acether on Gastric Mucosal Blood Flow

Blood flow in the gastric mucosa was determined by measurement of red blood cell velocity in the mucosal capillaries [8]. Male rats (200–300 g), deprived of food for 24 h but allowed water, were anaesthetized with pentobarbitone and maintained at 37°C. The abdomen was opened via a mid-line incision to expose the stomach, and the gastric contents were washed out with isotonic saline through an incision in the fore-stomach. A needle was inserted into a femoral vein for the infusion of vehicle or drug.

The in vivo microscopy technique described previously in detail by Guth and colleagues [9] was used to expose the mucose for the study of blood flow in the capillaries. A long incision was made in the anterior wall of the fore-stomach, just proximal and parallel to the limiting ridge. A portion of the posterior wall of the corpus was then everted through the incision, thus exposing the mucosal surface to direct visualization. The stomach wall was transilluminated with cool light from a high-intensity source through a fibre-optic light carrier rod with an attached mirrored prism. After the surgical preparation, the animal was left undisturbed for 15 min to ensure vessel diameter stability. A microscope equipped with long-working-distance objectives (× 6 and × 20) permitted visualization of blood flow through the mucosal superficial capillaries.

A shallow concave light-brass disk (2.5 cm diameter and 5 mm deep) with a small hole (5 mm diameter) in the centre was sealed fluid-tight to the mucosal tissue with a silicone plastic adherent. Krebs' solution (pH 7.4 at 37°C) was continuously superfused over the tissue to maintain temperature and moisture of the exposed area. The appearance of the exposed area of microvasculature was recorded on videotape, before and during the infusion of vehicle and drug, and analyses were performed on playback of the videotapes. The final magification on the TV screen was × 760. For the determination of red blood cell velocity (RBCV) in the capillaries, the voltage output at two points on a capillary was monitored on the playback of the videotape, and the signals were fed into a velocity tracking correlator. Since the voltage varies as red blood cells pass each point, the correlator can determine the time-lag of similar patterns between the upstream and downstream signals. By continuously dividing this time-lag into the preset distance between the two points, the correlator can continuously compute the RBCV. The lowest detectable level of RBCV in this system was 0.05 nm s^{-1}. In these studies, capillaries located close to a collecting venule were studied. One vessel in each preparation was selected for study which was clearly in focus and straight in the control period. The vessel was followed throughout the experiment, with the centre-line velocity measured for 1-min periods [10].

In control experiments, resting RBCV (0.63 ± 0.02 nm s^{-1}; $n = 19$) was stable throughout the observation period. Intravenous infusion of the vehicle or lyso-PAF (200 ng kg^{-1} min^{-1} for 20 min) had no significant effect on RBCV. A small fall in RBCV was observed 20 min after the start of the low-dose PAF infusion (25 ng kg^{-1} min^{-1}). At the higher doses of PAF (50 and 100 ng kg^{-1} min^{-1}), a significant fall in RBCV was obtained 2–3 min after commencing the infusion (Fig. 5); sluggish flow and sludging of blood cells along the capillary walls were observed. At the highest dose of PAF used (100 ng kg^{-1} min^{-1}), RBCV fell to non-detectable levels within 5 min of the start of infusion, and no flow could be detected during the remainder of the infusion period (Fig. 5). Stasis of flow in the capillaries could clearly be observed on the video-recordings.

In further studies using in vivo microscopy techniques, the effect of intravenous infusion of PAF-acether on the gastric submucosal microvasculature was evaluated [10]. During PAF-acether infusion (25–100 ng kg^{-1} min^{-1} for 20 min), no significant change in the calibre of the arterioles (resting diameter 26 ± 0.2 μm) or venules (56 ± 1 μm) could be detected. However, showing of

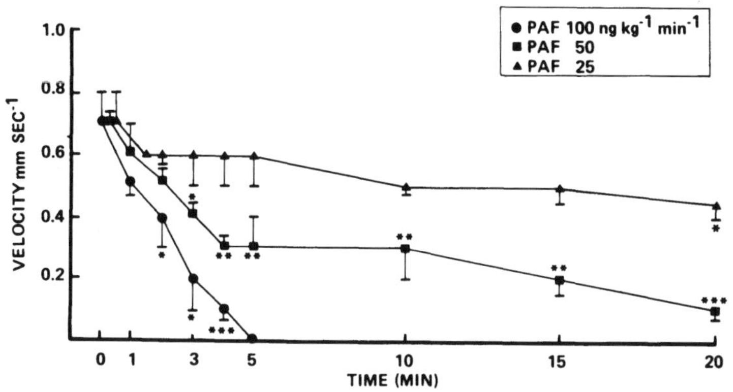

Fig. 5. Effect of PAF-acether (25–100 ng kg^{-1} min^{-1}) on capillary blood flow in the rat gastric mucosa during a 20-min intravenous infusion, as determined by red blood cell velocity. *Results*, shown as velocity (mm s^{-1}), are means ± SE means of four experiments for each dose, where level of statistical difference from basal velocity is shown by $^{*}P<0.05$, $^{**}P<0.01$, $^{***}P<0.001$. Data adapted from Whittle et al. [10]

flow could clearly be observed during administration of PAF-acether, with stasis of flow being observed in 50% of arterioles and 58% of the venules with the highest dose investigated.

Using hydrogen gas clearance as a further index of gastric mucosal blood flow [11], a dose-dependent reduction in blood flow with a concurrent fall in systemic arterial BP was determined during the intravenous infusion of PAF-acether [10]. With the highest doses of PAF-acether investigated (100 ng kg^{-1} min^{-1}), clearance reached an abrupt plateau within 4 min, indicating that blood flow had ceased.

Mechanisms Underlying the Microvascular Actions of PAF-Acether

The intravenous infusion of nanamole doses of PAF-acether induces extensive hyperaemia and focal haemorrhage in the gastric microcirculation. Histological evaluation revealed substantial vasocongestion within the microvasculature, which suggested that microcirculatory stasis may be a major factor precipitating the mucosal damage. Although such stasis could have resulted from direct vasoconstriction in the submucosal arterioles and venules, in the vessels that regulate mucosal blood flow no change in vessel diameter could be detected during administration of PAF-acether. This is in contrast to the effects of the other proulcerogenic lipid mediators, thromboxane A_2 and leukotriene C_4, which induce focal vasoconstriction in both arterioles and venules of the submucosa following local application [12].

The fall in gastric perfusion pressure following intravenous infusion of PAF-acether, resulting from the lowering of systemic BP, would contribute to the decreased blood flow through the mucosa. However, this alone is unlikely to explain completely the reduced mucosal blood flow, determined by RBCV and hydrogen gas clearance nor underlie the microvascular stasis or the gastric damage. Thus, in previous studies, intravenous administration of vasodilator agents, which reduced BP to a level comparable with that obtained with PAF-acether, did not lead to significant mucosal damage [3]. Furthermore, local intra-arterial infusion of PAF-acether can induce extensive mucosal damage in the absence of any substantial change in systemic BP.

Deposition of blood cells along the walls of the vessels was observed during the periods of sluggish blood flow in the gastric microcirculation induced by PAF-acether. These cells were not platelets, since despite its name, PAF-acether is only weakly active in stimulating platelet aggregation in the rat. Indeed, extensive mucosal damage can be induced by PAF-acether in platelet-depleted rats [3]. However, the presence of neutrophil aggregates was observed on histological examination of the rat gastric mucosal microvasculature [6] and systemic neutropenia was determined [13, 14] after PAF-acether infusion. These aggregates, by initially blocking the smaller capillaries, may contribute to the reduction in mucosal blood flow. Such effects would be enhanced by the concurrent marked haemoconcentration resulting from systemic extravasation of plasma protein that follows administration of PAF-acether [13, 14]. Thus, the changes in the rheological properties of the blood as a consequence of such haemoconcentration, coupled with the presence of aggregated cells, could account for the sluggish flow and eventual stasis observed in the gastric microcirculation.

The release of endogenous PAF-acether has been demonstrated in gastro-intestinal tissue during endotoxin shock [5] and is likely to be involved in the pathogenesis of the associated gastro-intestinal damage [3]. The hypoxia observed in the subepithelial microcirculation after septic shock [15] could thus be brought about by PAF-acether release. The observed aggregation of neutrophils in the microcirculation following PAF-acether administration would also be accompanied by the release of free radical and lysosomal enzymes, which would aggravate the damage to the gastric microvasculature and subepithelial tissue. PAF-acether may directly damage the endothelial cell lining of the microcirculation, provoking white cell-endothelium interaction and adhesion and allowing the extravasation of erythrocytes. Such events would lead to the subsequent development of gastric mucosal vasocongestion and haemorrhage.

References

1. Braquet P, Shen TY, Touqui L, Vargaftig BB (1987) Perspectives in platelet-activating factor research. Pharmacol Rev 39: 97–145
2. Bessin P, Bonnet J, Apffel A, Soulard C, Desgroux L, Pelas I, Benveniste J (1983) Acute circulatory collapse caused by platelet-activating factor (PAF-acether) in dogs. Eur J Pharmacol 86: 403–413
3. Rosam AC, Wallace JL, Whittle BJR (1986) Potent ulcerogenic actions of platelet-activating factor on the stomach. Nature 319: 54–56
4. Wallace JL, Whittle BJR (1986) Prevention of endotoxin-induced gastrointestinal damage by CV-3988, an antagonist of platelet-activating factor. Eur J Pharmacol 124: 209–210
5. Whittle BJR, Boughton-Smith NK, Hutcheson IR, Esplugues JV, Wallace JL (1987) Increased intestinal formation of Paf in endotoxin-induced damage in the rat. Br J

Pharmacol 92: 3–4
6. Wallace JL, Whittle BJR (1986) Picomole doses of platelet-activating factor predispose the gastric mucosa to damage by topical irritants. Prostaglandins 31: 989–998
7. Esplugues JV, Whittle BJR (1988) Gastric mucosal damage by local intra-arterial administration of Paf in the rat. Br J Pharmacol 93: 222–228
8. Holm-Rutili L, Obrink KJ (1985) Rat gastric microcirculation in vivo. Am J Physiol 248: G741–746
9. Guth PH, Paulson C, Nagata H (1984) Histologic and microcirculatory changes in alcohol-induced gastric lesions in the rat: Effect of prostaglandin cytoprotection. Gastroenterology 87: 1083–1090
10. Whittle BJR, Morishita T, Ohya Y, Leung FW, Guth PH (1986) Microvascular actions of platelet-activating factor on the rat gastric mucosa and submucosa. Am J Physiol 251: G772–778
11. Leung FW, Guth PH, Scremin OU, Golanska EM, Kauffman GL (1984) Regional gastric mucosal blood flow measurements by hydrogen-gas clearance in the anaesthetized rat and rabbit. Gastroenterology 87: 28–36
12. Whittle BJR, Oren-Wolman N, Guth PH (1985) Gastric vasoconstrictor actions of leukotriene C_4, $PGF_{2\alpha}$, and thromboxane mimetic U-46619 on rat submucosal microcirculation in vivo. Am J Physiol 248: G580–586
13. Doebber JW, Wu WS, Shen TY (1984) Platelet activating factor intravenous infusion in rats stimulates vascular lysosomal hydrolase secretion independent of blood neutrophils Biochem Biophys Res Comm 125: 980–987
14. Wallace JL, Whittle BJR (1986) Effects of inhibitors of arachidonic acid metabolism on PAF-induced gastric mucosal necrosis and haemoconcentration. Br J Pharmacol, 89: 415–422
15. Payne JG Bowen JC (1981) Hypoxia of the canine gastric mucosa caused by *Escherichia coli* sepsis and prevented by methyl prednisolone therapy. *Gastroenterology* 80: 84–93

Gastric Microcirculatory Changes Associated with Physicochemical and Ionic Mediators

SUNAO KAWANO[1], NOBUHIRO SATO[1], SHINGO TSUJI[1], TAKENOBU KAMADA[1], HIROSHI SATOH[2], and NOBUHIRO INATOMI[2]

Introduction

The mechanism of stress-induced acute gastric mucosal lesions (AGML) has been investigated for some time. We have reported that in hemorrhagic shock, the decrease of gastric mucosal blood flow, volume, and its oxygenation precedes the gastric ulceration which appears usually after infusion of blood or at the recovery stage in rats and humans. It is believed that the microcirculatory disturbance resulting in hypoxia in the gastric mucosa produced an incipient mucosal state for ulcerogenesis and that in this hydrochloric acid and histamine played an aggressive role. The precise mechanism leading to cell death after ischemia is, however, obscure. In this symposium, we presented a movie film which showed the process of gastric mucosal microcirculatory disturbance and bleeding caused by indomethacin, leukotriene C4 (LTC4), platelet-activating factor (PAF) and HCl and also reported the role of chemical and ionic factors in the repefusion state in the etiology of gastric ulceration.

Materials and Methods

In Vivo Microscopic Observation of Gastric Mucosal Microcirculation

Figure 1 shows a block diagram of the in vivo microscopic observation system for gastric mucosal microcirculation. Spragne-Dawley (S-D) male rats were deprived of food for 24 h and anesthetized with pentobarbital sodium (35 mg·kg i.p.) and the abdomen was opened with a midline incision. A small incision along the greater curvature with a thermoknife was made and the stomach was gently extended on a special stage under the microscope (BH2, Olympus Co, Tokyo).

After observation of normal blood flow, 10 μl indomethacin (10 mg/ml), LTC4 (10μg/ml), or PAF (12.5 μg/ml) was added topically with a microsyringe.

[1]First Department of Medicine, Osaka University Medical School, 1–50, Fukushima 1-chome, Fukushima-ku, Osaka, 553 Japan
[2]Central Research Division, Takeda Chemical Industries Ltd., 17–85, Juso-honmachi 2-chome, Yodogawa-ku, Osaka, 532 Japan

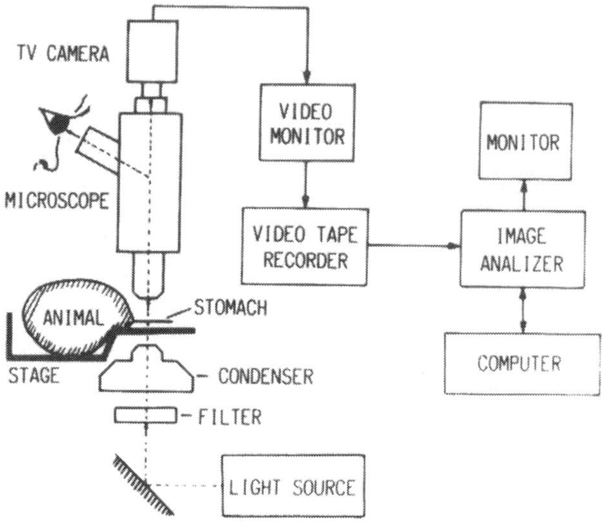

Fig. 1. Blockdiagram of in vivo microscopic system

The changes in the gastric mucosal microcirculation and gastric mucosa were observed and recorded with a movie camera or tape recorder throughout the experiments.

Effect of Chemical Mediators (Prostaglandins, LTC4, or PAF) in Conjunction with Acid on Gastric Ulceration

Indomethacin experiment. S-D male rats were deprived of food for 24 h. Indomethacin, 10 mg/kg, was injected subcutaneously. One hour later, 2 ml 0.2 *N* HCl was given orally. The rats were killed to examine the ulcer index expressed as millimeters (total length of lesions) 1 h after HCl administration.

LTC4 experiment. S-D male rats were deprived of food for 24 h. LTC4, 30 μg/kg, was injected i.v. via the caudal vein. One minute later, 1 ml 0.1 5*N* HCl and/or 20 m*M* taurocholate was given intragastrically. Rats were killed 1 h after HCl administration.

PAF experiment. S-D male rats were deprived of food for 24 h. At first, 1 ml 0.2 *N* HCl was given orally and 5 min later, 12.5 μg/kg PAF was injected intravenously. The rats were killed 1 h after PAF administration.

Role of Calcium Ion and Lipid Peroxidation in Gastric Ulceration

Effect of calcium antagonists on gastric ulceration in hemorrhagic shock rats. S-D male rats were deprived of food and anesthetized with pentobarbital sodium (35 mg/kg, i.p.). To remove the blood and monitor the systemic blood pressure, a polyethylene cannula was inserted into a carotid artery. Hydrochloric acid (2 ml, 0.2 *N*) was given orally. The blood was removed and the mean arterial blood pressure was maintained at 40 mmHg for 60 min using a reservoir. The blood was reinfused over a period of 15 min and ten minutes later the stomach was removed to examine the ulcer index, expressed as mm^2 (length × width). Using reflectance spectrophotometry, the indices of gastric mucosal blood volume (GMBV) and oxygen saturation of hemoglobin (SO_2) were estimated from the spectra taken every 15 min, as reported previously [1]. A calcium antagonist (diltiazem, verapamil, or flunaridine) was infused at the rate of 1 mg/kg/h via a caudal vein throughout the experiment.

Lipid peroxidation in hemorrhagic shock rats. With the same protocal as in the previous experiment on calcium artagonists, the gastric mucosa was obtained before hemorrhage, just before and after reinfusion of blood. Lipid peroxidation in the gastric mucosa was measured using the thio barbituric acid (TBA) method.

Results

In Vivo Microscopic Observation of Gastric Mucosal Microcirculation

With the in vivo microscopic system, gastric mucosal blood flow around the gastric pits was clearly seen. At first, 10 μl indomethacin was administered topically; gastric mucosal blood flow in the capillaries decreased. Three minutes later, the blood flow in the collecting venule became slower, and at the some parts around the gastric pits the blood flow disappeared and the gastric mucosa looked pale.

LTC4 and PAF caused a decrease in mucosal blood flow in the collecting venules and capillaries. The mucosal blood flow stopped within 10 min after LTC4 or PAF administration. These agents caused mucosal ischemia with partial congestion resulting in mucosal hypoxia in the stomach.

Under such ischemic and congestive conditions, an additive effect was induced by HCl, causing much greater ischemic changes in the gastric mucosa. Finally, the blood flow stopped completely in certain areas. The gastric pits then became difficult to identify and the gastric mucosa turned yellowish, suggesting degeneration of the surface mucosal cell layer. In the yellowish area around the collecting venule, hemorrhage began from a collecting venule. Red blood cells were clearly observed leaking out through the capillary wall. The bleeding became progressively bigger and finally a massive hemorrhage occurred.

Effect of Indomethacin, LTC4, or PAF in Conjunction with Acid on Gastric Ulceration

Indomethacin or HCl alone produced a very low ulcer index (1.6 ± 0.6 and 0, respectively). However, the combination of indomethacin and HCl caused significantly greater gastric lesions (ulcer index 19.4 ± 7.2) than those induced by indomethacin or HCl.

LTC4 or HCl caused no gastric ulceration when given alone. Taurocholate alone caused a small ulcer (0.1 ± 0.1). But again, the combined administration

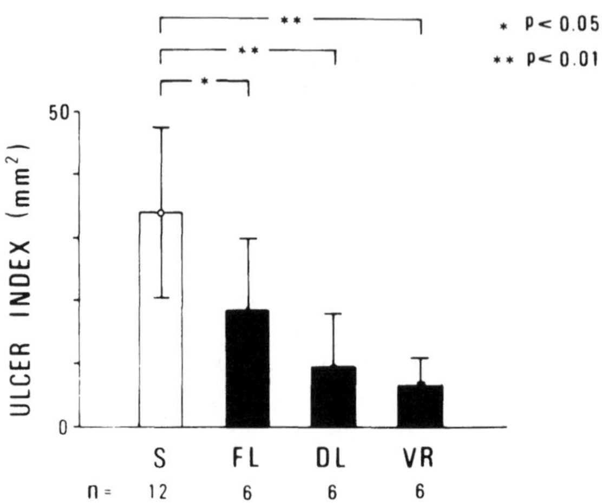

Fig. 2. Effect of calcium antagonists on gastric ulceration induced by gastric hemorrhagic shock in rats. *S* saline, *FL* flunaridine, *DL* diltiazem, *VR* verapamil

of these three substances caused significantly greater ulcers (102.4 ± 17.1).

The ulcer index induced by PAF and HCl alone was 37.8 ± 16.0 and 0, respectively. The combined administration of PAF and HCl again caused a significantly higher ulcer index (83.7 ± 10.6).

Role of Calcium Ion and Lipid Peroxidation in Gastric Ulceration

In both the control and calcium antagonist groups, the systemic blood pressure was maintained at 40 mmHg during hemorrhagic shock. After hemorrhage, the index of GMBV decreased by 50% and the index of SO_2 decreased from 45% to 4%. There were no significant differences in these parameters between the control and calcium antagonist groups. Figure 2 shows the effect of various calcium antagonists on the hemorrhagic shock-induced gastric ulceration. Pretreatment with calcium antagonists decreased the ulcer index significantly.

Table 1 shows the lipid peroxide level in the gastric mucosa and ulcer index in hemorrhagic shock rats treated with and without calcium antagonists. In the group without calcium antagonists, before hemorrhage and before reinfusion of blood, ulceration was not seen and lipid peroxide was 269.7 ± 33.9 and 298.0 ± 114.7 pmol MDA/mg protein, respectively. However, after reinfusion of blood, the ulcer index and lipid peroxide increased significantly (ulcer index 2.4 ± 1.6, lipid peroxide 719.0 ± 214.7 pmol MDA/mg protein). In the group treated with calcium antagonists, before hemorrhage and before reinfusion of blood, no ulceration was found and the lipid peroxide level was almost the same as in the group without calcium antagonist treatment. After reinfusion of blood, the calcium antagonist group showed a significantly lower level of the lipid peroxide (386.5 ± 115.9 pmol MDA/mg protein) and ulcer index (0.3 ± 0.5).

Figure 3 shows the relationship between ulcer index and lipid peroxide level in rats maintained under hemorrhagic shock with and without 0.2 *N* HCl. With

Table 1. Lipid peroxide and gastric ulceration in hemorrhagic shock rats treated with and without a calcium antagonist

	Without calcium antagonist		With calcium antagonist	
	Lipid peroxide	Ulcer index	Lipid peroxide	Ulcer index
Before hemorrhage	269.7 ± 33.9	0	282.0 ± 75.6	0
Before reinfusion	298.0 ± 114.7	0	315.4 ± 75.6	0
After reinfusion	719.0 ± 214.7[a]	2.4 ± 1.6	386.5 ± 115.9	0.3 ± 0.5

[a] Significantly different from other values ($P < 0.05$)

HCl, the ulcer index showed a remarkable increase linearly with the lipid peroxide level. Moreover, the calcium antagonist treatment caused a linear decrease in the ulcer index and lipid peroxidation.

Discussion

Many authors have reported the important role of gastric mucosal microcirculation in the etiology of stress-induced gastric ulceration. We previously reported that mucosal ischemia and hypoxia precede gastric ulceration. In our experiments, the ulcer size showed a good correlation with the extent of tissue hypoxia, and we found that histamine and hydrochloride aggravated the gastric ulceration significantly.

In the present study, using an in vivo microscopic system, the events in the gastric mucosal microcirculation leading to gastric bleeding were analyzed to elucidate the role of chemical mediators in gastric ulceration. Although the precise mechanism is unclear, the topical administration of indomethacin, LTC4, and PAF caused the gastric mucosal capillaries to shrink and slowed the velocity of erythrocyte flow. All the data obtained in the present study indicated that chemical mediators such as prostaglandins (PGs), LTC4, and PAF influenced the gastric microcirculation. LTC4 and PAF caused microcirculatory disturbance, resulting in ischemia with partial congestion and mucosal hypoxia. It was also shown that the acid showed an additive effect on microcirculatory disturbance and acted as an aggravating factor, causing greater mucosal ulceration and bleeding.

On the other hand, the mechanism of cell death after ischemia is still obscure. Stress ulceration occurs as the ischemia-reperfusion syndrome and recently it has been emphasized that free radicals in the reperfusion state play a role in the etiology of stress ulceration in the stomach. To investigate the events in reperfusion, we measured the lipid peroxide in the stomach of rats with hemorraghic shock. Furthermore, to elucidate the role of calcium ions in reperfusion, the effect of calcium antagonists on lipid peroxidation and the development of gastric ulceration was also investigated.

In hemorrhagic shock, the systemic blood pressure was maintained at 40 mmHg with a reservoir. GMBV and SO_2 measured by reflectance spectrophotometry showed a similar decrease in the control and calcium antagonist groups,

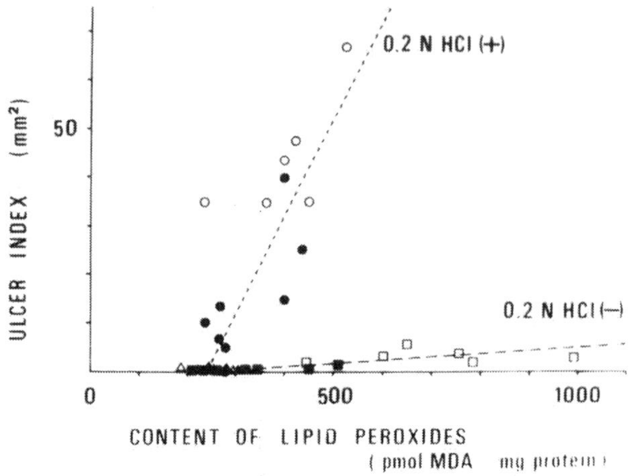

Fig. 3. Relationship between ulcer index and lipid peroxide. *Open circles* and *squares* signify the control group, and *closed circles* and *squares* the group treated with a calcium antagonist

indicating that the same level of ischemia and tissue hypoxia in the gastric mucosa was induced in both groups. Under such conditions, gastric ulceration and lipid peroxidation were significantly lowered in the calcium antagonist group in both the presence and absence of acid. These results suggest that in reperfusion, calcium ion influx through the damaged membrane may play a role in the etiology of gastric ulceration and that lipid peroxidation after reperfusion also strongly affects gastric ulceration.

In conclusion, gastric mucosal ischemia and hypoxia disintegrate the gastric mucosa and in reperfusion chemical factors, including lipid peroxide and calcium ions, affect gastric ulceration and bleeding.

References

1. Sato N, Kamada T, Shichiri M, Kawano S, Abe H, Hagihara B (1979) Measurement of hemoperfusion and oxygen sufficiency in gastric mucosa in vivo. Gastroenterology 76: 814–819
2. Kamada T, Sato N, Kawano S, Fusamoto H, Abe H (1982) Gastric mucosal hemodynamics after thermal or head injury. Gastroenterology 83: 535–540
3. Sato N, Kawano S, Kamada T, Takeda M (1986) Hemodynamics of the gastric mucosa and gastric ulceration in rats and in patients with gastric ulcer. Dig Dis Sci 31: 35S–41S
4. Hase T, Moss BJ (1973) Microvascular changes of gastric mucosa in the development of stress ulcer in rats. Gastroenterology 65: 224–234
5. Szabo S, Trier JS, Brown A, Schnoor J (1985) Early vascular injury and increased vascular permiability in gastric mucosal injury caused by ethanol in the rat. Gastroenterology 88: 228–236
6. Itoh M, Guth PH (1985) Role of oxygen-derived free radicals in hemorrhagic shock-induced gastric lesions in the rat. Gastroenterology 88: 1162–1167

Metabolic and Myogenic Control of Gastric Mucosal Blood Flow

J.W. KIEL, G.L. RIEDEL, and A.P. SHEPHERD[1]

Introduction

Previous studies of local circulatory control in the stomach showed that total gastric blood flow is regulated by metabolic and possibly myogenic mechanisms [1–3]. However, because of the limitations of previously available blood flow-measuring techniques, similar studies have not been extended to the gastric mucosa. Given the heterogeneity of the gastric circulation and the functional stratification of the gastric wall, it is possible that blood flow within the different layers of the stomach may be regulated independently and possibly by different mechanisms. This possibility is supported by our recent demonstration of mucosal blood flow autoregulation in the absence of autoregulation of total blood flow [4]. We designed the present study to identify the mechanism responsible for the pronounced autoregulation of gastric mucosal blood flow and determine whether metabolic or myogenic mechanisms regulate the mucosal circulation.

Methods

Animal Preparation

The chambered canine stomach preparation developed by Moody and Durbin [5] was used in all of the experiments. Mongrel dogs deprived of food for 24–48 h were anesthetized with pentobarbital sodium (30 mg/kg, supplemented as necessary) and given heparin (500 units/kg) as an anticoagulant. To prepare the chambered stomach flap, the splenic artery and vein were cannulated proximal to the left gastroepiploic artery and vein. The nerves and remaining connective tissue were severed during the cannulation procedure. The arterial cannula was connected to a pressurized reservoir filled with blood pumped from the left femoral artery. The venous cannula was connected to a second reservoir used to collect the venous outflow, which was then pumped back into the animal via the left

[1]Department of Physiology, University of Texas Health Science Center, San Antonio, TX 78284, USA

femoral vein. The region of the gastric corpus perfused by the left gastroepiploic artery was then excised and quickly clamped between two Lucite rings. Perfusion pressure and venous pressure were maintained at 120 and 0 mmHg, respectively. The temperature of the preparation was maintained at 37°C by an infrared heat lamp and by superfusing the mucosal surface with warm Ringer's solution.

Mucosal and muscularis blood flow were monitored with two laser-Doppler blood flowmeters [6, 7] and total blood flow was monitored by an extracorporeal electromagnetic flow probe (Zepeda Instruments) at the outlet of the pressurized reservoir. Arterial and venous pressures were measured with Statham pressure transducers. Arteriovenous oxygen difference was also monitored spectrophotometrically. Oxygen consumption was later calculated as the product of the arteriovenous oxygen difference and total blood flow. In some experiments, mucosal surface pH was measured as a index of gastric acid secretion.

Experimental Protocols

To elicit a functional hyperemic response, pentagastrin (Peptavlon, Ayerst Laboratories Inc., NY, USA was used to stimulate acid secretion and increase the metabolic rate ($n = 10$). Pentagastrin was administered by adding 2 ml pentagastrin (0.25 mg/ml) to 500 ml blood in the pressurized reservoir, giving a final pentagastrin concentration of 1 μg/ml.

To assess the reactive hyperemic responses in total and mucosal blood flow, complete arterial occlusions of 30, 60, and 90 s were performed in random sequence ($n = 6$). The hyperemic response was analyzed by integrating the area of the tracing above the preceding control flow level to obtain the volume of the hyperemia. Because the muscularis rarely exhibits a reactive hyperemic response [7], muscularis blood flow was not monitored in this series of experiments.

Autoregulation was studied by raising perfusion pressure from the control pressure of 120 mmHg to 180 mmHg and then lowering the perfusion pressure in 30-mmHg steps to a final pressure of 30 mmHg ($n - 10$). Autoregulation was assessed by calculating the gain factor (GF) for each pressure step [8]:

$$GF = 1 - [(\Delta F/F)/(\Delta P/P)]$$

where F and P are the blood flow and perfusion pressure immediately before the step-change in pressure, and ΔP and ΔF are the imposed change in pressure and the resultant change in flow, respectively. A positive GF value results when the change in flow is proportionately less than the change in pressure and was taken as evidence of autoregulation.

To test for myogenic reactivity, the venous pressure was elevated from 0 to 20 mmHg ($n = 13$). Venous pressure was maintained at 20 mmHg until all measured variables reached a steady state and was then lowered to 0 mmHg. Vascular resistance was later calculated by dividing the pressure gradient at each venous pressure by the respective blood flow.

Results and Discussion

Metabolic Control of Gastric Mucosal Blood Flow

The metabolic theory of local circulatory control states that the oxygen flux to the tissues is the regulated variable rather than blood flow per se [9]. In response to decreased oxygen availability or increased oxygen demand, the metabolic model predicts that a feedback signal originating within the tissue causes vasodilation of resistance vessels and relaxation of precapillary sphincters, thus maintaining oxygen delivery to the capillaries and optimized blood-tissue oxygen exchange.

Functional Hyperemia. The metabolic theory predicts that oxgyen extraction and blood flow both increase to meet the increased oxygen demand associated with elevated metabolic activity. In the stomach, this prediction is readily verified by stimulating acid secretion to elevate the metabolic rate. As shown in Fig. 1, when acid secretion was stimulated with pentagastrin, there was a corresponding increase in oxygen consumption mediated by increases in both oxgyen extraction and total gastric blood flow. Mucosal surface pH decreased from 5.63 ± 0.27 to 4.67 ± 0.33 ($P < 0.01$), indicating a significant increase in acid secretion. The concomitant increase in total oxygen consumption (1.09 ± 0.07 to 1.90 ± 0.13 ml/min/100 g, $P < 0.001$) was made possible by increased oxygen extraction (arteriovenous oxygen difference rose from 3.06 ± 0.27 to 4.25 ± 0.44 ml/100 ml, $P < 0.001$) and a functional hyperemia in total blood flow

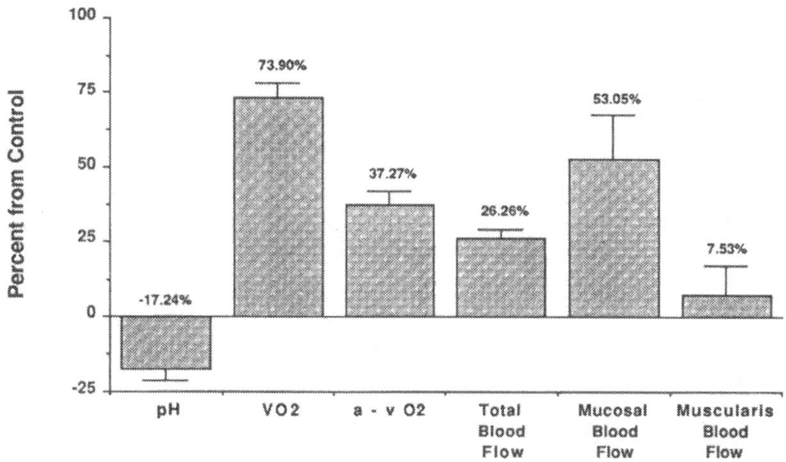

Fig. 1. Gastric functional hyperemia. Pentagastrin increased acid secretion as indicated by the decrease in mucosal surface pH. Increased acid secretion was accompanied by increased oxygen consumption (*VO_2*) made possible by increased oxygen extraction, as shown by the arteriovenous oxygen difference (*a–v O_2*), and functional hyperemia in total gastric blood flow. The increase in blood flow was limited to the mucosa since blood flow in the muscularis was not significantly different from control. Reprinted with permission from Kiel et al. [13]. Copyright 1987 by The American Gastroenterological Association

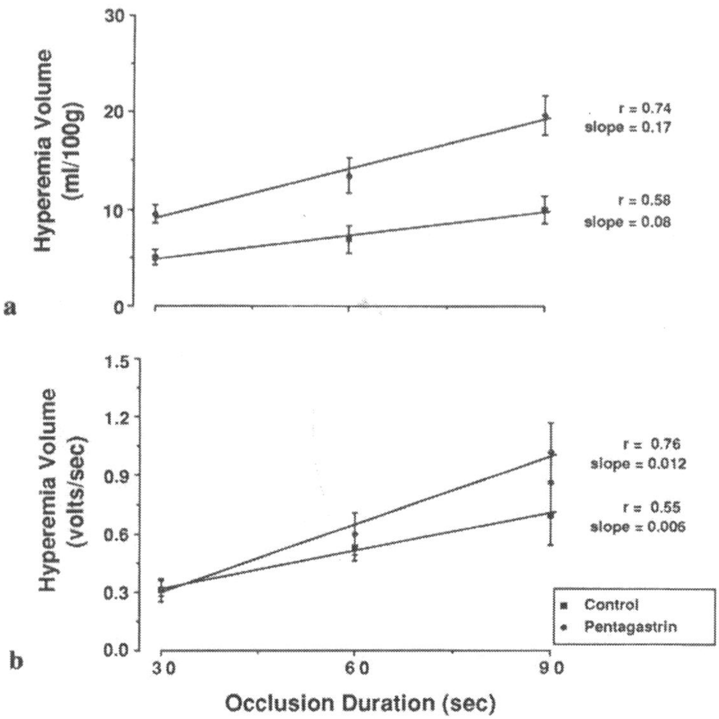

Fig. 2a, b. Gastric reactive hyperemia. Volume of reactive hyperemia in **a** total and **b** mucosal blood flow was dependent on the duration of the arterial occlusion and the prevailing metabolic state. Reprinted with permission from Kiel et al. [13]. Copyright 1987 by The American Gastroenterological Association

(37.52 ± 3.07 to 47.45 ± 4.39 ml/min/100 g, $P<0.001$). The functional hyperemia in total blood flow was confined to the actively secreting mucosa, where blood flow increased by 53.05% ± 14.74% ($P<0.01$) but was absent in the muscularis where blood flow was not significantly different from control (7.53% ± 9.72%, $P>0.05$).

Reactive Hyperemia. Although the feedback signal in the metabolic model is unknown, both a tissue-generated vasodilator (e.g., adenosine) and a circulating vasoconstrictor (e.g., oxygen) have been proposed [9]. Given either signal, the model predicts that the magnitude of the reactive hyperemic response following a partial or complete arterial occlusion will depend on the duration of the occlusion and the prevailing metabolic rate. As shown in Fig. 2, the volume of the hyperemic response in total blood flow was directly dependent on the length of the arterial occlusion (Fig. 2a) both under resting conditions (slope = 0.08 ml/min/100 g/s, $r=0.58$, $P<0.05$) and during metabolic stimulation (slope = 0.17 ml/min/100 g/s, $r=0.74$, $P<0.001$). However, the slope of the relationship between the volume of the hyperemia and occlusion duration was significantly greater during metabolic stimulation ($P<0.001$). Similarly, the volume of the mucosal reactive hyperemic response was also dependent on the length of the

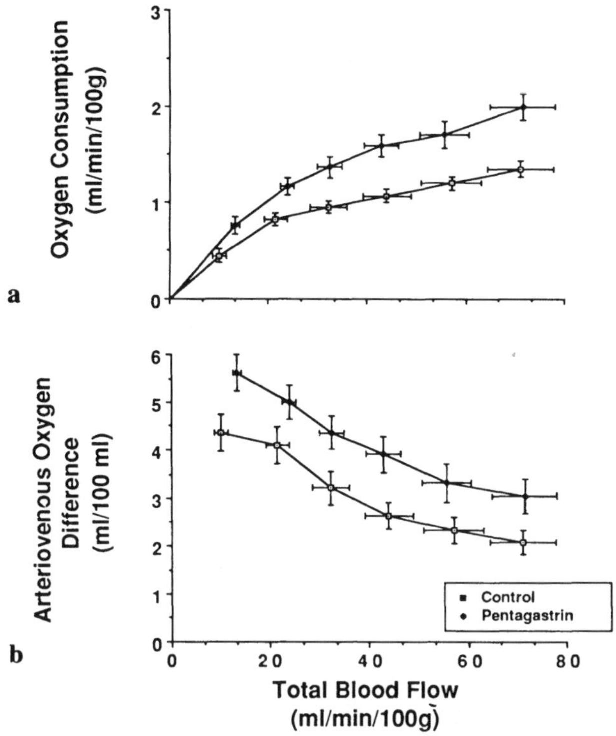

Fig. 3. **a** Gastric oxygen consumption and **b** oxygen extraction as perfusion pressure was reduced from 180 to 30 mmHg in 30-mmHg steps. Oxygen consumption was blood flow-independent over most of the pressure range during control and following pentagastrin but elevated above control at each perfusion pressure after pentagastrin. Oxygen extraction progressively increased following each reduction in perfusion pressure and each consequent decrease in total blood flow under both conditions but was increased above control at each perfusion pressure following pentagastrin. Reprinted with permission from Kiel et al. [13]. Copyright 1987 by The American Gastroenterological Association

occlusion both before and after metabolic stimulation (slope = 0.006 v/s, $r = 0.55$, $P < 0.05$ and 0.012 v/s, $r = 0.76$, $P < 0.001$, respectively). The gradient between the mucosal hyperemic volume and occlusion duration was also significantly steeper at the higher metabolic rate ($P < 0.001$).

Autoregulation. The metabolic theory further predicts that oxygen uptake should remain relatively constant following a drop in perfusion pressure because of the combined action of increased oxygen extraction and blood flow autoregulation. As shown in Fig. 3a, total oxygen consumption was reasonably well maintained when perfusion pressure was decreased stepwise from 180 to 30 mmHg, both during control and metabolic stimulation. The relative constancy of oxygen consumption under both conditions and the increased oxygen consumption following pentagastrin were mediated in part by appropriate increases in oxygen extraction (Fig. 3b). Parallel with the increases in oxygen extraction, the gain values for total blood flow became progressively less negative as perfusion

a

b

c

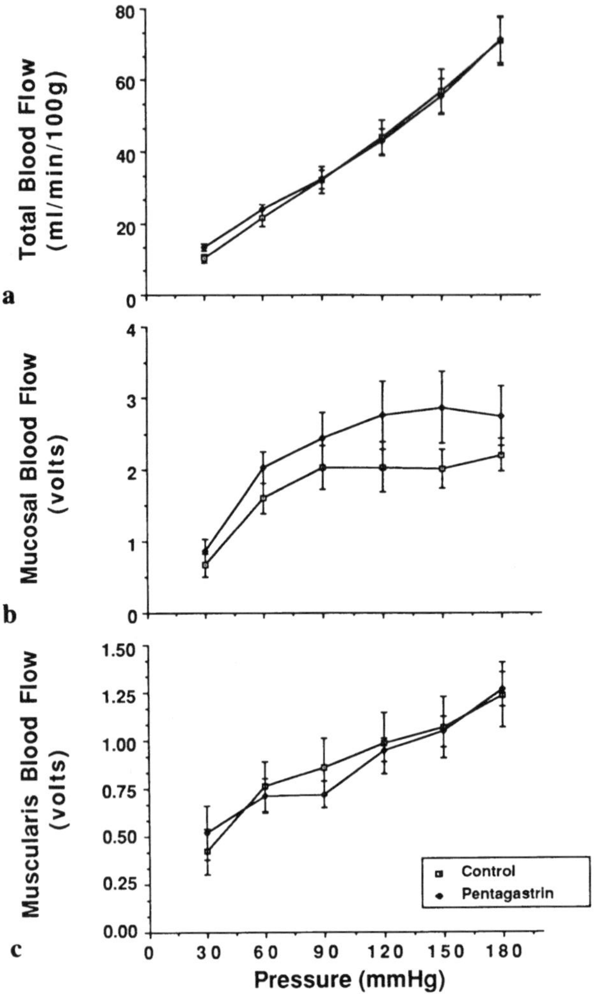

Fig. 4a–c. Pressure-flow relationships for **a** total gastric blood flow, **b** mucosal blood flow, and **c** muscularis blood flow. During stepwise reductions in perfusion pressure both before and after pentagastrin, neither total blood flow nor muscularis blood flow was particularly well maintained. However, mucosal blood flow was relatively constant over most of the perfusion pressure range during control and following pentagastrin. Reprinted with permission from Kiel et al. [13]. Copyright 1987 by The American Gastroenterological Association

pressure was reduced both before and after pentagastrin, suggesting that the tendency for autoregulation increased with the depletion of the venous oxygen reserve (Fig. 5a). However, it should be noted that total blood flow was not autoregulated during control and that even during metabolic stimulation, a positive gain value indicative of active autoregulation occurred only at the 90- to 60-mmHg-pressure-step ($P < 0.01$).

Unlike total blood flow, mucosal blood flow was particularly well maintained over most of the perfusion pressure range both before and after pentagastrin

a
b
c

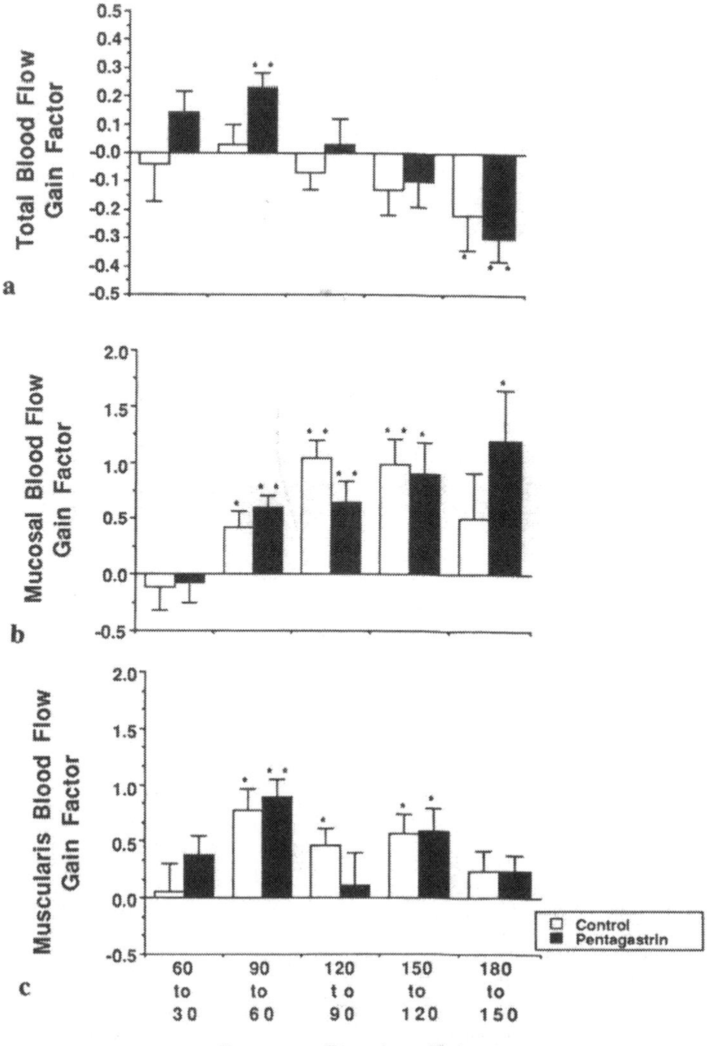

Fig. 5a–c. Gain values calculated at each pressure step for **a** total gastric blood flow **b** mucosal blood flow, and **c** muscularis blood flow. Except at the lowest pressure step, the gain values for total gastric blood flow increased progressively with each drop in perfusion pressure during control. The same trend occurred after pentagastrin but to a greater extent so that the gain value was positive at the 90- to 60-mmHg pressure step. The gain values for mucosal blood flow were positive at all but the lowest pressure step before and after pentagastrin; however, the gain values were not significantly different at any pressure step. Similarly, the gain values for muscularis blood flow were not significantly different at any pressure step before and after pentagastric. Reprinted with permission from Kiel et al. [13]. Copyright 1987 by The American Gastroenterological Association

(Fig. 4b). The fact that the mucosal gain values were positive at all but the lowest pressure step under both conditions (Fig. 5b) further substantiates the pronounced ability of the gastric mucosa to autoregulate its blood flow. Although mucosal blood flow tended to be higher at each perfusion pressure following pentagastrin, the mucosal gain values were not significantly different at any pressure step before and after pentagastrin, indicating that mucosal autoregulation was not enhanced by metabolic stimulation. However, both before and after pentagastrin, the pronounced autoregulation of mucosal blood flow coincided with the plateau portion of the oxygen uptake curve (Fig. 3a, 4b). Furthermore, oxygen consumption became blood flow-dependent when the mucosa failed to autoregulate at the lowest pressure step. The pronounced autoregulation of mucosal blood flow and the lack of autoregulation in total blood flow suggest that blood flow was preferentially redistributed to the more metabolically active mucosa and that mucosal autoregulation contributes significantly to the maintenance of total gastric oxygen consumption. The results in the muscularis were less striking. As shown in Figs. 4c and 5c, there was no significant difference in either muscularis blood flow or the gain values at any perfusion pressure before and after pentagastrin.

Myogenic Control of Gastric Mucosal Blood Flow

Although both oxygen homeostasis and blood flow autoregulation are predicted by the metabolic theory, autoregulation can also be explained by a myogenic mechanism [10, 11]. According to the myogenic theory, vascular wall tension is actively regulated by vascular smooth muscle. Thus, in response to increased transmural pressure and passive vascular distension following an increase in arterial pressure, vascular smooth muscle actively contracts, increasing vascular resistance and minimizing the increase in blood flow which would have occurred in a passive system. The metabolic and myogenic theories differ in their predicted response to venous pressure elevation—vasodilation and vasoconstriction, respectively. Although the myogenic response is well documented in the intestinal circulation [11, 12], it has not been thoroughly investigated in the stomach.

As shown in Fig. 6a, elevating venous pressure from 0 to 20 mmHg elicited a significant fall in total (39.62 ± 4.23 to 30.76 ± 3.10 ml/min/100 g, $P<0.001$) and mucosal blood flow (2.32 ± 0.26 to 1.49 ± 0.25 v, $P<0.001$) but only a slight decrease in muscularis blood flow (0.98 ± 0.14 to 0.98 ± 0.19 v). Oxygen consumption underwent a slight but statistically significant decrease despite an increase in oxygen extraction. Arteriovenous oxygen difference increased significantly (2.95 ± 0.33 to 3.37 ± 0.43 ml/100 ml, $P<0.001$) so that oxygen consumption fell by only 6.05% (1.05 ± 0.08 to 0.96 ± 0.07 ml/min/100 g, $P<0.05$). As shown in Fig. 6b, total vascular resistance increased slightly but significantly (3.45 ± 0.35 to 3.68 ± 0.39 mmHg/ml/min/100 g, $P<0.05$), indicating a myogenic response. The myogenic response was confined to the mucosa, where vascular resistance increased dramatically (59.55 ± 6.47 to 96.16 ± 18.29 mmHg/v, $P<0.01$), but was absent in the muscularis, which generally did not respond to venous pressure elevation or showed only a slight increase in vascular resistance (148.83 ± 19.01 to 171.15 ± 41.67 mmHg/v, $P>0.05$).

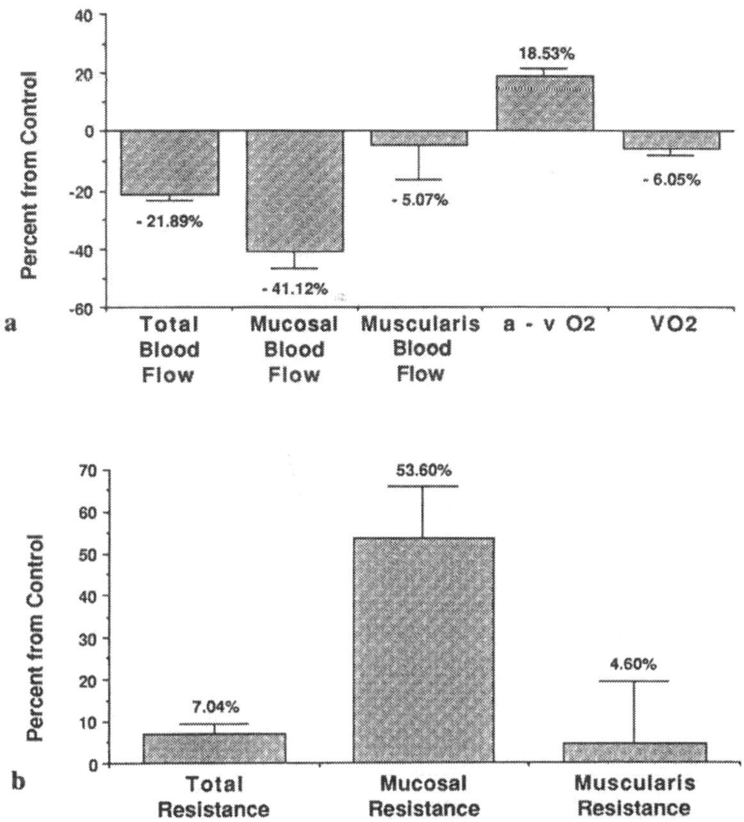

Fig. 6a, b. Gastric myogenic response. **a** When venous pressure was elevated from 0 to 20 mmHg, total and mucosal blood flow decreased but muscularis blood flow was not significantly different from control. In conjunction with the fall in perfusion, oxygen extraction increased significantly as shown by the arteriovenous oxygen difference (a–v O_2); however, oxygen consumption (VO_2) was still slightly but significantly decreased. **b** Total and mucosal vascular resistances were both significantly increased but muscularis resistance was not. Reprinted with permission from Kiel et al. [13]. Copyright 1987 by The American Gastroenterological Association

Conclusions

The following observations are evidence of a metabolic mechanism controlling the gastric mucosal circulation: (a) the mucosa exhibited functional hyperemia when oxygen consumption was elevated during stimulated acid secretion; (b) the volume of mucosal reactive hyperemia was directly dependent on the duration of the arterial occlusion and the prevailing metabolic state; (c) mucosal blood flow was well autoregulated; and (d) mucosal blood flow and total oxygen consumption were both relatively constant over the same range of perfusion pressures. Each of these observations was predicted by a purely metabolic model of local circulatory control [9]. By contrast, the one observation consistent with a myogenic mechanism was the mucosal vasoconstriction that occurred during venous pressure elevation. Thus, these results indicate that both metabolic and myogenic mechanisms participate in the regulation of gastric mucosal blood flow.

References

1. Holm-Rutilli L, Perry MA, Granger DN (1981) Autoregulation of gastric blood flow and oxygen uptake. Am J Physiol 241: G143–G149
2. Perry MA, Murphree D, Granger DN (1982) Oxygen uptake as a determinant of gastric blood flow autoregulation. Dig Dis Sci 27: 675–679
3. Lutz J, Biester J (1971) Die Reaktion der Magengefäße auf venöse und arterielle Druckreize und ihr Vergleich mit Werten von Milz- und Intestinalstrombahn. Plügers Arch 330: 230–242
4. Kiel JW, Riedel GL, Shepherd AP (1987) Autoregulation of canine gastric mucosal blood flow. Gastroenterology 93: 12–20
5. Moody FG, Durbin RP (1965) Effects of glycine and other instillates on concentration of gastric acid. Am J Physiol 209: 122–126
6. Bonner R, Nossal R (1981) Model for laser-Doppler measurements of blood flow in tissue. Appl Opt 20: 2097–2107
7. Kiel JW, Riedel GL, DiResta GR, Shepherd AP (1985) Gastric mucosal blood flow measured by laser-Doppler velocimetry. Am J Physiol 249: G539–G545
8. Norris CP, Barnes GE, Smith EE, Granger HJ (1979) Autoregulation of superior mesenteric flow in fasted and fed dogs. Am J Physiol 237: H174–H177
9. Shepherd AP, Granger HJ (1973) Autoregulatory escape in the gut: a systems analysis. Gastroenterology 65: 77–91
10. Folkow B (1964) Description of the myogenic hypothesis. Circ Res 14 (Suppl. 1): 279–285
11. Johnson PC (1965) Effect of venous pressure on mean capillary pressure and vascular resistance in the intestine. Circ Res 16: 294–300
12. Shepherd AP (1977) Myogenic responses of intestinal resistance and exchange vessels. Am J Physiol 233: H547–H554
13. Kiel JW, Riedel GL, Shepherd AP (1987) Local control of canine gastric mucosal blood flow. Gastroenterology 93: 1041–1053

Leukocyte Adherence in Hepatic Microcirculation in Ischemia Reperfusion

ANTHONY KOO[1], GREGORY BREIT[2], and MARCOS INTAGLIETTA[2]

Introduction

The pathophysiological problem of ischemia and reperfusion in the liver is clinically encountered in liver transplantation [1] and in hemorrhagic shock [2]. Vascular complications of liver transplantation occur in the early postoperative period and are unrelated to graft rejection, which may occur at a later stage. To understand the underlying pathogenetic mechanisms, it is important to consider the following two conditions. First, the donor liver is not perfused by blood and is an ischemic organ during storage. Second, the transplanted liver is reperfused after the surgical anastomoses of blood vessels have been completed. Thus, the liver transplant undergoes the pathophysiological consequences of ischemia and reperfusion. Similarly, in circulatory shock, the liver is rendered ischemic, and reperfusion occurs when the systemic hypotension is corrected.

In general, ischemia to an organ occurs when there is a reduction in microcirculatory flow to levels insufficient to maintain cellular metabolism and function. Reperfusion is the reconstitution of flow which may occur following either incomplete or complete ischemia [3]. In many vascular beds, reperfusion after a period of ischemia only results in a transient return of blood flow, to be followed by a reduction or complete cessation of blood flow (the "no reflow" phenomenon). It is logical to postulate that ischemia and reperfusion in the liver also result in a "no reflow" situation. It is, therefore, pertinent to study this phenomenon.

In the liver, experimental global or lobar ischemia can be produced by clamping hepatic vessels for a specified period of time [4, 5]. Reperfusion of the liver is accomplished by removing these clamps. However, there have been few studies of the liver microcirculation under the conditions of ischemia and reperfusion [5]. The aim of the present study was to apply in vivo video microscopic methods [6] to investigate the microcirculatory disturbances which contribute to the "no reflow" phenomenon in the ischemic and reperfused liver.

[1] Department of Medicine, University of California, Los Angles, School of Medicine, Center for Ulcer Research and Education, V.A. Wadsworth Medical Center, Los Angeles, CA 90073, USA
[2] Department of AMES-Bioengineering, University of California, San Diego, La Jolla, CA 92093, USA

It has been increasingly recognized that in conditions characterized by reduced blood flow, leukocytes tend to adhere to the endothelium of capillaries and postcapillary venules of the microcirculation. In the dog myocardium [7, 8], it has been demonstrated that leukocytes which are trapped in the myocardial capillaries at the time of reperfusion following a period of ischemia are responsible for the microcirculatory flow obstruction (the "no reflow" phenomenon). However, there is little documentation by direct in vivo microscopic observation [9, 10] of the occlusion of vascular lumen by leukocyte plugging in the microcirculation.

Recently, we have developed a technique to study the dynamics of leukocytes in the liver microcirculation. We use fluorochrome acridine orange to label the leukocytes in vivo and use the fluorescence video microscopy to follow the movement of the fluorescent leukocytes. Thus, it is now feasible to quantify the in vivo dynamics of the leukocytes and to correlate the leukocyte dynamics with the microcirculatory disturbances in the ischemia reperfusion of the liver. Hitherto, such aspects of leukocyte dynamics have not been studied.

Materials and Methods

Animal Preparation

All experiments were performed on male Sprague-Dawley rats (250–300 g). The rats were deprived of food for 24 h but were allowed free access to water prior to the experiment. The rats were anesthetized with sodium pentobarbital (45 mg/kg i.m.). The body temperature (rectal) was monitored and maintained between 37°C and 38°C by a heating pad. The femoral vein was cannulated for intravenous administration of supplementary doses of anesthesia and for systemic administration of the fluorochrome.

Preparation of Liver Microcirculation

The abdomen of the rat was opened by a midline incision to expose the liver. The falciform and coronary ligaments of the liver were severed to free the liver from its attachments to the diaphragm. A metal "shield," molded to the shape of the lower thoracic cage and the diaphragmatic surface of the liver [11], was inserted between the diaphragm and the liver in order to eliminate movements of the liver due to respiratory excursions and heart beats. For in vivo microscopic observation, the liver surface was covered with a polyethylene wrap except the area where the liver was epi-illuminated with incident light.

In Vivo Fluorescence Video Microscopy

The liver microcirculation was observed by an American Optical microscope, which utilized the nosepiece as the focusing device. Epi-illumination was delivered via a vertical illuminator (American Optical, Buffalo, NY, USA) from a 100-W mercury vapor lamp (Osram, Berlin, Germany). The objective lens (x60/0.65, American Optical) also served as the condenser lens since both the incident and reflected lights passed through the same lens. For observing the fluorescent leukocytes after the administration of the fluorochrome, a combination of excitor (BG 12 + KV 418, or 490 nm), dichroic (500 or 510 nm), and barrier (OG 515 or 520 nm) filters was used. In order to obtain a better image of the fluorescent leukocytes, a silicon-intensified-target video camera (Cohu Electronics, San Diego, CA, USA) was used. The closed-circuit video system also consisted of a cassette video recorder (Panasonic, Tokyo, Japan) and video monitor (Panasonic, Tokyo, Japan).

In Vivo Labeling of Leukocytes

A 1% solution of acridine orange was injected intravenously (1 mg/100 g) in the rat. This fluorochrome (also called a fluorescent dye) was taken up by the leukocytes in vivo. Upon excitation by the mercury vapor lamp, the dye emitted fluorescence at a shorter wavelength. Using the optical filter system described above, the fluorescent leukocytes were recorded by the video camera and visualized on the monitor.

Production of Liver Ischemia

Ischemia to the left and median lobes of the liver was induced by placing a miniature clamp around the left portal vein, left hepatic artery, and left hepatic duct [5]. The blood supply to the omental and right lateral lobes was left uninterrupted and portal blood flow was maintained through them. Usually, there was no evidence of vascular congestion in the alimentary tract. The rats in which vascular congestion was seen were discarded. After 30 min, the miniature clamp around the obstructed vessels was removed so that blood began to reperfuse the left and median lobes.

Measurement of Leukocyte Velocity

The leukocyte velocity in a liver sinusoid was analyzed during the playback of the videotape. In this off-line method, the x- and y-coordinates of a fluorescent leukocyte on the video monitor was determined frame by frame using a video densitometer (Instrument for Physiology and Medicine, Inc. San Diego, CA, USA). The distance traversed by the moving leukocyte in the time interval between two video frames (i.e., 1/30 s) was calculated from the two sets of x- and y-coordinates (Fig. 1). The leukocyte velocity was the quotient of distance over time. Within the visible length of a liver sinusoid, approximately five to ten measurements were made for one particular fluorescent leukocyte until the leukocyte disappeared on the video monitor. The measurement was repeated on the same liver sinusoid for another 10–20 leukocytes. The mean leukocyte velocity was estimated statistically from all the measurements (Fig. 2). Determination of the x- and y-coordinates from the video monitor was performed manually, but the calculation of distance and velocity and the statistical estimation of mean velocity were performed using a microcomputer system. In the present method, since we calculated the distance traversed by a leukocyte from the two sets of x- and y-coordinates from two consecutive video frames, it was pertinent to ensure that there was no movement of the background image (except the leukocytes) during this interval.

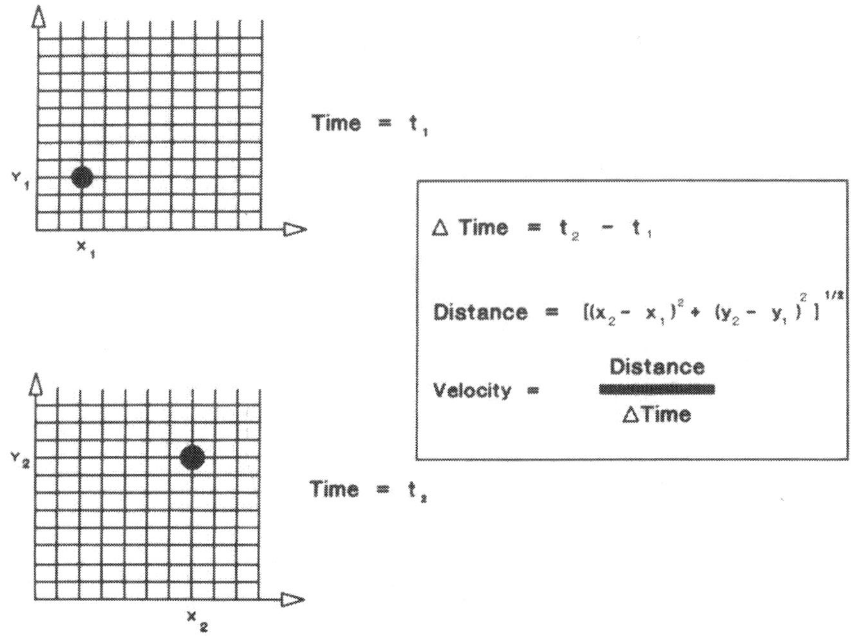

Fig. 1. Calculation of leukocyte velocity from two sets of x- and y-coordinates in two consecutive video frames. The time interval between two video frames ($t_2 - t_t$) is 1/30 s

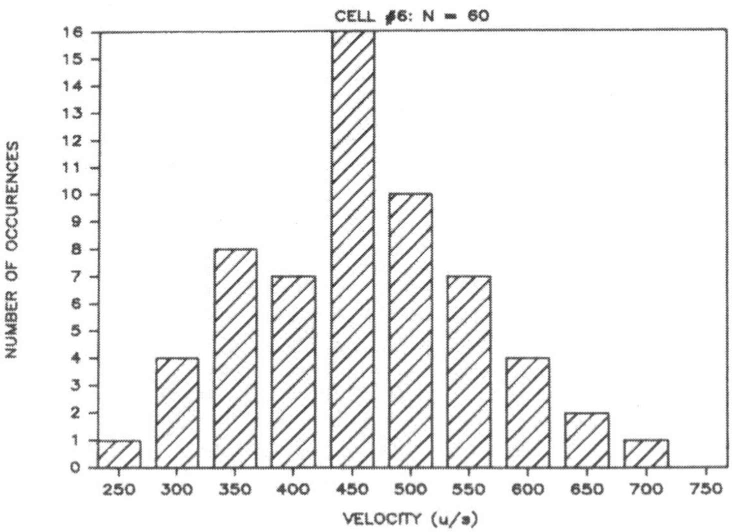

Fig. 2. Frequency distribution plot of leukocyte velocities in a liver sinusoid. In this example, 60 measurements of velocities were obtained from six leukocytes, which were visualized to pass through the sinusoid during the observation period. The bell-shaped frequency pattern is suggestive of a normal distribution of leukocyte velocities

Distribution of Leukocyte Velocity

The leukocyte velocity in a hepatic venule was estimated in a similar manner to that in the liver sinusoid. Since a hepatic venule is much longer than a liver sinusoid, it was feasible to estimate the distribution of leukocyte velocity along the length of the venule. Thus, the leukocyte velocity was plotted versus the position along the length of the venule. During ischemia reperfusion, when the leukocytes were observed to adhere to the wall of the venule, the exact site of leukocyte adherence (zero leukocyte velocity) was determined from the velocity-position plot.

Comparison of Leukocyte and Erythrocyte Velocities

On the same liver sinusoid or hepatic venule in which the leukocyte velocity was estimated, the erythrocyte velocity was also measured using the two-window video densitometric and cross-correlation computation technique [2]. The leukocyte velocity was plotted versus the erythrocyte velocity. The ratio of leukocyte velocity to erythrocyte velocity was also estimated.

Results

In Vivo Fluorescence Microscopy

In the pilot study in 30 rats, the application of the fluorescence epi-illumination microscopic technique to quantitate the leukocyte dynamics was confirmed in the liver microcirculation. Labeling the leukocytes in vivo with acridine orange enabled direct recording of leukocyte movements in the microcirculation. In the liver microcirculation, the acridine orange was also taken up by the hepatic parenchymal cells, which became fluorescent. Presumably, the fluorescent dye was metabolized by the hepatocytes. Thus, in the liver microcirculation, there was a good optical contrast between the bright background (the fluorescent liver cell mass) and the dark liver sinusoids and hepatic microvessels, in which bright (fluorescent) leukocytes were easily visualized (Fig. 3).

Leukocyte Plugging in Liver Sinusoids

Preliminary data indicated that during the reperfusion period following the 30-min ischemia in the liver, there was an increased incidence of intravascular plugging by leukocytes, causing complete cessation of blood flow in some liver sinusoids. Figure 3 shows a typical example of the plugging of liver sinusoids by the adherent leukocytes. Figure 3C was taken at a time lapse of 0.23 s (14 video fields or $14 \times 1/60$ s = 0.23 s) after Fig. 3B. One of the fluorescent leukocytes (marked with an asterisk in Fig. 3) remained adherent to the wall of the liver sinusoid while the other leukocyte (marked with two asterisks), which had moved to a new position, adhered to the sinusoid itself. It was much easier to observe leukocyte adherence to the liver sinusoids from the video monitor by

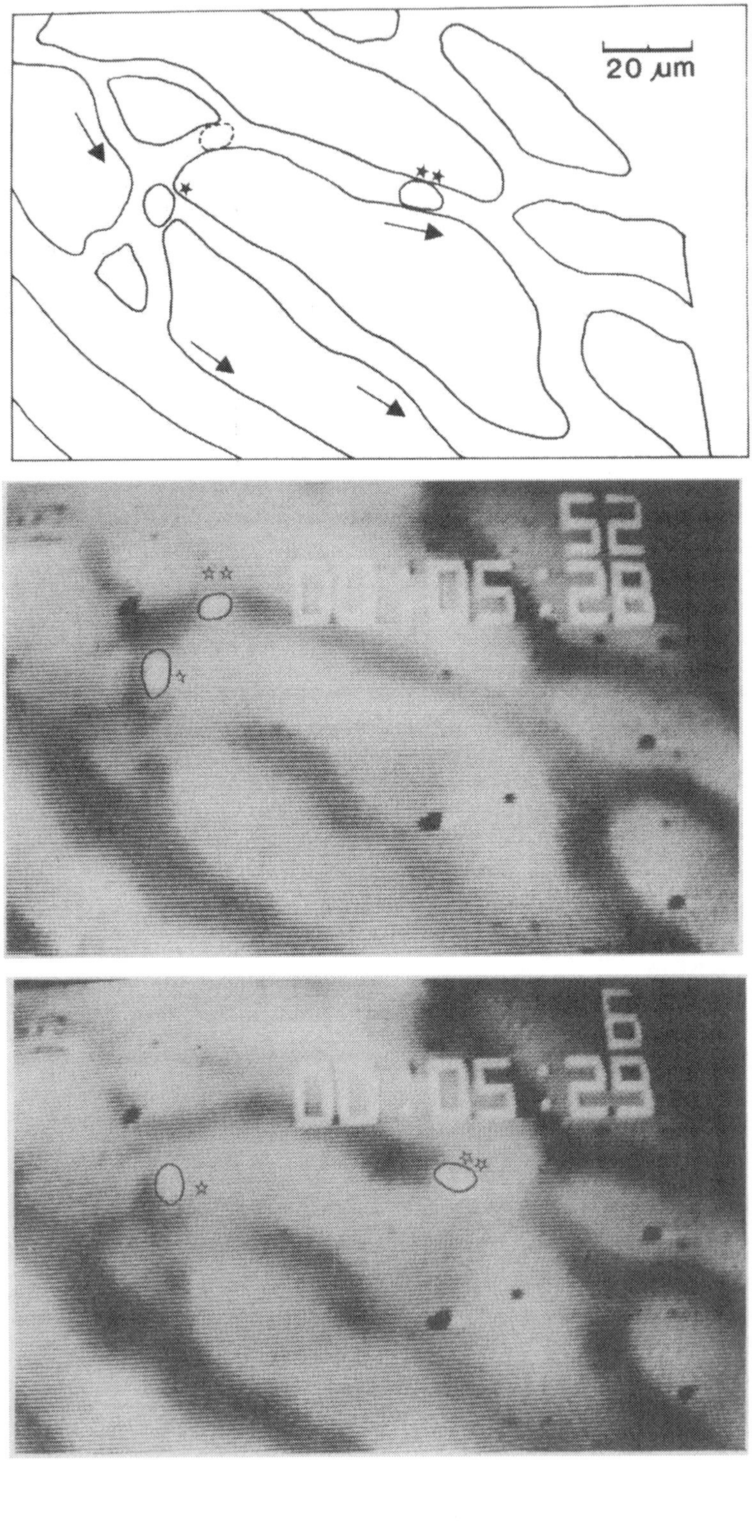

a

b

c

Fig. 3

playing back the videotape than from still pictures as in Fig 3. However, as shown in Fig. 3, the absence of a column of erythrocytes (which appeared as a dark and nonfluorescent shadow) in the liver sinusoid in front of the fluorescent leukocyte indicated that the leukocyte had adhered to the sinusoid and produced an obstruction to blood flow. Reviewing the videotape confirmed that these two leukocytes did not move even at the end of 30 min when the experiment was terminated.

Leukocyte and Erythrocyte Velocities in Liver Sinusoids

As described above, by playing back the videotape the leukocyte velocity in a liver sinusoid was determined by calculating the distance traversed by the fluorescent leukocyte from consecutive video frames. The erythrocyte velocity in the same liver sinusoid was determined by calculating the average transit time of the passage of the erythrocytes between two video windows which had a fixed separation distance. Figure 4 shows a pilot study in 13 liver sinusoids in one rat, in which both leukocyte and erythrocyte velocities were determined. Only the mean values of the velocities are shown. Thus, in this experiment, during the reperfusion phase following 30-min ischemia of the liver, the leukocyte velocity was approximately 80% of the corresponding erythrocyte velocity in the liver sinusoids.

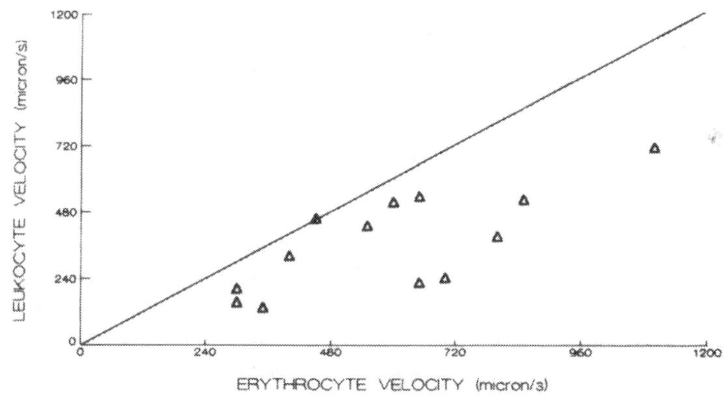

Fig. 4. Cross-plot of leukocyte and erythrocyte velocities in the same sinusoids in the reperfusion phase after a period of ischemia to the liver. Each *triangle* represents the mean value of the corresponding leukocyte and erythrocyte velocities. The *straight line* is the line of identity

←

Fig. 3a–c. Photographs taken from video monitor, showing liver microcirculation observed under fluorescence microscopy. **a** Line drawing of the liver microcirculation approximately 5½ min after starting reperfusion of the liver following a 30-min period of ischemia. *Arrows* indicate direction of blood flow. The two fluorescent leukocytes indicated by *asterisks* in **b** and **c** are outlined to enhance their visibility. Video field counts are shown above the video timer (hours: minutes: seconds)

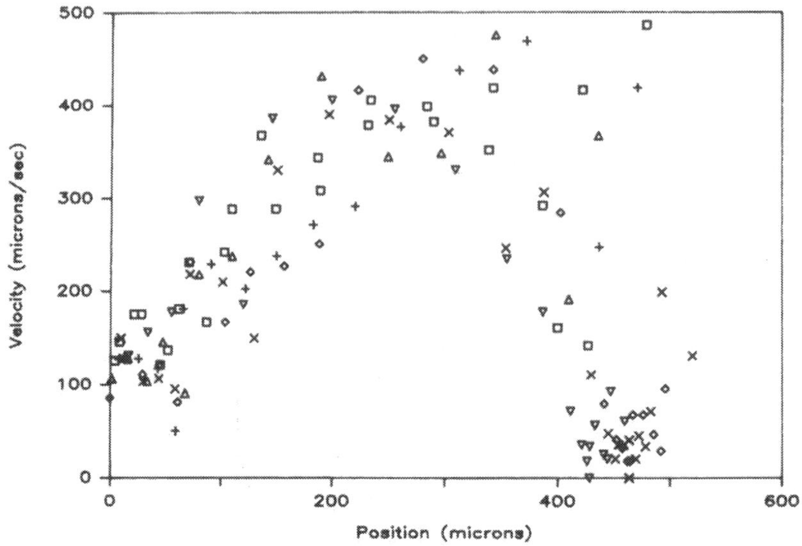

Fig. 5. Cross-plot of leukocyte velocity versus leukocyte position in a hepatic venule. The position at 0 μm indicates the point where the liver sinusoid enters the hepatic venule. Zero leukocyte velocity indicates that the leukocyte has become adherent to the wall of the venule. Each *symbol* indicates one fluorescent leukocyte

Leukocyte Velocity in Hepatic Venule

The distribution of the leukocyte velocity along the length of a hepatic venule was analyzed during the reperfusion phase following 30-min ischemia of the liver. By playing back the videotape, the position of the fluorescent leukocyte (in respect to the point where the liver sinusoid entered the hepatic venule) and the velocity of the leukocyte were determined as described above. Figure 5 summarizes the velocity distribution of six leukocytes in one hepatic venule. Thus, when the leukocyte began to enter the hepatic venule (position 0 μm), its velocity (100–150 μm) was only one-third of the maximum velocity (about 400 μm/s), which was detected at a point about 300 μm downstream from the entrance of the sinusoid into the venule. Further downstream along the venule, the leukocyte significantly decelerated (i.e., decreasing velocity) until a point 450 μm from the entrance of the sinusoid, where the leukocyte became adhered to the wall of the venule (i.e., zero velocity).

Discussion

Preliminary results from the present study demonstrate several aspects of the quantitative analysis of leukocyte dynamics in the liver microcirculation. In particular, our results confirm the contention that plugging of the microcirculation by adherent leukocytes occurs during the reperfusion phase following a period of ischemia of the liver. Adherence of leukocytes to the hepatic venule did not completely occlude blood flow but undoubtedly reduced the effective lumen of the venule and enhanced the resistance to flow. In contrast, adherence of leukocytes to the wall of the liver sinusoid completely obstructed blood flow through the sinusoid. The above features inevitably have a profound impact on liver transplantation. Since ischemia and reperfusion are features of liver transplantation, this area warrants further investigation in the future development of liver transplantation.

References

1. Starzl TF (1984) Liver transplantation. Hepatology 4 (Suppl): S47–49
2. Koo A, Liang IYS (1977) Blood flow in hepatic sinusoids in experimental hemorrhagic shock in the rat. Microvasc Res 13: 315–325
3. Arfors KE (1986) Free radicals in microcirculation. Acta Physiol Scand Suppl 548: 7
4. Atalla SL, Toledo-Pereyra LH, MacKenzie GH, Cederna JP. (1985) Influence of oxygen-derived free radical scavengers on ischemic livers. Transplantation 40: 584–590
5. Clemens MG, McDonagh PF, Chaudry IH, Baue AE (1985) Hepatic microcirculatory failure after ischemia and reperfusion: Improvement with ATP-$MgCl_2$ treatment. Am J Physiol 248: H804–811
6. Koo A (1984) Current methods and concepts on the visceral microcirculation. Prog Appl Microcirc 6: 54–68
7. Engler R, Schmid-Schombein GW, Pavelec RS (1983) Leukocyte capillary plug-ging in myocardial ischemia and reperfusion in the dog. Am J Pathol 111: 98–111
8. Engler R, Dahlgren MD, Morris DD, Peterson MA, Schmid-Schonbein GW (1986) Role of leukocytes in response to acute myocardial ischemia and reflow in dogs. Am J Physiol 251: H314–322
9. Bunnag SC, Bunnag S, Warner NE (1963) Microcirculation in the islets of Langerhans of the mouse. Anat Rec 146: 117–124
10. Warner NE, Bunnag S, Bunnag SC (1965) Microcirculation of the islets of Langerhans in experimental endotoxemia in mice. Biblthca Anat 7: 449–452
11. Koo A (1986) Liver microvascular flow in rats: Quantitation by laser Doppler flowmetric technique and effects of sodium dehydrocholate. J Gastroenterol Hepatol 1: 347–358

Role of the Hepatic Microcirculation in the Pathogenesis and Development of Alcoholic Liver Disease: Possible Involvement of Hypercatecholaminemia in Alcoholic Liver Damage

Nobuhiro Sato, Sunao Kawano, Takakatsu Matsumura, Harumasa Yoshihara, Taizo Hijioka, Hiroshi Eguchi, and Takenobu Kamada[1]

Summary

The effect of adrenaline on the hepatic microcirculation and hepatic oxygenation was investigated in normal and alcoholic rats. The intraperitoneal administration of adrenaline (0.25-mg, 0.5-mg/kg body weight) to rats decreased regional hepatic hemoglobin (Hb) concentration, an index of regional hepatic blood volume, and reduced the oxygen saturation of Hb in the regional hepatic tissue. A rise of serum glutamic-pyruvic transaminase (GPT) activity resulted. The reduction of hepatic Hb oxygenation was closely correlated with an elevation of serum GPT activity.

The adrenaline treatment caused a remarkable drop in sinusoidal blood flow velocity in hepatic lobules as measured by a TV monitor using the dual-slit photometric method.

The chronically ethanol-treated rats (20% ethanol for 3 months) showed a more severe hepatic hypoxia and higher elevation of serum GPT level in response to adrenaline treatment than normal control rats.

These findings support the possible involvement of hypercatecholaminemia in the development and progression of alcoholic liver damage through microcirculatory disturbance.

Introduction

The involvement of hypoxia in the pathogenesis of alcoholic liver damage still remains inconclusive. The acute ingestion of alcohol stimulates hepatic oxygen consumption [1, 2], which appears to be compensated by enhanced oxygen supply to the tissue through an increase in portal and hepatic arterial blood flow [2–4]. On the other hand, alcoholic patients show elevated blood catecholamine levels, such as adrenaline and noradrenaline [5], and we previously demonstrated a close relationship between hypercatecholaminemia and hepatic

[1] Department of Medicine, Osaka University Medical School, 1–50, Fukushima 1-chome, Fukushima-ku, Osaka, 553 Japan

damage evidenced by the rise of serum transaminase activity [6]. Alpha-agonists of catecholamine is characteristic of vasoconstrictive effect to decrease hepatic blood flow [7, 8]. Thus, this study was conducted to examine if hypercatecholaminemia induces hepatic hypoxia, leading to liver cell damage.

Materials and Methods

Sprague-Dawley rats were used. The alcoholic state was induced in rats by the administration of ethanol (20% v/v) in the drinking water for 3 months. The normal control and alcoholic rats were anesthetized with pentobarbital (37.5 mg/kg intraperitoneally).

Analysis of Hepatic Hemodynamics by Reflectance Spectrophotometry

The index of regional hepatic Hb concentration and the oxygen saturation of regional hepatic Hb were determined with reflectance spectrophotometry as previously reported [1]. The abdomen of anesthetized rats was incised along the midline. A flexible fiber-optic bundle (6 mm in diameter, Sumitomo Elect. Ind., Osaka, Japan) was introduced and kept in gentle contact with the liver surface at the point of measurement. The regional hepatic tissue Hb content was determined from the difference in absorbance between 569 nm and 650 nm (ΔEr569–650), since this parameter has a good correlation with local tissue Hb concentration [1]. The oxygen saturation of regional hepatic tissue blood hemoglobin was estimated from the hepatic spectrum at three different wavelengths (569, 577, and 586 nm) as described previously [1]. The following equaton was used:

$$SO_2 = [0.673\,(\Delta Er(577-586) - 9/17 \times \Delta Er(569-586))/\Delta Er(569-586)] \times 100\%.$$

In Vivo Microscopic Observation and Measurement of Sinusoidal Erythrocyte Flow Velocity

Sinusoidal blood flow velocity was measured as described elsewhere [9]. The liver of anesthetized rats was exposed by making a left subcostal incision and positioned over a window in a specially designed microscope stage. The liver was examined with a Leitz water-immersion objective (x23) and the optical image was recorded with a Nubicon camera (Hitachi HR-34) and videotape recorder (Sony U-matic). Sinusoidal blood flow velocity was measured from a video monitor using a dual-slit photometric method. Two photodiodes were put on the measuring sinusoid in the video monitor and the signal data for 1 min were stored in a personal computer (TEAC PS-9000). One value was determined from 5-s signal data and the mean blood flow velocity for 1 min at one sinusoid was calculated from 12 values. The sinusoidal blood flow velocity was determined before and 15 min after intraperitoneal administration of adrenaline at the dose of 0.25 mg/kg body weight. Statistical analysis was performed with Student's *t*-test.

Results

Adrenaline was administered intraperitoneally at the dose of 0.25 mg or 0.50 mg/kg body weight. Figure 1 shows the change in regional hepatic tissue Hb concentration following the administration of adrenaline. The regional hepatic Hb concentration decreased by approximately 10%–20% in the initial 15 min and the decrease lasted for 2 h after administration. Treatment with 0.5 mg/kg adrenaline produced a greater decrease in regional hepatic Hb concentration than with 0.25 mg/kg. As shown in Fig. 2, the oxygen saturation of regional hepatic Hb declined to the lowest degree between 15 and 45 min, and then it returned gradually to the basal level 120 min after the treatment. The decrease in the Hb-oxygen saturation was greater after administration of 0.50 mg/kg adrenaline than after 0.25 mg/kg adrenaline. When alcoholic rats were treated with adrenaline, the oxygen saturation of hepatic tissue Hb dropped to a lower level and the low hepatic oxygenation lasted longer than in normal rats (Fig. 2).

Figure 3 presents the values of serum GPT and its relation to mean hepatic Hb oxygenation following adrenaline administration. The elevation of serum GPT was closely related to the reduction of hepatic Hb oxygenation. In comparison with normal controls, alcoholic rats showed a lower mean hepatic Hb oxygenation and, consequently, more elevated serum GPT activity. The effect of adrenaline (0.50 mg/kg) on sinusoidal blood flow velocity is shown in Fig. 4. Sinusoidal blood flow velocity varied between 0.10 and 0.26 mm/s before adrenaline administration and it was reduced remarkably. In some areas of the sinusoids with a lower steady state blood flow velocity, the blood flow completely stopped 30 min after administration.

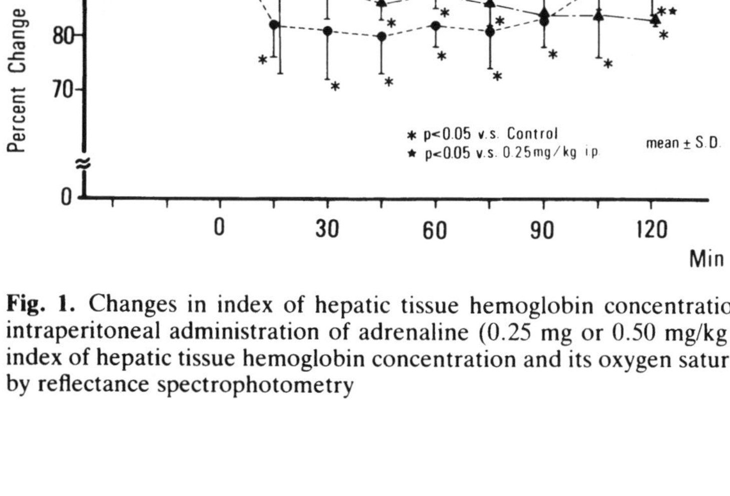

Fig. 1. Changes in index of hepatic tissue hemoglobin concentration in rats following intraperitoneal administration of adrenaline (0.25 mg or 0.50 mg/kg body weight). The index of hepatic tissue hemoglobin concentration and its oxygen saturation were assessed by reflectance spectrophotometry

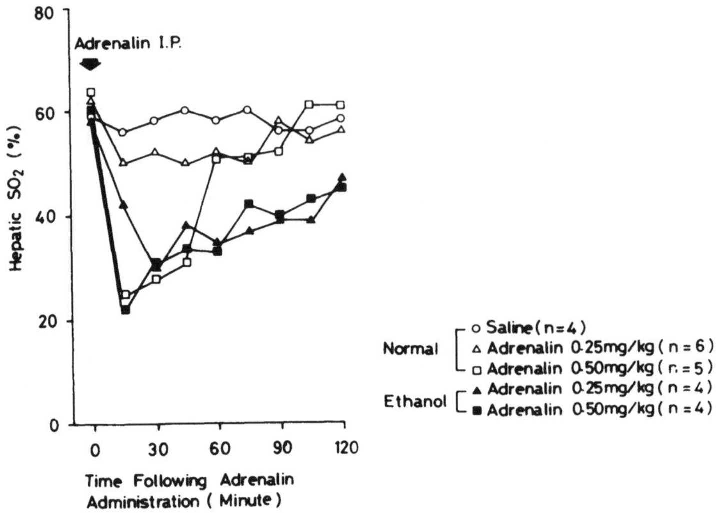

Fig. 2. Changes in hepatic tissue hemoglobin oxygenation level following intraperitoneal administration of adrenaline in control and alcoholic rats

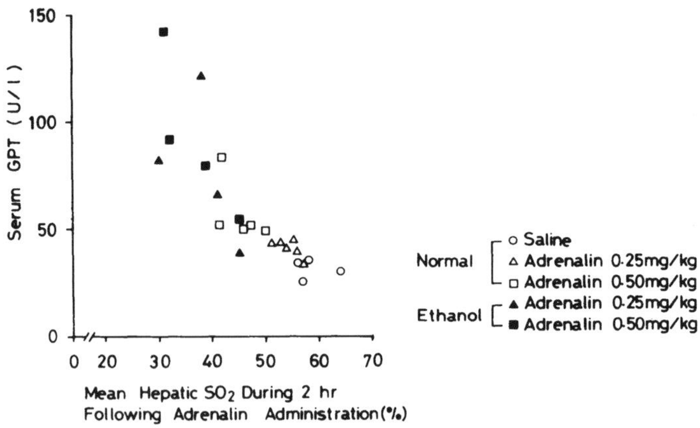

Fig. 3. Effect of intraperitoneal administration of adrenaline (0.05 mg/kg body weight) on sinusoidal blood flow velocity. Sinusoidal blood flow velocity was measured from images on TV monitor by dual-slit method

Discussion

Adrenaline is a vasoactive hormore [7, 8]. The infusion of low-dose adrenaline produces hepatic arterial vasodilatation, although a large dose causes vasoconstriction of both the hepatic arterial and portal venous vascular beds [7, 8]. The intraperitoneal administration of adrenaline at the dose of 0.25 mg/kg or 0.50 mg/kg decreased the regional hepatic Hb concentration (Fig. 1). Since the regional hepatic Hb concentration reflects the hepatic vascular bed containing the erythrocytes, the dose of adrenaline administered in this study was shown to

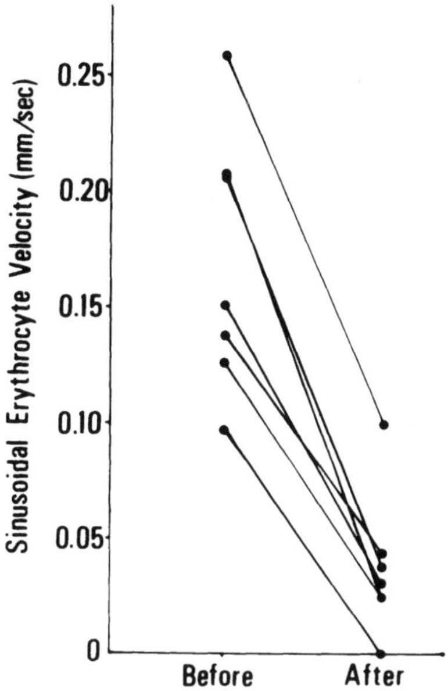

Fig. 4. Relation between serum GPT activity and mean hepatic oxygenation level over 2 h following intraperitoneal administration of adrenaline. Blood was withdrawn from rats 2 h after adrenaline treatment

have a vasoconstrictive effect on the hepatic vasculature. Indeed, the sinusoidal blood flow velocity was reduced remarkably and, in part, completely ceased (Fig. 4). These decreases in hepatic vascular beds and sinusoidal blood flow could be attributed to the decrease in hepatic blood flow due to adrenaline-induced vasoconstriction. In addition to these microcirculatory effects, adrenaline is known to stimulate hepatic oxygen consumption [10, 11]. Thus, the vasoconstrictive and stimulatory effects on hepatic oxygen consumption seem to contribute to the hepatic tissue hypoxia, which was suggested by the lowering of oxygen saturation of tissue Hb (Fig. 2). In response to adrenaline administration, hepatic blood Hb oxygenation level greatly decreased to about 20%. Hepatic oxygenation assessed by reflectance spectrophotometry expresses the mean value of Hb oxygenation within the liver lobule. Our recent study using an in vivo microscopic system coupled with spectrophotometry confirmed the presence of an oxygen gradient along the liver lobule, demonstrating a heterogeneous oxygenation distribution in both periportal and pericentral regions of the liver lobule [12]. Thus, it seems likely that an ischemic region occurs downstream along the sinusoid of the liver lobule when the mean hepatic tissue Hb oxygenation shows a large decrease. These considerations are consistent with the finding that some sinusoids show complete cease of blood flow after adrenaline administration. Lemaster et al. [13] demonstrated that hepatocytes exposed to ischemia and hypoxia develop bleb formation in the cell surface membrane, through which intracellular components such as enzymes are released into blood stream. The adrenaline-induced elevation of serum GPT is related to the degree of hepatic hypoxia (Fig. 3). Consequently, it is considered that adrenaline treatment produces hepatic ischemia and hypoxia, which result in hepatic cell damage.

Alcoholic patients frequently reveal the symptoms of hypercatecholaminemia such as elevated blood pressure, tachycardia, and elevated serum free fatty acid level. We previously demonstrated the close relationship between plasma catecholamine concentration and liver damage [6]. The present study has shown that the intraperitoneal administration of adrenaline is capable of producing hepatic damage. Therefore, hypercatecholaminemia found in alcoholic patients may be involved in the development of hepatic cell damage through a microcirculatory disturbance.

References

1. Sato N, Matsumura T, Shichiri T, Kamada T, Abe H, Hagihara B (1981) Hemoperfusion, rate of oxygen consumption and redox levels of mitochondrial cytochrome c(+c1) in liver in situ of anesthetized rat measured by reflectance spectrophotometry. Biochem Biophys Acta 634: 1–10
2. Jauhonen P, Baraona E, Miyakawa H, Lieber CS (1982) Mechanism for selective perivenular hepatotoxity of ethanol. Alcoholism 3: 350–357
3. Sato N, Kamada T, Kawano S, Hayashi N, Kishida Y, Meren H, Yoshihara H, Abe H (1985) Effect of acute and chronic ethanol consumption on hepatic tissue oxygen tension in rats. Alcohol 2: 463–468
4. Yoshihara H, Sato N, Sasaki Y, Uchima E, Inoue A, Matsumura T, Hayashi N, Kawano S, Kamada T, Abe H (1985) Effect of alcohol ingestion on portal venous blood flow in healthy volunteers: Comparison between the subjects with and without ALDH I isozyme. Alcohol 2: 463–468
5. Ogata M, Mendelson JH, Mello NK (1971) Adrenal function and alcoholism: II. Catecholamines. Psychosomat Med 33: 159–180
6. Yoshihara H, Kawano S, Hayashi N, Kishida Y, Matsumura T, Meren H, Kamada T (1981) A study on plasma catecholamine level in alcoholics—its relation to liver injury. Jpn J Alcohol Studies Drug Dependence 16: S74–S75
7. Greenway CV, Stark RD (1971) Hepatic vascular bed. Physiol Rev 51: 23–65
8. Richardson PDI, Withrington PG (1981) Liver blood flow: II. Effect of drug and hormones on liver blood flow. Gastroenterology 81: 356–375
9. Sato N, Eguchi H, Inoue A, Matsumura T, Kawano S, Kamada T (1986) Hepatic microcirculation in Zucker fatty rats. Adv Exp Med Biol 200: 477–483
10. Scholz R, Schwabe U (1980) Stimulation of ethanol metabolism by catecholamines. In: Thurman RG (ed.) Alcohol and aldehyde metabolizing system. Plenum, New York, pp-601–618
11. Bernstein J, Videla L, Israel Y (1975) Hormonal influences in the development of the hypermetabolic state of the liver produced by chronic administration of ethanol. J Pharmacol Exp Therapeut 192: 583–591
12. Eguchi H, Sato N, Matsumura T, Kawano S, Kamada T (1988) In vivo estimation of oxygen saturation of hemoglobin in hepatic lobules in rats. Oxygen Transport to Tissue X (in press)
13. Lemaster JJ, Stemkowski CJ, Ji S, Thurman RG (1983) Cell surface changes and enzyme release during hypoxia and reoxygenation in the isolated perfused rat liver. J Cell Biol 97: 778–786

Abnormalities in the Hepatic Sinusoids: Pathological Basis of Self-perpetuation of Liver Cirrhosis

Masaya Oda[1], Nobuhiro Tsukada[1], Hirokazu Komatsu[1], Koya Honda[1], Kotaro Kaneko[1], Toshifumi Azuma[1], Mayumi Ueno[1], Norihito Watanabe[1], Masahiko Nakamura[1], Isao Okazaki,[2] and Masaharu Tsuchiya[1]

Introduction

The hepatic microcirculatory system consists of four microvascular components: the terminal portal venule and hepatic arteriole as two afferent vessels, the sinusoids corresponding to the capillary bed, and the terminal hepatic venule as an efferent vessel. This microvascular unit is the basis for the simple liver acinus, which has been proposed as the smallest functional unit of the hepatic lobule [1]. The major components among these microvessels are the hepatic sinusoids, which are characterized by the presence of the sieve-like pores [2], i.e., the sinusoidal endothelial fenestrae (SEF), and by the absence of the basement membrane beneath the sinusoidal endothelial cells. These ultra-structural characteristics reflect the active exchange of metabolites between the sinusoidal blood and the hepatocytes, maintaining constant liver cell functions. In this respect, impairment of the sinusoidal blood flow directly leads to a variety of liver cell dysfunction.

According to in vivo and in vitro studies, the contraction and dilatation of the SEF contributes to the dynamic regulation of sinusoidal blood flow mainly by control of the transport of plasma components from the sinusoid into the perisinusoidal space (the space of Disse) [3–10]. The aim of the present paper is to review our recent studies [3, 7] on the adrenergic and cholinergic control of the dilatation and contraction of the SEF and on the alterations of hepatic sinusoids in cirrhosis, particularly the changes in the SEF and the formation of the basement membrane components, type IV collagen, laminin, and glycosaminoglycans in the perisinusoidal space; we shall also show how these sinusoidal abnormalities contribute to the progression of liver cirrhosis.

Department of Internal Medicine[1] and Department of Preventive Medicine and Public Health[2], School of Medicine, Keio University, 35 Shinanomachi, Shinjuku-ku, Tokyo, 160 Japan

Hepatic Sinusoidal Responses to Aminergic Receptor Agonists in Normal Liver

Intravital Microscopic Alterations of Hepatic Microcirculation

By intravital microscopy using the transillumination method, the hemodynamics of the hepatic microcirculatory system on the surface of the rat liver has been clearly demonstrated [3]. The blood is seen flowing radially from the terminal portal venules (TPV) into the anastomosing sinusoids surrounding the portal tract. The sinusoidal blood flow is uniform and rapid, draining into the terminal hepatic venules (THV), corresponding to the periphery of the hepatic lobule. It has been observed that the blood leaves the terminal hepatic arterioles directly emptying into the sinusoids in a jetlike manner but such observations are extremely rare.

Infusion of an α-adrenergic receptor agonist, norepinephrine, via a catheter inserted into a mesenteric vein or abdominal aorta causes a remarkable contraction of the TPV followed by a variety of microcirculatory disturbances, such as the sludge phenomenon and regurgitation in the sinusoidal blood flow [3]. The sinusoids are also found to be contracted simultaneously, leading to complete stasis of the blood stream in some sinusoids and no red blood cell supply to others—plasma skimming. Although there is no contraction of the THV in the early stage of norepinephrine infusion, the blood flow in the THV in an extremely low-flow state frequently accompanies the sludge phenomenon and regurgitation. These hepatic microcirculatory disturbances are more intense with norepinephrine infusion via the portal vein than via the hepatic artery. In contrast, infusion of muscarinic acetylcholine receptor agonists, acetylcholine and bethanechol, and a β-adrenergic receptor agonist, isoproterenol, enhances the sinusoidal blood flow. The TPV and sinusoids appear to be dilated, and the blood flow becomes more rapid.

Quantitative Changes in Hepatic Intralobular (Sinusoidal) Blood Flow

The hepatic sinusoidal blood flow measured by the hydrogen gas clearance method is markedly reduced by norepinephrine infusion, while it is significantly increased by acetylcholine, bethanechol, and isoproterenol infusion [3, 5]. Histamine and endotoxin infusion also decreases the sinusoidal blood flow [11].

Scanning Electron-Microscopic Alterations in Sinusoidal Endothelial Fenestrae

Two types of the sinusoidal endothelial fenestrae (SEF), sievelike small pores and relatively large scattered pores, are evident within the hepatic sinusoidal endothelium in the periportal area (zone 1) [3, 5, 6]. Only sievelike pores are present within the sinusoidal endothelium in the perivenular area (zone 3) surrounding the terminal hepatic venule. Both large and small latex particles, 0.26 and 0.09 μm in diameter, infused through a mesenteric vein catheter, are seen to enter the perisinusoidal space in zone 1, while only small latex particles enter the persinusoidal space in zone 3 [4], indicating that both small and large pores exist within the periportal sinusoidal endothelium in the normal state.

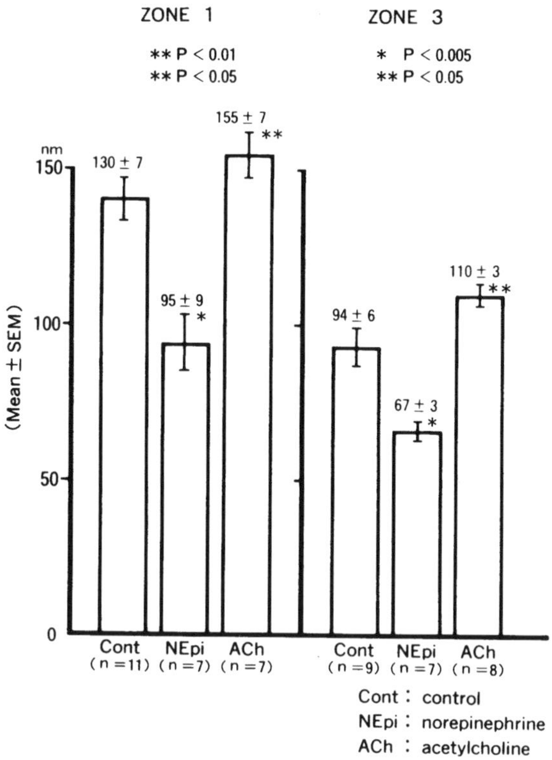

Fig. 1. Effects of biogenic amines on the diameter of the sinusoidal endothelial fenestrae in a normal rat liver

Morphometric analysis reveals that the SEF are significantly larger in diameter in zone 1 (129 ± 5 nm, $n = 13$) than in zone 3 (93 ± 4 nm, $n = 13$; $P < 0.001$), while there are fewer SEF in zone 1 (4.36 ± 0.53/μm^2, $n = 13$) than in zone 3 (7.39 ± 0.53/μm^2, $n = 13$; $P < 0.001$). The presence of relatively large scattered pores as well as sievelike small pores is also proved in the primary cultured sinusoidal endothelial cells isolated from the rat liver [6].

By norepinephrine infusion via a mesenteric catheter, the SEF are reduced in diameter in zone 1 (95 ± 9 nm, $n = 7$) and in zone 3 (67 ± 3 nm, $n = 7$) in comparison with those in controls (130 ± 7 nm, $n = 11$, 94 ± 6 nm, $n = 9$), while they are increased in zone 1 (155 ± 7 nm, $n = 7$) and zone 3 (110 ± 3nm, $n = 8$) by acetylcholine infusion ($P < 0.05$; Fig. 1). The SEF are also found to be increased in diameter by the infusion of isoproterenol, a β-adrenergic receptor agonist, and they tend to be decreased in diameter by histamine and serotonin infusion.

All these contraction and dilatation responses of the SEF to the exogenous administration of the biogenic amines are reproduced in the primary cultures of the isolated sinusoidal endothelial cells [7], implying that these amines directly act on the endothelial cells via the cell surface receptors. In the intracellular regulatory mechanism of this contraction and dilatation of the SEF, actin filaments in the sinusoidal endothelium may play an important role in the presence of calcium ions and calmodulin, Ca^{2+}-binding protein [8–10, 12].

Alterations in Hepatic Microcirculatory System in Liver Cirrhosis

Changes in Hepatic Sinusoidal Blood and Bile Flow

The hepatic sinusoidal blood flow measured by the hydrogen gas clearance method is significantly reduced in CCl_4-induced rat liver cirrhosis (42.1 ± 4.2 ml/min/100 g, mean $\pm$ SEM, $n = 17$) compared with controls (58.9 ± 3.0 ml/min/100 g, $n = 11$; $P < 0.005$). The bile flow measured by the common bile duct cannulation method is also decreased in CCl_4-induced liver cirrhosis (2.25 ± 0.18 μl/min/100 g body weight) compared with controls (2.68 ± 0.10 μl/min/100 g body weight; $P < 0.05$).

Morphological Alterations in Hepatic Sinusoids

Liver cirrhosis is morphologically characterized by the formation of fibrous septa and regenerative nodules concomitant with disorganization of the hepatic lobule. In the process of hepatic fibrosis, collagen fibers extend into the parenchyma from the perivenular areas as well as from the portal tracts, particularly along the vacuolated hepatocytes; this leads to the formation of fibrous septa between the portal tracts themselves, the portal tracts and tributaries of the hepatic venules, or between the hepatic venules themselves. In these fibrous septa, microvascular shunts are formed between the portal venules and the hepatic venules, resulting in the escape of portal blood from the sinusoids into the efferent microvessels.

Deposition of proteoglycans in perisinusoidal space. Digestive PAS(periodic acid-Schiff)-positive and toluidine blue-metachromatic substances are abnormally accumulated in the fibrous tissue and around the degenerated hepatocytes. Electron microscopically, in the ruthenium red (RR) en bloc stained preparations, the RR-positive, electron-dense amorphous substances, largely corresponding to proteoglycans, i.e., glycosaminoglycans protein complex, are excessively deposited in the perisinusoidal space, where collagen fibrils are rarely present (Fig. 2a). These substances are also closely associated with unstriated collagen fibrils formed in the perisinusoidal space in the early stage of fibrosis. In the progression of perisinusoidal fibrosis, the RR-positive globular or band-like substances are periodically bound to the outer surface of mature collagen fibers formed in the perisinusoidal space, largely in accordance with the periodic cross bands [13].

Immunohistochemical and immunoelectron-microscopic localization of type I, IV collagen and laminin. Immunohistochemical observations using anti-type I, IV collagen and laminin antibody have been made on control and CCl_4-induced cirrhotic rat liver. The specific immunofluorescence-positive or immunoperoxidase-positive substances showing the presence of type I collagen are largely confined to the portal tract and perivenular portion in controls (Fig. 3a), whereas they are noted on mature collagen fibers in the fibrous septa and partly along the sinusoids in the cirrhotic liver (Fig. 3b). Electron microscopically, the immunoperoxidase-positive, electron-dense substances showing the presence of

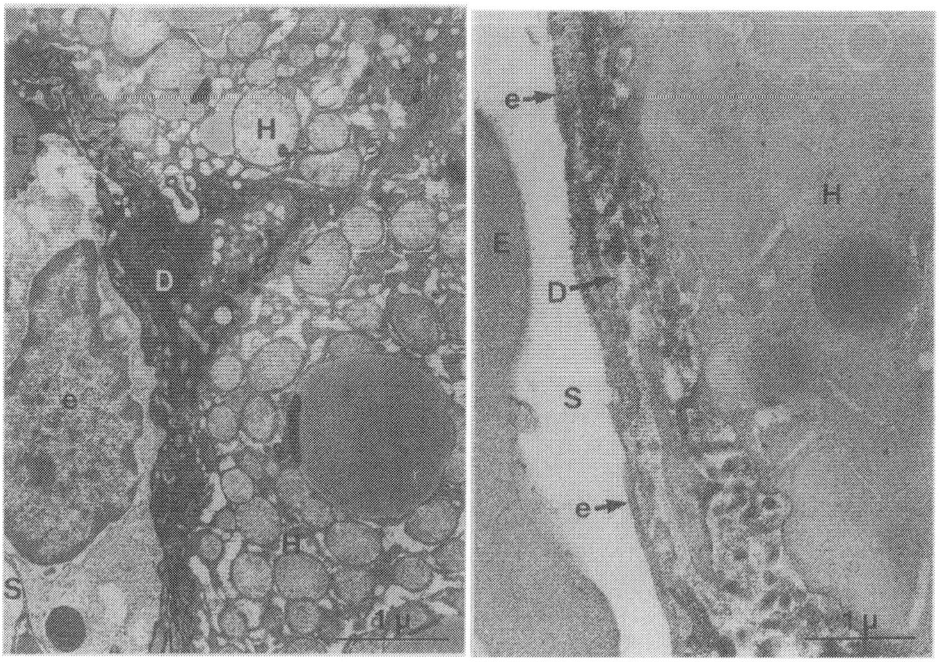

a b

Fig. 2a, b. Transmission electron micrographs demonstrating the deposition of glycosaminoglycans and type I collagen in the perisinusoidal space in CCl_4-induced rat liver cirrhosis. **a** The ruthenium red(RR)-positive, electron-dense amorphous substances corresponding to glycosaminoglycans (GAG) are heavily deposited in the perisinusoidal space (*D*). RR en bloc stain, × 15000. **b** Immunoperoxidase-positive, electron-dense substances showing the presence of type I collagen are noted in the perisinusoidal space (*D*). *e* endothelium, *H* hepatocyte, *E* erythrocyte, *S* sinusoid, Noncounterstained, × 15000

type I collagen are deposited in the perisinusoidal space, particularly near the fibrous septum (Fig. 2b).

Type IV collagen is located around blood vessels, such as portal, hepatic venules and arterioles, and bile ducts in the portal tract of control rat livers (Fig. 4a), whereas it is extensively distributed not only around the proliferated microvessels and bile ductules in the fibrous seputum, but also along the sinusoids, particularly in the parenchyma surrounded by the fibrous septum in the CCl_4-induced cirrhotic liver (Fig. 4b). The distribution of laminin is largely similar to that of type IV collagen both in control and cirrhotic livers (Fig. 4c, d). By immunoelectron microscopy, the immunoperoxidase-positive type IV collagen and laminin are found to be heavily deposited in the perisinusoidal space in the cirrhotic liver parenchyma (Fig. 5a, b). These immunoreactive type I, IV collagen and laminin are most frequently found in the dilated lumina of the rough endoplasmic reticulum and Golgi apparatus in Ito cells (fat-storing cells) and partly in those of hepatocytes in cirrhotic livers, indicating that these connective tissue components are synthesized mainly by Ito cells and partly by hepatocytes in the process of perisinusoidal fibrosis. The immunoelectron-microscopic

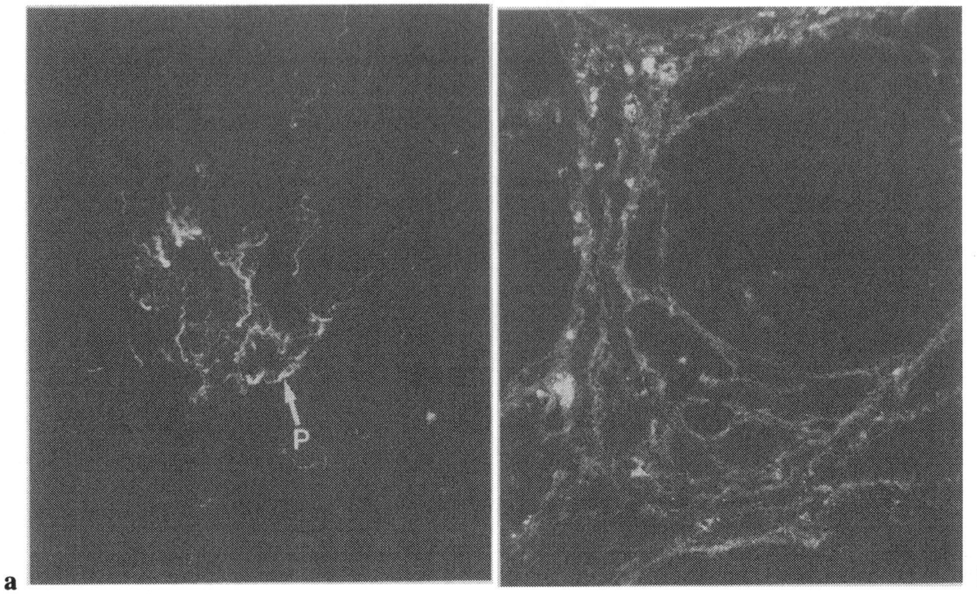

Fig. 3a, b. Immunofluorescence micrographs demonstrating the changes in the distribution of type I collagen in CCl_4-induced rat liver cirrhosis. **a** Specific immunofluorescence showing the presence of type I collagen is restricted to the portal tract (*P*) and around the tributaries of the hepatic venules in the control rat liver. **b** In the cirrhotic liver, the immunopositive type I collagen is distributed extensively in the fibrous septum and partly extends into the parenchyma along the sinusoids, surrounding the hepatocytes

findings also indicate that type IV and laminin would be partly produced by the sinusoidal endothelial cells.

Formation of basement membrane in perisinusoidal space (capillarization of hepatic sinusoids). As described, the basement membrane components, type IV collagen, laminin, and glycosaminoglycans (GAG) are seen to be deposited in the perisinusoidal space in CCl_4-induced liver cirrhosis. Transmission and scanning electron microscopy reveals the presence of small pores within the sinusoidal endothelium and small gaps between the adjacent sinusoidal endothelial cells without the basement membrane in the normal liver (Fig. 6a, c). By transmission electron microscopy, the basement membrance is observed to be formed both discontinuously and continuously beneath the sinusoidal endothelial cells (Fig. 6b). This morphological alteration of the hepatic sinusoids is termed capillarization of sinusoids [14].

Alterations of hepatic sinusoidal endothelial fenestrae. By scanning electron microscopy, the SEF are found to be significantly reduced both in number and diameter in the cirrhotic liver (Fig. 6d). Based on morphometric analysis, the SEF are markedly reduced both in number ($3.76 \pm 0.23/\mu m^2$, $n = 8$, $P < 0.001$)

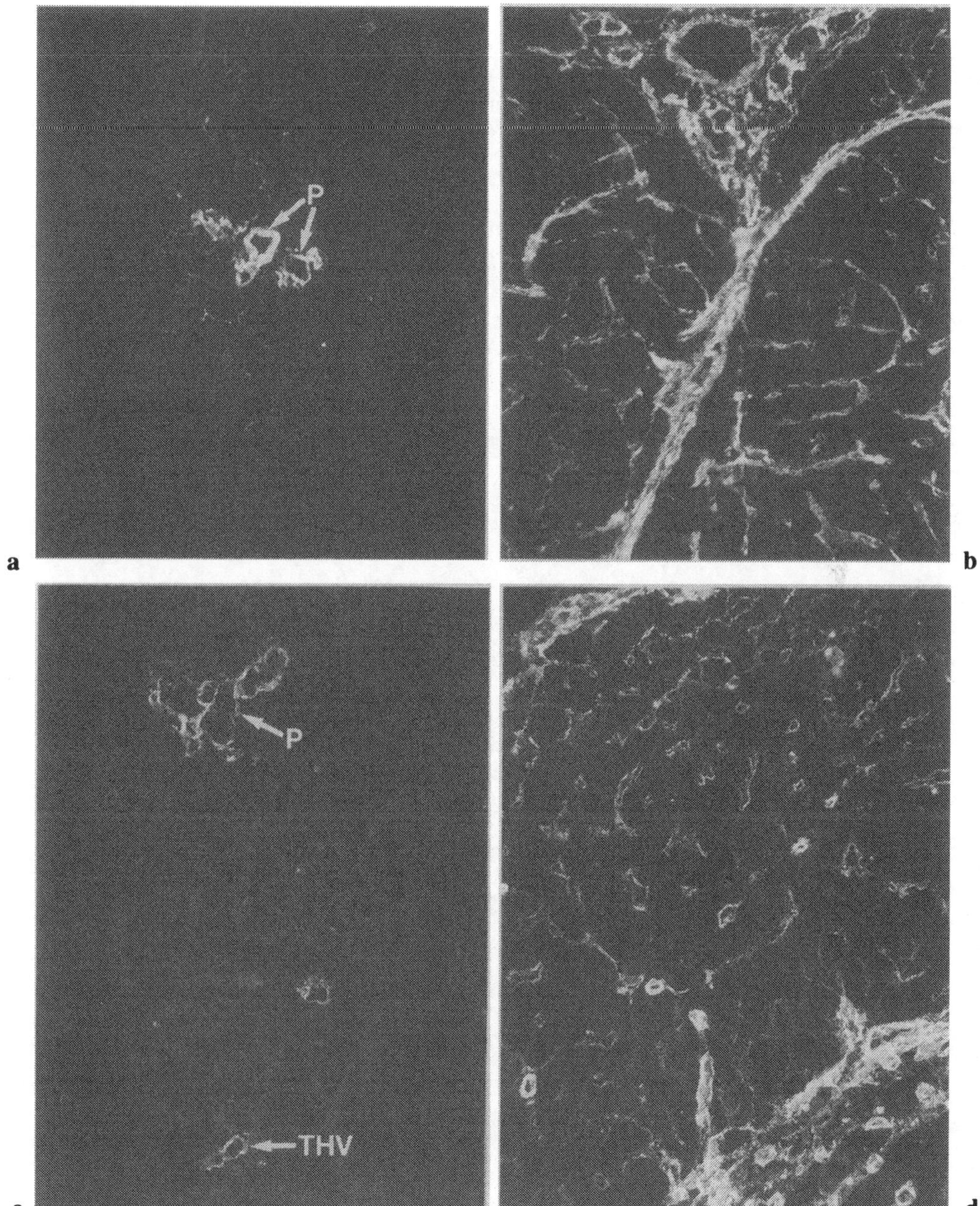

Fig. 4a–d. Immunofluorescence micrographs demonstrating the changes in the distribution of type IV collagen and laminin in CCl_4-induced rat liver cirrhosis. **a** Specific immunofluorescence for type IV collagen is localized around blood vessels and bile ducts in the portal tract (*P*) and around the tributaries of the hepatic venules in the control liver. **b** Immunopositive type IV collagen is deposited not only around the proliferated bile ductules and microvessels in the fibrous septum, but also along the sinusoids particularly near the fibrous septum. **c** Distribution of laminin in the control liver is similar to that of type IV collagen (cf. Fig. 4a). *P* portal tract, *THV* terminal hepatic venule. **d** Distribution of laminin in the CCl_4-induced cirrhotic liver is also similar to that of type IV collagen (cf. Fig. 4d). Note the sinusoidal pattern

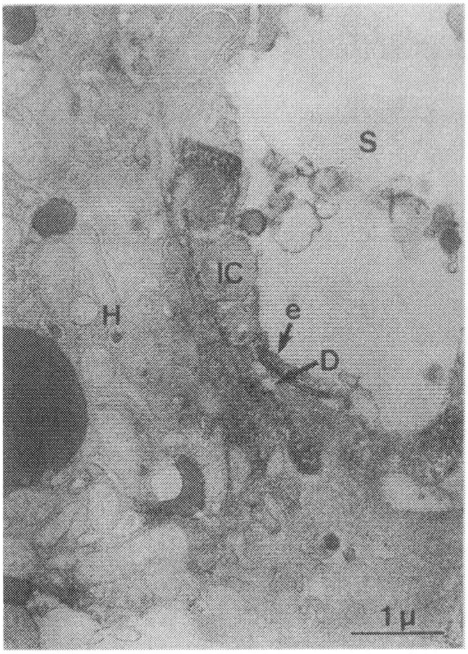

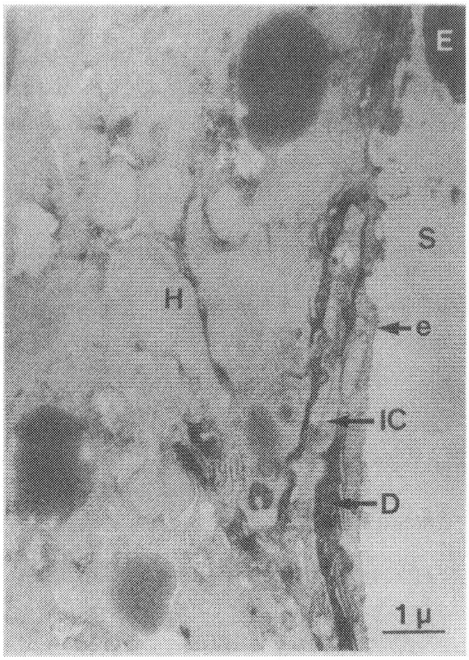

a b

Fig. 5a, b. Immunoelectron micrographs demonstrating the localization of type IV collagen and laminin in the CCl_4-induced rat cirrhotic liver. **a** Immunoperoxidase-positive type IV collagen is deposited in the perisinusoidal space (*D*). Immunoreactive substances are also evident in the cisternae of the rough endoplasmic reticulum in the hepatocyte (*H*) as well as in the Ito cell (*IC*). *S* sinusoid, *e* endothelium, Counterstained with lead citrate, × 12000. **b** Ultrastructural distribution of the immunoperoxidase-positive laminin is similar to that of type I collagen. Note that laminin is more densely deposited in both the perisinusoidal space (*D*) and the cisternae of the rough endoplasmic reticulum in the Ito cell (*IC*), in the hepatocyte (*H*), and also in the sinusoidal endothelium (*e*). *S:* sinusoid, *E* erythrocyte, Noncounterstained, × 8000

Fig. 6a–d. Ultrastructural alterations of the sinusoids in CCl_4-induced rat liver cirrhosis. **a** Transmission electron micrograph of control liver. There are small gaps (*arrowheads*) in or between the sinusoidal endothelial cells (*e*). *S* sinusoid, *H* hepatocyte. Uranyl acetate and lead citrate stain, × 14500. **b** Transmission electron micrograph of cirrhotic liver. The basement membrane (*BM*) is formed beneath the sinusoidal endothelial cells (*e*) with the prominent deposition of collagen fibers (*Co*) in the widened perisinusoidal space (*D*). Small gaps appear to be decreased in number. *S* sinusoid. Uranyl acetate and lead citrate stain, × 10700. **c** Scanning electron micrograph showing the luminal surface of the sinusoidal endothelium in a control liver. Sieve like small pores, one of the two types of the sinusoidal endothelial fenestrae, are evident in the sinusoidal endothelium in zone 3 of the hepatic lobule × 11000. **d** As **c** in a cirrhotic liver. Note that the sinusoidal endothelial fenestrae are markedly reduced both in number and in diameter. × 11000

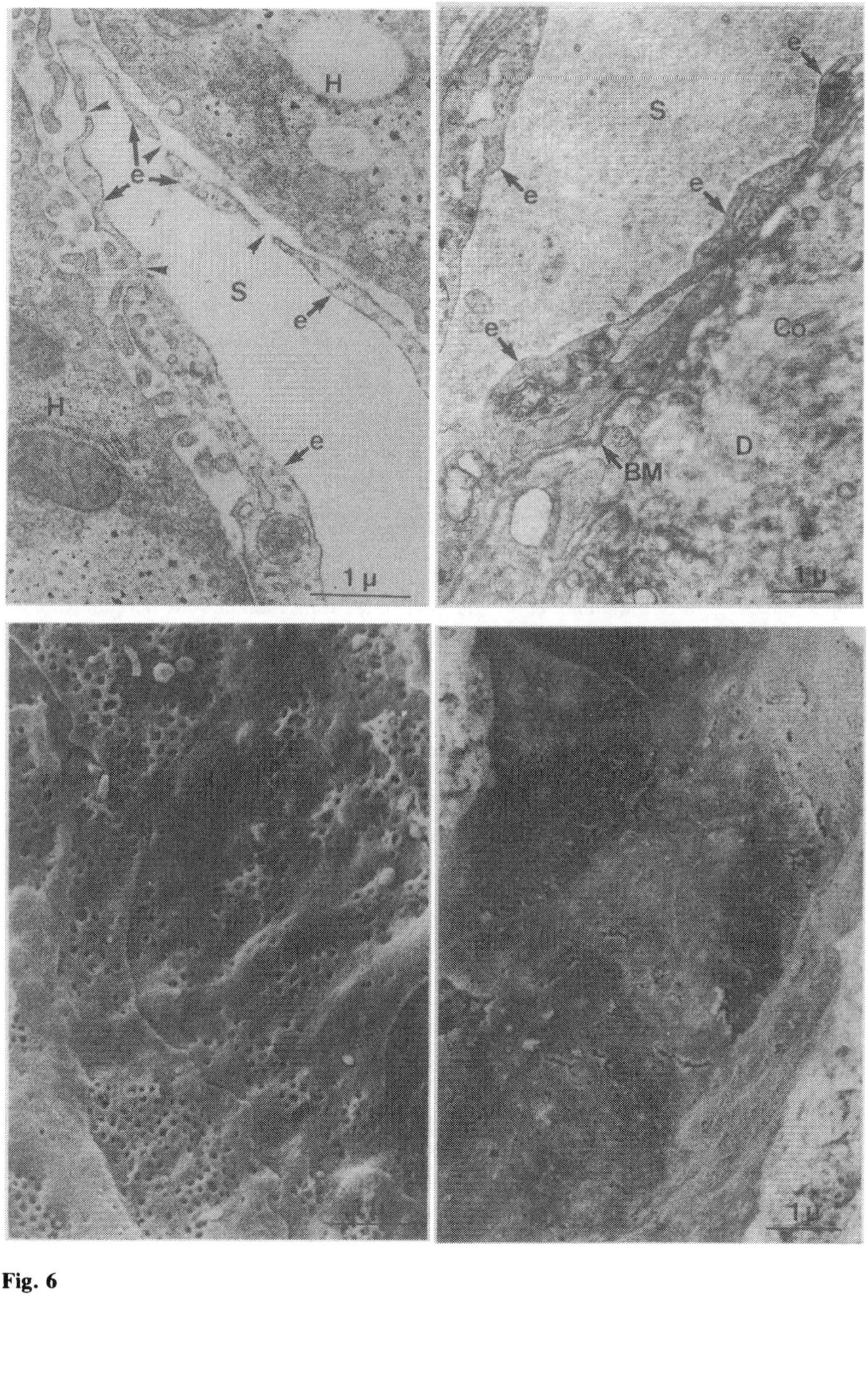

Fig. 6

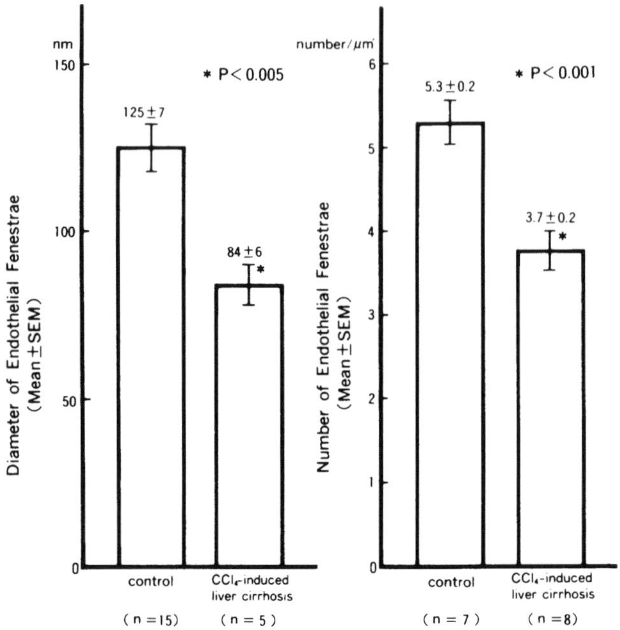

Fig. 7. Alterations of the diameter and number of the sinusoidal endothelial fenestrae in CCl_4-induced liver cirrhosis in rats

and diameter (84 ± 6 nm, $n = 5$, $P < 0.01$) in CCl_4-induced liver cirrhosis compared with the SEF in controls ($5.30 \pm 0.24/\mu m^2$, $n = 7$; 126 ± 8 nm, $n = 13$, respectively; Fig. 7) [15]. Similar results are obtained in the human cirrhotic liver; the number of the SEF ($2.80 \pm 0.35/\mu m^2$, $n = 5$) as well as the diameter (46 ± 6 nm, $n = 5$) are significantly smaller than in control livers ($6.57 \pm 0.88/\mu m^2$, $n = 8$, $P < 0.05$; 70 ± 5 nm, $n = 8$, respectively; $P < 0.01$) [15]. Thus, the decrease of the SEF in number and diameter concomitant with the accumulation of type IV collagen, laminin, and GAG in the cirrhotic liver, resulting in the formation of the basement membrance surrounding the sinusoidal endothelial cells, would inhibit free exchange of metabolites between the sinusoidal blood and hepatocytes, enhancing perisinusoidal fibrosis and impairment of hepatocyte functions.

Elevation of Norepinephrine, Histamine, and Endotoxin Content

Norepinephrine in the plasma, measured by high-performance liquid chromatography (HPLC), tends to be elevated in CCl_4-induced liver cirrhosis (0.55 ± 0.12 ng/ml, $n = 5$) compared with controls (0.31 ± 0.08 ng/ml, $n = 5$; $P < 0.1$). Histamine, measured by a modification of the method of Shore, is also increased (103.5 ± 20.5 ng/ml, $n = 5$) in liver cirrhosis compared with controls (59.9 ± 8.6 ng/ml, $n = 5$; $P < 0.1$). The chromogenic quantitative endotoxin assay reveals a significant increase in endotoxin content in the plasma of CCl_4-

induced cirrhotic rats (11.72 ± 1.23 pg/ml, $n = 10$) compared with controls (3.56 ± 0.57 pg/ml, $n = 10$; $P < 0.005$). Norepinephrine is released from the adrenergic nerve terminals, while histamine is derived from the mast cell granules, under the pathological conditions of liver cirrhosis. An elevation of endotoxin in the plasma may be attributable to an impairment of Kupffer's cell functions. As described, all these substances elevated in the plasma may be involved in the changes of the SEF and sinusoidal blood flow in liver cirrhosis.

Summary

The endothelial cells of the hepatic sinusoids, the major component of the hepatic microcirculatory system, possess a large number of small pores, i.e., SEF, but are not surrounded by the basement membrane. These ultrastructural features

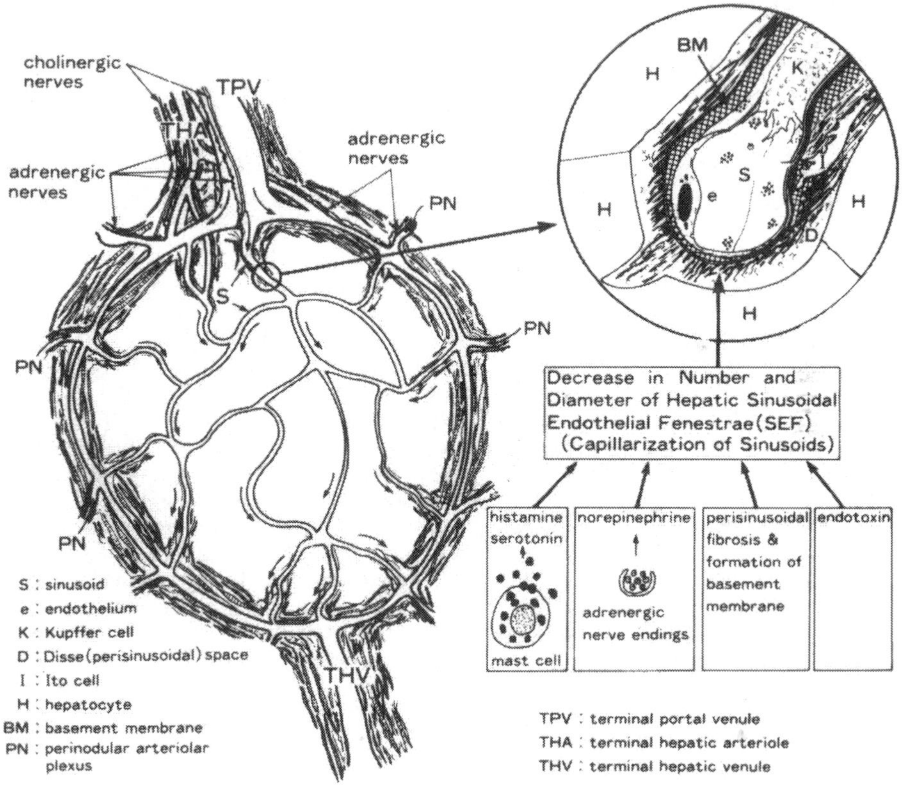

Fig. 8. Schematic illustration of the hepatic microcirculatory alterations in liver cirrhosis. Not only the deposition of glycosaminoglycans, type I, IV collagen, and laminin in the perisinusoidal space, but also the decrease of the sinusoidal endothelial fenestrae (SEF) both in number and diameter would interrupt the transition of sinusoidal plasma into the perisinusoidal space, contributing to the development of a self-perpetuating progression of liver cirrhosis

reflect the free and rapid metabolic exchange between the sinusoidal blood and hepatocytes, facilitating a variety of liver functions as a central organ in the body metabolism. Recent in vivo and in vitro studies imply that the contraction and dilatation of the SEF in response to changes in the sinusoidal blood flow and to the exogenous administration of a variety of biogenic amines contribute to the regulatory mechanism of sinusoidal blood flow and blood-hepatocyte exchange by controlling the transition of plasma components from the sinusoids into the perisinusoidal space. In experimental and human liver cirrhosis, the SEF are significantly reduced both in diameter and number with the deposition of GAG, type I, IV collagen, and laminin in the perisinusoidal space, resulting in the formation of the basement membrance beneath the sinusoidal endothelial cells. These sinusoidal alterations interrupt the supply of plasma components and oxygen to the hepatocytes via the SEF, leading to a self-perpetuating condition of liver cirrhosis, as schematically illustrated in Fig. 8. Not only a certain type of biogenic amines, such as norepinephrine and histamine, but also endotoxin are increased in the plasma in liver cirrhosis, possibly involving the abovementioned alterations of the hepatic sinusoids (Fig. 8).

Acknowledgment. This study was supported by the Grants-in-Aid for Scientific Research of the Ministry of Education, Science and Culture (#60570337 and #62570335).

References

1. Rappaport AM (1973) The microcirculatory hepatic unit. Microvasc Res 6: 212–228
2. Wisse E (1970) An electron microscopic study of fenestrated endothelium lining of rat liver sinusoids. J Ultrastruct Res 31: 125–150.
3. Oda M, Nakamura M, Watanabe N, Ohya Y, Sekizuka E, Tsukada N, Yonei Y, Komatsu H, Nagata H, Tsuchiya M (1983) Some dynamic aspects of the hepatic microcirculation—Demonstration of sinusoidal endothelial fenestrae as a possible regulatory factor—. In: Tsuchiya M, Wayland H, Oda M, Okazaki I (eds) Intravital observation of organ microcirculation. Excerpta Medica, Amsterdam, pp 105–138
4. Oda M, Tsukada N, Watanabe N, Tsuchiya M (1983) Heterogeneity of hepatic lobule—Some ultrastructural aspects of hepatic microcirculation system—. J Clin Electron Microscopy 16: 437–438
5. Oda M, Tsukada N, Watanabe N, Komatsu H, Yonei Y, Tsuchiya M (1984) Functional implications of the sinusoidal endothelial fenestrae in the regulation of the hepatic microcirculation. Hepatology 4: 754
6. Tsukada N, Oda M, Nakamura M, Ichikawa E, Watanabe N, Akaiwa Y, Yonei Y, Komatsu H, Kaneko K, Tsuchiya M, Kiryu Y, Fujiwara T (1984) Ultrastructural characteristics of liver sinusoidal endothelial fenestrae—An in vivo and in vitro study—. J Clin Electron Microscopy 17: 619–620
7. Tsukada N, Oda M, Yonei Y, Honda K, Akaiwa Y, Kiryu Y, Tsuchiya M (1986) Alterations of the hepatic sinusoidal endothelial fenestrae in response to vasoactive substances in the rat—In vivo and in vitro studies. In: Kirn A, Knook DL, Wisse E (eds) Cells of the hepatic sinusoid. The Kupffer cell foundation, Rijswijk, pp 515–516
8. Oda M, Tsukada N, Komatsu H, Kaneko K, Nakamura M, Tsuchiya M (1986) Electron microscopic localizations of actin, calmodulin and calcium in the hepatic sinusoidal endothelium in the rat. In: Kirn A, Knook DL, Wisse E (eds) Cells of the hepatic sinusoid. The Kupffer cell foundation, Rijswijk, pp 511–512
9. Oda M, Tsukada N, Komatsu H, Yonei Y, Honda K, Tsuchiya M (1986) Mechanism

of contraction and dilatation of sinusoidal endothelial fenestrae in the liver. Hepatology 6: 771
10. Tsukada N, Oda M, Azuma T, Kaneko K, Ishii M, Komatsu H, Honda K, Akaiwa Y, Nakamura M, Funatsu K, Mizuno Y, Kiryu Y, Tsuchiya M (1987) Involvement of calcium ions in the contraction of the sinusoidal endothelial fenestrae—An in vitro study—. In: Tsuchiya M, Asano M, Mishima Y (eds) Microcirculation annual 1987. Nihon-Igakukan, Tokyo, pp 95–96
11. Tsukada N, Oda M, Kaneko K, Komatsu H, Yonei Y, Honda K, Akaiwa Y, Ichikawa E, Nakamura M, Funatsu K, Mizuno Y, Kiryu Y, Tsuchiya M (1986) Possible involvements of mast cells and sinusoidal endothelial fenestrae in endotoxin-induced hepatic microcirculatory disturbances—An in vivo and in vitro study. In: Tsuchiya M, Asano M, Hayashi H, Kambara T (eds) Microcirculation annual 1986. Nihon-Igakukan, Tokyo, pp 35–36
12. Oda M, Tsukada N, Honda K, Komatsu H, Kaneko K, Azuma T, Nishizaki Y, Watanabe N, Tsuchiya M (in press) Hepatic sinusoidal endothelium—Its functional implications in the regulation of sinusoidal blood flow. Symposium on Hepatic Microcirculation. In: Tsuchiya M, Asano M, Mishima Y, Oda M (eds) Proceedings of Fourth World Congress for Microcirculation, July 27–30, 1987, Tokyo
13. Oda M, Funatsu K, Maruyama K, Okazaki I, Kamegaya K, Tsuchiya M (1982) Electron microscopic studies on collagen formation and degradation in the liver. In: Tsuchiya M, Tamayo RP, Okazaki I, Maruyama K (eds) Collagen degradation and mammalian collagenase. Excerpta Medica, Amsterdam, pp 174–197
14. Schaffner F, Popper H (1963) Capillarization of hepatic sinusoids in man. Gastroenterology 44: 239–242
15. Tsukada N, Oda M, Kaneko K, Komatsu H, Yonei Y, Honda K, Akaiwa Y, Ichikawa E, Nakamura M, Fujiwara T, Kiryu Y, Tsuchiya M (1985) Ultrastructural observations of sinusoidal endothelial fenestrae in rat and human cirrhotic liver. J Clin Electron Microscopy 18: 606–607

Observation of Microcirculatory Disorders of the Hemorrhagic Rat Liver by Use of Fluorescence-Stained Gamma Globulins

Hermann P. Metzger and Michael Schywalsky[1]

Summary

Using two different fluorescent dyes coupled to serum albumin, the sinusoids of the rat liver ($n = 36$, ketamine-xylazin anesthesia) were first stained red with an RB-200 infusion. The spreading of the yellow-green plasma front in the acinus following FITC bolus application was then fixed by means of liquid N_2 and investigated with the background of the red-marked sinusoidal network (7 μm cryostat cuts).

Under normovolemia, the convective front had a sharply defined, regular contour which spread over all of the acinus sections with an increasing perfusion period.

Some liver acini showed asymmetrical coloring toward the terminal branch, which was probably caused by vasomotion and flow redistribution as well as through the course of sinusoids situated perpendicular to the observation plane. Compared with intravital microscopic observations of superficial acini, a wider variety of sinusoidal network architecture can be observed within deeper tissue layers where groups of sinusoids run perpendicular to each other.

Under hemorrhagic hypotension (mean arterial pressure = 40 mmHg, lasting 90 min), plasma-perfused and nonplasma-perfused sinusoids lie adjacent to one another; the distinct contour of the convective front is absent. Despite intrasinusoidal erythrocyte aggregation and break-down of hepatic O_2 transport (91% of the liver surface has a Po_2 value of 0 mmHg), the remaining circulation during hemorrhage is about 25% that of normal and is mainly established through the sinusoidal plasma flow.

Introduction

Intravital microscopic investigations of the blood flow within the liver acinus under normovolemic and hemorrhagic conditions have primarily been made on superficial sinusoids of the peripheral part of the largest liver lobe [1–3]; the

[1]Department of Physiology, Medizinische Hochschule Hannover, Postbox 610180, 3000 Hanover, Federal Republic of Germany

microcirculatory perfusion pattern of the deep layers of the three-dimensional sinusoidal network could not, however, be observed. Furthermore, there is some information regarding the extent of plasma flow occuring during hemorrhage, which in the case of slowed down or stagnant erythrocyte flow is of special importance in the transport of substances to and from the inadequately supplied liver parenchyma.

At predetermined time intervals of 5, 10, and 20 s, the spreading of the convective front was investigated by means of fluorescent albumin in the liver acinus. The flow of the spread was fixed by freeze-stopping. Fluorescence-microscopic observation of frozen cuts enabled us to document the yellow-green convective front against the background of the red sinusoidal network of the acinus by adding both colors photographically. Typical differences of the microcirculatory perfusion patterns within the acinus, i.e., the distributional velocity of the flow of erythrocytes and plasma within the sinusoidal network, were examined under the conditions of normovolemia and initial and prolonged hemorrhage with and without prophylactic applications of heparin.

To compare sinusoidal flow distribution with integrative methods of liver blood flow determination, hepatic blood flow was measured using hydrogen clearance. Oxygen transport to the normal and ischemic liver tissue was analyzed by means of PO_2 surface electrodes.

Materials and Methods

Animals and Anesthesia

White rats ($n = 36$, Wistar-Frömter strain, pathogen-free, 160–220 g body weight) were anesthetized with ketamine (Ketavet) 15 mg/100 g bw and xylazin (Rompun) 0.5 mg/100 g bw i.p., cannulated and laparotomized. A catheter within the arteria carotis sinistra was used to determine mean arterial pressure (MAP), PaO_2, $PaCO_2$, arterial pH (pHa), hemoglobin (Hb), and hematocrit (Hct) as well as for the injection of fluorochromized serum proteins. During the experiments, the animals were monitored under controlled respiration and heart rates and rectal temperature. Surface PO_2- and H_2-clearance measurements were made on the lobus sinister. To avoid circadian fluctuations in the investigated parameters, experiments were conducted between 9 a.m. and 1 p.m.

The experimental animals were classified into four groups: group I, control group ($n = 9$), untreated for 90 min; group II ($n = 9$), adjusted to MAP = 40 mmHg after initial stabilizing by slowly withdrawing blood (0.5 ml/min); group III ($n = 9$), kept at 40mmHg MAP for 90 min; group IV ($n = 9$), treated with 200 international units/100 g bw heparin prior to bleeding.

Visualization of Perfusion Patterns

To demonstrate the sinusoidal network, 0.3 ml/100 g bw RB-200 gamma globulin (6% solution) was infused 5 min before ending the experiment. Immediately before stopping the microcirculation by freezing the tissue probe, FITC gamma globulin was applied; intervals of 5, 10, and 20 s between dye application and freezing were tested in order to obtain an optimal FITC colored convective front. A piece of the lobus sinister measuring about 1 cm^3 was quickly excized, precooled in isopentane (−80°C) and freeze-fixed in liquid N_2. Later, frozen sections (7 μm thick) were prepared, counterfixed with absolute ethanol and embedded in Entellan (Merck, Darmstadt, West Germany). Using filter systems I_2 (FITC) or M_2 (RB-200) with x100 magnification (oil immersion), the specimens were screened for functional units in a fluorescent microscope (Dialux, Leitz Wetzlar, West Germany) and photographed (Agfa-chrome 50L). To obtain optimal colored double exposure, the lighting time relation was 120:40 s for FITC to RB-200.

Dye Preparation

Serum proteins were prepared with fluorochrome as previously described [4–6] but with the following modifications. Fluorescein isothiocyanate (FITC, Sigma, St. Louis, USA) was coupled to bovine serum gamma globulin (molecular weight = 169 000, Serva, Heidelberg, West Germany) and added to a 2% protein solution (pH = 9.0) as a dry substance. Following 24-h incubation in an ice bath, the stain solution was centrifuged and separated from the uncoupled stain on Sephadex G25. The substance was then concentrated in a dialysis tube, against polyethylene glycol (molecular weight = 20 000), and made up to a 6%–7% concentration. For the preparation of RB-200 gamma globulin, lissamine-rhodamine (RB-200, Ferak, Berlin, West Germany) was ground together with double the amount of PCl_5. The activated stain was extracted from the mixture with acetone as RB-200 sulfonyl-chloride and a 2.5% gamma globulin solution was added following evaporation. Additional preparations were done in similar fashion to FITC gamma globulin. Both dyes showed different spectra, which reached a maximum at 595-nm for RB-200 gamma globulin and 525 nm for FITC gamma globulin.

Surface Electrodes for PO_2- and H_2-Clearance Measurements

Specially developed electrodes, 5 mm in diameter and weighing 2 g, were placed on the surface of the liver in a "riding" position. In making these electrodes, six gold wires (15 μm in diameter) or four platinum-iridium wires (100 μm in diameter; Heraeus, Hanau, West Germany) were placed on small 3×3 mm^3 printed plates, soldered, and sealed with Hysol (Dexter Corp., New York, USA), a resin used in cardiac pacemakers. The PO_2 electrode had a central Ag/AgCl wire as its reference electrode; an external calomel electrode served as reference for the H_2-clearance measurements. The polarization voltage of the O_2 measurement was −800-mV and that of the H_2 measurement +150-mV. A small thermistor (K292B, Siemens, Munich, West Germany) was used to monitor the surface temperature and fitted into the tip of the electrodes. The PO_2 electrode was covered with a polypropylene membrance 6 μm thick; the H_2 electrode was used without a protective covering. The PO_2 electrode was calibrated with gas mixtures of known O_2 content; the H_2-clearance curves were plotted as relative values on a semilogarithmic scale. The steepest slope of the straight part of the curve was used to calculate the liver blood flow (LBF), according to the formula $LBF = 0.692/t_{1/2}$, $t_{1/2}$, as the period up until half of the initial H_2 concentration. Stability of the electrodes was less than 1%/h (PO_2 electrode) or 5%/h (pH_2 electrode).

Results

The yellow-green FITC-marked convective front spread from the portal areas and terminal branches through the sinusoidal network of the acinus to the central vein following the arterial bolus injection and is shown against the background of the red RB-200-stained microvascular system of the liver in Fig. 1. Portal fields and sinusoids reached by the convective front form a larger enclosed field, the longer the period of perfusion, from the bolus injection to the point of freeze-stop. When the circulation was stopped after 5 s following the FITC gamma globulin bolus, the terminal branches originating from the traversely cut portal areas and related sinusoids, i.e., simple acini, were primarily observed. After

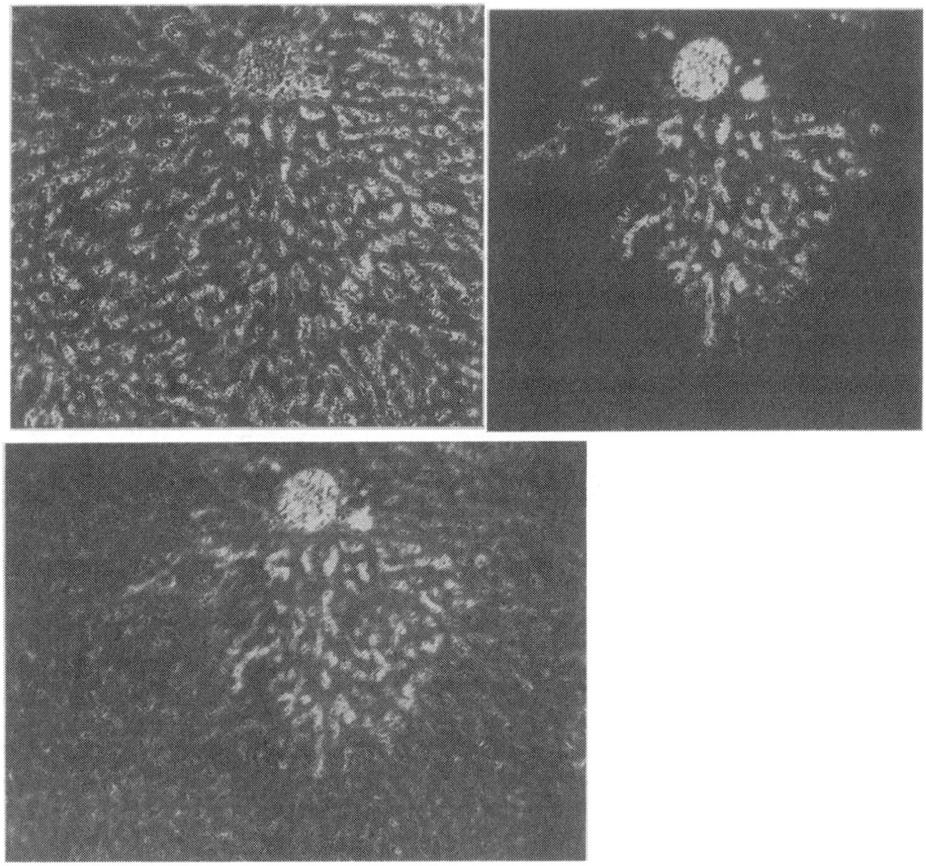

a b c

Fig. 1a–c. Staining of the sinusoidal network by **a** 4-min infusion of RB-2oo and **b** spreading of the convective front in response to FITC-bolus application. Photographic addition of **a** and **b** was performed **c** by use of different filters. The figure shows the triangle of the portal field (*upper middle*) with bile duct and biliary plexus as well as the corresponding arteriolar input. Terminal portal branches are running in a vertical direction. × 100

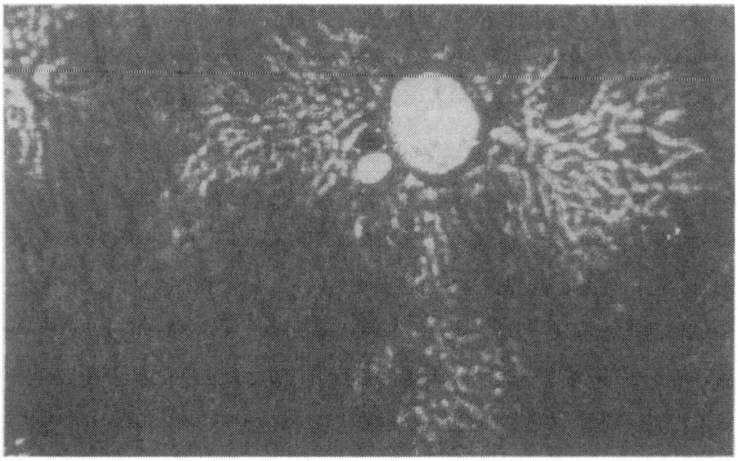

Fig. 2. Complex acinus composed of three acini. Three terminal venules branch from a preterminal parent stem; each venule with its sinusoids irrigates a simple acinus. × 100

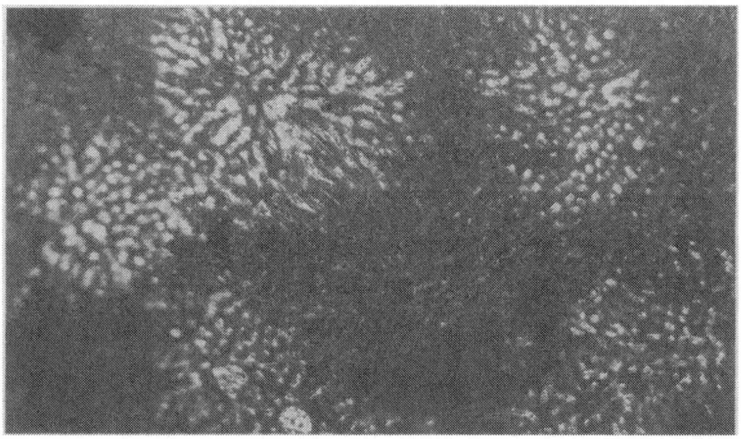

Fig. 3. Staining of five complex acini which already show confluent border zones arising from their corresponding terminal branches. The five complex acini are arranged concentrically around the draining vein and form the classic hexagonal structure as already described by Koo and Liang [3]. × 60

10 s, the number of FITC-stained portal areas and acini increased; the acini reached by the convective front formed a complex acinus (Fig. 2), from which subsequently a clover leaf pattern developed after 20 s through the confluence of serveral acini (Fig. 3).

In addition to the standard perfusion patterns, yellow-green areas, lines, and points, reflecting the different degrees of heterogeneity of flow in the sinusoidal network, formed resulting from the velocity differences of the corresponding sinusoids.

Perfusion Pattern of Acinus Under Normovolemia

Small arteries, arterioles of the portal areas, and the capillaries surrounding the biliary plexus are the first to be reached by the light yellow-green convective front. In some acini, the terminal branches and the beginnings of the sinusoids are marked. The portal areas and related terminal branches only form punctate or linear sources of the acinus network, while conducting and distributing veins as a rule do not supply sinusoids.

As the convective front continues to spread, the early perfused sinusoids belonging to the same acinus are completely stained. At this stage, the junctions of the discharging venous system can be observed at all levels of the venous vascular network.

Related sinusoidal groups within an acinus can be identified, each of which is traversed length- or crosswise. Adjacent sinusoids running per pendicular to the sectional plane partly retain the same direction for more than 30–40 μm and are supplied from a deeper terminal branch. This observation has been confirmed on the basis of serial sections from selected tissue areas but still requires further investigation.

An asymmetrical pattern of the yellow-green convective front on the sides of the terminal branches appears in approximately 25%–30% of all acini. This one-sided development of the convective front was observed in all sinusoids drained from the same central vein.

Perfusion Patterns of Acinus Under Hemorrhagic Hypotension

All the topographical variations of the acinus perfusion pattern already described in normovolemic animals were found under hemorrhagic conditions in the same manner. In addition, there were changes induced by flow reduction. These changes were determined by intrasinusoidal erythrocyte aggregation and also by flow redistribution resulting from changes in the hydrodynamic resistance. At the start of hemorrhage, the convective front moving from the terminal branches showed an irregular development, which was brought on by velocity differences in neighboring sinusoids (Figs. 4, 5). With continual hemorrhage (90 min duration), the acinus perfusion became more and more irregular, as both adjacent sinusoids and segments within single sinusoids were stained irregularly or alternately, so that perfused and nonperfused sinusoids were observed side by side. The convective front was no longer evident; the contour that was clearly recognizable under normovolemia had disappeared. Consequently, the acinus perfusion pattern was exceptionally heterogeneous and, thereby, clearly differed from the homogeneous pattern under normovolemia.

Perfusion patterns were observed following the prophylactic application of heparin and 90 min of hemorrhage. They did not differ from the patterns without heparin application.

Liver Surface PO_2

The liver surface PO_2 (sPO_2) values were characterized by a Gaussian frequency distribution (mean value $\pm$ SD $= 27 \pm 4.5$ mmHg, $n = 68$ measurements) under normovolemia. At the start of hemorrhagic hypotension, a parallel drop to the

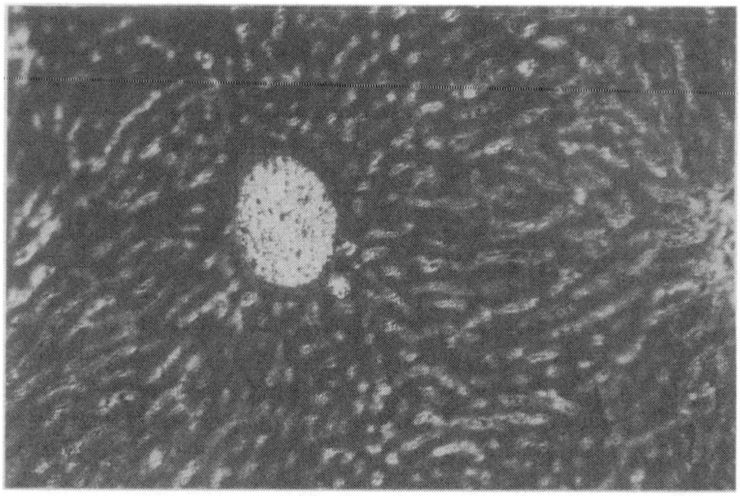

Fig. 4. Microcirculatory perfusion pattern of the liver acinus under hemorrhagic hypotension (40 mmHg MAP, 90 min). The sharp contour of the convective front disappears. Neighboring sinusoids are stained alternately. Within single sinusoids, stained and unstained segments are observed

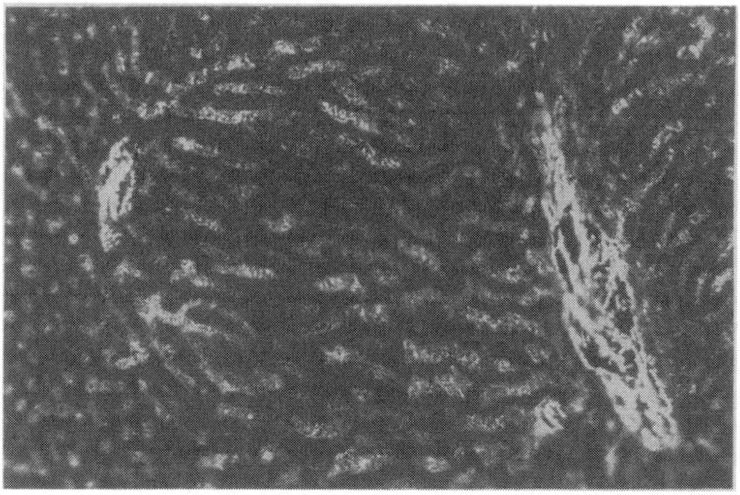

Fig. 5. The perfusion pattern of the acinus is drastically changed under hemorrhagic hypotension. Stained sinusoidal segments are observed within the same sinusoid as well as in neighboring blood vessels. The defined contour seen in normovolemia disappears under hemorrhage; heterogeneous distribution of fluorescence is seen

MAP of the sPO_2 curves was registered. A marked left shift was noted in the sPO_2 histogram (mean value 9 mmHg, median = 3.5 mmHg, modul = 0 mmHg), whereby 24% of the sPO_2 values are at 0 mmHg. Anoxia of the liver parenchyma intensified more (mean value = 1.6 mmHg, median = 0 mmHg, modul = 0 mmHg) after 45 min of continual hemorrhagic hypotension (MAP = 40 mmHg) and included nearly the whole liver surface after 90 min with 91% of the sPO_2 values at 0 mmHg. The normovolemic control group also showed a Gaussian frequency distribution of sPO_2 values (mean value ± SD = 29 ± 5.0 mmHg, $n = 48$) and switched over to a left-shifted histogram (mean value = 19 ± 7.0 mmHg) following a 90-min of hemorrhage. The left-shift was determined by the influence of anesthesia, surgical trauma, and redistribution of the blood volume into the brain, heart muscle, and adrenal cortex.

Liver Blood Flow

H_2-clearance curves were registered by means of four electrodes in a measuring field of about 100 μm in diameter per electrode, which evaluated the desaturation period according to the degree and duration of hemorrhagic hypotension. The normal liver blood flow of the animal in the normovolemic state was—mean value ± SD = 1.2 ± 0.4 ml/g·min ($n = 68$). At the beginning of hemorrhagic hypotension (MAP = 40 mmHg), about half the initial liver blood flow (mean value = 0.57 ml/g·min) was determined. Following prolonged hemorrhage lasting 90 min, about one-fourth of the initial value was recorded (0.28 ml/g·min).

Blood Gas amd Hematocrit

During hemorrhage, a slight decrease of pHa and $PaCO_2$ values was observed as well as an increase in the PaO_2 value. The reduction of hematocrit by 20% of the initial value within 30 min was due to the migration of plasma from the extravasal to the intravasal space (Table 1).

Discussion

The liver acinus perfusion pattern was investigated in three dimensions by analyzing the spread of the convective front of fluorochrome-marked FITC gamma globulin following an arterial bolus injection and freeze-stopping after 5–10s of circulation. Through the spread of the FITC fluorescence, characteristics of the flow distribution within a large RB-200-marked section of the terminal vascular bed, 200–400 μm in diameters, could be visualized and documented by means of an overlay photograph. The pictures showed the yellow-green convective front against the background of the red RB-200-stained sinusoidal network of the acinus. Earlier intravital-microscopic observations had concentrated exclusively on the superficial sinusoidal networks [1–3]. The validity of the acinus concept as a microcirculatory unit according to Rappaport [2] is also confirmed in the third dimension. Compared with the two-dimensional acini of the liver surface, the three-dimensional arrangement of the sinusoids and bile ducts is impressive in the way that the group- or cord-shaped bundles of parallel sinusoids with the perpendicular or parallel arrangement bear obvious similiarity with technical counter- and cross-current heat and mass exchangers.

Drainage to and from the acinus was very clearly observed with the applied fluorescence technique. Punctate or linear sources belonging to the same acinus were exclusively formed by portal fields and terminal branches. They received

Table 1. Arterial blood gas, pH, and hematocrit values under the conditions of hemorrhagic hypotension

	Before bleeding	30 min after bleeding	85 min after bleeding
pHa	7.38 ± 0.04	7.37 ± 0.06	7.36 ± 0.04
$PaCO_2$ (mmHg)	45 ± 4	36 ± 6	33 ± 5
PaO_2 (mmHg)	72 ± 5	89 ± 16	84 ± 6
Hct (%)	47 ± 2	38 ± 2	34 ± 2

pHa arterial pH, *Hct* hematocrit

the inflow from conducting and distributing veins, which in turn did not show any direct sinusoidal connections and were even characterized by a nearby sinusoidal-free outer zone. Conversely, on the outflowing venous side, sinusoids can lead into larger veins, as described by Gershbein and Elias [7].

Vasomotive effects could be indirectly studied by the registration of sPO_2- and H_2-clearance curves. The rhythmic activity indicated slow fluctuations in the midrange with an amplitude of 5%–25% in the frequency range of 0.2--6/min. The origin of the vasomotive activity in liver sinusoids is not yet clear; it may be located within pre-, intra-, and postsinusoidal sphincter-like structures, as originally hypothesized by McCuskey [8]. Moreover, the oscillatory sPO_2- and H_2-clearance registrations might reflect the precapillary smooth muscle activity of the hepatic arterial system, which feeds the acinus and influences its flow and pressure distribution.

Postsinusoidal changes of resistance, which according to Greenway and Stark [9] comprise the principal part of the hepatic resistance, may cause the phenomenon of asymmetry of fluorescence distribution in relation to the terminal branches. The phenomenon is to be observed in 25%–30% of all acini. Asymmetrical staining is to be seen about 5–10 s after arterial FITC gamma globulin application and disappears after 20 s, since all sinusoids have become plasma-perfused once in the meantime even though erythrocyte flow is stagnant within most of the sinusoids of the acinus under observation. Asymmetrical FITC distribution is also in part conditioned by a group of sinusoids running perpendicular to the terminal branches of the observation plane. These sinusoids belong to the portal fields and terminal branches not yet marked with FITC gamma globulin. Whether postsinusoidal flow control and/or presinusoidal influences from acini supplied by portal fields from deeper areas is responsible for the asymmetry cannot be answered at the moment; this has to be further clarified by means of intravital-microscopy.

The microcirculatory perfusion pattern and O_2 transport under hemorrhage are drastically altered: Heterogeneity of the acinus perfusion increases with the duration of hemorrhage and is characterized by a completely irregular flow pattern with intrasinusoidal changes of erythrocyte aggregates and plasma sections. Fluorescent-free sections mainly correspond to erythrocyte aggregations, while FITC gamma globulin-stained spots are identical with plasma segments. The increase in heterogeneity of the liver acinus perfusion pattern causes a reduction of liver blood flow at one-fourth of the initial value after 90 min of hemorrhage.

The progressive ischemia induces tissue anoxia with 91% of the sPO_2 values at 0 mmHg.

Under these conditions, the plasma flow gains significance as it counteracts further spreading of intrahepatic acidosis by removing protons and metabolic by-products from anoxic parenchymal areas. The existing plasma flow explains why retransfusion and regeneration of impaired liver function is possible despite a long period of parenchymal ischemia [10]. Even though an intensified plasma migration from the extravasal space (Hct = 38%) occurs and sinusoidal flow and substance removal improve, the hemoconcentration in the sinusoidal network remains. Erythrocyte aggregation is so pronounced that even a prophylactic heparin application prior to hemorrhage bears no influence on the microcirculatory perfusion pattern of the acinus, just as with O_2 transport.

References

1. Vanecko RM, Szanto PB, Shoemaker WC (1969) Microcirculatory changes in primate liver during shock. Surg Gynecol Obstet 129: 995–1004
2. Rappaport AM (1973) The microcirculatory hepatic unit. Microvasc Res 6: 212–228
3. Koo A, Liang IYS (1977) Blood flow in hepatic sinusoids in experimental hemorrhagic shock in the rat. Microvasc Res 13: 315–325
4. Coons AH, Kaplan MH (1950) Localization of antigen in tissue cells. J Exp Med 91: 1–13.
5. Nairn RC, Chadwick CS, McEntegart MG (1958) Fluorescent protein tracers in the study of experimental liver damage. J Pathol Bact 76: 143–152
6. Vetterlein F, Heinz dal Ri, Schmidt G (1982) Capillary density in rat myocardium during timed plasma staining. Am J Physiol 242: H133–H141
7. Gershbein LL, Elias H (1954) Observations on the anatomy of the rat liver. Anat Rec 120: 85–98
8. McCuskey RS (1966) A dynamic and static study of hepatic arterioles and hepatic sphincters. Am J Anat 119: 455–478
9. Greenway CV, Stark RD (1971) Hepatic vascular bed. Physiol Rev 51: 23–65
10. Scherf M, Oestern HJ, Metzger HP (1984) Studies of hemorrhagic and traumatic shock influence on liver oxygen tension: effects of a single large dose of dexamethasone. Adv Exp Med Biol 169: 571–582

Chapter 4
Cerebral Ischemia and Hyperemia

Cerebral Hemoconcentration Following Blood Flow Reduction in the Gerbil

Hiroaki Naritomi[1], Masahiro Sasaki[1], Shi-yao Bao[1], Yoshihiro Kuriyama[2], and Tohru Sawada[2]

Introduction

In minute vessels, the average speed of red blood cells (RBC) is greater than that of plasma. This velocity difference leads to reduction in hematocrit (Ht) of minute vessels (Fahraeus effect), and for this reason, the Ht measured in organs is generally lower than large-vessel Ht [1].

The brain contains rich capillary beds. Several workers measured the Ht in the normal brain and reported it to be 15%–30% lower than large-vessel Ht [2–7]. This Ht reduction in the brain is likely to be attributable to Fahraeus effect. Little is yet known, however, as to whether this cerebral/large-vessel Ht ratio stays the same irrespectively of flow condition.

In the present study, the unilateral or bilateral common carotid artery was occluded in Mongolian gerbils, and the cerebral Ht changes following flow reduction were investigated.

Methods

Eighty-five male Mongolian gerbils weighing 60–80 g were anesthetized with intraperitoneal injection of pentobarbital (40 mg/kg). PE-10 catheters were introduced into the femoral veins and arteries. Arterial blood pressure and blood gases were monitored. The animals were divided into three groups, and the following three experiments were performed. In one group, RBC volume, plasma volume, and cerebral Ht were measured in the control state ($n = 16$), 1 min after bilateral carotid artery occlusion ($n = 19$), or 10 min after bilateral carotid artery occlusion ($n = 19$). In another group, the right common carotid artery was occluded, and 10 min thereafter, cerebral Ht and cerebral blood flow (CBF) were measured in occluded and nonoccluded hemispheres, respectively. The relationship between CBF and cerebral Ht was assessed in this group. In the third group, the extent of tracer extravasation was measured in the control state or 10 min after bilateral carotid artery occlusion, and the influence of blood-brain

Cerebral Circulation Laboratory[1] and Department of Neurology[2], National Cardiovascular Center, 7–1, Fujishirodai 5-chome, Suita, Osaka, 565 Japan barrier disruption on cerebral Ht measurement was estimated.

RBC volume and plasma volume were measured using 99m-Tc-labeled RBC and 131-I-labeled serum albumin. The mixture of the two tracers was injected from the femoral vein, and 15 min thereafter both common carotid arteries or the right common carotid artery were occluded. After 1 min or 10 min of occlusion, the animals were put into a freon chamber and frozen at −40°C. The brain was removed, and the temporal-parietal cortex of both hemispheres was sampled as a representative area. Visible large vessels were removed from the samples as recommended by Cremer and Seville [5]. RBC volume and plasma volume were calculated according to the following equations:

$$\text{RBC volume } (\mu\text{l/g brain}) = \frac{\text{99m-Tc activity/g brain}}{\text{99m-Tc activity/}\mu\text{l blood}} \times \text{Ht}$$

$$\text{Plasma volume } (\mu\text{l/g brain}) = \frac{\text{131-I activity/g brain}}{\text{131-I activity/}\mu\text{l blood}} \times (1 - \text{Ht})$$

Total cerebral blood volume (CBV) was calculated as a sum of the RBC volume and plasma volume. Cerebral Ht was calculated from the ratio of the RBC volume and CBV.

In the unilateral occlusion group, CBF was measured simultaneously with the cerebral Ht at 10 min after the occlusion. First, 99m-Tc RBC and 131-I albumin were injected from one femoral vein; 15 min later, the right common carotid artery was occluded. Ten minutes after the occlusion, 20 μCi 14-C iodoantipyrine was injected from the other femoral vein over 30 s, and after injection the animals were decapitated. The brain was removed quickly and frozen in freon at −40°C. The temporal-parietal cortex of each hemisphere was then sampled. The 99m-Tc and 131-I activity of the brain and peripheral blood were assayed, and the cerebral Ht was calculated. The samples were stored in a deep freezer for 2 months to allow for depletion of 99m-Tc and 131-I activities. The 14-C activity in the brain and blood were then assayed, and CBF in each hemisphere was calculated according to the method described by Sakurada et al. [8].

The extent of extravasation of the tracers was estimated in 13 other animals. In these animals, 99m-Tc RBC and 131-I albumin were injected intravenously. In seven animals, both common carotid arteries were occluded; in the other six, neck manipulation alone was performed without the occlusion. After 10 min, the brain was perfused with normal saline through a catheter inserted into the left ventricle of the heart. After 30 min of the perfusion, the temporal-parietal cortex was sampled, and the residual tracer activities were measured. The residual activities were calculated as blood volume per gram of brain, and the values were compared with the RBC volume and plasma volume obtained in the control state and 10 min of occlusion.

Results

As shown in Table 1, mean arterial blood pressure (MABP) began to increase 1 min after the bilateral carotid artery occlusion and was significantly elevated 10 min after the occlusion ($P < 0.01$). However, no significant blood gas changes occurred after the occlusion. Following bilateral carotid artery occlusion, RBC

Table 1. Changes in blood pressure, blood gases, and hemodynamic parameters after bilateral carotid artery occlusion

Parameters	Control ($n = 16$)	1 min of occlusion ($n = 19$)	10 min of occlusion ($n = 19$)
MABP (mmHg)	70 ± 12	73 ± 15	86 ± 18*
PaO_2 (mmHg)	101 ± 21	99 ± 19	94 ± 15
$PaCO_2$ (mmHg)	37 ± 8	38 ± 10	42 ± 11
pH	7.28 ± 0.08	7.24 ± 0.08	7.24 ± 0.06
RBC vol (μl/g)	3.74 ± 0.42	3.82 ± 0.55	3.91 ± 0.72
Plasma vol (μl/g)	6.30 ± 0.69	5.70 ± 0.52*	5.75 ± 0.90
CBV (μl/g)	10.04 ± 1.01	9.52 ± 0.99	9.66 ± 1.47
Cerebral Ht (%)	37.3 ± 2.4	40.0 ± 2.6*	40.4 ± 3.3*
Large-vessel Ht (%)	48.9 ± 2.6	48.4 ± 1.9	49.3 ± 2.4
Cereb/LV Ht (%)	76.3 ± 2.4	82.5 ± 5.2**	81.9 ± 5.4**

MABP mean arterial blood pressure, *Cereb/LV Ht* cerebral/large-vessel Ht ratio
Values are means ± SD
*$P < 0.01$, significant difference compared with control values
**$P < 0.001$

volume showed little change, while plasma volume decreased significantly 1 min after occlusion ($P < 0.01$), as indicated in Table 1. The CBV exhibited some tendency toward reduction after occlusion, though the changes were not significant. Cerebral Ht measured in the control state was 37.3% and was significantly lower than large-vessel Ht ($P < 0.001$). The cerebral/large-vessel Ht ratio in the normal control state was 76.3%. After bilateral carotid artery occlusion, cerebral Ht increased significantly ($P < 0.01$), while large-vessel Ht remained unaltered. The cerebral/large-vessel Ht ratio increased significantly after occlusion ($P < 0.001$).

In the 13 animals perfused with the saline after tracer injection, some 99m-Tc and 131-I activity remained in the brain. The extravasated 99m-Tc and 131-I activity was 0.08 μl/g brain and 0.08 μl/g brain in the control state and 0.16 μl/g brain and 0.27 μl/g brain 10 min after the occlusion, respectively, calculated as the blood volume. These extravasated tracers corresponded to 2.1% of the RBC volume and 1.3% of plasma volume in the control state, and 4.1% of RBC volume and 4.7% of plasma volume 10 min after the occlusion. Extravasation of the tracers 10 min after the occlusion was, thus, small and had little influence on blood volume measurements.

In the unilateral carotid artery occlusion group, MABP increased from 70 ± 8 mmHg to 82 ± 19 mmHg 10 min after occlusion. Arterial blood gases exhibited no significant changes after occlusion. The CBF measured in the nonoccluded hemisphere was 0.48 ± 0.10 ml/g brain/min, while that in the occluded hemisphere was 0.23 ± 0.18 ml/g brain/min. The CBF values in the occluded hemisphere widely varied from 0.01 to 0.53 ml/g brain/min, probably because of a difference in the extent of collaterals through the circle of Willis in each animal. Cerebral Ht in the nonoccluded hemisphere was 35.8% ± 1.6%, while that in the occluded hemisphere was 37.6% ± 2.4%. The latter was significantly higher than the former ($P < 0.001$). There was a significant correlation between the grade of CBF reduction and the extent of increase in cerebral/large-vessel Ht ratio (Spearman's rank correlation coefficient $r = -0.49$, $P < 0.01$). The relationship between CBF and cerebral/large-vessel Ht ratio was, however, not monoexponential. The cerebral/large-vessel Ht ratio increase was small when the CBF reduction was moderate. The cerebral/large-vessel Ht increase suddenly became large when CBF was reduced below 0.10 ml/g brain/min.

Discussion

Cerebral Ht was first measured by Gibson et al. [9] in dogs in 1946 and shown to be approximately 50% lower than large-vessel Ht. Later, several workers measured cerebral Ht in rats [2, 5], cats [4], and humans [3, 6, 7] and reported it to be 16%–31% lower than large-vessel Ht. Excluding the report of Gibson et al. [9], there is close agreement in the cerebral/large-vessel Ht ratio reported by these workers and it is in the range of 69%–84%. The cerebral/large-vessel Ht ratio obtained in our normal control gerbils was also within this range. The cerebral/large-vessel Ht ratio may be approximately the same irrespective of species if measured in the normal circulatory condition.

The present study has clearly demonstrated the increase in cerebral Ht after carotid artery occlusion in gerbils. It is obvious that the increase is not attributable to a systemic hemoconcentration or overestimation of Ht resulting from extravasation of tracers. As shown in the unilateral carotid artery occlusion group, there was a significant correlation between the degree of CBF reduction and the extent of cerebral Ht increase. This strongly suggests that blood flow reduction is an important factor in causing cerebral Ht increase after carotid artery occlusion.

Pappenheimer and Kinter [10] measured renal Ht in two groups of cats, one with normal blood pressure and the other with severe hypotension. Renal Ht was significantly higher in the hypotensive group than in the normotensives. Several workers observing cerebral pial vessels through a skull window reported that the hemoconcentration or RBC sludging was often visualized in pial vessels soon after cerebral artery occlusion [11]. These observations are in accordance with the results obtained in the present study.

On the other hand, Mchedlishvili and Varazashvili reported in a microcirculation study of frog retrolingual vessels that the number of RBC circulating in minute vessels decreased after blood flow reduction [12]. Their results concerning Ht reduction after blood flow reduction are at odds with the present results. This dissociation may, however, be explained by an inhomogeneity of local Ht in ischemic organs. As reported by Yoshimine et al. (Chap. 4) local Ht changes in ischemic organs seem to be enormously nonhomogeneous. If measurement is performed in a very small area or in a certain restricted vascular territory, biased results may be obtained. On the other hand, if the measurement is carried out in a large area, as in the present study, more representative Ht changes are likely to be observed.

Two types of hemorheological Ht change are known to occur in in vitro circulation models when the blood is circulated from a feed reservoir to a discharge reservoir through a capillary tube. One type is a reduction of the capillary tube Ht compared with the feed reservoir Ht or discharge reservoir Ht. This Ht reduction occurs within the capillary tube due to the velocity difference between RBC and plasma, and the phenomenon is usually termed the "Fahreus effect" [1, 13, 14]. The other type is a reduction of the discharge reservoir Ht compared with the feed reservoir Ht. This Ht reduction occurs at the orifice of the capillary tube due to the screening of cells; this phenomenon is usually termed the "screening effect" [13, 14]. The screening effect is manifest more markedly in smaller capillary tubes than in larger capillary tubes [13] and occurs more prominently in a lower than in a higher flow state [13, 14]. Therefore, if the measurement is performed in small capillaries, Ht may be underestimated due to enhancement of the screening effect. Gaehtgens et al. studied the effect of capillary flow reduction on the screening effect and Fahreus effect in an in vitro circulation model [14]. They found that the flow reduction enhanced the screening effect but diminished the Fahreus effect. As a consequence, capillary Ht was elevated.

It is obvious that complete arrest of the circulation abolishes hemorheological effects, such as the Fahreus effect or screening effect, and finally cancels the difference between large-vessel and minute-vessel Ht. It is probable in extremely low-flow states that hemorheological effects are abolished, resulting in an increase of the cerebral/large-vessel Ht ratio toward 100%.

References

1. Fahreus R (1929) The suspension stability of the blood. Phys Rev 9: 241–274
2. Everett NB, Simmons B, Lasher EP (1956) Distribution of blood (Fe^{59}) and plasma (I^{131}) volumes of rats determined by liquid nitrogen freezing. Cir Res 4: 419–424
3. Oldendorf WH, Kitano M, Shimizu S, Oldendorf SZ (1965) Hematocrit of the human cranial blood pool. Cir Res 17: 532–539
4. Sklar FH, Burke EF-Jr, Langfitt TW (1968) Cerebral blood volume: values obtained with ^{51}Cr-labeled red blood cells and RISA. J Appl Phys 24: 79–82
5. Cremer JE, Seville MP (1983) Regional brain blood flow, blood volume, and hematocrit values in the adult rat. J Cereb Blood Flow Metabol 3: 254–256
6. Lammertsma AA, Brooks DJ, Beaney RP, Turton DR, Kensett MJ, Heather JD: Marshall J, Jones T (1984) In vivo measurement of regional cerebral hematocrit using positron emission tomography. J Cereb blood Flow Metabol 4: 317–322
7. Sakai F, Nakazawa K, Tazaki Y, Ishii K, Hino H, Igarashi H, Kanda T (1985) Regional cerebral blood volume and hematocrit measured in normal human volunteers by single-photon emission tomography. J Cereb Blood Flow Metabol 5: 207–213.
8. Sakurada O, Kennedy C, Jehle J, Brown JP, Carbin GL, Sokoloff L (1978) Measurement of local cerebral blood flow with [14C]-iodo-antipyrine. Am J Physiol; 234: H59–H66
9. Gibson JG, Seligman AM, Peakock WC, Aub JC, Fine J, Evans RD (1946) The distribution of red blood cells and plasma in large and minute vessels of the normal dog, determined by radioactive isotopes of iron and iodide. J Clin Invest 25: 848–857
10. Pappenheimer JR, Kinter WB (1956) Hematocrit ratio of blood within mammalian kidney and its significance for renal hemodynamics. Am J Phys 185: 377–390
11. Meyer JS (1958) Localized changes in properties of the blood and effects of anticoagulant drugs in experimental cerebral infarction. New Engl J Med 258: 151–159
12. Mchedlishvili G, Varazashvili M (1981) Red cell/plasam ratio in blood flowing in microvascular beds under control and ischemic conditions. Micro Res 21: 302–307
13. Cokelet GR (1976) Macroscopic rheology and tube flow of human blood. In: Grayson J, Zingg W (eds) Microcirculation, vol. 1. Plenum, New York, pp-9–31
14. Gaehtgens KH, Albrecht KH, Kreutz F (1978) Fahreus effect and cell screening during tube flow of human blood: I. Effect of variation of flow. Biorheology 15: 147–154

Plasma and Red Blood Cell in Focal Cerebral Ischemia: Differential Visualization with Double-Fluorescence Technique

Toshiki Yoshimine, Toru Hayakawa, and Heitaro Mogami[1]

Method

We recently developed a method to study the microvascular perfusion within the brain parenchyma using fluorescence-labeled plasma [1]. The method was extended in the present study to visualize circulated plasma as well as red blood cells (RBC) simultaneously in the same brain slice [2]. After centrifugation and repeated washing with glucose-saline-barbiturate buffer, RBC of normal gerbils were labeled with dichlorotriazinil aminofluorescein-2HC1 (DTAF) at pH 9.0 for 1 h at room temperature. The gerbil plasma was similarly labeled with tetramethyl rhodamine isothiocyanate (TRITC). The RBC suspension and the plasma were mixed (4:1) to make up double-labeled blood. The posterior communicating artery of a gerbil was occluded [3], producing ischemia in the ipsilateral hippocampus and thalamus [4–6]. From 30 min to 3 h after occlusion, 0.5 ml of the double-labeled blood was injected in 5 s from the femoral vein. Thirty seconds after the injection, the brain was removed and fixed in 95% ethanol. Coronal sections, 25 μm thick, were mounted in glycerol and examined under the fluorescence microscope.

Results

Using two different excitation modes, the labeled RBC and plasma could be distinguished as green spots and red arborizations, respectively. In the hippocampus at 30 min of occlusion, the RBC circulation was markedly disturbed in contrast to the minimal defect in the plasma circulation (Fig. 1). At 3 h of ischemia, the plasma perfusion was also disturbed, resulting in disappearance of the dissociation of RBC and plasma circulation (Fig. 2).

[1]Department of Neurosurgery, Osaka University Medical School, 1-50, Fukushima 1-chome, Fukushima-ku, Osaka, 553 Japan

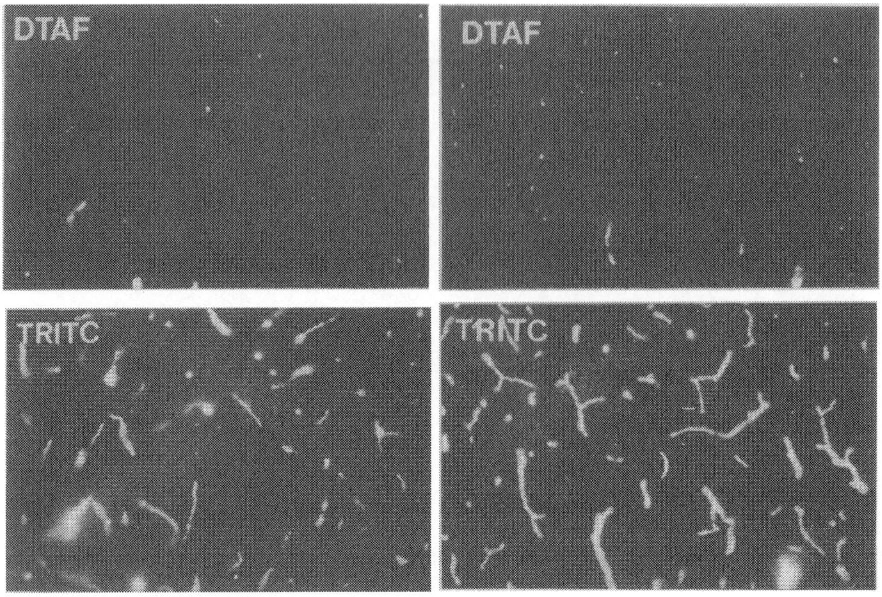

Fig. 1a–d. In the ischemic hippocampus at 30 min of occlusion, **a** DTAF-labeled RBC perfusion was significantly disturbed compared with **b** the opposite side. **c** TRITC-labeled plasma was, however, well preserved when compared with **d** the opposite side. Double-fluorescence microscopy, original magnification × 100

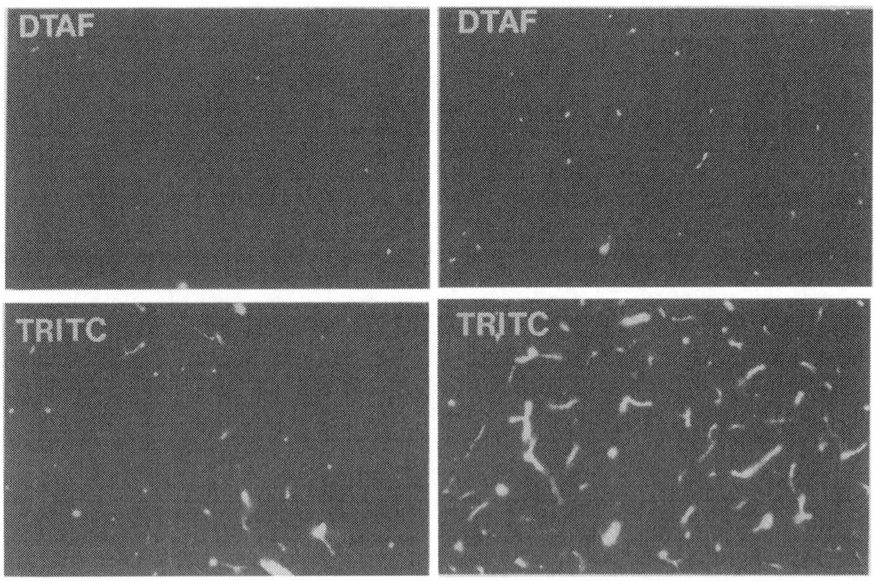

Fig. 2a–d. At 3 h of ischemia, the circulation of both **a** DTAF-labeled RBC and **c** TRITRC-labeled plasma was disturbed in the ischemic hippocampus as compared with **b**, **d** the opposite side. Double-fluorescence microscopy, original magnification × 100

Discussion

The present findings suggest that the circulatory disturbance of RBC may precede that of the plasma in the early period of focal cerebral ischemia. Considering the vital role of the RBC circulation in the maintenance of the functional and morphological integrity of the brain, the disturbance in RBC circulation seems to be critically important in understanding the pathophysiology of cerebral ischemia and in seeking new therapeutic measures.

References

1. Yoshimine T, Kato A, Hayakawa T, Ushio Y, Mogami H (1987) Deterioration and recovery of microcirculation during cerebral ischemia and recirculation. J Cereb Blood Flow Metabol 7: S337
2. Yoshimine T, Hayakawa T, Mogami H (1988) Plasma and RBC circulation in focal cerebral ischemia. Differential visualization with double fluorescence technique. In: Tomita M, Sawada T, Naritomi H, Heiss W-D (eds) Excerpta Medica International Congress Series. Cerebral Hyperemia and Ischemia. From the standpoint of cerebral blood volume, Elsevier, Amsterdam, pp 65–72
3. Yoshimine T, Yanagihara T (1983) Regional cerebral ischemia by occlusion of the posterior communicating artery and the middle cerebral artery in gerbils. J Neurosurg 58: 362–367
4. Yamamoto K, Yoshimine T, Homburger HA, Yanagihara T (1986) Immunohistochemical investigation of regional cerebral ischemia in the gerbil; occlusion of the posterior communicating artery. Brain Res 371: 244–252
5. Yoshimine T, Hayakawa T, Yamada K, Takemoto O, Kato A, Ushio Y, Mogami H (1986) Regional cerebral ischemia in the gerbil. Measurement of regional cerebral blood flow by quantitative autoradiography. J Cereb Blood Flow Metabol 6: 348–357
6. Yoshimine T, Hayakawa T, Kato A, Yamada K, Matsumoto K, Ushio Y, Mogami H (1987) Autoradiographic study of regional protein synthesis in focal cerebral ischemia with TCA wash and image subtraction techniques. J Cereb Blood Flow Metabol 7: 387–393

Cerebral Blood Volume Reactivity to Hypercapnia Measured by ^{11}C-Labeled Carboxyhemoglobin and Positron Emission Tomography

IWAO KANNO, KAZUO UEMURA, MATSUTARO MURAKAMI, FUMIO SHISHIDO, SHUICHI MIURA, HIDEHIRO IIDA, KAZUHIRO TAKAHASHI, HIROSHI SASAKI, and ATSUSHI INUGAMI[1]

The purpose of this study was to examine regional reactivity of cerebral blood volume (CBV) to changes in $PaCO_2$. CBV was measured using an ^{11}CO-inhalation method and positron emission tomography (PET) [1].

Six subjects with minor stroke were examined. Each subject inhaled about 40 mCi ^{11}CO. After 5-min equilibrium of ^{11}C-labeled carboxyhemoglobin, serial scans of 1-min frame were started and continued for 20 min [2]. During the measurement, forced hypercapnia was induced on the subject by CO_2 inhalation. The PET scanner [3] measured five cross-sectional image planes with 15-mm intervals simultaneously and with 10-mm full width at half-maximum spatial resolution. Arterial blood was sampled every minute from the radial artery and was measured for radioactivity and $PaCO_2$. CBV/100-ml brain tissue was calculated by the equation: CBV = 100 Ct / 0.85 Cb, where Ct and Cb were the radioactivity concentrations per unit volume in the brain tissue and blood, respectively (measured by PET and well counter), and 0.85 was the hematocrit ratio between the large vessel and the capillary. CBV reactivity to $PaCO_2$ change (ReCBV) was given by CBV change in ml/100-ml per $PaCO_2$ change in mmHg, i.e., ml/100-ml/mmHg $PaCO_2$ [4]. The CBV measurement was preceded by the CBF measurement as an anatomical reference in the data analysis.

ReCBV in the intracerebral tissue (0.038 ml/100-ml/mmHg) was significantly higher than that of the extracerebral tissue (0.032 ml/100ml/mmHg). CBV in the venous sinus showed a slight, negative response to $PaCO_2$ increase. In the cerebral parenchymal tissues of the cerebellum, basal ganglia, frontal cortex, temporal cortex, parietal cortex, and centrum semiovale, regional CBVs were 3.4, 4.7, 2.6, 4.0, 3.4, and 2.1 ml/100-ml, respectively, and regional ReCBV were 0.043, 0.053, 0.031, 0.041, 0.041, and 0.028 ml/100-ml/mmHg, respectively. The CBVs were slightly smaller than reported previously [5], because owing to the accurate anatomical location of regions of interest in this study, the CBV contained less contamination of the CBV in the extracerebral tissue. ReCBVs were revealed to be almost proportional to the resting state CBV in each region. Therefore, when the CBV reactivity to $PaCO_2$ change was represented by relative change per unit CBV, it became fairly uniform throughout the brain parenchymal tissue.

[1] Department of Radiology and Nuclear Medicine, Research Institute of Brain and Blood Vessels, 6–10, Kubota, Senshu, Akita, 010 Japan

References

1. Phelps ME, Huang SC, Hoffman EJ, Kuhl DE (1979) Validation of tomographic measurement of cerebral blood volume with C-11 labeled carboxyhemoglobin. J Nucl Med 20: 328–334
2. Kanno I, Murakami M, Miura M, Iida H, Takahashi K, Sasaki H, Uemura K (1987) Cerebral blood volume measurement using radioactive carboxyhemoglobin and positron emission tomography. In: Tomita N, Sawata T, Naritomi H (eds) Cerebral ischemia and hyperimia. Elsevier, Tokyo
3. Kanno I, Miura S, Yamamoto S, Iida H, Murakami M, Takahashi K, Uemura K (1985) Design and evaluation of a positron emission tomograph: HEADTOME III. J Comput Assist Tomogr 9: 931–939
4. Kanno I, Uemura K, Murakami M, Shishido F, Tomura N (1987) Cerebral blood volume reactivity to hypercapnia measured by ^{11}C-labeled carboxyhemoglobin and positron emission tomography. In: Tomita N, Sawata T, Naritomi H (eds) Cerebral ischemia and hyperimia. Elsevier, Tokyo
5. Greenberg JH, Alavi A, Reivich M, Kuhl D, Uzzell B (1978) Local cerebral blood volume response to carbon dioxide in man. Circ Res 43: 324–331

Capillary Density in Stroke Regions of the Living Human Brain

Albert Gjedde, Curt Beil, Ernst Meyer, Alan C. Evans, and Antoine M. Hakim[1]

The regional density of capillaries varies in the brain, some regions having more capillaries per unit weight, other regions having fewer. This arrangement is anatomical and does not reflect a functional coupling of flow, capillary permeability, or cerebral metabolic rate. The total number of capillaries in any one region is a reflection of the normal average energy requirement of the region and of the fact that individual capillaries have similar properties (radius, length, permeability) in different regions. This observation does not address the question of how many capillaries actually are perfused at any one time and how this number varies with the changing energy requirements of individual regions.

In order to prove a functional relationship between the number of perfused capillaries and the energy requirements of the tissue (recruitment), it is necessary to verify parallel adjustments of flow, density of perfused capillaries, and capillary diffusion capacity when metabolism is subject to change in a region of interest.

The hypothesis of recruitment explains how the diffusion-limited transfer of oxygen from the blood to the brain can be rate-limiting for oxygen utilization in the brain and responsible for the negligible oxygen tension there. Increasing the linear velocity of the blood perfusing the brain does not significantly improve the delivery of oxygen. Hence, increases of the capillary surface area are necessary to explain increases of oxygen utilization during activation. Likewise, during deactivation, decreases of capillary surface area must parallel decreases of metabolic rate and blood flow.

Positron emission tomography can measure most of these variables in the living human brain. However, it is usually a problem to establish conditions of activation or deactivation that are sufficiently stable to allow several measurements in the same subject. Initially, therefore, we did not examine the issue of activation and turned to the depression of brain function associated with ischemic insults. Although this is not a deactivation in the physiological sense, further insight into capillary reactions in ischemia may provide clues to more general mechanisms of regulation of capillary function in the brain. Also, the depression associated with stroke is sufficiently stable over a period of a few hours to allow

---

[1]Brain Imaging Centre, Montreal Neurological Institute, Montreal, Quebec, H3A 2B4, Canada

Table 1. Capillary bed in regions of cerebral cortex affected by an ischemic insult and in the contralateral mirror images

Subject	Region	(n)	$CMRO_2$ (μmol/hg/min)	CBF (ml/hg/min)	FRC (%)	T_{cap} (s)	N_{cap}
1	1 day poststroke						
	Control	6	118	30	9	0.9	360
	Stroke	6	51	11	9	1.7	253
2	1 day poststroke						
	Control	8	131	36	8	0.6	295
	Stroke	8	57	21	4	1.0	247
2	8 days poststroke						
	Control	8	148	49	10	0.6	384
	Stroke	8	87	51	5	0.4	271

$CMRO_2$ regional oxygen utilization, *CBF* regional blood flow, *FRC* fraction of total vascular bed represented by capillaries, T_{cap} mean capillary transit time, N_{cap} number of cross sections of perfused capillaries per mm^2

comparisons to be made between the different variables.

We scanned the brains of two stroke patients within 36 h of the insult and compared measurements of blood flow, blood volume, unidirectional and net glucose uptake, and oxygen utilization in regions affected by the stroke and in contralateral normal regions. From the direct measurements, we computed and compared the fraction of capillaries in the vascular bed, the mean capillary transit time, and the average number of perfused capillaries in regions of stroke and in contralateral normal regions.

The regional oxygen utilization was calculated from the initial uptake of labeled oxygen, the regional blood flow from the initial uptake of water, and the capillary surface area from the initial uptake of labeled fluorodeoxyglucose. The fraction of the total vascular bed represented by capillaries was calculated from the ratio between the cerebral blood volume, measured by labeled carbon monoxide, and the capillary surface area. The mean capillary transit time was calculated from the ratio between capillary volume and blood flow, and the number of cross sections of perfused capillaries per square millimeter section of tissue from the capillary volume, assuming a fixed capillary radius. Details of these measurements are given in Table 1.

In both patients, capillaries represented 8%–10% (v/v) of the total vascular bed. The most pronounced change after the stroke was the 50% decline of oxygen (and glucose) utilization in stroke regions, in spite of which the number of perfused (i.e., glucose-transporting) capillaries declined less than 30%. In both patients, the mean transit time through the capillary bed almost doubled after the stroke. In one patient, 8 days after the cerebrovascular incident, blood flow, oxygen utilization, and the number of perfused capillaries all increased in the normal control regions. In the stroke regions, however, only blood flow improved, while oxygen utilization and the number of perfused capillaries remained low. For this reason, the mean transit time through the capillaries declined markedly. Figure 1 illustrates the recruitment of capillaries in nor-

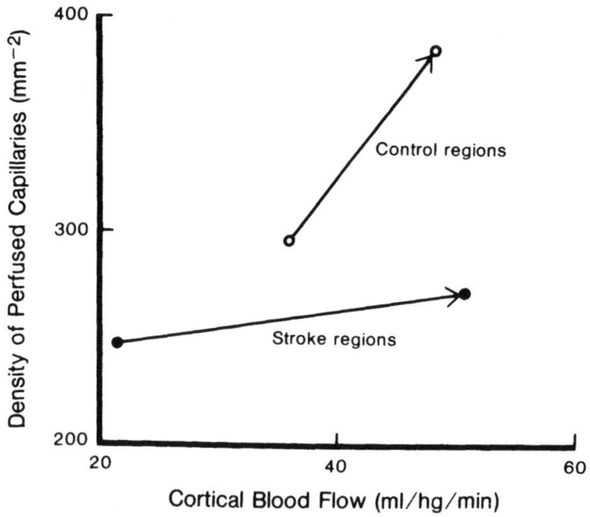

Fig. 1. Change of density of perfused capillaries as function of cortical blood flow changes of ischemia. *Arrow* indicates direction of change 1–8 days poststroke. *Closed circles* indicate stroke regions, *open circles* control mirror regions

mal brain regions and the absent recruitment during reperfusion of the stroke regions.

We concluded that the initial ischemic reduction of blood flow was followed by marked decline of oxygen utilization and some reduction of the number of perfused capillaries. The reduced ratio between capillaries and other vessels indicated a shift of blood from capillaries to venules and arterioles. The inability of stroke regions to increase capillary density during reperfusion may reflect sphincter depolarization elicited by potassium ions seeping from the ischemic nerve cells, or reperfusion in excess of actual metabolic needs by denervation of resistance vessels ("luxury perfusion") and deactivation of long or short stretch reflex circuits. This study, therefore, confirmed the separate control of blood flow and capillary recruitment.

SPECT Measurements of Regional Cerebral Blood Flow, Blood Volume, and Hematocrit in Stroke

FUMIHIKO SAKAI, HISAKA IGARASHI, SYUICHI SUZUKI, and YOSHIAKI TAZAKI[1]

Introduction

In the present study, single-photon emission computed tomography (SPECT) was used for the measurement of regional cerebral blood flow (CBF), blood volume (CBV), and cerebral hematocrit (Hct) in normal subjects and patients with occlusive cerebral vascular diseases. Using these three cerebral hemodynamic parameters, regional pathophysiology during the acute stages of cerebral infarction and transient ischemic attack (TIA) was investigated.

Subjects and Methods

Twenty-one neurologically normal subjects aged 32–43 years, 34 patients with cerebral infarction, and five patients with TIA due to severe stenosis or occlusion of internal carotid or middle cerebral arteries were studied.

The SPECT system used for the present study was the GE Maxi 400T camera connected to the Informatec Simis 3 computer or GE Starcam 400AC/T camera system.

Regional CBF was measured using N-isopropyl-p-I-123-iodoamphetamine (IMP). SPECT scans of the head were performed three times following the intravenous injection of IMP at 15 min, 2 h, and 4 h. Arterial and jugular venous blood was sampled serially and each sample was subjected to the octanol extraction to measure the proportion of IMP to its metabolites. Arterial IMP input curves were used for calculating regional CBF values [1].

CBV was measured using both a red blood cell (RBC) tracer and a plasma tracer [2]. For the RBC volume study, a sample of the subject's RBC was labeled with 20 mCi Tc-99m, using stannous pyrophosphate as a reducing agent. In the plasma volume study, 20 mCi Tc-99m-labeled human serum albumin (HSA) was used as a plasma tracer.

The RBC volume study and plasma volume study were performed either separately with an interval of 48 h or serially on the same day.

---

[1]Department of Medicine, School of Medicine, Kitasato University, 15-1, Kitasato 1-chome, Sagamihara, Kanagawa, 228 Japan

Results

After the intravenous injection of IMP in normal subjects, arterial activity made an initial peak within 5 min. Jugular venous activity also showed a smaller but similar initial peak. After an initial peak, the arterial activity continued but gradually approached an equilibrium with jugular venous activity at around 45 min, indicating a balance between washin and washout of cerebral activities. After 2 h, jugular venous activity exceeded the arterial activity, indicating the washout of the tracer from the brain. Mean CBF in normal subjects corrected for the extraction ratio was 44.8 ± 6.4 ml/100 g brain/min.

During the acute stages of cerebral infarction, the reduction of CBF in the ischemic hemisphere measured by early scan was seen in larger areas than the low density on the CT scan. In patients with good clinical recovery, the area of low flow in the early image showed a late accumulation of IMP. Hemispheric asymmetry became minimal in images at 2 h and 4 h. Late filling reached an equilibrium within 2–3 h.

The mean hemispheric CBV values in normals was 4.81 ± 0.37 ml/100 g brain. The mean of the RBC volume in the resting state was 1.50 ± 0.09 ml/100 g brain. This was significantly smaller than the mean of the plasma volume, which was 3.4 ± 1.8 ml/100 g brain. The mean cerebral Hct calculated from these values was $31.3\% \pm 1.8\%$, and the cerebral/large vessel Hct ratio was $75.9\% \pm 2.1\%$.

CBV increased in the ischemic hemisphere corresponding to the zone of reduced flow compared with the nonischemic hemisphere. Cerebral Hct did not show significant hemispheric asymmetry in patients with good clinical recovery. In patients with poor clinical prognosis, cerebral Hct was higher in the ischemic hemisphere during the acute stage.

Discussion

Our study has demonstrated that the use of SPECT enables us to measure CBF, CBV, and cerebral Hct in humans. It also suggests that the method can reveal variations in cerebral Hct during different physiological and pathological conditions. The cerebral/large vessel Hct ratio in the present study was 75.9%, which is lower than the previously reported standard value of 85% [3–5]. It is likely that cerebral Hct measured by three-dimensional resolution [6] presents more regional values closer to the true tissue Hct level, which is known to be lower in large-diameter vessels [7, 8].

In the present study, low CBF was associated with increased CBV during the acute stage of cerebral infarction and during symptom-free intervals of TIA. It is also suggested that cerebral Hct is increased in ischemic regions of poor prognosis. In the region of cerebral ischemia, if the CBV is maximally increased the blood viscosity assumes greater importance in the determination of cerebral perfusion. The question of whether the increase of cerebral Hct in the ischemic tissue could predict further reductions in CBF or simply shows the result of completed stroke with blood stasis should be answered in larger series of studies.

References

1. Kuhl DE, Barrio JR, Huang SC, et al. (1982) Quantifying local cerebral blood flow by N-isopropyl-p-iodo amphetamine tomography. J Nucl Med 23: 196–203
2. Sakai F, Nakazawa K, Tazaki Y, et al. (1985) Regional cerebral blood volume and hematocrit measured in normal human volunteers by single-photon emission computed tomography. J Cereb Blood Flow Metabol 5: 207–213
3. Phelps ME, Grubb RL, Ter-Pogossian MM (1973) Correlation between Pa CO2 and regional cerebral blood volume by X-ray fluorescence. J Appl Physiol 35: 274–280
4. Oldendorf WH, Kitano M, Shimizu S, Oldendorf SZ (1965) Hematocrit of human cerebral blood pool. Circ Res 17: 532–539
5. Larsen OA, Lassen NA (1964) Cerebral hematocrit in normal man. J Appl Physiol 19: 571–574
6. Lammertsma AA, Brooks DJ, Beaney RP, Turton DR, Kensett MJ, Heather JD, Marshall J, Jones T (1984) In vivo measurement of regional cerebral hematocrit using positron emission tomography. J Cereb Blood Flow Metabol 4: 317–322
7. Fahraeus R (1929) The suspension stability of fluid. Physiol Rev 9: 241–274
8. Barbee JH, Cokelet GR (1971) The Fahraeus effect. Microvasc Res 3: 6–16

Endothelium-Dependent Relaxing Factors in Brain Microvessels

William I. Rosenblum[1]

Introduction

A pathological decrease in local or general cerebral blood flow may have many causes, several of which can act at the same time. In recent years, a significant addition has been made to the number of ways by which the flow may be increased. This addition is the result of a new discovery concerning the importance of endothelial cells in some forms of vasodilation. The new understanding began with the discovery that acetylcholine (ACh) produces dilation in many blood vessels, not by activating muscarinic receptors in vascular smooth muscle, but by activating such receptors in the endothelium. The endothelium in turn produces and releases a relaxing factor that penetrates the muscle and produces relaxation. This substance has become known as endothelium-dependent relaxing factor (EDRF). This entire area has been extensively reviewed [1–4], and the evidence for multiple EDRFs has been supported by additional publications [5–7].

The original technique for demonstrating endothelium dependence was based on the loss of the dilating response in large vessels in vitro following the removal of large numbers of endothelial cells. The questions remain whether resistance vessels also have EDRFs, whether putative dilator substances other than those traveling in the bloodstream can release EDRF, and whether EDRF can be manifest in vivo. As the following data show, we have answered these questions in the affirmative, at least for the resistance vessels on the surface of the brain.

Methods

Our methods for exposing and observing the pial vessels of mice and our two techniques for injuring in situ microvessels in vivo have been described elsewhere in detail [8–12]. With the first method, injury to all vessels in a microscopic field is caused by exposing the field to filtered light from a mercury lamp after sensitizing the microvascular bed by intravenous injection of sodium fluorescein

[1]Neuropathology, Medical College of Virginia, Virginia Commonwealth University, Box 17 MCV Station, Richmond, VA 23298-0017, USA

[10, 11]. With the second method, injury is produced only at a single point, 18 or 36 μm wide, by the beam of a 6-mW HeNe laser, following sensitization of the microvascular bed with an intravenous injection of Evans' blue [12].

Electron-microscopic study of vessels in which EDRFs were lost or of vessels treated in an identical manner to those with attenuated EDRF revealed only mild damage to the endothelial cells and no damage to the smooth muscle. More severe damage occurred only after platelet aggregates had formed. Such aggregates were recognized as "white bodies" during our intravital microscopic monitoring of the vessels. Mice in which aggregates appeared were discarded and not used for studies of EDRF.

Results

Injury by Hg Light/Fluorescein

Prior to injury, 12 arterioles were monitored (one arteriole per mouse); they were 30–45 μm in diameter. ACh chloride (80 μg/ml) dilated the arterioles to 117% ± 4% (mean ± SD) of baseline diameter. After injury, the average response to ACh was constriction to 91% ± 6% of the baseline value (pre-vs. postinjury removal; $P < 0.01$, Wilcoxon test).

Five arterioles (mean diameter 36 ± 4 μm) were examined in five additional mice. Before injury, 80-μg/ml bradykinin triacetate relaxed them to 116% ± 3% of the baseline value. After injury, they constricted on average to 87% ± 4% of the baseline diameter (pre-vs. postinjury response; $P < 0.01$, paired Student's t'-test after log transformation of data).

Papaverine HC1 (320 μg/ml) successfully dilated all damaged vessels in each study; in the first, papaverine relaxed the vessels to 120% ± 7%, in the second to 117% ± 6% of baseline values. The diameter in each study was unchanged by the noxious light or dye.

Injury by HeNe Laser/Evan's blue

At the center of the laser, 80 μg/ml ACh Chloride caused relaxation to 127% ± 5% of baseline diameter before injury and constriction to 97% ± 5% after injury (pre-vs. postinjury response; $P < 0.01$, Wilcoxon test). With progression 25, 55, or 80 μm upstream, increasing degrees of relaxation were observed after injury to 106% ± 14%, 110% ± 14%, and 116% ± 11% of baseline values, respectively. Relaxation was also decreased downstream, for example to 109% ± 3% of baseline diameter at a point 80 μm from the laser center. The spread of injury is thought to be due to diffusion of the damaging heat.

To test the selectivity of the effects of laser/Evan's blue, we performed five separate studies using sodium nitroprusside, a dilator whose action has been found in large vessels to be independent of the endothelium. The laser injury had absolutely no effect on the response to $10^{-4}M$ sodium nitroprusside.

Nature of EDRF

The EDRF for ACh must differ from that for bradykinin. This was shown by testing the effects of each dilator in the presence of 60 units/ml superoxide dismutase (SOD). No effect was observed against ACh, the dilation being identical with or without SOD. However, dilations to bradykinin were significantly reduced by SOD, from 113% ± 7% to 96% ± 7% of baseline diameter ($P < 0.01$, Wilcoxon test).

The effect of SOD on response to bradykinin suggested that the relaxing action of bradykinin was dependent upon an oxygen-centered free radical. This was substantiated by separate studies with 46 units/ml catalase and deferoxamine (0.1 or 0.2 mmoL). The former scavenges H_2O_2, while the latter prevents hydroxyl radical formation from the superoxide reaction with H_2O_2 by chelating the iron that catalyzes this reaction [13]. In each case, dilation by bradykinin was significantly inhibited [6].

Discussion

Our data establish that in cerebral resistance vessels, endothelium-dependent relaxation is a phenomenon that regulates tone. Loss of endothelium-dependent relaxation would deprive these vessels of a relaxing mechanism in disease states. Moreover, like ACh, endothelium-dependent relaxants may be potent constrictors once EDRF is eliminated. Therefore, loss of EDRF also provides us with a new mechanism for vasospasm.

References

1. Vanhoutte PM, Houston DS (1985) Platelets, endothelium and vasospasm. Circ 72: 728–734
2. Busse R, Trogisch G, Bassenge E (1985) The role of endothelium in control of vascular tone. Basic Res Cardiol 80: 475–490
3. Furchgott RF (1983) Role of endothelium in responses of vascular smooth muscle. Circ Res 53: 557–573
4. Peach MJ, Singer HA, Loeb AL (1985) Mechanisms of endothelium dependent vascular smooth muscle relaxation. Bioch Pharm 34: 1867–1874
5. Kontos HA, Wei EP, Povlishock JT, Christmann CW (1984) Oxygen radicals mediate the cerebral arteriolar dilation from arachidonate and bradykinin in cats. Circ Res 55: 295–303
6. Rosenblum WI (1987) Hydroxyl radical mediates the endothelium dependent relaxation produced by bradykinin in mouse cerebral arterioles. Circ Res
7. Griffith TM, Edwards DH, Lewis MJ, Newby C, Henderson AH (1984) The nature of endothelium derived relaxant factor. Nature 308: 645–647
8. Rosenblum WI (1975) Constriction of pial arterioles by prostaglandin F_{α}. Stroke 6: 293–297
9. Rosenblum WI, Zweifach BW (1963) Cerebral microcirculation in the mouse brain. Arch Neurol 9: 414–423
10. Povlishock JT, Rosenblum WI, Sholley MM, Wei EP (1983) An ultrastructural

analysis of endothelial change paralleling platelet aggregation in a light/dye model of microvascular insult. Am J Pathol 110: 148–160
11. Rosenblum WI (1986) Endothelial dependent relaxation demonstrated in vivo in cerebral arterioles. Stroke 17: 494–497
12. Rosenblum WI, Nelson GH, Povlishock JT (1987) Laser induced endothelial damage inhibits endothelium dependent relaxation in the cerebral microcirculation of the mouse. Circ Res 60: 169–176
13. Gutteridge JMC, Richmond R, Halliwell B (1979) Inhibition of the iron catalyzed formation of hydroxyl radicals from superoxide and of lipid peroxidation by desferrioxamine. Biochem J 184: 469–472

Role of Oxygen Free Radicals in Focal Brain Ischemia

REGINALD J. DAVIS[1], GREGORY B. BULKLEY[2], and RICHARD J. TRAYSTMAN[3]

Oxygen-derived free radicals have been implicated in a wide variety of disease states [1,2] and have been postulated to mediate an element of cerebral ischemic injury. We tested the hypothesis that neutralization of oxygen free radicals using superoxide dismutase (SOD) ameliorates the cerebral ischemic injury produced by temporary occlusion of the middle cerebral artery.

Twenty-four cats (2.7–4.1 kg) were anesthetized with ketamine (5–10 mg/kg) and acepromazine (0.5 mg/kg) and maintained with a constant infusion of fentanyl (2–5 μg/kg) and inhalation of nitrous oxide and oxygen (70%/30%). Femoral arterial and venous catheters were placed for monitoring arterial blood pressure, blood gases, and infusion of fluids and drugs. Somatosensory evoked potentials (SEP) were obtained and monitored using the CA 1000 Evoked Potential Monitor and needle electrodes. Regional cerebral blood flow (CBF) was measured using the radiolabeled microsphere technique. Microspheres were injected into the left ventricle and reference organ blood flow was obtained by constant withdrawal of blood from a right axillary artery catheter. Regional cerebral ischemia was induced by occlusion of the left middle cerebral artery (MCA). The MCA was microsurgically exposed by exoneration of the left orbit and enlargement of the optic foramen. The MCA was occluded using a microvascular clip. This procedure produces a reproducible ischemic injury. The region of the MCA was reperfused upon release of the clip. Two control measurements, consisting of duplicate bilateral SEPs and a microsphere injection, were taken 15 min apart. The MCA was then occluded for 30 min and a third measurement was taken at the end of the occlusion but before reperfusion. Subsequent measurements were made at 15, 60, and 120 min following reperfusion. At the end of each experiment, the animals were killed by injection of KC1. The brains were removed, fixed, and later sectioned and counted in a gamma counter. The animals were divided into four groups: group I ($n = 6$) received saline, group II ($n = 7$) received SOD (Sigma 30000 units/h) prior to MCA occlusion, group III ($n = 6$) received SOD (Sigma) prior to reperfusion, and group IV ($n = 5$) received ultrapure SOD prior to reperfusion. In group I, CBF decreased from 110 ± 12 to 38 ± 8 ml/min/100 g with 30-min MCA occlu-

Departments of Neurosurgery[1], Surgery[2], and Anesthesiology/Critical Medicine[3], The Johns Hopkins Medical Institutions, Baltimore, MD 21205, USA sion. CBF was 98 ± 23, 49 ± 14, and 46 ± 13 ml/min/100 g at 15, 60, and 120 min, respectively, following reperfusion. SEP was reduced to 5% of control values during MCA occlusion, and was 39% ± 17%, 15% ± 8% and 7% ± 5% of control at 15, 60, and 120 min of reperfusion. In SOD-treated groups (II-IV), CBF was reduced similarly with MCA occlusion, but CBF was 142 ± 13, 93 ± 9, and 77 ± 8 ml/min/100 g at 15, 60, and 120 min after reperfusion. SEP was also reduced similarly with MCA occlusion in SOD-treated groups but was 58% ± 8%, 55% ± 5%, and 48% ± 6% of control values at 15, 60, and 120 min following reperfusion.

Thus, both CBF and SEP were improved after SOD treatment and it made little difference whether Sigma SOD or the ultrapure SOD was used. These data suggest that a component of the injury produced by focal brain ischemia is mediated by the superoxide radical and that this injury occurs at the time of reperfusion. This injury can be partially prevented by SOD. These studies also implicate the delayed hypoperfusion in the injury resulting from MCA occlusion. SOD resulted in higher CBF in the reperfusion period (better cerebral perfusion) and this might account for the improved cerebral function with SOD. Finally, the injury is probably one of reperfusion, not ischemia, since SOD exerted positive effects when administered at reperfusion only. While much still remains to be done with ischemia-reperfusion injury in the brain, these preliminary experiments offer some information concerning the potential mechanism of injury with ischemia and potentially offer ideas for therapeutic intervention.

References

1. Fridovich I (1978) The biology of oxygen radicals. Science 201: 875–880
2. Weiss SJ (1986) Oxygen, ischemia and inflammation. In: Del Maestro RF, Arfors KE (eds) Free radicals in microcirculation. Acta Physiol Scand [Suppl] 548: 9–37

Microcirculatory and Ionic Responses to Ischemia in the Mongolian Gerbil

Avraham Mayevsky[1]

Introduction

The Mongolian gerbil (*Meriones unguiculatus*) is a very useful animal model for studying brain responses to partial or complete ischemia [1–5]. Various aspects of brain functions and responses have been studied in this model exposed to ischemic conditions. When cerebral blood flow diminished due to the ischemia [6], inhibition of the Na^+K^+ATPase occurred and, as a result, extracellular K^+ level increased [7, 8]. In 1978, we described the effects of ischemia on the metabolic activity in the gerbil brain using the surface fluorometry technique to monitor reduced nicotinamide adenine dinucleotide (NADH) redox state [9]. In ischemia, we described a new phenomenon defined as secondary reflectance increase (SRI), [10]; this event is associated with ionic homeostasis disturbances which occur under energy deprivation conditions. To study this microcirculatory phenomenon under ischemia, the multiparametric monitoring approach [8] was used. Metabolic activity was measured by monitoring tissue surface O_2 tension by a surface electrode. Intramitochondrial NADH redox state was evaluated by the surface fluorometry reflectometry technique described in detail previously [11]. The reflected light at the excitation wavelength (336 nm) measured simultaneously with the fluorescence light (450 nm) was used to correct the fluorescence signal for hemodynamic artifacts. This signal is largely dependent upon blood volume at the measurement site. Extracellular K^+ activity was measured by a surface valinomycine electrode located in the multiprobe assembly.

Methods

All probes used were located in the multiprobe assembly (MPA) constructed according to the principles described previously [8, 11, 12]. The probes were mounted in a Lucite holder (cannula) cemented directly to the skull. The holes accommodating the specific sensory electrodes converged at the implantation site, occupying less space on the brain, and diverged at the top of the cannula to leave maximum room for mounting and replacing the electrodes.

[1]Department of Life Sciences, Bar-Ilan University, Ramat-Gan 52100, Israel

The intramitochondrial NADH redox state was monitored by a light guided DC fluorometer/reflectometer [11]. The joined part of the Y-shaped light guide was cemented inside the multiprobe assembly in the same way as the other electrodes. The gerbil was anesthetized, and the MPA implanted above the brain as described previously [8, 12].

Results and Discussion

To clarify the unusual microcirculatory response to ischemia, the effects of bilateral carotid artery occlusion in the gerbil are presented in Fig. 1. In this gerbil, the PO_2 trace showed a decrease followed by a small recovery during the occlusion. The NADH reached a stable high level (CF in Fig. 1) due to the depletion of oxygen. Extracellular K^+ started to accumulate immediately after the occlusion. The electrocorticogram (ECoG) disappeared almost completely after the occlusion, although the DC steady potential was not initially affected. About 2 min after the occlusion, a massive depolarization occurred, seen as a negative shift in the DC potential (20 mV), as well as a large increase in extracellular K^+ levels (from 3 to 30 mmol/l). During this depolarization, the optical properties

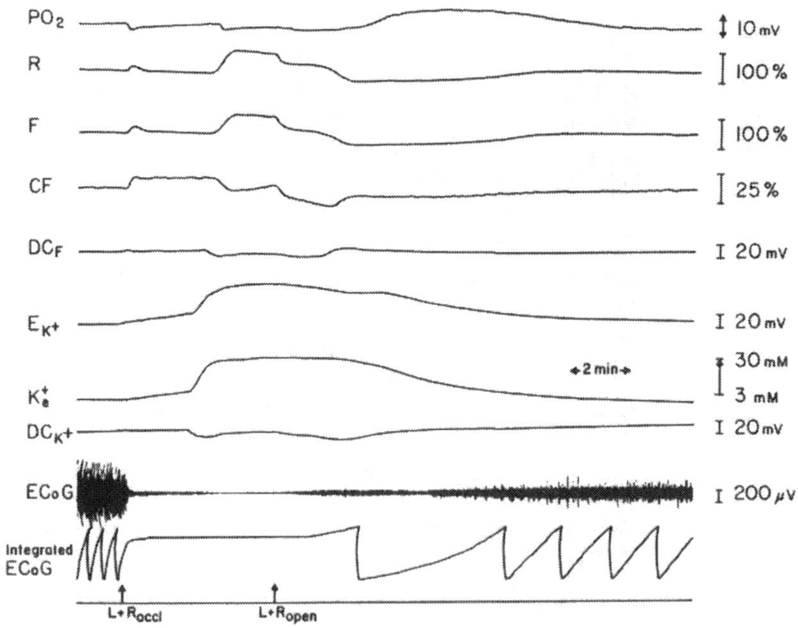

Fig. 1. The effects of bilateral carotid artery on the metabolic ionic and electrical activities in the gerbil brain. PO_2 tissue surface O_2 levels, *R* 366-nm reflectance, *F* 450 nm fluorescence, *CF* NADH-corrected fluorescence, DC_F, $DC_K{}^+$ DC steady potential around the optical fibers and the K^+ electrode, respectively, $E_K{}^+$, $K_e{}^+$ uncorrected extracellular K electrode potential and corrected (for DC changes) K^+ levels, respectively, *ECoG* electrocorticogram, $L + R_{occl}$ left and right carotid artery occlusion, $L + R_{open}$ left and right carotid artery open

of the tissue were changed and a large increase in the reflectance trace (R) was recorded. This change in the R signal was secondary to the initial response to the occlusion itself and wad defined by us as SRI [10]. The change in the R signal led to an apparent decrease in the NADH-corrected fluorescence trace due to the inability of the correction factor to handle such a large change which included optical changes in the tissue besides the hemodynamic ones. The PO_2 trace showed a further decrease during depolarization, suggesting a vasoconstriction event. This further decrease in PO_2 may suggest that the level of ischemia was below 100% and the vasoconstriction led to a complete ischemia. The recovery of the K^+ and DC steady potential was very fast compared with the ECoG, which was partially depressed for a longer period of time. The PO_2 trace showed an overshoot during the recovery period, correlating to the large blood volume in the tissue as seen by The NADH redox state showed a large undershoot during the recovery period due to the extra pumping activity done by the Na^+-K^+-ATPase to shift the K^+ into the cellular compartment.

As shown by various investigators, the Mongolian gerbil is a good model for studying the effects of partial as well as complete ischemia on the brain [13–15]. One of the problems in using any model of ischemia is evaluating the level of the ischemic insult developed, which can be done by monitoring the NADH redox state.

Acknowledgments. This study was supported in part by a grant from the Chief Scientist's Office, Ministry of Health, Israel and the Health Science Research Center, Dept. of Life Sciences, Bar-Ilan University, Ramat-Gan, Israel.

References

1. Levine S, Payan H (1966) Effects of ischemia and other procedures on the brain and retina of the gerbil. Exp Neurol 16: 255–262
2. Kahn K (1972) The natural course of experimental cerebral infarction in the gerbil. Neurology 22: 510–515
3. Berry K, Wisniewski HM, Svarzbein L, Baez S (1975) On the relationship of brain vasculature to production of neurological deficit and morphological changes following acute unilateral common carotid artery ligation in gerbils. J Neurol Sci 25: 75–92
4. Molinari GF, Laurent JP (1976) A classification of experimental models of brain ischemia. Stroke 7: 14–17
5. Robinson DG (1980) The gerbil stroke model. Gerbil Digest 7 (2): 1–4
6. Kelly RA, Halsey JH (1976) Comparison of local blood flow and oxygen availability at the same locus in the ischemic gerbil brain. Stroke 7: 274–278.
7. Mayevsky A, Crowe W, Mela L (1980) The interrelation between brain oxidative metabolism and extracellular potassium in the unanesthetized gerbil. Neurol Res 1: 213–226
8. Friedli CM, Sclarsky DL, Mayevsky A (1982) A new multiprobe assembly for surface monitoring of ionic metabolic and electrical activities in the awake brain. Am J Physiol 243: R 462–R469
9. Mayevsky A, Bar-Sagie D, Levy N, Amosi, M (1978) The effects of ischemia on the metabolic response of the cerebral cortex of the gerbil. Fed Proc 37: 497 (Abstr 1495)
10. Zarchin N, Mayevsky A (1981) The effects of age on the metabolic and electrical responses to decapitation in the awake anesthetized rat brain. Mechan Aging Devel 16: 285–294
11. Mayevsky A (1984) Brain NADH redox state monitored in vivo by fiber optic surface

fluorometry. Brain Res Rev 7: 49–68
12. Mayevsky A (1983) Multiparameter monitoring of the awake brain under hyperbaric oxygenation. J Appl Physiol 54: 740–748
13. Levy DE, Brierley JB (1974) Communications between vertebrobasilar and carotid arterial circulations in the gerbil. Exp Neurol 45: 503–508
14. Ginsberg MD, Mela L, Wrobel-Kuhl K, Reivich M (1977) Mitochondrial metabolism following bilateral cerebral iscehmia in the gerbil. Ann Neurol 1: 519–527
15. Mayevsky A (1978) Pyridine nucleotide oxidation-reduction state of the cerebral cortex in the awake gerbil. J Neurosci Res 3: 369–374

Postischemic Hyperemia

Wolf-Dieter Heiss, Rudolf Graf, and Gerhard Rosner[1]

Postischemic hyperperfusion is a heterogeneous phenomenon of variable pathophysiological origin and divergent prognostic implications. Even the nomenclature is not clear, with various names and definitions for this state, i.e., hyperperfusion, hyperemia, luxury perfusion, and vasomotor paralysis. Postischemic hyperperfusion is quite a common finding in transient perfusion disturbances in animal experiments, but it can be also observed with permanent arterial occlusion and spontaneous collateral reperfusion. While postischemic hyperperfusion often develops after ischemia lasting up to 30 min and is usually followed by normal perfusion and fast recovery of function (as recorded in evoked responses), it can be observed regularly after 60-min transient ischemia but then often leads to postischemic hypoperfusion and impaired function [1]. With 2-h ischemia, postischemic hypoperfusion with permanently impaired function often develops without postischemic hyperperfusion. Autoregulation and CO_2 reactivity are disturbed during postischemic hyperperfusion in the center as well as in the periphery of the middle cerebral artery (MCA) territory. Therefore, with impaired vascular reactivity, neither the vessels in the center nor in the periphery are able to compensate for pressure changes. As hyperperfusion after ischemia of 60 or 120 min duration is usually followed by postischemic hypoperfusion and pressure gradients are changed concomitantly, alternating cycles of hyper- and hypoperfusion may occur and spread over the brain. Therefore, hyperperfusion may contribute to the extension of ischemic damage into primarily unaffected brain regions. It is important to note that functional regulation of cerebral blood flow (CBF) seems to be more resistant than the other regulatory mechanisms and may still be present when autoregulation and CO_2 reactivity are impaired during postischemic hyper- and hypoperfusion.

Spontaneous or stimulus-related cellular activity recovered after short-term ischemia often at the same time as postischemic hyperperfusion was normalized; longer lasting and more severe ischemia led to irreversible impairment of neuronal function [2]. Recovery of evoked responses after ischemia of up to 60 min was nearly complete in the border-zone and poor or only partial in the core of the ischemia. In the experiments with 2-h ischemia, persistent neurological

[1]Max-Planck-Institut für neurologische Forschung, Joseph-Stelzmann-Straße 9, D-5000 Köln 41, Federal Republic of Germany

deficits and disturbances of the energy-producing metabolism, as demonstrated by the low regional ATP content, were significantly correlated to the severity of the ischemia but not to the level of reperfusion [3]. Recovery of function was poor in the ischemic core (auditory-evoked responses in MCA occlusion in cats) and variable in the borderzone of ischemia (somatosensory-evoked responses), and this functional course was related to water accumulation and disruption of the blood-brain barrier [4].

In permanent MCA occlusion in cats, postischemic hyperperfusion developing spontaneously due to collateral circulation during the first 4 h was always followed by early death as a result of tentorial herniation, which was a sequel of severe brain edema and large infarcts [5]. In contrast, hyperperfusion occurring after several days (late hyperperfusion) indicated a favorable prognosis with resolution of the neurological deficits and small infarcts. Similar observations were also made in some stroke patients, in whom hyperperfused regions developing in previously ischemic areas were found 7–12 days after the ischemic attack [6]. The clinical course in these cases was characterized by fair resolution of the neurological deficits, and later studies demonstrated improved flow in the primarily disturbed regions. With positron emission tomography, uncoupling of flow, oxygen consumption, and glucose metabolism may be observed early after an ischemic episode [7], and increased local blood volume in an area of decreased blood flow may indicate a compensatory mechanism (low-perfusion hyperemia) [8]. With decreased oxygen consumption and oxygen extraction rate as indicators of morphological tissue damage, increased flow is a sign of luxury perfusion [9] without beneficial effects on prognosis. When hyperperfusion is combined with increased uptake of glucose, these compartments may survive and be present as viable tissue within infarcted regions [10].

All these data from various experimental and clinical observations indicate that postischemic hyperemia is not a uniform phenomenon with a defined pathophysiological cause and clear prognostic implication. While it is a functional overshoot after short-term ischemia on the way to normalization, it is a pathogenetic mechanism leading to additional tissue damage and to late hypoperfusion after longer lasting transient ischemia. In subacute stages, it might be an indicator of beneficial collateral flow or of excessive vasodilatation in necrotic tissue. In these instances, the state of the nervous tissue can only be evaluated by additional studies of metabolism and oxygen consumption.

References

1. Traupe H, Kruse E, Heiss WD (1982) Reperfusion of focal ischemia of varying duration: Postischemic hyper- and hypoperfusion. Stroke 13: 615–622
2. Heiss WD, Rosner G (1983) Functional recovery of cortical neurons as related to degree and duration of ischemia. Ann Neurol 14: 294–301
3. Paschen W, Sato M, Pawlik G, Umbach C, Heiss WD (1985) Neurologic deficit, blood flow and biochemical sequelae of reversible focal cerebral ischemia in cats. J Neurol Sci 68: 119–134
4. Kataoka K, Graf R, Rosner G, Heiss WD (1987) Experimental focal ischemia in cats: Changes in multimodality evoked potentials as related to local cerebral blood flow and ischemic brain edema. Stroke 18: 188–194

5. Heiss WD, Hayakawa T, Waltz AG (1976) Patterns of changes of blood flow and relationships to infarction in experimental cerebral ischemia. Stroke 7: 454–459
6. Heiss, WD, Zeiler K, Turnheim M, Podreka I (1976) Flow and compartmental weight in relation to the course of stroke. Stroke 7: 399–403
7. Wise RJS, Bernardi S, Frackowiak RSJ, Legg NJ, Jones T (1983) Serial observations on the pathophysiology of acute stroke. The transition from ischaemia to infarction as reflected in regional oxygen extraction. Brain 106: 197–222
8. Tomita M, Gotoh F, Amano T, Tanahashi N, Tanaka K (1980) "Low perfusion hyperemia" following middle cerebral arterial occlusion in cats of different age groups. Stroke 11: 629–636
9. Lassen NA (1966) The luxury-perfusion syndrome and its possible relation to acute metabolic acidosis localized within the brain. Lancet II: 1113–1115
10. Heiss WD, Herholz K, Böcher-Schwarz HG, Pawlik G, Wienhard K, Steinbrich W, Friedmann G (1986) PET, CT, and MR imaging in cerebrovascular disease. J Comput Assist Tomogr 10: 903–911

Remote Hyperemia After Focal Cerebral Ischemia: Disinhibition Mechanism of Remote Hyperemia

Akira Tamura[1], Hitoshi Nakayama[1], Takaaki Kirino[1], Noriko Tomukai[1], Keiji Sano[1], and Ichiro Kanazawa[2]

Introduction

Hyperemia after focal cerebral ischemia generally develops in two situations. Hyperemia in the surrounding area of infarction is sometimes observed in clinical cases accompanied by local hypometabolism. Hyperemia in the ischemic focus, on the other hand, usually results from recanalization to an area damaged by ischemia and may cause hemorrhagic infarction.

Using the left middle cerebral artery (MCA) occlusion model in the rat, we have previously reported both a marked reduction of cerebral blood flow (CBF) in the territory of the occluded artery and increased CBF in the ipsilateral globus pallidus and substantia nigra [1, 2]. Both areas lie outside the ischemic area but have transsynaptic connections with the ischemic focus, i.e., the caudate nucleus. Our hypothesis is, thus, as follows: The hyperemia in these remote areas may be explained as a reflection of altered neuronal function and increased metabolism, which is caused by diminished inhibitory output from the ischemic region. The aim of the present study was to elucidate the mechanism of this remote transsynaptic disinhibition hyperemia after focal cerebral ischemia.

Methods and Results

Measurement of Neurotransmitters

Adult male Sprague-Dawley rats were anesthetized by halothane inhalation. The left MCA was permanently occluded via the transretro-orbital approach. The animals were decapitated on the 1st, 2nd, 3rd, 7th, 14th, and 28th days following MCA occlusion. The brains were quickly removed and frozen. Then, 150-μm-thick serial coronal sections were prepared with a cryostat. From these sections, the substantia nigra, globus pallidus, and caudate nucleus were removed using a microdissection technique. Amino acid neurotransmitters were

[1]Department of Neurosurgery, Teikyo University School of Medicine, 11–1, Kaga 2-chome, Itabashi-ku, Tokyo, 173 Japan.
[2]University of Tsukuba, 1-1, Tennodai 1-chome, Sakura-mura, Ibaragi, 305 Japan

measured by an enzymatic-fluorometric method [3], and the protein content of the specimens by Lowry's method.

Gamma-aminobutyric acid (GABA) significantly decreased to about 60% of the control value in the ipsilateral substantia nigra from days 3 through 28. Aspartate also decreased significantly in the ipsilateral substantia nigra from days 3 through 28. Glutamate remained within normal range. In the contralateral substantia nigra, GABA increased significantly from day 1 through 28, whereas glutamate and aspartate showed no significant change. The same, although less pronounced, tendency was observed in the globus pallidus.

Neuropathological Study

A total of 29 rats were perfusion-fixed 2 days, 7 days, 3 weeks, and 3 months following MCA occlusion. Histological studies were carried out using the sections, including the substantia nigra. Neuropathological studies invariably showed infarction of the cortex and the lateral part of the neostriatum 2 days after MCA occlusion. No pathological change was revealed in the substantia nigra. One week after MCA occlusion, there was necrosis of the cortex and the lateral part of the striatum within the distribution area of the MCA. The edge of the necrotic tissue was clearly delineated from normal tissue. There were reactive changes in the ipsilateral globus pallidus but none in the substantia nigra. However, 3 weeks after the operation, neuronal loss, gliosis, and atrophy were observed in the ipsilateral substantia nigra in all animals. Three months thereafter, marked atrophy and gliosis were noticed in this area in all six animals.

Discussion

The efferent fibers of the caudate nucleus have a restricted distribution, projecting only to two ipsilateral structures—the globus pallidus and pars reticularis of the substantia nigra. The caudate nucleus of the rat contains high concentrations of several neurotransmitters, such as acetylcholine, dopamine, glutamate, substance P, and GABA. The neuroinhibitory transmitter GABA plays an important functional role in the striatonigral pathway [4]. The long-term decrease of GABA and aspartate can be explained by ischemic damage to the afferent tracts and subsequent degeneration of synaptic terminals in the substantia nigra. It is probable that the decrease of GABA renders the substantia nigra neurons liable to fire spontaneously, thus leading to the coupled increase of CBF and glucose use [1, 2, 5]. The persistent increase of GABA in the contralateral substantia nigra may indicate the compensation for the decrease of GABA in the ipsilateral substantia nigra.

In our neuropathological study, neuronal loss, gliosis, and then marked atrophy were observed in the ipsilateral subatantia nigra in the chronic phase. These histological changes may be slowly progressive.

In conclusion, our findings reveal that hyperemia resulting from alterations in neuronal function and metabolic activity in the ipsilateral substantia nigra may be caused by a loss of inhibition. Since the increase of CBF is considered to arise by a transsynaptic disinhibition mechanism, it could be termed "disinhibition hyperemia."

References

1. Tamura A, Graham DI, McCulloch J, Teasdale GM (1981) Focal cerebral ischemia in the rat: 2. Regional cerebral blood flow determined by [14-C] iodoantipyrine autoradiography following middle cerebral artery occlusion. J Cereb Blood Flow Metabol 1: 61–69
2. Tamura A, Orii H, Nagashima T, Matsutani M (1983) Fundamental study for imaging diagnostic medicine: I. Cerebral infarction. Nippon Acta Radiologica 43: 377–380
3. Miyata Y, Otsuka M (1975) Quantitative histochemistry of γ-aminobutyric acid in cat spinal cord with special reference to presynaptic inhibition. J Neurochem 25: 239–244
4. Kelly PT, Graham DI, McCulloch J (1982) Specific alterations in local cerebral glucose utilization following striatal lesions. Brain Res 233: 157–172
5. Tamura A, Matsutani M, Orii H (1984) Fundamental study for image diagnostic medicine: II. Local cerebral glucose metabolism in cerebral infarction. Nippon Acta Radiologica 44: 1546–1548

Cerebral Hyperemia and Breakthrough During Hypertension

SEIZO SADOSHIMA and MASATOSHI FUJISHIMA[1]

Introduction

Cerebral blood flow is maintained relatively constant with variations of perfusion pressure. This autoregulatory function is adapted to higher levels of blood pressure in hypertensive humans and animals than in normotensives [1, 2]. The present study was designed to elucidate the effect of sympathetic denervation on the autoregulatory capacity in the cortex and thalamus during the development of hypertension.

Materials and Methods

Male spontaneously hypertensive rats (SHR), aged 1, 3, or 6 months, were anesthetized with Isomytal (amobarbital, 100-mg/kg-i.p.), and superior cervical ganglionectomy was performed on one side or bilaterally to examine the acute effect of denervation on autoregulation. Another group of rats was prepared for chronic unilateral denervation at 4 weeks of age and kept alive for 2 or 5 months thereafter. Cerebral blood flow to the cortex and thalamus was measured with the hydrogen clearance technique during stepwise increases in the blood pressure by infusion of phenylephrine. The effect of rising blood pressure with advancing age and chronic sympathetic denervation on vascular hypertrophy was examined with the freeze-substitution technique [3] at 2 or 5 months after denervation.

Results

Cerebral Blood Flow Autoregulation

The mean resting blood pressure elevated from 89 mmHg at 4 weeks of age to 165 mmHg at 6 months. The baseline cerebral blood flow averaged 45–50 ml/100

[1] Second Department of Internal Medicine, Kyushu University, School of Medicine, 1-1, Maidashi 3-chome, Higashi-ku, Fukuoka City, 812 Japan

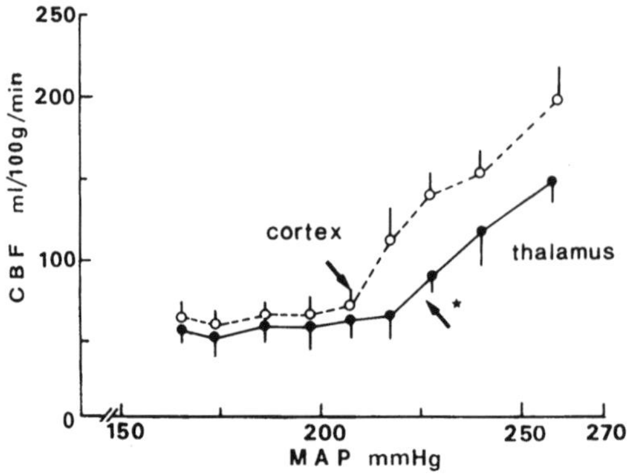

Fig. 1. Cerebral blood flow (*CBF*)-blood pressure curve in the cortex and thalamus. The breakthrough point is significantly higher in the thalamus than cortex. *$P < 0.05$ vs. cortex

g/min to the cortex and 50–55 ml/100 g/min to the thalamus; these values were not different between the groups of rats. In the innervated cortices, the upper limits of autoregulation, breakthrough points, were 118, 180, and 208 mmHg at 1, 3, and 6 months of age, respectively. In the acutely denervated cortices, the upper limits were lowered to 105, 162, and 185 mmHg, respectively. The upper limits of autoregulation were also reduced by 13 to 15 mmHg in the cortices ipsilateral to the chronic ganglionectomy. Acute bilateral, but not unilateral, denervation in the thalamus also lowered the upper limits from 226 mmHg in the control rats to 202 mmHg in the denervated rats at 6 months of age ($P < 0.05$). The cerebral blood flow-blood pressure curves in the cortex and thalamus are shown in Fig. 1. The upper limit is about 20 mmHg higher in the thalamus than in the cortex.

Wall/Lumen Ratio

In 3-month-old SHR, the ratio in the cortical and pial arteries was 0.128 and 0.170 in the denervated and innervated hemispheres, respectively (25%, $P < 0.02$). At 6 months, the ratio was 0.161 and 0.223, respectively (28%, $P < 0.05$)

Discussion

The present results demonstrate that the wall/lumen ratio enhances with advancing age and hypertension and that the upper limits are shifted to higher levels concomitant with increases in basal blood pressure. Age- and hypertension-related structural alterations in the vessel wall may significantly influence the responsiveness of the cerebral arteries during the development of hypertension [1, 2, 4].

The superior cervical ganglion was dissected acutely or chronically to examine whether sympathetic tonic or trophic influences are more important in regulating cerebral blood flow during acute elevation of blood pressure. Breakthough points were significantly lowered after acute and chronic denervation and the wall/lumen ratio was reduced by chronic ganglionectomy. Thalamic autoregulation was also altered by bilateral ganglionectomy [5].

In conclusion, the upper limit of cerebral blood flow autoregulation is clearly related to the resting blood pressure levels, and sympathetic innervation plays an important role in the maintenance of reactivity of cortical and thalamic blood vessels in response to rises in arterial pressure.

References

1. Strandgaards S, Olesen J, Skinhoj E, Lassen NA (1973) Autoregulation of brain circulation in severe arterial hypertension. Br Med J 1: 507–510
2. Vinall PE, Simenone FA (1981) Cerebral autoregulation. An in vitro study. Stroke 12: 640–642
3. Sadoshima S, Fujishima M, Tamaki K, Nakatomi Y, Ishitsuka T, Ogata J, Omae T (1980) Response of cortical and pial arteries to changes of arterial CO_2 tension in rats—A morphometric study. Brain Res 189: 115–120
4. Sadoshima S, Yoshida F, Ibayashi S, Shiokawa O, Fujishima M (1985) Upper limit of cerebral autoregulation during development of hypertension in spontaneously hypertensive rats—Effect of sympathetic denervation. Stroke 16: 477–481
5. Sadoshima S, Fujii K, Kusuda K, Shiokawa O, Yao Y, Ibayashi S, Fujishima M (1987) Importance of bilateral sympathetic innervation on cerebral blood flow autoregulation in the thalamus. Brain Res 413: 297–301

Maintenance of Constant Cerebral Blood Volume by Veni-Arterial Reflex

GEORGE MCHEDLISHVILI[1]

The constancy of cerebral blood volume (CBV) was originally conjectured to be dependent solely upon mechanical factors, e.g., the rigidity of the skull, incompressibility of intracranial ingredients. Subsequently, however, a physiological regulatory mechanism was discovered to be responsible for active maintenance of constant CBV [1]. This physiological mechanism was first found under experimental conditions when the CBV was increased and the resistance in major arteries of the brain was simultaneously monitored. A significant increase in CBV was easily achieved in animal experiments, whereby a large opening was made in the skull and the hyperemic brain could readily expand out of the hole.

Experimental procedures aimed at increasing the CBV consisted of artificial reduction of blood outflow from the brain via the jugular veins. This was achieved by: (a) simultaneous occlusion of all four jugular veins in the neck of the experimental animal (rabbits); (b) rapid infusion of blood or blood-substituting fluid into the cerebral venous bed (rabbits and dogs); or (c) acute occlusion of the cranial vena cava (in dogs).

Alternatively, CBV was experimentally increased by means of widespread dilatation of the pial arteries, which was produced in rabbits: (a) by a temporary (about 1-min) obstruction of the trachea, causing asphyxia; (b) under postischemic hyperemia in the whole brain, i.e., following a 1- to 2-min complete drop of the systemic arterial pressure induced by the exsanguination from the arteries, the blood was reinfused into the animal's circulation, and the arterial pressure returned to normal; (c) during generalized seizure activity in the cerebral hemispheres, brought about by the injection of strychnine solution into the internal carotid artery.

Constrictor responses of all the brain's major arteries (internal carotid and vertebral arteries) were monitored according to the following techniques: (a) recording the blood outflow from the circle of Willis via one of the internal carotid arteries, with the systemic arterial pressure maintained at a constant level; (b) simultaneous recording of the arterial pressures in the aortic branches and circle of Willis (pressure-gradient changes along the major arteries of the brain were indicative of resistance variations in these arteries under otherwise

[1]Microcirculation Research Center, I. Beritashvili Institute of Physiology, Georgian Academy of Sciences, 14 Gotua Street, 380060 Tbilisi, USSR

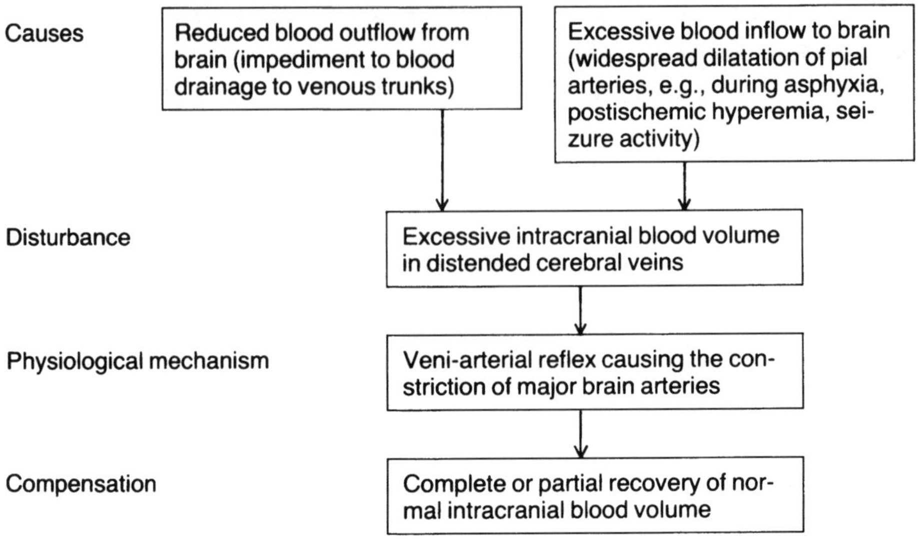

Fig. 1. Physiological mechanism maintaining constant cerebral blood volume

constant conditions); (c) computing the resistance in the major arteries of the brain from their pressure gradient and blood flow rate.

Thus, it was shown under various experimental conditions that the brain's major arteries (internal carotid and vertebral arteries) became constricted with the increase of CBV (Fig. 1).

Of the three feasible physiological feedback mechanisms operating during CBV regulation—myogenic, humoral (metabolic), and neurogenic—the latter seems to be the most likely candidate responsible for this particular type of cerebral blood flow regulation, since the information is transmitted from the distended cerebral veins to the major arteries of the brain. Alternatively, direct myogenic response of the arteries cannot be assumd to be involved in this case, since, firstly, the intraluminal pressure distending primarily the arterial walls cannot be considerably increased under actual circumstances (a decrease in the blood pressure was detected only in the circle of Willis); secondly, the actual myogenic effects were found to be inadequate to provide the necessary arterial constriction, even during a significant rise in the intravascular pressure [1]. Similarly, the humoral effect on the major arteries of the brain cannot be involved in this case: The substances would not be able to reach the arteries from cerebral tissue by diffusion. Metabolic substances in the venous blood surrounding the walls of the major arteries inside the sinuses released in the cerebral tissue during deficient blood supply could cause dilatation rather than constriction of cerebral arteries [1].

During cerebral blood volume regulation, the feedback mechanism is triggered in all probability by the information relayed from the distended walls of cerebral veins, stretched due to an increase in the blood volume. Cerebral veins are supplied with a variety of mechanoreceptors [1]. Owing to the great distensibility of their walls, cerebral veins with their receptors thus appear to be perfectly arranged to detect blood volumetric changes. However, little is known so far about the localization and function of the nervous centers involved in the mechanism of control of CBV described above.

Reference

1. Mchedlishvili G (1986) Arterial behavior and blood circulation in the brain. Plenum, New York

Bordering Zone Hyperemia and Glucose Metabolism in Experimental Cerebral Ischemia

Junichiro Choki[1], Yasuhiro Hasegawa[1], Kazuo Minematsu[2], and Takenori Yamaguchi[1]

Areas of increased blood flow (hyperemia) at the periphery of ischemic foci have been noted in experimental animals [1]. Experiments using ^{14}C-2-deoxyglucose (2-DG) for the measurement of local cerebral glucose utilization (LCGU) have also demonstrated increased uptake of 2-DG in the bordering zone of focal ischemia [2]. The present study was designed to elucidate the relationship between hyperemia and increased 2-DG uptake in gerbils with unilateral common carotid artery (CCA) occlusion.

Mongolian gerbils were briefly anesthetized with halothane and the left CCA was ligated. Only animals showing "circling movement" continuously for 2 h were selected for further experiments. Eight animals were used for measurement of local cerebral blood flow (LCBF), and nine for LCGU by autoradiographic methods. Both measurements were done under pentobarbital anesthesia at various times ranging from 5 to 27 h after ligation. In the remaining two animals, a double-tracer (^{131}I-iodo-antipyrine and ^{14}C-2-DG) technique was applied at 2 and 21 h after ligation.

The cerebral cortex supplied by the anterior cerebral artery (ACA cortex) on the side ipsilateral to CCA ligation was spared ischemia in all but one animal. Increased 2-DG uptake was found in the ACA cortex and ischemic hypothalamus of four animals studied at times ranging from 5 to 9 h after CCA ligation (early stage). In three animals after 23 to 27 h ischemia, increased 2-DG uptake was not present in the ACA cortex, but it was demonstrated in the ischemic hypothalamus of two animals. In the early stage, hyperemic foci were seen in the ACA cortex of the ischemic and hypothalamus of the nonischemic hemisphere in all animals. In three animals studies later than 23 h, hyperemia was not observed in either brain region.

Thus, we found two different types of hyperemia—one in the ACA cortex of the ischemic and the other in the hypothalamus of the nonischemic hemisphere.

Hyperemia in the early stage of ischemia may be caused by two mechanisms: (a) diffusion of lactate into the nonischemic region from the ischemic focus, and (b) damage of mitochondrial function in the ACA cortex by transient ischemia.

Since hyperemia was present in regions adjacent to the ischemic focus, diffu-

Cerebrovascular Division[1] and Research Institute[2], National Cardiovascular Center, 7-1, Fujishirodai 5-chome, Suita, Osaka, 565 Japan sion of lactate into nonischemic from ischemic regions must have been the main cause of hyperemia where increased 2DG uptake was absent. The pathophysiological mechanism of hyperemia in the ACA cortex, however, has to be explained in another way, which is as follows. Most Mongolian gerbils lack the anterior communicating artery, and the pericallosal artery originates from the unilateral ACA, making a common trunk that supplies bilateral ACA cortices. It is possible to speculate that the ACA cortex became transiently ischemic immediately after ligation of the CCA contralateral to the ACA, which branches off the pericallosal artery, since the pericallosal artery works as a collateral pathway into the ischemic region, resulting in a "steal phenomenon." Thus, mitochondrial aerobic glucose metabolism may have been impaired for a certain time. This damage to the mitochondria would make the ACA cortex hyperemic due to the production of lactate.

References

1. Blair RD, Waltz AG (1970) Regional cerebral blood flow during acute ischemia. Correlation of autoradiographic measurements with observations of cortical microcirculation. Neurology 20: 802–808
2. Welsh FA, Greenberg JH, Jones SC, Ginsberg MD, Reivich M (1980) Correlation between glucose utilization and metabolic levels during focal ischemia in cat brain. Stroke 11: 79–84

Chapter 5
Myocardial Ischemia

Influence of Myocardial Contraction on Coronary Microcirculation: Techniques and Results

Stephen H. Nellis and Larry Whitesell[1]

Introduction

For several years, our laboratory has been examining the hemodynamics of the coronary microcirculation with particular emphasis on the effect of myocardial contraction on these small vessels. The initial goals of the laboratory were to measure flow, diameter, and pressure in small vessels and relate the phasic characteristics of these measurements to each other.

Materials and Method

Since myocardial contraction was a major component of our investigation, we attempted to allow the heart to beat freely with as few restraints as possible. The free-motion technique utilized in our laboratory was based on a simple procedure and took advantage of the cyclic nature of heart activity [1]. The heart was visualized for a brief period of time, but at the same time point during each consecutive cycle so that, as viewed through the microscope, the heart appeared stationary. This was accomplished with a xenon flash synchronized with the cardiac cycle.

This free-motion technique demanded that cardiac motion be synchronized with the heart rate; thus, respiratory motion artifacts needed to be eliminated. Our approach was to synchronize respiration and the motion imparted to the heart by the respiration with the heart cycle. Respiratory motion then effectively became another component of myocardial contraction. A schema of the apparatus is shown in Fig. 1.

Recording an image on a videotape recorder demanded that the cardiac cycle, respiration, xenon flash, and video camera be synchronized. The basic approach was to pace the heart at some subinterval of the video framing rate so that the heart could be examined at any of these subintervals. The sequence of events then was to provide a pacing stimuli to the heart, a jet of air to the lungs, wait M intervals after the pacing signal to activate the xenon light strobe, and command

[1]The Section of Cardiology, The University of Wisconsin Medical Center, 600 Highland Avenue, H6/339 Madison, WI 53792, USA

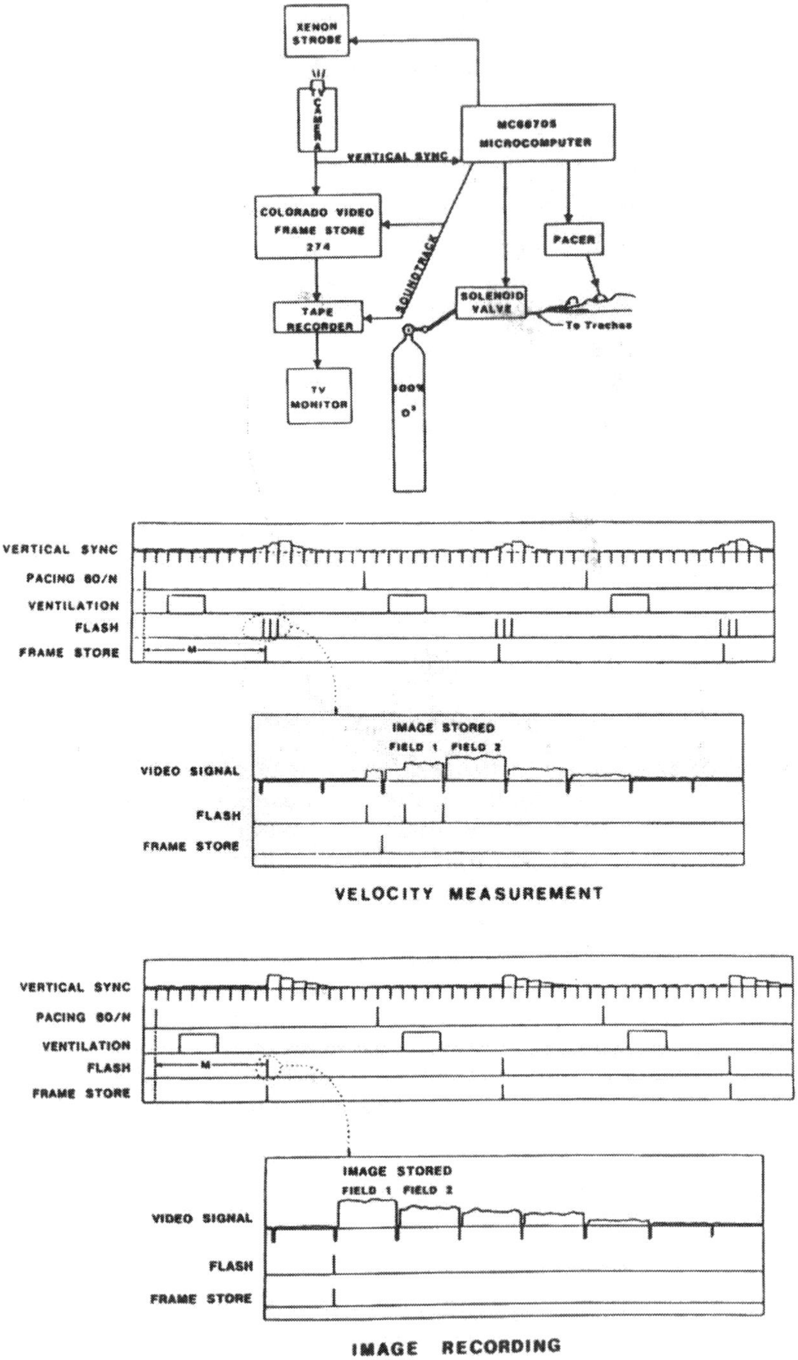

Fig. 1. Schema of apparatus used to capture a video image of the beating heart. The time of the flash for a single image recording and timing of flashes for velocity measurements are shown

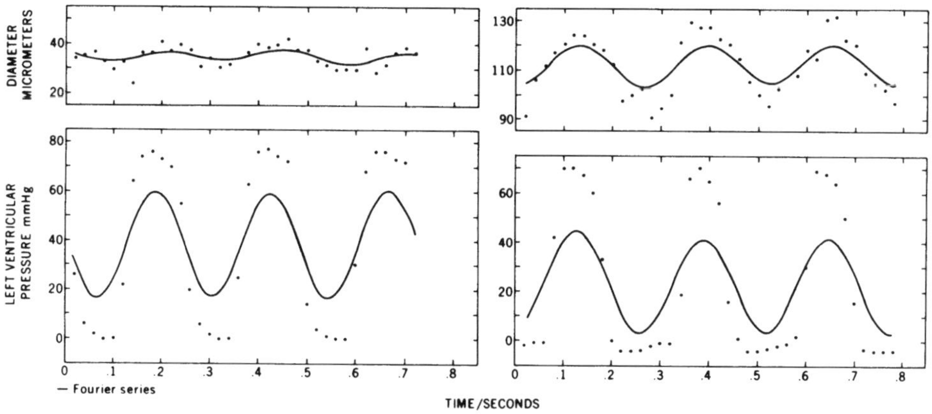

Fig. 2. The diameters of two different vessels at several different times during different cardiac cycles are shown by *points*. The left ventricular pressure at the time the image was acquired is also shown by points in the *bottom panel*. The *solid line* represents the first three harmonics resulting from discrete Fourier analysis

a Colorado videodigitizer to capture and redisplay the next frame of video information for recording on the videotape recorder. This image was continually redisplayed until a new image was captured during the next cardiac cycle. The timing for image capture is shown in Fig. 1.

Diameter measurements could be made directly from the recorded images. Changing M allowed the examination of any part of the cardiac cycle. The diameter of two veins at several different times in the cardiac cycle are shown as points in the upper panels of Fig. 2. The images from which these diameters were measured were obtained by slowly advancing the flash through the cardiac cycle. In this examination, the flash was advanced through the cycle three times to obtain a composite of three cardiac cycles. The left ventricular pressure is shown as dots in the bottom panels of Fig. 2.

Discrete Fourier analysis provided an objective technique to evaluate the temporal relationship between the cardiac cycle and the phasic diameter variation. The angles were calculated such that a positive angle indicated that the diameter change occurred late in the cardiac cycle, whereas a negative angle indicated the diameter changed earlier. An angle of 0° indicated that the diameter reached its maximum value in left ventricular systole.

Results and Discussion

The maximum diameter changes encountered in our investigation were 60%, but for the most part the changes were smaller and averaged 12%. As shown in Fig. 2, large-vessel diameters had small phase shifts, while small vessels lagged behind pressure, so that the maximum diameter occurred in late left ventricular systole or early diastole. Our original assumption was that diameters passively followed luminal pressure. As the heart contracted, blood was forced out of the

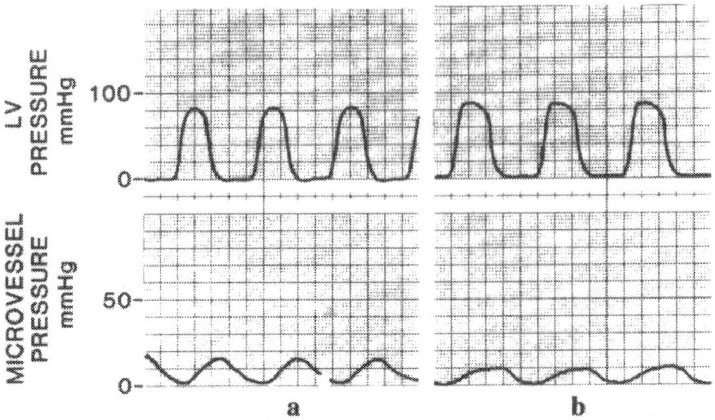

Fig. 3a, b. The *bottom panels* are the pressures recorded from **a** an 80-μm vein on the left and **b** a 150-μm vein of the right. The *upper panels* are left ventricular pressure measurements

endocardial vessels, increasing the pressure in the epicardial vessels so that the diameter passively increased.

Figure 3 shows the pressure recorded from veins. The most striking feature about pressures recorded from small veins was the magnitude of their phasic components. The minimum pressures in these vessels averaged slightly above zero. We have recorded peak pressures as high as 16 mmHg. The average pulsatile component in our laboratory was 12 mmHg. Other investigators have reported even higher values.

The other surprising feature was that these peak pressures reach a maximum value late in the cardiac cycle. Again, these tracings were subjected to Fourier analysis to determine their timing in the cardiac cycle.

The phasic relationship of pressure as related to diameter is shown in Fig. 4. If diameter passively followed pressure, the diameter should have increased with pressure or slightly after pressure increased. Instead, exactly the opposite appeared to happen, i.e., diameter increase preceded that of pressure.

Increasing pressures resulting from decreasing diameters could have resulted from two possible mechanisms. Pressure could have increased simply because resistance increased, resulting from vessel narrowing. Spaan et al. [2], however, suggested the existence of an intramyocardial pump. As the vessels narrow, blood volume is displaced from the vessels, increasing blood flow and thus increasing pressure.

The next step was to examine the phasic changes of flow in these vessels. Because of the poor contrast and inherent motion of the thick myocardium, we elected to track the motion of fluorescent particles as opposed to other more conventional means for measuring microvessel blood flow.

We used a low-light-level camera to record images with fluorescent microscopy. The image in Fig. 5a was produced utilizing a double-intensified Newvicon camera to record particle positions in the rabbit omentum in conjunction with a strobed xenon light source operating at 60 flashes/s. The Newvicon tube has a particularly high persistence so that the location of particles revealed by several

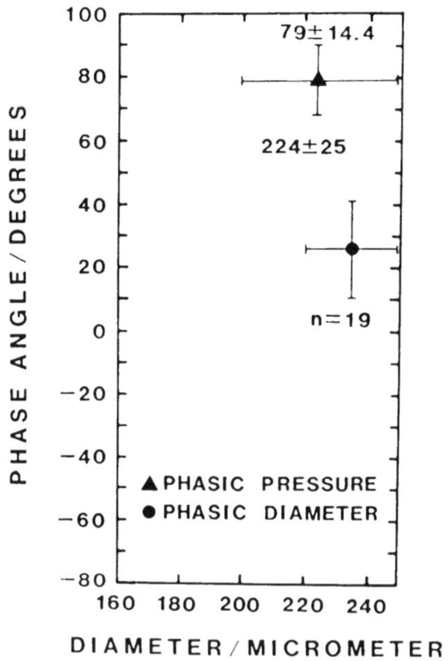

Fig. 4. Phase angle of diameter compared with phase angle of vessel pressure. The *bars* represent SEM. Positive angles represent delays

flashes can be identified in one image. Two particles traveling through two different vessels were captured in this image. The spots at the heads of the comet like images are the locations of particles at the last flash. Traveling down the tails we can identify the location of the spheres at several of the previous flashes of light. The time interval between flashes is known, the distance traveled can be measured, and so the velocity of the particle can be determined. The trapped particles appear at only one location. Continual illumination, however, could not be utilized on the heart with our technique.

We modified our technique to provide three flashes of light in rapid succession, but at the same point in the cardiac cycle, so that the heart still appeared stationary although somewhat blurred. The interval between flashes ranged from 16 to 4 mm/s. The timing of the flash (Fig. 1 velocity measurement) was such that the third flash occurred between the first and second fields recorded, so that the third image was seen on only the last captured video field. The captured images were recorded on a video-recorder for later analysis. A signal which indicated the capture of two new fields was also recorded on the sound track of the videotape so that the images could be recaptured from the tape recorder for analysis after the experiment.

The result of this timing sequence was the capture of two fields of video information shown in Fig. 5b. The first field has the images resulting from the first two flashes, while the last field has the images which result from all three flashes. Thus, a particle was recorded at three different positions as it moved through a vessel, and the last position was recorded on only one of the video fields; it could thus readily be identified and the direction of motion determined. The last position is marked with an arrow.

The vessels shown in Fig. 6 were located on the epicardial surface of the left ventricle of a cat. The vessel to the left is a 70-μm vein, which branches into two

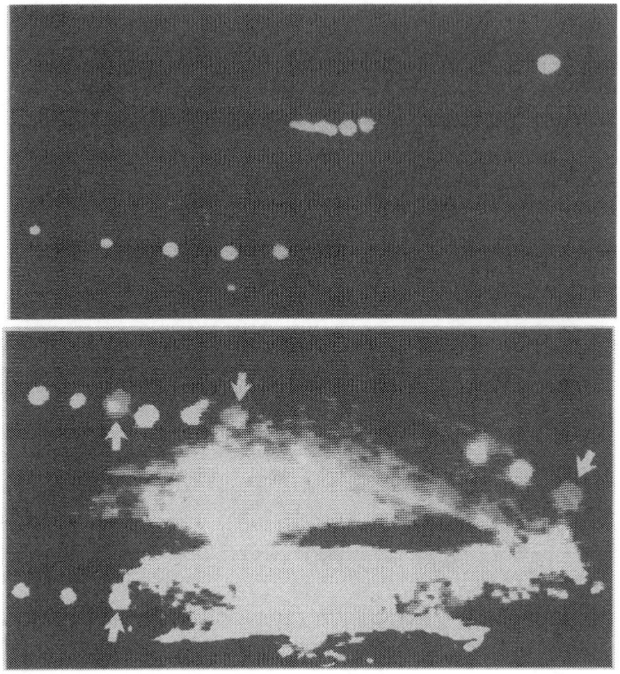

a

b

Fig. 5a, b. These images were obtained from the rabbit omentum after the injection of 2.5-μm latex fluorescent sphere with **a** a xenon flash operating at 60 flashes/s and **b** after a three-flash burst. The timing of the flashes is shown in Fig. 1. The position of the sphere in the last flash is marked with an arrow

smaller veins. The large particles in the upper right are 10-μm spheres and were injected so they would become trapped to reveal the epicardial motion. The vector of motion of the epicardial surface must be subtracted from the motion of the particles flowing through the vessels to reveal relative motion or flow. These points in the cardiac cycle were specifically selected because heart motion was minimal; therefore, the large spheres appear at only one location. The image in Fig. 6a was captured when the heart was at end diastole. Approximately 700 images were recorded at each point in the cardiac cycle and this one was selected since, by chance, three particles were captured which dramatically demonstrate the flow pattern at this point in the cardiac cycle. The three particle positions are marked with arrows. The last position of each sphere is marked with a solid arrow. As these three particles reveal, blood flows out of the larger vessels into the smaller veins.

Figure 6b shows the flow pattern found in mid-systole. Blood was flowing from the smaller veins into the larger vessel. There was also an acceleration of particle velocity in the forward direction as indicated because the distance traveled between the first and second flashes was less than the distance traveled between the second and third flashes. The velocity in late systole and early diastole is represented by the particle seen in Fig. 6c. There was a continual acceleration in the forward direction. The displacement vector of approximately 20 different

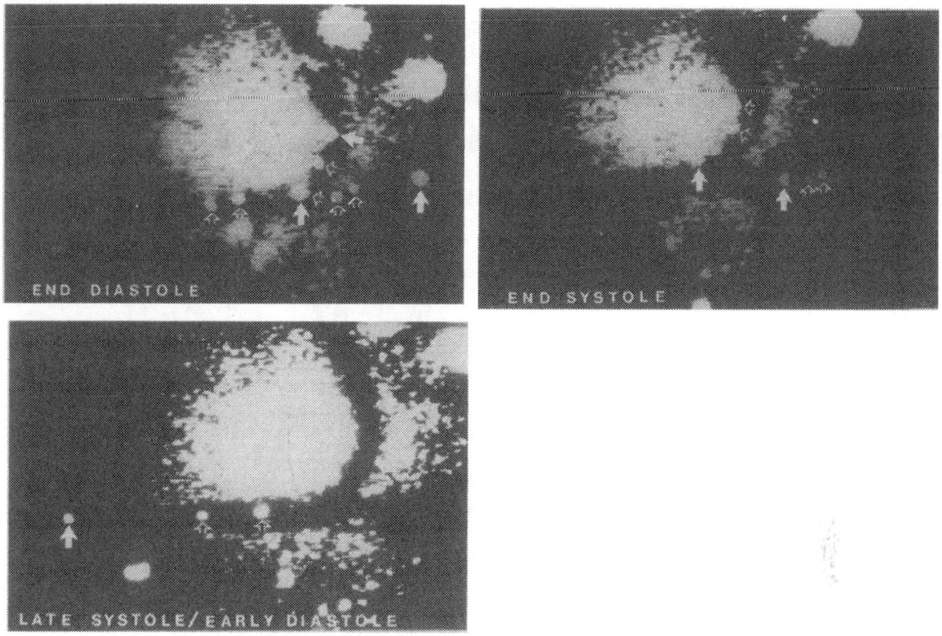

a b c

Fig. 6a–c. Image resulting from the heart after a three-flash burst with timing as demonstrated in Fig. 1. The three positions of the 2.5-μm sphere are marked with *arrows*. The last position is marked with a *solid arrow*. Two trapped 10-μm spheres can be seen in the *upper right* of **a–c**

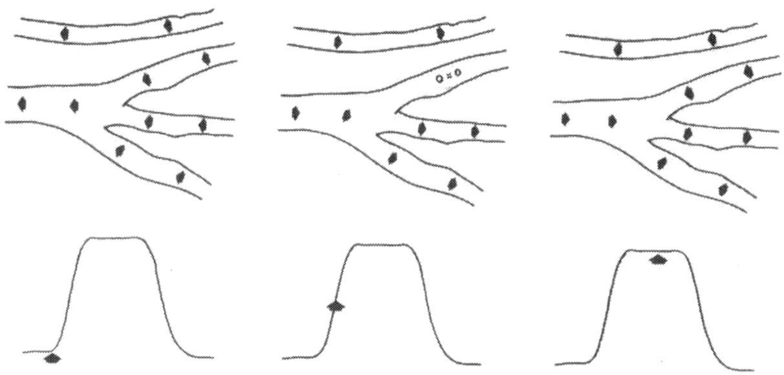

Fig. 7. The direction of blood flow in veins with right ventricular epicardium is shown at three different times in the cardiac cycle

particles was measured at each point in the cardiac cycle to acquire an average particle velocity.

Flow patterns found in veins appeared to be more complicated than originally anticipated. Figure 7 represents a venous network found on the right ventricular surface. The arrows represent the direction of flow. The three panels represent

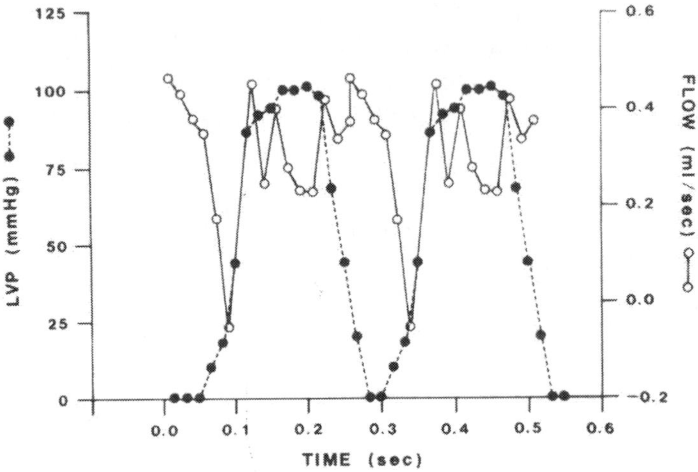

Fig. 8. Phasic flow through a small (50-μm) epicardial artery

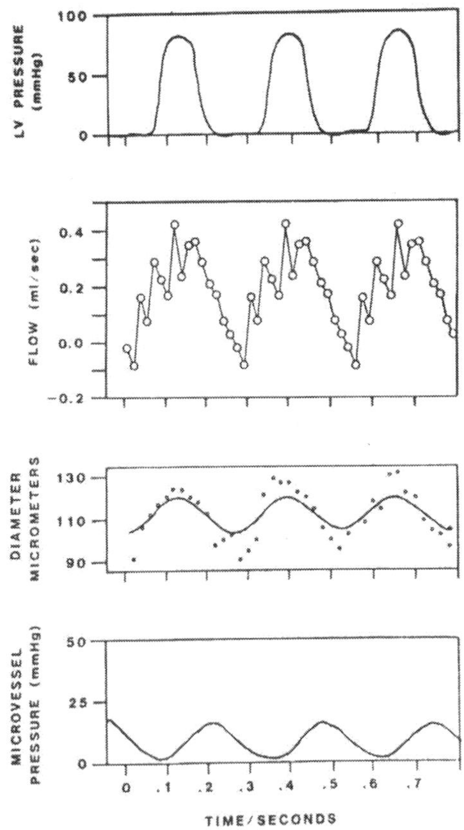

Fig. 9. Representation of the phasic flow, pressure, and diameter in epicardial veins larger than 100 μm in the right ventricle

the direction of blood flow at three different points in the cardiac cycle. The time in the cardiac cycle is indicated by arrows in the lower panels. As can be appreciated, the flow pattern in these small vessels was quite complicated and depended on the particular vessel under investigation. All of these vessels were less than 100 μm in diameter. Arteries (Fig. 8) did not show the major flow reversals seen in veins. There was usually a sharp, brief perturbation, which occurred at or around left ventricular isovolumetric contraction and sometimes resulted in particles briefly reversing direction. For the most part, however, flow remained in a forward direction in arteries and the pattern was independent of vessel size.

Although flow patterns in small veins were complex, larger veins appeared to have a predictable phasic pattern, with flow reaching a peak in left ventricular systole and approaching zero in diastole. Figure 9 represents the phasic relationship between pressure, flow, and diameter found in those veins with diameters between 100 and 200 μm.

It is difficult to determine the exact phasic flow relationship with so few measurements; however, at this time, it appears that pressure and flow are in phase and dictated by smaller and/or endocardial vessels. The diameter of these vessels are responding to something besides luminal pressure, probably myocardoal strain.

Acknowledgment. This work was supported by a National Heart, Lung, and Blood Institute Grant #HL29917.

References

1. Nellis SH, Liedtke AJ, Whitesell L (1981) Small coronary vessel pressure and diameter in an intact beating rabbit heart using fixed-position and free-motion techniques. Circ Res 49: 342–353
2. Spaan JAE, Breuls NPW, Laird JD (1981) Diastolic-systolic coronary flow differences are caused by intramyocardial pump action in the anesthetized dog. Circ Res 49: 584–593

Changes in Coronary Microcirculation in Acute Ischemia

TAKASHI YAMAKAWA, SABURO YAMAGUCHI, and HIDEYUKI NIIMI[1]

Introduction

Blood cells flowing in the coronary microvascular network are responsible for oxygen supply to myocardial cells. Among these cells, white cells (WBCs) are more spherical, larger, and less deformable than red cells (RBCs) [1]. For this reason, WBCs may have an important influence on the microcirculation, especially at a low perfusion pressure. In fact, according to intravital microscopic observation of microcirculation in the skeletal muscle, one or several WBCs may block the capillary flow during hemorrhagic shock [2]. There is also histological evidence that WBC plugging may cause mechanical obstruction of coronary capillaries in myocardial ischemia [3].

All the RBCs flowing in one capillary are not the same in deformability, shape, and volume. A large decrease in perfusion pressure may greatly affect the passage time of individual RBCs through capillaries, so that the cells may be distributed non-uniformly along a capillary.

To elucidate changes in blood flow and cell distribution along a capillary in acute ischemia, we directly observed the behavior of individual cells in the coronary network of the left atrial muscle in the cat [4, 5].

Material and Methods

Experiments were performed on 19 cats of either sex weighing 2.0–3.0 kg. Anesthesia was intravenously induced with pentobarbital sodium (20 mg/kg body weight).

A flexible catheter was inserted into the aorta through the femoral artery to monitor blood pressure and blood gases. A tracheotomy was performed and the cat was ventilated artificially with room air and supplemental oxygen. After a left-sided thoracotomy was performed and the ribs were retracted, the pericardium was incised and the heart was kept moist with frequent applications of Krebs-Henseleit solution bubbled with 5% CO_2 and 95% O_2 at 37.0°C.

---

[1]National Cardiovascular Center Research Institute, 7-1, Fujishirodai 5-chome, Suita, Osaka, 565 Japan

A transillumination technique was used to observe blood flow in the capillary network of the left atrial muscle. A small portion of the tip of the left atrial appendage was clamped with a Pott's clamp. A small incision was made at the tip of the atrial appendage to insert a light pipe through its opening. A suture was quickly tightened around the light pipe to prevent leakage of blood. An appropriate amount of tension was applied to the atrial wall to prevent the light pipe from interfering with the blood supply to myocardial tissues.

Acute ischemia was induced by occluding a left atrial branch of the left circumflex artery (or an artery on the atrial surface) using a Scovile clip. We used a custom-made intravital microscope system, which consisted of a light source, the transilluminator (light pipe), and a vital microscope (Sankei Co., Tokyo, Japan) equipped with an animal stage, a TV camera, and a high-speed 16-mm cinecamera (Photo-Sonics 1PL, Burbank, CA, USA). To illuminate the microcirculation in the atrial muscle, we used a transilluminator as a light guide, which was modified from Hellberg's type [6]. One end of the optical fiber was cut at a right angle and the other end at 45°; the angle end was aluminized to reflect the light from the light source upward through the tissue. The light source was a pulsed short-gap 300-W xenon illuminator (varian AVL, San Carlos, CA, USA); its power supply could provide a strobe impulse to boost the xenon arc at a rate of 500/s, which was triggered by operation of the cinecamera. A glass fiber conduit was used from the xenon illuminator to the light pipe. The color pictures (Kodak Ektachrome) were taken on 16-mm cinefilm by the high-speed cinecamera at a rate of 500 frames/s at an open shutter time of 1/3000–1/5000.

The data recorded on the 16-mm cinefilm were analyzed using a photo optical analyzer (L-W International, Woodland Hills, CA, USA). The optical magnification on the projection screen was approximately ×3000. The behavior of cells in the capillaries could be observed clearly on the projection screen; the WBCs could be observed as cylinders with a low, white contrast in the capillary lumen.

To estimate the capillary hematocrit (Hcap), we counted the number of RBC (n) in a segment of capillary (length: l) and multiplied it by the mean corpuscular volume (MCV) to obtain the total volume of RBC existing in the segment. Then, the Hcap value was calculated as follows:

$$\mathrm{Hcap} = \mathrm{n} \times \mathrm{MCV}/\pi \mathrm{r}^2 \mathrm{l} \times 100\ (\%)$$

where r is the capillary radius.

The velocity of RBCs (Vrbc) was measured by frame-by-frame analysis of the RBC movement on a projection screen. The heterogenous arrangement of flowing RBCs along a capillary was estimated in terms of "inter-RBC distance" (IRD), which is defined as the distance between two adjacent cells. The standard deviation (SD) of IRD was used as a quantity representing the intensity of heterogeneity or "nonuniformity."

Results

Under control conditions, the Hcap in the contracting left atrial muscle was 31.2% ± 5.2% (SD) at the mean atrial pressure of 95–115 mmHg. Most of the

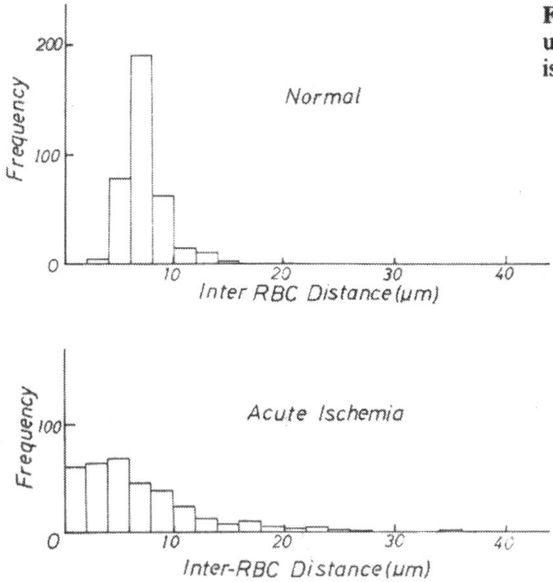

Fig. 1. Inter-RBC distance measured under normal conditions and acute ischemia

capillaries (approximately 95%) were perfused with respect to RBCs. The average velocity of the RBCs was 960 ± 365 (mm/s. Some stationary RBCs appeared in a few capillaries (approximately 5%) in which the flow velocity was very slow. There were no capillaries containing plasma only.

The IRD and its distribution measured under the control condition are shown in Fig. 1. The IRDs were almost constant under normal conditions, showing a uniform distribution along a capillary. The present result indicates that RBCs passed through the capillary entrance for a short time such that they might flow in a uniform arrangment.

We observed the microcirculatory network in the heart muscle during acute ischemia. The main changes were as follows (Figs. 2, 3): (a) Immediately after ischemia, capillary blood flow was slowed down, accompanied by high Hcap (60%–80%). Some of the capillaries became low in Hcap after several minutes. (b) Following the ischemia, RBC flow velocity decreased in arterioles, capllaries, and venules. A small degree of ischemia could stop the flow in most venules but did not stop arteriolar flow until all venular and the capillary flows had stopped completely. (c) WBCs were observed in the microcirculatory network after several minutes of ischemia. Several WBCs plugged the capillary branching. Once a WBC plugged the capillary entrance, RBCs accumulated upstream and were absent downstream (an RBC-depleted region downstream). The abnormal flow pattern may be a reflection of the different rheological behavior between RBCs and WBCs in capillaries, especially at the entrance. In fact, a WBC becomes lodged at the entrance to a capillary branch longer than RBCs owing to the rheological difference between the two types of cells.

We examined the effect of ischemia on the RBC distribution along a capillary by comparing the IRDs before and after acute ischemia. The histogram in Fig. 4 shows that the IRD became scattered widely during acute ischemia. The mean IRD and SD^2 changed from 7.6 and 0.27 to 7.7 and 0.78, respectively (Fig. 4). It

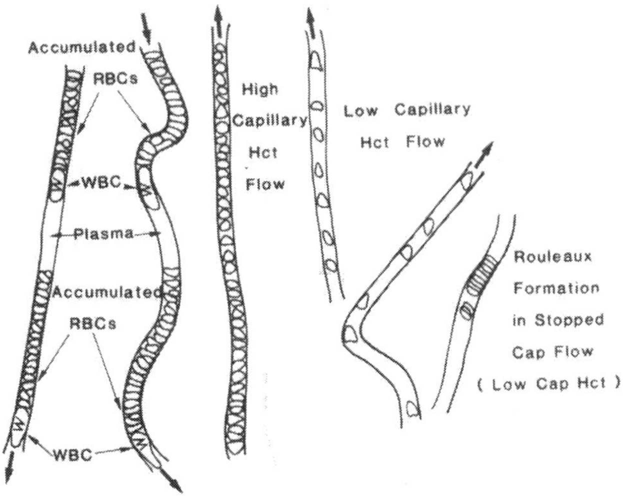

Fig. 2. Cells flowing in the coronary capillary network during acute ischemia

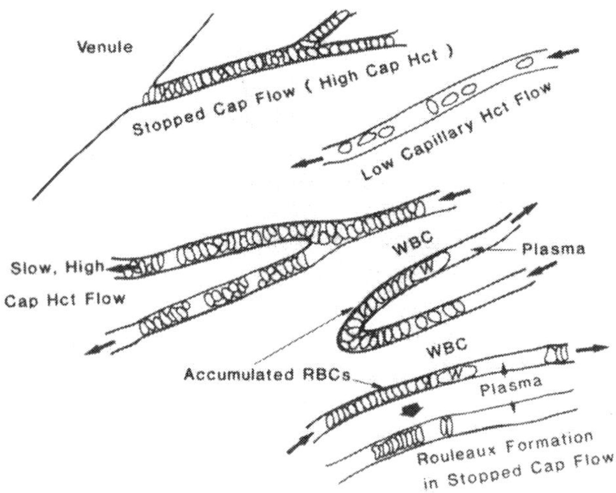

Fig. 3. Clustered RBCs and plasma-WBC-accumulated RBCs in the capillaries (acute ischemia)

is noticeable that the RBC arrangement changed markedly with the mean IRD unchanged. Under normal conditions, the RBCs were arranged uniformly along a capillary. Acute ischemia induced two types of nonuniform distribution—plasma-WBC-accumulated RBCs flow pattern and "clustered" RBCs but WBC-free flow pattern (Fig. 5).

Discussion

Many investigators have reported that the hematocrit in capillaries (Hcap) may be smaller than that in large vessels. According to Lipowsky and Zweifach, the

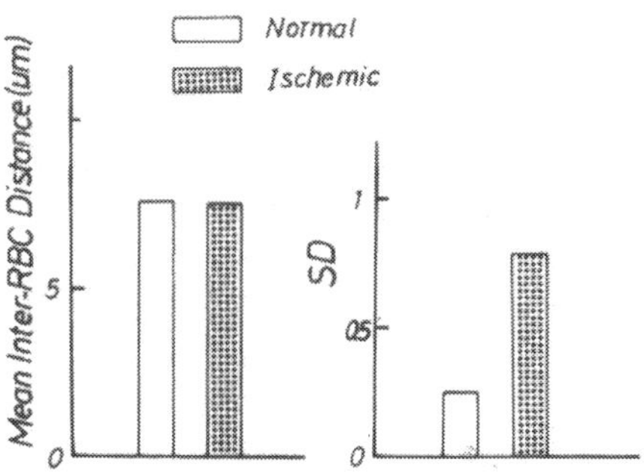

Fig. 4. Mean and standard deviation (*SD*) of inter-RBC distance under normal conditions and acute ischemia

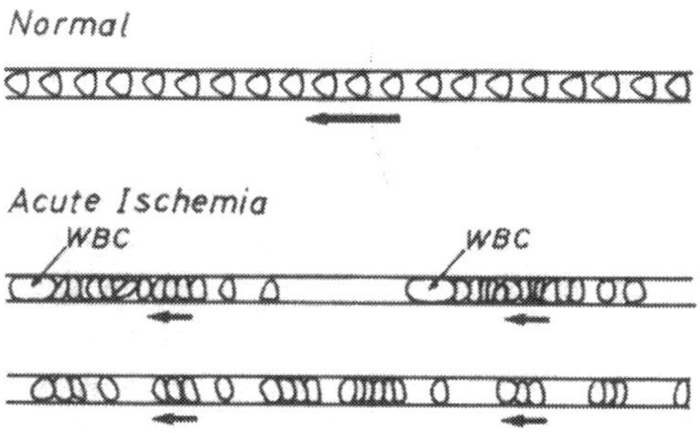

Fig. 5. Cells flowing in arrangement through capillaries under normal conditions and acute ischemia

Hcap in the cat mesentry averages 8.2% ± 0.4% [7]. Klitzman and Duling reported that the Hcap in striated muscle was 10.4% ± 2.9% at rest, but that its level increased to 18.5% ± 2.4% during muscle contraction [8]. In heart muscle, however, the Hcap value has been hitherto rarely investigated experimentally.

We have measured the Hcap in perfused capillaries of normal and ischemic heart muscle and obtained experimental evidence of the reduced coronary Hcap. It is interesting to note that Hcap in the contracting heart muscle is larger than that reported in other organs. This is probably connected with the oxygen demand of heart muscle being greater than that of other organs.

Our observations have showed the appearance of slow capillary blood flow with Hcap higher than the systemic hematocrit immediately after ischemia. It may be speculated that this increased hematocrit could reflect the leakage of plasma components from the capillary. In fact, Leinberger et al. showed that acute ischemia could increase the albumin permeability when RBCs were retained in the capillaries [9]. It should be mentioned here that such high Hcap observed in ischemia is never advantageous for regaining flow after reperfusion. This is because the perfusion pressure will be decreased by ischemia though blood viscosity is increased with an increase in Hcap, so that the pressure difference between both ends of the capillary may be small enough not to allow blood flow.

The present observations have demonstrated how some capillaries with low Hcap appeared among capillaries with high Hcap. Such low Hcap will be favorable for maintaining blood flow even under a small pressure difference.

The RBC velocity was decreased in the microvessels (Fig. 2). Arteriolar blood flow was not stopped until all venular and capillary flow had stopped completely. These changes in flow depend upon the ratio of arteriole to venule distribution per area; its value was approximately 6.9%.

WBCs appeared in the slow capillary flow after several minutes of ischemia. The passage time of a WBC through the capillary branch was much longer than that of an RBC. Furthermore, WBCs often plugged the capillary entrance; numbers of RBCs then accumulate upstream of the WBC plugging and, consequently, an RBC-depleted region was formed downstream. Once a WBC was dislodged and entered the capillary, the flow pattern of plasma-WBC-accumulated RBCs was formed. In general, WBCs have to be deformed remarkably to pass through capillaries. However, the cells are lower in deformability than RBCs and so they may plug the entrance of a capillary. This plugging phenomenon appears only when the perfusion pressure is reduced under pathological conditions such as ischemia. The WBC plugging has been observed in vivo in skeletal muscle capillaries under hemorrhagic shock [2] and in the cat brain cortex during acute hemorrhagic hypotension [10]. The WBC plugging phenomenon may be responsible for the increased number of unperfused capillaries in heart muscle in acute myocardial ischemia. It has been shown that WBCs may increase the flow resistance substantially in the skeletal muscle microcirculation and cause permanent plugging of capillaries [2, 11]. Engler et al. have provided morphological evidence in myocardial ischemia indicating that WBCs may cause mechanical obstruction in capillaries and thereby play a key role in "no reflow" phenomena [3, 12].

The present result has shown that the IRDs remained almost constant under normal conditions. This indicates that RBCs could pass through the capillary entrance. The passage time of individual cells through the entrance is generally dependent on their own deformability as well as on the pressure difference between both ends of the capillary. Under normal conditions, where the pressure difference is large enough, the difference in deformability between individual cells has no significant influence on their passage time and, thus, on the IRD. Acute myocardial ischemia induced two types of nonuniform distribution—plasma-WBC-accumulated RBCs flow pattern and "clustered" RBCs without WBC. While the former flow pattern is due to WBC rheology, the latter may be closely connected with RBCs through different volume and deformability in individual cells or abnormal rheological behavior, such as RBC aggregation, in very slow flow.

Due to the different rheological behavior between RBCs and WBCs, acute ischemia induced abnormal blood flow in the coronary microcirculation. WBCs greatly affected the capillary flow during acute ischemia. Since the coronary microcirculation is closely related to the oxygen supply to heart muscle, the abnormal capillary flow may have an important influence not only on the oxygen myocardial transport process but also on the pathophysiology of the ischemia.

References

1. Schmid-Schonbein GW, Sung K-LP, Tozeren H, Skalak R, Chien S (1981) Passive mechanical properties of human leukocyte. Biophys J 36: 243–256

2. Bagge U, Amundson S, Lauritzen C (1980) White blood cell deformability and plugging of skeletal muscle capillaries in hemorrhagic shock. Acta Physiol Scand 108: 159–163
3. Engler, RL, Schmid-Schonbein GW, Pavelec RS (1983) Leukocyte plugging in myocardial ischemia and reperfusion in the dog. Am J Pathol 111: 98–111
4. Yamakawa T, Niimi H (1983) Intravital microscopic study of coronary microcirculation during acute ischemia. In: Tsuchiya M, Wayland H, Oda M, Okazaki I (eds) Intravital observation of organ microcirculation. Excerpta Medica, Amsterdam, pp 205–219
5. Yamakawa T, Niimi H (1986) Analysis of coronary micro-circulation using transillumination-intravital microscope-high speed cine system. In: Kitamura K, Abe H, Sagawa K (eds) New approaches in cardiac themselves. Japan Scientific Societies Press, Tokyo, pp 315–325
6. Hellberg K, Wayland H Richart AL, Bing RJ (1972) Studies on the coronary microcirculation by direct visualization. Am J Cardiol 29: 593–597
7. Lipowsky HH, Zweifach BW (1977) Methods for the simultaneous measurement of pressure differentials and flow in single unbranched vessels of the microcirculation for rheological studies. Microvasc Res 14: 345–361
8. Klitzman B, During BR (1970) Microvascular hematocrit and red cell flow in resting and contracting striated muscle. Am J Physiol 237: H481–H490
9. Leinberger H, Tillmanns H, Hoppe S, Kubler W (1982) Microcirculatory impairment following transit myocardial ischemia. In: Tillmanns H, Kubler W, Zebe H (eds) Microcirculation of the heart. Springer, Berlin Heidelberg New York, pp 98–103
10. Yamakawa T, Yamaguchi S, Niimi H, Sugiyama I (1987) White cell plugging and blood flow maldistribution in the capillary network of cat cerebral cortex in acute hemorrhagic hypotension. Circ Shock, 22: 323–332
11. Braide M, Amundson B, Chien S, Bagge U (1984) Quantitative studies on the influence of leukocytes on the vascular resistance in a skeletal muscle preparation. Microvasc Res 27: 331–352
12. Engler RL, Dahlgren MD, Peterson MA, Dobbs A, Schmid-Schonbein GW (1986) Accumulation of polymorphonuclear leukocytes during 3-h experimental myocardial ischemia. Am J Physiol 251: H93–H100

Flow Characteristics in Poststenotic Regions of the Human Coronary Artery Assessed by 20-MHz 80-Channel Pulsed Doppler Velocimetry

FUMIHIKO KAJIYA[1], YOSHIFUMI WADA[1], and TAKASHI FUJIWARA[2]

Introduction

A detailed assessment of flow dynamics in coronary stenosis is essential for better understanding of the pathophysiology of the obstructive coronary artery disease. However, measurements of phasic blood flow velocity and velocity distribution in a native human coronary artery have been hampered by methodological limitations. The ultrasound pulsed Doppler method is useful for measuring local blood flow velocity in vessels noninvasively. However, a conventional single-channel pulsed Doppler velocimeter with low carrier frequencies cannot obtain detailed blood velocity profiles of small vessels like the coronary artery. Recently, we have developed an 80-channel 20-MHz pulsed Doppler velocimeter [1–3], which detects Doppler signals from 80 channels by a zero-cross method and analyzes Doppler signals from one optional channel by a fast Fourier transform method, both in real time.

In the present study, using this device, we examined the flow characteristics in the human coronary artery with severe stenosis during coronary artery bypass graft surgery. The purposes of our study were: (a) to analyze the characteristics of the coronary artery flow-velocity profile distal to severe stenosis before bypass grafting and (b) to investigate the change in the diastolic and systolic blood flow velocities in a native distal coronary artery by the grafting.

Methods

Principle of 80-Channel 20-MHz Pulsed Doppler Velocimeter

The basic principle of our system is outlined in Fig. 1. The transducer consists of a $\pi \times 0.5^2$ mm^2 piezoelectrical crystal with a 20-MHz carrier frequency. The pulse repetition period is 20 μs and the sampling pulse width is 0.25 μs. Since the depth resolution is 0.2 mm, the sample volume for each sampling point

Department of Medical Engineering and Systems Cardiology[1] and Department of Thoracic Surgery[2], Kawasaki Medical School, 577 Matsushima, Kurashiki, Okayama, 701-01 Japan

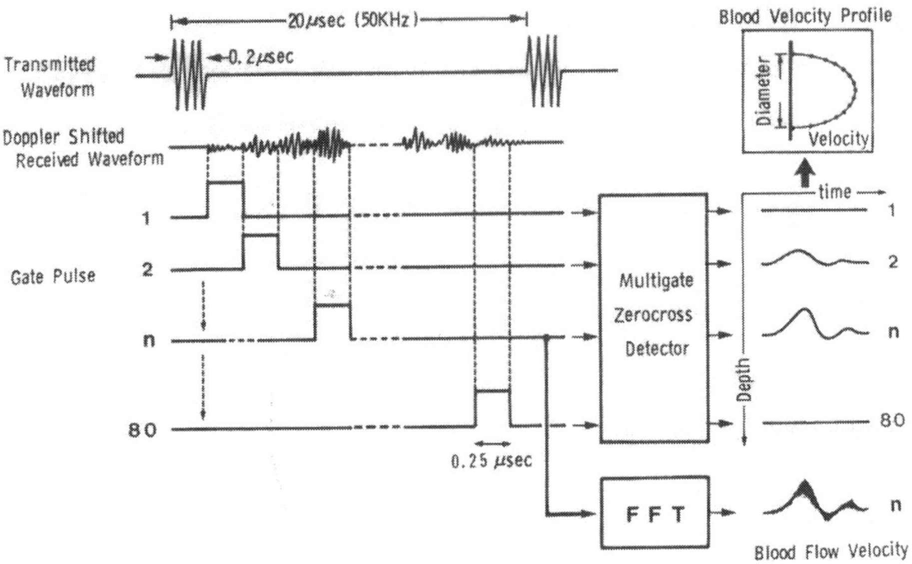

Fig. 1. Principle of the 80-channel 20-MHz pulsed Doppler velocimeter with zero-cross and Fourier transform methods. From Kajiya et al. [2] with permission

is $\pi \times 0.5^2 \times 0.2$ mm^3. The system has 80 sampling gates and Doppler signals from the multigated circuit are analyzed by a zero-cross method. Since the sample volume of our system is small, a zero-cross can precisely detect Doppler signals in the sample volume for nondisturbed blood velocity fields. For disturbed flow, as expected in poststenotic flow, however, velocity detection is inaccurate even with the use of a 20-MHz transducer. In our system, therefore, a fast Fourier transform (FFT) is performed for an optional channel by means of a computer. The unit data length of the Fourier analysis is 128 data points. The frequency resolution, temporal resolution, and maximum detectable frequency of our system are 290 Hz, 2.56 ms, and 25 kHz, respectively.

Intraoperative Measurements of Blood Flow Velocity in Human Coronary Artery

Blood flow velocities in human coronary arteries were measured by our method during a saphenous vein bypass operation. A total of 11 patients aged 39–68 years who had been admitted to the Department of Thoracic and Cardiovascular Surgery were studied. All patients underwent coronary arteriography and opacification of the left ventricle within 2 months before the surgical procedure. Each patient had 75%–99% stenosis in the diameter of the left anterior descending coronary artery (LAD). Two cases had stenosis only in the LAD and nine cases had additional stenosis of the other major branches. None of the patients had a history of previous myocardial infarction in the LAD perfusion area.

A specially designed probe holder was used to place the transducer on the LAD without dissection of the vessel. This probe holder was made of silicon and a transducer was mounted in it at an angle of 60° to the bottom surface. The

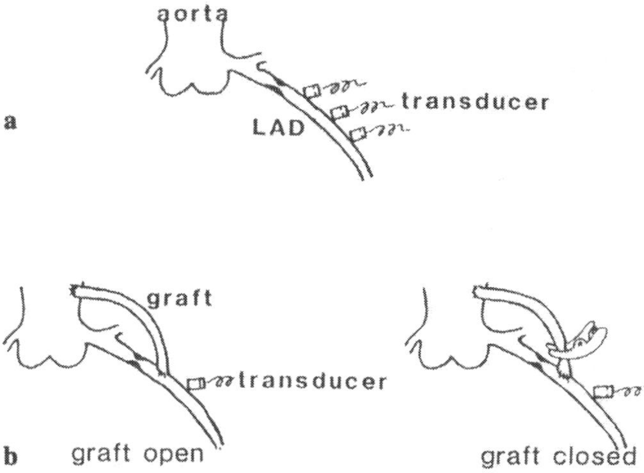

Fig. 2a, b. Protocol of study. **a** Before induction of extracorporeal circulation, blood flow velocities were measured at several locations distal to the stenosis. **b** After bypass grafting, the blood flow velocities in the distal left anterior anterior descending artery (*LAD*) were compared before and during transient graft occlusion. From Kajiya et al. [3] with permission

bottom was rough to avoid slippage of the holder on the cardiac surface. A linear groove was made on the bottom to avoid compression of the coronary artery by the holder. The operator takes the grip of the holder with his fingers and places it on the epicardial coronary artery.

Protocol 1. Before induction of the extracorporeal circulation, phasic changes in the LAD blood velocity profile across the vessel were observed at several locations distal to the stenosis by using the 80-channel zero-cross method (Fig. 2a). The velocity waveforms near central axial regions were analyzed by an FFT method.

Protocol 2. After bypass grafting, the velocity profile and central axial velocity at several centimeters distal to the graft insertion in the LAD were measured before and during a transient graft occlusion (Fig. 2b). Brief graft occlusion was accomplished by obstructing a distal portion of the graft with vascular forceps for about 20 s. Velocity measurements were performed after the velocity waveform became stable. The blood velocity waveforms were compared between the time before graft closure and that during graft clamping.

Results

By employing multichannel detection and our probe holder, we have succeeded in measurements of native LAD flow velocity in all cases studied. However, the number of measuring points along the poststenotic coronary artery was limited in those cases in which the artery was partly covered with thick adipose tissue.

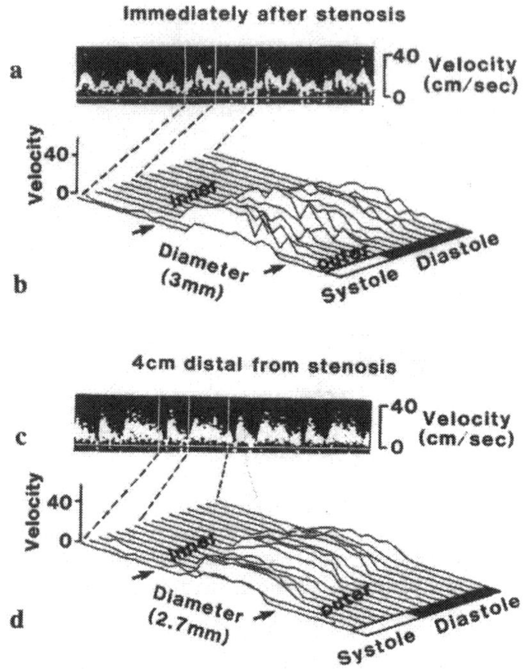

Fig. 3a–d. Representative tracings of poststenotic flow velocities **a, b** at the portions immediately distal and **c, d** about 4 cm distal to the stenosis in the LAD. **a** and **c** are velocity waveforms obtained at the central region of the vessel by FFT, and **b** and **d** are the velocity profiles across the vessel by the zero-cross method. From Kajiya et al. [3] with permission

Flow Characteristics in Poststenotic Regions

Figure 3 shows a representative tracing of the velocity waveforms in the distal portion of a 90% stenosis. Figure 3a, b illustrates the downstream velocities immediately distal to the stenosis. Figure 3c, d shows the velocities about 4 cm distal to the exit of the stenosis. The traces in Fig. 3a, c are velocity waveforms obtained by FFT at the central region of the vessel; those of Fig. 3b, d are the velocity profiles across the vessel obtained by 80-channel zero-cross analysis. The coronary artery velocity waveform through a severe stenosis was characterized by augmentation of the systolic velocity component and a relatively small diastolic velocity component. These characteristics distinctly contrasted with normal coronary artery flows, which showed a predominantly diastolic pattern. The broadening of the velocity spectrum was observed at each sampling point in the poststenotic region. The velocity spectrum, however, was rather wider in the distal portion than near the exit of the stenosis.

The velocity pattern in the vicinity of the vessel wall was more irregular in the immediately distal portion than in the far distal portion. Reverse flow velocities were frequently observed near the vessel wall at the portion close to the stenosis, although it was not clear in the case in Fig. 3. An example with a reverse flow is

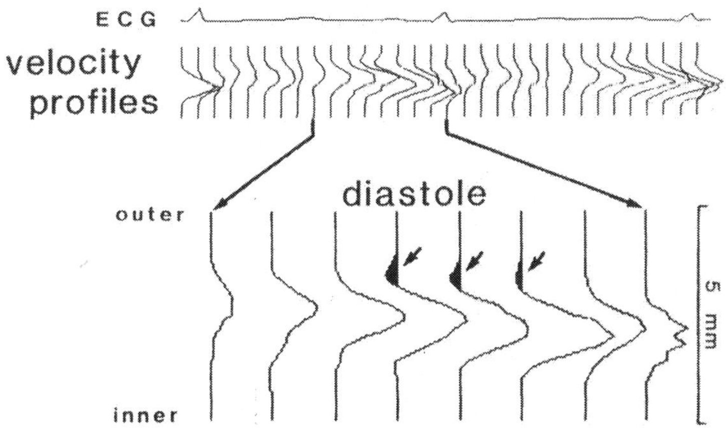

Fig. 4. An example of a poststenotic velocity profile across a vessel in which reverse flow was clearly noted near the outer vessel wall (probe side) during mid-diastole

shown in Fig. 4. In this case with 90% stenosis, the reverse velocity component was clearly noted near the outer vessel wall (probe side) during mid-diastole, which is indicated by arrows.

Comparison of Coronary Artery Velocity Waveforms Before and During Transient Graft Occlusion

Figure 5 shows typical tracings of the distal LAD velocities in a patient with 90% stenosis before and during a transient graft occlusion. Before graft occlusion, the LAD velocity distal to the graft insertion displayed a predominantly diastolic pattern. In contrast, a transient graft occlusion caused a marked reduction in the diastolic velocity component, while the systolic velocity component remained almost unchanged. To quantify the changes in the phasic velocity waveform before and during graft occlusion, the LAD velocities were integrated during systole, during diastole, and throughout one cardiac cycle. As shown in Fig. 6, the total and diastolic velocity areas decreased significantly by graft occlusion, but the systolic velocity area remained almost unchanged. Thus, the systolic to diastolic velocity area ratio increased significantly following graft occlusion. Heart rate and systolic and diastolic blood pressures did not change as a result of graft occlusions.

Discussion

The major contributions of our studies are: (a) description of the characteristics of poststenotic blood velocity in the native human coronary artery, and (b) evaluation of the changes in the velocity waveform in a distal coronary artery after saphenous vein bypass graft operations.

For this study, we employed the 80-channel 20-MHz dual-mode (zero-cross and FFT) pulsed Doppler velocimeter developed in our own laboratory [1–3].

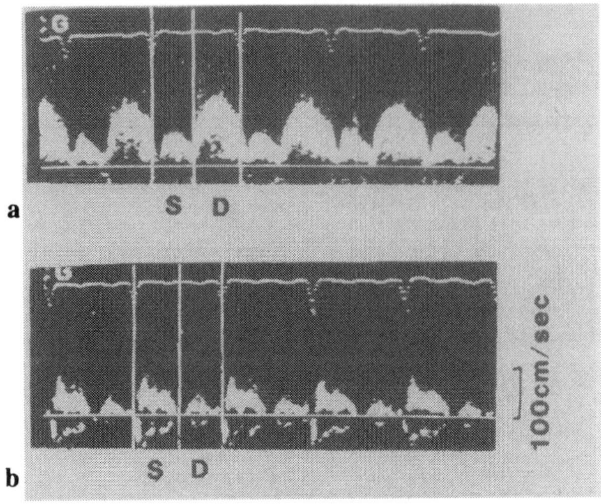

Fig. 5a, b. Comparison of blood velocities in a distal LAD beyond a bypass insertion before and during transient graft occlusion. It should be noted that the transient graft occlusion caused a marked reduction in the diastolic velocity component. **a** Graft open; **b** graft closed. *S* systole, *D* diastole

Eighty channels were used to allow evaluation of a detailed blood flow velocity profile across the vessel and for easier detection of a coronary artery covered with tissue. Marcus et al. [4] first succeeded in measuring coronary arterial flow velocity without surgical dissection of the artery by introducing a unique suction cup. They used a 20-MHz transducer with zero-cross Doppler shift detection, which was developed by Hartley and Cole [5]. The zero-cross method with a high-frequency transducer can detect Doppler signals from undisturbed flow precisely. When the flow is disturbed as in poststenotic flows, however, velocity distribution may occur even with a small sample volume. Our dual-mode Doppler detection (zero-cross and FFT) is indispensable to the analysis of poststenotic flow dynamics.

We observed reverse flow velocities near the vessel wall in the poststenotic coronary arteries (Fig. 4) and/or an irregularity in the velocity configuration in the vicinity of the wall (Fig. 3) in all cases, indicating the existence of flow separation and recirculation, which dissipate energy. This study is the first to demonstrate the occurrence of such phenomena in the poststenotic portion of an in vivo coronary artery. The broadening of the velocity spectrum measured at central axial regions in the poststenotic coronary artery indicates the presence of flow disturbance, although a clear-cut distinction between normal and disturbed flow is difficult. In our cases with more than 75% stenosis, the velocity spectrum was wider in the distal portion than near the exit of stenosis (Fig. 3). This finding is consistent with those obtained in model experiments [6, 7].

Before graft occlusion in the second protocol (Figs. 5, 6), the LAD flow velocity distal to the graft insertion represented a predominantly diastolic pattern, indicating that sufficient perfusion into the myocardium was achieved by the bypass grafting. In contrast, a transient graft occlusion caused a marked reduc-

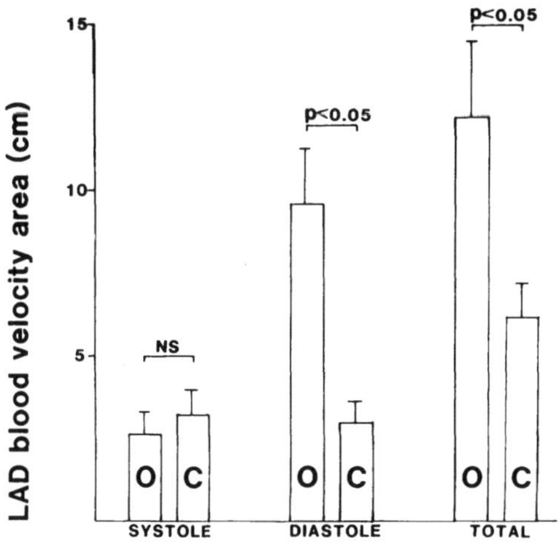

Fig. 6. Comparison of the LAD blood velocity areas in systole, diastole, and throughout the cardiac cycle before and during transient graft occlusion. Note that the diastolic and total velocity areas were reduced significantly by the graft occlusion, whereas the systolic velocity area was unchanged. *O* graft open, *C* graft closed

tion in the diastolic velocity, while the systolic velocity remained almost unchanged. These findings indicate that there was impaired myocardial perfusion before grafting. Why does a transient graft occlusion (stenotic flow) induce a remarkable reduction in diastolic coronary flow without a significant change in systolic flow? This could be mainly due to the change in the relative importance of stenotic resistance against distal (intramyocardial) vascular resistance between systole and diastole. Since distal vascular resistance is low during diastole, stenotic resistance may predominantly limit the flow, but during systole, in which distal vascular resistance becomes high due to myocardial compression, the stenotic resistance is much less important than distal vascular resistance. Although not significant statistically, a slight increase in the systolic flow component was observed during the bypass graft occlusion. The increase may result from a localized reduction in myocardial contractility and/or local distal vasodilation in the myocardium, especially in the epimyocardium. The latter would be expected to favor blood flow to the subepicardium, where perfusion may also occur during systole.

Acknowledgments. We are grateful to the American Heart Association for permission to reproduce in part or papers published in Circulation 74 (suppl 3): 53, 1986 and Circulation 76: 1092, 1987.

References

1. Ogasawara Y, Hiramatsu O, Kagiyama M, Tsujioka K, Tomonaga G, Kajiya F, Yanashima T, Kimura Y (1984) Evaluation of blood velocity profile by high frequency

ultrasound pulsed Doppler velocimeter by a multigated zerocross method together with a Fourier transform method. IEEE Comput Cardiol 447
2. Kajiya F, Ogasawara Y, Tsujioka K, Nakai M, Goto M, Wada Y, Tadaoka S, Matsuoka D, Mito K, Fujiwara T (1986) Evaluation of human coronary blood flow with an 80 channel pulsed Doppler velocimeter and zero-cross and Fourier transform methods during cardiac surgery. Circulation 74 (suppl 3): 53
3. Kajiya F, Tsujioka K, Ogasawara Y, Wada Y, Matsuoka S, Kanazawa S, Hiramatsu O, Tadaoka S, Goto M, Fujiwara T (1987) Analysis of flow characteristics in poststenotic regions of the human coronary artery during bypass graft surgery. Circulation 76: 1092
4. Marcus ML, Write CB, Doty DB, Eastham CL, Laughlin D, Krumm P, Fastenow C, Brody MJ (1981) Measurements of coronary velocity and reactive hyperemia in the coronary circulation of humans. Circ Res 49: 877
5. Hartley CJ, Cole JS (1974) An ultrasound pulsed Doppler system for measuring blood flow in small vessels. J Appl Physiol 37: 626
6. Young DF, Tsai FY (1973) Flow characteristics in models of arterial stenosis: I. Unsteady flow. J Biomech 6: 547
7. Khalifa AMA, Giddens DP (1981) Characterization and evolution of poststenotic flow disturbances. J Biomech 14: 279

Coronary Collateral Circulation in Acute and Chronic Myocardial Ischemia

BERND WINKLER, THOMAS SCHMIDT, and WOLFGANG SCHAPER[1]

We have recently demonstrated in different animal species that myocardial infarct (MI) size depends mainly on the amount of acute coronary collateral blood flow and time of occlusion (TOC) [1]. In these experiments, myocardial infarction was produced by occlusion of a branch of the left anterior descending artery (LAD). Coronary blood flow was measured by the tracer microsphere technique. The amount of infarcted tissue was determined histochemically by negative pNBT staining and related to the size of the myocardium which was supplied by the occluded coronary vessel. Animals with very low acute residual blood flow develop myocardial infarction rapidly and to a larger extent (rats, rabbits, and pigs) than animals with a noticeable acute collateral blood flow (cats and dogs). No myocardial infarction could be detected in guniea pigs even after an occlusion of 24 h. These results are summarized in Table 1 and Fig. 1. In Table 1, the imbalance between blood flow in the occluded myocardial tissue and tissue perfused by normal coronary arteries is expressed as the supply/demand ratio (SDR).

The development of myocardial infarction was suppressed in dogs experimentally by chronic occlusion of a coronary artery [2]. Recently, we could demonstrate similar results in pigs. Chronic occlusion was produced by implantation of an ameroid constrictor around the left circumflex artery. The pro-

Table 1. Experimental results with myocardial infarction, time of occlusion, and supply/demand ratio

	Rat	Rabbit	Pig	Cat	Dog	Guinea pig
SDR	0.01	0.01	0.03	0.04	0.05	1.00
TOC	< 45 min	< 90 min	< 90 min	6 h	12 h	24 h
MI (%)	95	90	85	80	75	No infarction

SDR supply/demand ratio, *TOC* time of occlusion, *MI* myocardial infarct

[1] Department of Experimental Cardiology, Max-Planck Institute, Benekestrasse 2, 6350 Bad Nauheim, Federal Republic of Germany

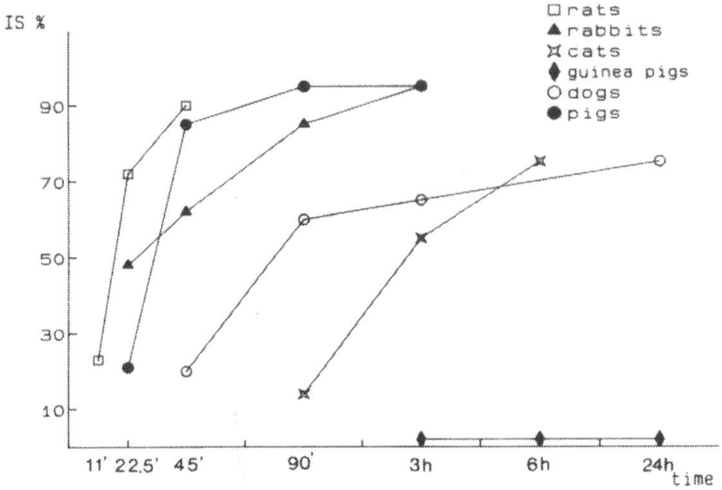

Fig. 1. Development of infarct size (*IS*) with time of occlusion. Infarct size is related to the total occluded vasculatory bed

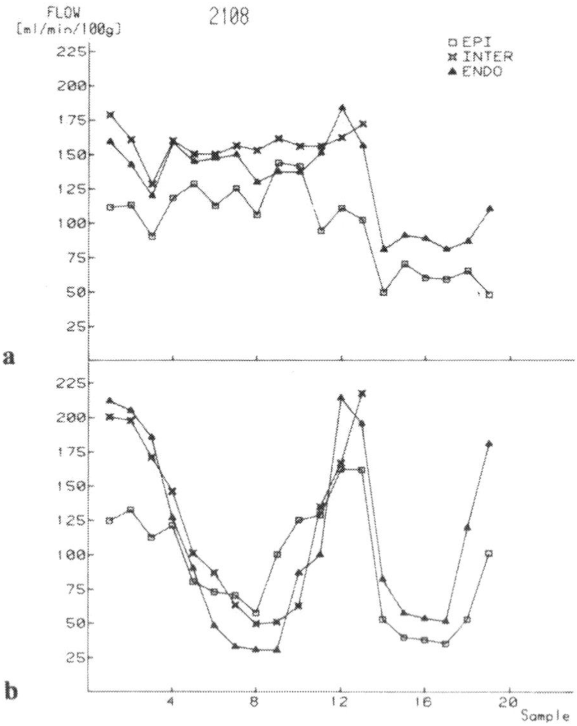

Fig. 2a, b. Blood flow distribution in a dog heart **a** during exercise and **b** during maximal vasodilation. Coronary circumflex artery and right coronary artery were occluded chronically by ameroid constrictors. Samples *1–3* belong to a slice of the left ventricle, samples *14–19* represent right ventricle in different layers (epi-, intermural, and endocardial)

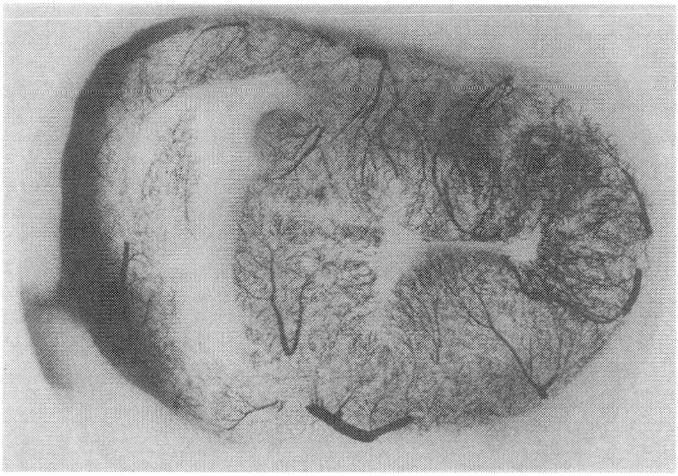

Fig. 3. Angiographic representation of a slice of a pig heart, which developed numerous microvessels in the region of the circumflex coronary artery within 2 months after implantation of an ameroid constrictor

gressively narrowing vessel produced a transient myocardial ischemia, which was considered to be a stimulus for the enlargement of the collateral circulation. The vessel was completely occluded within 2–3 weeks after implantation and the collateral circulation was maximally developed after about 8 weeks. Dogs increase the capacity of their collateral circulation by the formation of larger epicardial vessels. These vessels are so potent that even during heavy exercise, blood flow is matched to its demand, as demonstrated in Fig. 2. Figure 2a depicts the blood flow distribution in a heart slice of a dog running on a treadmill with no underperfusion in the occluded part of the myocardium. In contrast, underperfusion is visible in the same slice during maximal vasodilation produced by adenosine in an isolated heart preparation (Fig. 2b).

Pigs develop their collateral circulation by increasing the number of microvessels in the chronic ischemic tissue, as demonstrated in Fig. 3. Thus, their capacity can match normal resting myocardial blood flow by up to 60%, which is sufficient to prevent myocardial infarction. Coronary flow reserve is restricted during maximal vasodilation.

References

1. Winkler B, Sass S, Binz K, Schaper W (1986) Myokardiale Durchblutung und Myokardinfarkt in Ratten, Meerschweinchen, Kaninchen und Katzen. In: Burger OK, Grosdanoff P, Henschler D, Kraupp O, Schnieders B (eds) Aktuelle Probleme der Biomedizin. Gruyter, Berlin, pp 27–34
2. Schaper W (1979) (ed) The pathophysiology of myocardial perfusion. Elsevier/North-Holland, Amsterdam

Granulocyte Capillary Plugging in Myocardial Ischemia

GEERT W. SCHMID-SCHÖNBEIN[1] and ROBERT L. ENGLER[2]

Introduction

In spite of the relatively small numbers in the circulation, leukocytes have in recent years been recognized as playing a significant role in microvascular perfusion. As a result of their large volume and stiffness, leukocytes have to deform on their passage through the microcirculation. This could lead to a situation where they not only impose a relatively large vascular resistance, but also may obstruct the capillary lumen. In contrast, erythrocytes deform easily at the entrance to capillaries and do not cause obstruction. In addition, granulocytes regularly become attached to the vascular endothelium and, if activated, may release a spectrum of toxic substances to the surrounding tissue, which may lead to membrane damage, cell dysfunction, changes in vascular smooth muscle tone, increased permeability, and other defects. The traditional view that granulocytes participate in the inflammatory reaction and antimicrobal defense may represent only a limited aspect of leukocyte activity. These cells may in fact be the key elements in cell injury, organ dysfunction, necrosis, and death.

Capillary Kinetics

As leukocytes enter the terminal portion of the arterial circulation, they regularly encounter a strong hemodynamic interaction with the vascular endothelium. Nowhere is this more apparent than at the entrance to relatively narrow capillaries. At those sites, the granulocyte diameter exceeds that of the lumen so that they need to deform in order to fit into the lumen. The force for deformation is provided entirely by the local blood pressure. At such capillary entry regions, the cells come to a temporary stop for 1–3 s [1]; this is long compared with the entry time of erythrocytes, which is of the order of milliseconds. In the capillary,

[1] Department of Applied Mechanics and Engineering Sciences, Bioengineering, University of California, San Diego, La Jolla, CA 92093, USA
[2] Department of Medicine, University of California, San Diego and Research Service and Cardiology Section, Veteran's Administration Medical Center, San Diego, CA 92161, USA

the thickness of the plasma film between the leukocyte and endothelium is reduced to a distance of less than 1 μm [2], so that molecular forces between the two membrances may be exerted. Under normal flow conditions, the cell will only temporarily interrupt the flow and then pass relatively unhindered through the capillary lumen, although its velocity remains slightly lower than that of red cells. The consequence of this slight difference in axial cell velocity is the phenomenon of a white cell-red cell train formation along the length of the capillary and the ensuing postcapillary attachment of granulocytes to the endothelium [3]. However, under conditions of reduced perfusion pressure, the capillary lumen is decreased in diameter [4] and the force available for deformation of the leukocyte is reduced. Consequently, leukocytes may reside progressively longer periods of time in the capillary network. In particular, they may obstruct individual capillaries to the degree of complete flow cessation [5]. Under these conditions, few additional cells will enter the capillary at its upstream bifurcation, and only few leukocytes are present in a capillary network with obstructed vessels.

One of the consequences of progressive capillary obstruction is a gradual rise of the vascular resistance after occlusion of the left anterior descending coronary artery—in the canine heart typically about 10%–20% of total vascular resistance during the 1st h of ischemia. In other organs, such as the lung, with a dense capillary network, the whole organ resistance does not necessarily reflect the microvascular accumulation of the granulocytes unless a massive accumulation takes place. Besides the capillary accumulation of leukocytes, ischemic organs also show an accumulation of leukocytes in the collecting venules; these cells do not occlude the lumen but raise the vascular resistance. The two pools of granulocytes cannot readily be distinguished by the whole-organ approach but may be differentiated with intravital or histological techniques. Leukocytes in both capillary and postcapillary venules contribute to injury.

Capillary Occlusion and Capillary No-Reflow Phenomenon

One of the consequences of leukocyte entrapment in capillaries during hypotensive perfusion is the fact that the cell will develop a contact area with the endothelium. In this contact area, a molecular attractive force can be exerted. A cell which is attached to the endothelium in this way requires considerably higher transcellular pressures to break away. Depending on the exact magnitude of the adhesive energy, the pressure drop across a single capillary may be insufficient to remove the granulocyte, even after restoration of the arterial pressure to normal values [6].

Investigation of the no-reflow phenomenon in the canine heart with an intravascular tracer technique [7] shows that the only microvessels which are obstructed after acute ischemia and reperfusion are capillaries; arterioles or venules in the microcirculation still show flow and accept the tracer. This suggests that individual granulocytes obstruct the capillary network (Fig. 1), an observation that is confirmed by measurements of the granulocyte accumulation in the capillary network and by the observation that after perfusion with agranulocytic blood, the capillary no-reflow phenomenon is suppressed [8].

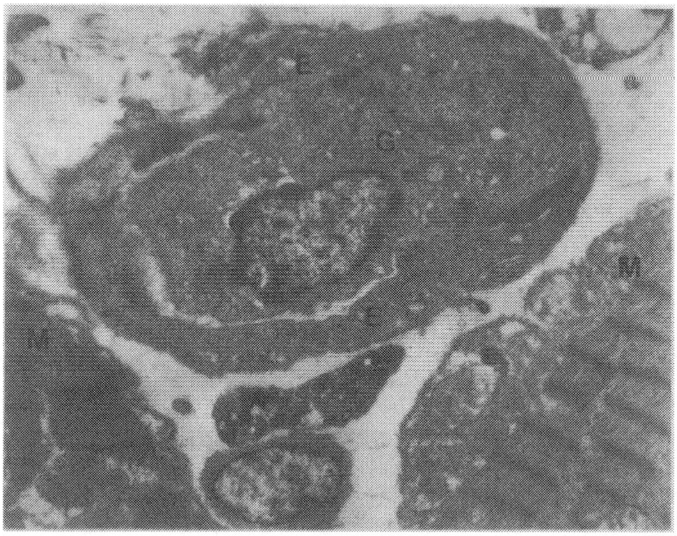

Fig. 1. Electron micrograph of a granulocyte (*G*) in a capillary in the heart after 5 h of ischemia followed by a 5-min reperfusion and transfusion with Ringer's lactate and ink tracer solution for about 3 min at 90 mmHg mean pressure. Note that the cell could not be removed by this procedure and that the cell is already partially degranulated (primary granules). The adjacent myocytes (*M*) exhibit swelling of their cytoplasm and mitochondria. The capillary lumen is almost entirely filled by the granulocyte and the endothelium (*E*) is still intact and shows limited evidence of swelling

Capillary no-reflow is a typical aspect of acutely ischemic conditions and may be accompanied by other manifestations in other organs or under other conditions [9–12].

Agranulocytic Perfusion

One of the key experiments to test the hypothesis that granulocytes may be involved in myocardial ischemic injury is the perfusion of an ischemic heart with agranulocytic blood. This raises the question of how to remove the granulocytes. Neutropenia can be achieved by whole-body radiation, administration of cytotoxins or other agents that interfere with hemopoiesis, and recently by the use of specific cell antiserum which can be directed at selected cell populations. The use of such techniques has often shown a limited degree of protection against ischemic and reperfusion injury [13], but few studies have shown a degree of protection that would unequivocally point toward any specific blood cell as the single major participant in ischemic and reperfusion injury. It should be kept in mind that some methods of inducing neutropenia, such as the use of antiserum, merely shift leukocytes from the circulating pool into the marginating pool. The marginating pool is largely uncontrolled and unmeasured. Trapping of the cells may occur in the lung, liver, and spleen but may occur in other organs depending on the manner of inducing neutropenia. Thus, in some experimental forms of neutropenia, the circulating blood may in fact be largely depleted of neutrophils, yet the organs under investigation may have, even prior to the experimental procedure, an abnormal accumulation of granulocytes. There is a need to evaluate neutropenic animal models not only with regard to the circulating cell density but also with respect to the marginating pool and tissue injury before ischemia.

Perfusion of the ischemic heart with agranulocytic blood by the use of a cotton-wick or nylon filter shows a remarkable degree of protection during 1 h of coronary occlusion and ischemia [8]. The capillary no-reflow phenomenon is eliminated, and the progressive rise in vascular resistance to collateral flow prevented. Instead, one observes a consistent decrease in resistance. These agranulocytic pefused hearts showed no significant edema formation, a reduced number of premature ventricular beats, and near complete suppression of ventricular tachycardia and ventricular fibrillation [8]. The effect of prolonged reperfusion with agranulocytic blood beyond 1 h of ischemia remains to be determined. Following 15 minutes of ischemia, postischemic dysfunction is completely suppressed in the absence of granulocytes (Fig. 2) [14]. There appear to be few other procedures that give such a high degree of protection against ischemia and reperfusion injury. However, every form of neutropenia employed experimentally has its limitations. The filter method removes some platelets as well and may cause adenosine release [14]. The interaction between platelets and granulocytes also needs further study.

Leukocyte Activation

One of the important factors for microvascular injury may be granulocyte activation. Cell activation may be accompanied by several phenomena, some of which may be regarded as disruptive to normal organ perfusion. Cell activation may include: (a) formation of pseudopodia, i.e., local regions of membrane-covered cytoplasm enriched with F-actin and with a stiffened cytoplasm; (b) production of free radicals (the oxygen burst); (c) release of lysosomes; and (d) expression of adhesion proteins and others [15, 16]. The question arises by what mechanisms granulocytes may become activated in the ischemic myocardium. There are currently several known mechanisms for activation: (a) activation through specific cell surface activator receptors, such as serum complement, leukotriene B_4, peptides, platelet-activating factor, lymphokines, and others; (b) activation via a negative feedback mechanism, e.g., the elimination of deactivators such as adenosine [17, 18]; (c) activation by mechanical shear; and (d) activation by contact with other cells, such as endothelial cells. The pathophysiologically significant mechanisms in the ischemic myocardium are currently largely unexplored.

Infusion of activated leukocytes into the coronary circulation with a normal perfusion pressure may cause a reduction of the active force developed by the myocytes and a detectable increase in coronary vascular resistance; both processes are irreversible if agents are used which permanently activate the granulocytes [19]. Activation of cells with shorter acting agents causes only a temporary increase in vascular resistance and reduced contraction [20].

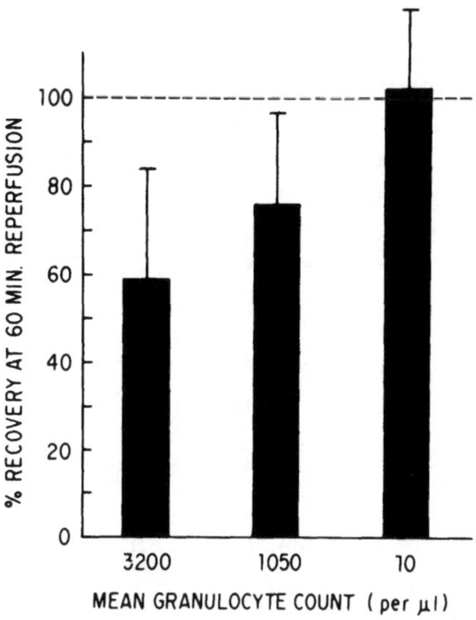

Fig. 2. Recovery of regional function measured by mid wall ultrasonic dimensions gauges in the ischemic area following 15 min of ischemia and 60 min of recovery in dogs. Function is normalized to percent shortening prior to ischemia; loading condition and heart rate were unchanged. *Left* control animals perfused with whole blood, *center* after 2 h of leukopak filtration when filters were removed, *right* during leukopak filtration

Source of O_2 Radicals

Superoxide is formed by the univalent reduction of oxygen. It is a potent oxidizing agent, which can lead to the formation of several other oxidizing agents and harmful cells in a variety of ways, including self-sustaining lipid chain peroxidation [21]. This process can cause lethal damage to biological membrances. One demonstration of the role of superoxide in ischemic and reperfusion injury involves the use of superoxide dismutase and catalase, scavengers of superoxide and the hydroxyl radical, to reducing the infarct size in dogs [22]. Superoxide is a mediator of reperfusion injury, as originally suggested by McCord based on data in isolated perfused hearts [23]. The major source of superoxide in McCord's experiments was presumed to be endothelial cell xanthine oxidase. In intestinal ischemia and reperfusion, xanthine oxidase appears to trigger granulocyte activation, which magnifies the injury [24].

In considering superoxide as a source of injury, it is important to keep in mind that the net superoxide is the sum of all sources. If there is a threshold for any particular marker of injury, then reduction of one source may decrease or eliminate apparent injury but leave other sources of superoxide just below the threshold for detection. In the intact heart, there are several potentially important sources for superoxide radicals during reperfusion: endothelial cells (xanthine oxidase), granulocytes (reduced nicotinamide adenine dinucleotide oxidase), mitochondrial leak due to physical or chemical damage (ubiquinone), arachidonate metabolism, catecholamine oxidation, and cytochrome P450.

Whether or not xanthine oxidase (which is converted from xanthine dehydrogenase by a calcium protease during or after ischemia) is quantitatively important under clinical conditions is unclear. First, xanthine oxidase has not been demonstrated in the endothelium of the human myocardium following ischemia, so that data from experimental models may not be directly applicable in man [25]. Second, the mitochondrial leak of superoxide is in the first approximation proportional to the level of pO_2; thus, when isolated perfused hearts with high pO_2 are used to study superoxide during reperfusion, an increase in mitochondrial sources may bias the data by raising the physiological level of superoxide. Third, based on results in isolated buffer-perfused hearts, subsequent in vivo experimental models in some animal species have shown that allopurinol treatment reduces infarct size; however, the results are not unanimous [26–29]. The drug allopurinol, or its derivative oxipurinol, are potent inhibitors of xanthine oxidase. It appears that pretreatment as well as the choice of species may be important factors for the success of allopurinol treatment. Allopurinol has also other effects on purine metabolism [30], and as such could possibly affect adenosine release, which inhibits granulocyte superoxide production as well as other manifestions of granulocyte activation [17]. However, small amounts of xanthine oxidase may produce chemoattractants, which could activate granulocytes [23, 24].

The other sources of superoxide, arachidonate metabolism and cytochrome P450, may not be quantitatively important in heart muscle. But in other organs these two may be significant [31].

Granulocytes Contribute to Oxygen Radical Injury

Granulocytes can generate large quantities of superoxide [15]. Evidence for granulocyte superoxide production in cardiac ischemia and reperfusion injury came from studying nonlethal reperfusion injury (the stunned myocardium). In dog hearts, reperfusion following 15 min of ischemia results in prompt, complete return of contractile function, followed quickly by a decline to 20%–60% of normal function [32]. All tissue goes on to complete recovery without necrosis, and function returns to normal after a period of more than about 6 h. Several investigators have shown that oxygen free radical scavengers such as superoxide dismutase and catalase can reduce myocardial stunning [33, 34]. Perfusion with agranulocytic blood can completely prevent the stunned myocardium in this model, indicating that granulocytes are a major source of superoxide radical causing stunning (Fig. 2) [14]. In other species or during longer periods of ischemia, other sources of free radical may be important. Granulocytes in both the capillary and postcapillary venules may be important sources of free radicals.

Endothelium, Edema, and Granulocytes

Edema is observed in the ischemic myocardium and, to a greater extent, upon reperfusion [35, 36]. The edema that occurs during ischemia is dramatically decreased by agranulocytosis [8]. With whole-blood perfusion, tissue water content during ischemia correlates with granulocyte content [37]. In other models of tissue injury, edema is also granulocyte dependent [16, 38], but no causal relationship has been established in cardiac ischemia.

Endothelial cell damage occurs in regions of infarction. The extent of endothelial damage is decreased concomitantly with a reduction in infarct size when interventions which inhibit granulocytes are used [39]. It is well established that endothelial damage and microvascular leakage are part of the inflammatory response. Activated granulocytes can damage the endothelium and, conversely, endothelial pretreatment may result in the expression of endothelial leukocyte adherence molecules [40]. However, the primary cause of the endothelial damage (ischemia or inflammation) has yet to be determined in cardiac muscle; it may be that endothelial activation triggers granulocyte activation during ischemia and reperfusion. Furthermore, it seems likely that this important relationship between endothelial injury, inflamatory cell activation, and ischemic damage to myocytes will be a function of the duration of ischemia.

Conclusion

Granulocytes accumulate in the microcirculation during ischemia and upon reperfusion and cause a capillary no-reflow phenomenon. The consequences of accumulation and concomitant activation during the acute phase of ischemia are significant for microvascular and organ function. Whether or not modifications of these events will alter long-term prognosis requires further study.

Acknowledgments. The investigations reported in this study were supported by grants from NHLBI Ischemic Heart SCOR HL 17682 and HL 10881.

References

1. Fenton BM, Wilson DW, Cokelet GR (1985) Analysis of the effects of measured white blood cell entrance times on hemodynamics in a computer model of a microvascular bed. Pflügers Arch 403: 396–401
2. Tözeren H, Skalak R (1979) The flow of closely fitting particles in tapered tubes. Int J Multiphase Flow 5: 395–412
3. Schmid-Schönbein GW, Usami S, Skalak R, Chien S (1980) The interaction of leukocytes and erythrocytes in capillary and postcapillary vessels. Microvasc Res 19: 45–70
4. Skalak TC, Schmid-Schönbein GW (1986) Viscoelastic properties of microvessels in rat spinotrapezius muscle. J Biomech Eng 108: 193–200
5. Bagge U, Amundson B, Lauritzen C (1980) White blood cell deformability and plugging of skeletal muscle capillaries in hemorrhagic shock. Acta Physiol Scand 108: 159–163
6. Schmid-Schönbein GW (1987) Mechanisms of granulocyte-capillary-plugging. Prog Appl Microcirc 12: 223–230
7. Engler RL, Schmid-Schönbein GW, Pavelec RS (1983) Leukocyte capillary plugging in myocardial ischemia and reperfusion in the dog. Am J Pathol 111: 98–111
8. Engler RL, Dahlgren MD, Morris D, Peterson M, Schmid-Schönbein GW (1986) Role of leukocytes in response to acute myocardial ischemia and reflow in dogs. Am J Physiol 252: H314–H322
9. Majno G, Ames A III, Chaing J, Wright RL (1967) No reflow after cerebral ischemia. Lancet 2: 569–570

10. Krug A, de Rochemont WM, Korb G (1966) Blood supply of the myocardium after temporary coronary occlusion. Circ Res 19: 57–62
11. Kloner RA, Ganote CE, Jennings RB (1974) The "no reflow" phenomenon after temporary coronary occlusion in the dog. J Clin Invest 54: 1496–1508
12. Ames A, Wright RL, Kowada M, Thurston JM, Majno G (1968) Cerebral ischemia: II The no-reflow phenomenon. Am J Pathol 52: 437–453
13. Romson JL, Hook B, Kunkel S, Abrams G, Schork MA, Lucchesi BR (1983) Reduction of the extent of ischemic myocardial injury by neutrophil depletion in the dog. Circulation 67: 1016–1023
14. Engler RL, Covell JW (1987) Granulocytes cause reperfusion ventricular dysfunction after 15-minute ischemia in the dog. Circ Res 61: 20–28
15. Babior BM (1978) Oxygen dependent microbial killing by phagocytes. N Engl J Med 288: 659–668, 721–725
16. Arfors K-E, Lundberg C, Lindbom L, Lundberg K, Beatty P, Harlan JW (1987) A monoclonal antibody to the membrane glycoprotein complex CD 18 inhibits polymorphonuclear leukocyte accumulation and plasma leakage in vivo. Blood 69: 338–340
17. Cronstein BN, Levin RI, Belanoff J, Weissman G, Hirschhorn R (1986) Adenosine is an endogenous inhibitor of neutrophil mediated injury to endothelial cells. J Clin Invest 78: 760–770
18. Engler RL (1987) Consequences of activation and adenosine mediated inhibition of granulocytes during myocardial ischemia. Fed Proc 46: 2407–2412
19. Semb AG, Ytrehus K, Vaage J, Mjos OD (1987) Intracoronary infusion of activated leukocytes causes functional depression of isolated rat hearts. 4th World Congress for Microcirculation, Tokyo, Abstract 317
20. Martin SE, Chenowith D, Engler RL, Roth DM, Longhurst J (1987) Reduced coronary flow and myocardial function by complement: implication of a granulocyte mechanism. Fed Proc 46: 640
21. Fridovich I (1983) Superoxide radical: an endogenous toxicant. Ann Rev Pharmacol Toxicol 23: 239–257
22. Jolly SR, Kane WJ, Bailie MB, Abrams GD, Lucchesi BR (1984) Canine myocardial reperfusion injury: its reduction by the combined administration of superoxide dismutase and catalase. Circ Res 54: 277–285
23. McCord JM (1985) Oxygen-derived free radicals in postischemic injury. N Eng J Med 312: 159–163
24. Hernandez LA, Grisham MB, Twohig B, Arfors KE, Harlan JM, Granger DN (1987) Role of neutrophils in ischemia-induced microvascular injury. Am J Physiol 253: H699–H703
25. Eddy LJ, Stewart JR, Jones HP, Engerson TD, McCord JM, Downey JM (1987) Free radical producing enzyme, xanthine oxidase, is undetectable in human hearts. Am J Physiol 253: H709–H711
26. Shatney CHO, MacCarter DJ, Lillehei RC (1976) Effects of allopurinol, propranolol and methyl prednisolone on infarct size in experimental myocardial infarction. Am J Cardiol 37: 572–580
27. Akizuki S, Yoshida S, Chambers D, Eddy L, Pamlely L, Yellon D, Downey J (1984) Blockage of the O_2 radical producing enzyme, xanthine oxidase, reduces infarct size in the dog. Fed Proc 43: 540
28. Reimer KA, Jennings RB (1985) Failure of the xanthine oxidase inhibitor allopurinol to limit infarct size after ischemia and reperfusion in dogs. Circulation 71: 1069–1075
29. Arnold WL, DeWall RA, Kezdi P, Zwart HHJ (1980) The effect of allopurinol on the degree of early myocardial ischemia. Am Heart J 99: 616–624
30. Fox IH, Wyngaarden JB, Kelley WN (1970) Depletion of erythrocyte phosphoribosyl pyrophosphate in man—a newly observed effect of allopurinol. N Eng J Med 282: 1177–1182
31. Kukreja RC, Kontos HA, Hess ML, Ellis F (1986) PGH synthase and lipoxygenase

generate superoxide in the presence of NADH or NADPH. Circ Res 59: 612–619
32. Heyndrickx GR, Baig H, Nellens P, Leusen I, Fishbein MC, Vatner SF (1978) Depression of regional blood flow and wall thickening after brief coronary occlusions. Am J Physiol 234: H653–H659
33. Gross GJ, Farber NE, Hardman HF, Warltier DC (1986) Beneficial actions of superoxide dismutase and catalase in stunned myocardium in dogs. Am J Physiol 250: H372–H377
34. Przyklenk K, Kloner RA (1986) Superoxide dismutase plus catalase improve contractile function in the canine model of the "stunned myocardium." Circ Res 58: 148–156
35. Powell WJ Jr, Dibona DR, Flores J, Leaf A (1976) The protective effect of hyperosmotic mannitol in myocardial ischemia and necrosis. Circulation 54: 603–615
36. Willerson JT, Powell WJ Jr, Guiney TE, Stark JJ, Sanders CA, Leaf A (1972) Improvement in myocardial function and coronary blood flow in ischemic myocardium after mannitol. J Clin Invest 51: 2989–2998
37. Engler RL, Dahlgren MD, Peterson M, Dobbs A, Schmid-Schönbein GW (1986) Accumulation of polymorphonuclear leukocytes during 3-hour experimental myocardial ischemia. Am J Physiol 251: H93–H100
38. Wedmore CV, Williams TJ (1981) Control of vascular permeability by polymorphonuclear leukocytes in inflammation. Nature 289: 646–650
39. Forman MB, Puett DW, Bingham SE, Virmani R, Tantengco MV, Light RT, Price R, Friesinger GC (1987) Preservation of endothelial cell structure and function by intracoronary perfluorochemical in a canine preparation of reperfusion. Circulation 76: 469–479
40. Bevilacqua MP, Pober JS, Wheeler ME, Cotran RS, Gimbrone MA Jr (1985) Interleukin-1 acts on cultured vascular endothelium to increase the adhesion of polymorphonuclear leukocytes, monocytes, and related cell lines. J Clin Invest 76: 2003–2011

Nonesterified Fatty Acid Metabolism and Membrane Disorders in Myocardial Ischemia and Reperfusion

Robert S. Reneman, Frits W. Prinzen, Marc Van Bilsen, Wim Engels, and Ger J. Van der Vusse[1]

Introduction

Under normal circumstances, 40%–60% of the circulatory nonesterified fatty acids (NEFAs) are extracted from the heart in a single transit time [1]. The majority of NEFAs are oxidized in the mitochondria for energy delivery. Such NEFAs as arachidonic acid, linoleic acid, and docosahexaenoic acid are mainly incorporated into phospholipids, a major constituent of cell membranes. In this respect, species differences and the effect of nutrition have to be appreciated. For example, in the dog, myocyte membranes mainly consist of arachidonic acid and linoleic acid, while membrane lipids of rat myocytes mainly consist of arachidonic acid and docosahexaenoic acid.

The myocardial NEFA content is extremely low under normoxic conditions [2–4] but increases significantly during myocardial ischemia [2, 5–7]. All NEFAs increase, but the NEFAs with the highest relative increase during myocardial ischemia are those incorporated in cellular membranes. Because NEFAs have been found to uncouple mitochondrial activity [8] and to block membrane-bound Na^+/K^+-ATPase activity [9], the NEFA accumulation during myocardial ischemia may have consequences for the performance of the heart. Since enzymatic oxidation of arachidonic acid leads to a variety of biochemically important products, such as leukotrienes (lipoxygenase pathway), prostaglandins, thromboxanes, and prostacyclin (cyclooxygenase pathway), the formation of these products, referred to collectively as eicosanoids, may be anticipated during myocardial ischemia and reperfusion. Since the situation may be different during ischemia, when oxygen supply is limited, and reperfusion, when oxygen is delivered to the myocardium in abundance, both conditions are considered.

In the present survey, we will consecutively discuss the NEFA content in normoxic myocardium, the accumulation of NEFA in ischemic myocardium in relation to, among others, the changes in myocardial blood flow and ATP content under these circumstances, the possible consequences of increased NEFA content for myocardial function and membrane integrity, and the formation, if any, of eicosanoids from the accumulated arachidonic acid in ischemic myocardial

[1] Departments of Physiology and Microbiology, University of Limburg, P. O. Box 616, 6200 MD, Maastricht, The Netherlands

tissue. Most of the data presented are derived from in situ dog hearts, subjected to regional, low-flow ischemia and isolated, working rat hearts perfused with Tyrode's solution. When studying the effect of reperfusion, in some animals ischemia was induced by total occlusion of the coronary artery. The observations were made during 1–2 h of ischemia, when the transition from reversible to irreversible myocardial damage is supposed to occur, followed by 1 h of reperfusion. These circumstances are of clinical importance because of the increasing number of methods developed to restore blood flow acutely to the jeopardized myocardium.

NEFA Content in Normoxic Myocardial Tissue

Although the values published range from 25 to at least 22000 $nmol.g^{-1}$ wet weight, recent studies have shown that the level of NEFAs in normoxic myocardial tissue is extremely low [2, 3] and that the high values reported may be considered to be artificial due to the use of unspecific assays or technical imperfections in the assay method [4]. In the dog heart, less than 0.1% of all fatty acids are likely to be present in the nonesterified form, only a small fraction of which (median values, about 1.4–3.0 $nmol.g^{-1}$ wet weight in the various experiments) can be attributed to arachidonic acid (Table 1). When corrections are made for the NEFAs present in blood and the interstitial space, the intracellular NEFA content can be estimated to be about 10 $nmol.g^{-1}$ wet weight [2], which means that the intracellular content of, for example, nonesterified (free) arachidonic acid will be extremely low. No significant differences in the free arachidonic acid content can be detected between the subepicardial, mesocardial, and subendocardial layers in normoxic conditions [10].

In the dog heart, the majority of fatty acids are incorporated in phospholipids (88.2%; Table 1). Palmitic acid and stearic acid are the main constituents of NEFAs. Oleic acid accounts for about 41% of all fatty acids incorporated in triacylglycerol. Linoleic acid and arachidonic acid are the main constituents of phospholipids. In this lipid group, phosphatidylcholine and phosphatidylethanolamine are the main phospholipid subclasses. Lysophospholipids are present in only small amounts.

NEFA Content in Ischemic Myocardial Tissue

A relatively high NEFA content is found in the ischemic myocardium. In general, the increase in total NEFA content during low-flow ischemia of the canine myocardium is caused by a rise of each individual fatty acid, but the longer chain, unsaturated fatty acids, such as linoleic acid (by about 600%) and arachidonic acid (by 600%–1000% in the various studies), show the highest relative increase. The accumulation of NEFAs during low-flow myocardial ischemia is a relatively slow process. No significant increase in NEFA content can be observed after 10 min of ischemia. During prolonged, low-flow myocardial ischemia, the NEFA content significantly increases, the highest values being found in the endo- and mesocardial layers, the layers with the lowest blood flow

Table 1. Lipid content and relative content of some fatty acids in the various lipid classes in normoxic dog myocardium. The values are as measured in the middle layer of the free wall of the left ventricle

	NEFA	Triacyl-glycerol	Cholesteryl-esters	Phospholipids
Content (nmol. g^{-1} net wt.)	28 ± 14	5530 ± 4384	203 ± 175	43068 ± 2048
Relative composition (%)				
Palmitic acid	29.8	21.5	9.8	8.6
Oleic acid	14.2	41.2	21.2	18.0
Linoleic acid	8.8	16.6	41.3	25.2
Arachidonic acid	5.0	0.7	14.4	28.3

Values are means ± SD (n = 6–10)

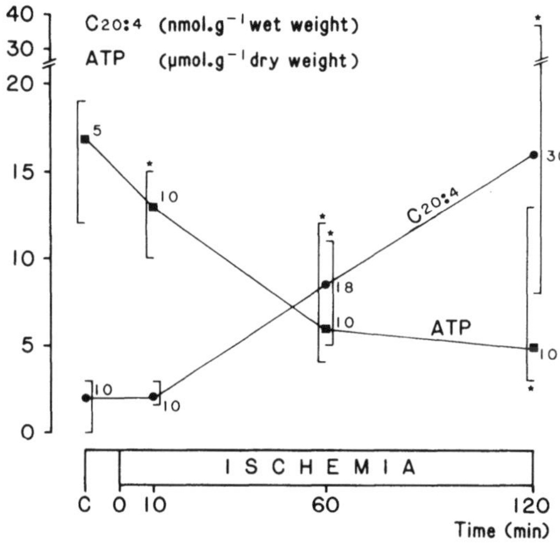

Fig. 1. Tissue content of free arachidonic acid (*C 20: 4*) and ATP in the inner layers of dog left ventricular myocardium in the control situation and at various intervals after induction of regional low-flow ischemia. Median values and 95% confidence limits are depicted. The *figures* near the *median values* refer to the number of observations. *Significantly different from the control situation ($P<0.05$). After Reneman et al. [10]

during ischemia [6].

From experiments on low-flow regionally ischemic dog hearts and isolated no-flow global ischemic rat hearts, it can be concluded that at least 30 min of oxygen deprivation are required before NEFA accumulation occurs. The myocardial free arachidonic acid and ATP content, as measured in the inner layers in the control situation and during prolonged ischemia, are presented in Fig. 1. The free arachidonic acid content increases with the duration of ischemia, reaching a median value of about 15 nmol.g^{-1} wet weight after 120 min. These data clearly show that the ATP content falls before an increase in free arachido-

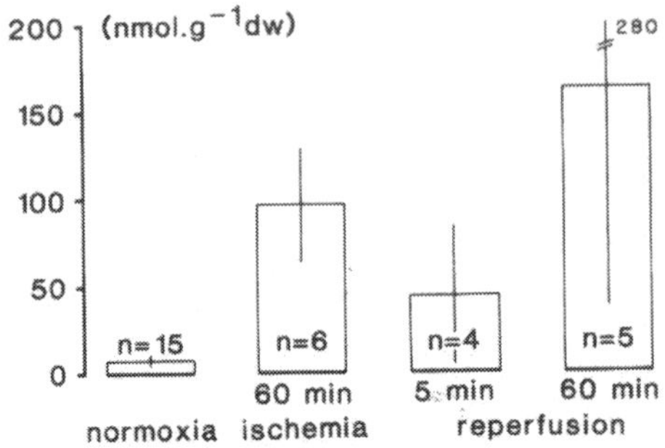

Fig. 2. Free arachidonic acid content (nmol.g^{-1} dry weight) in normoxic, ischemic (total coronary artery occlusion), and reperfused subendocardial tissue in the dog (means ± SD). Ischemia and reperfusion data are derived from different experiments. *Significantly different from normoxic value ($P<0.05$)

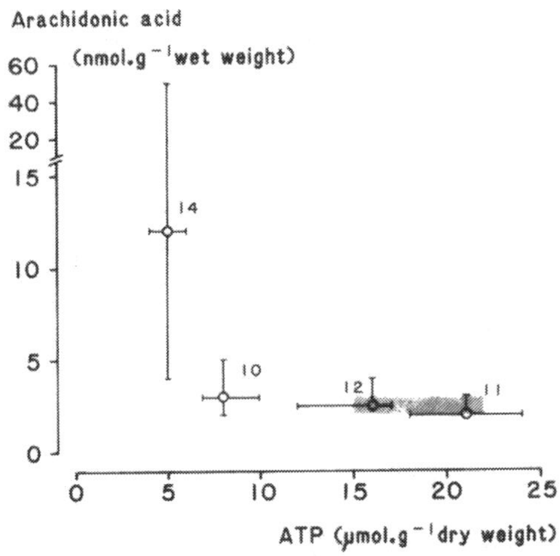

Fig. 3. Relation between content of free arachidonic acid and ATP in samples taken from ischemic and nonischemic dog left ventricular myocardium 120 min after onset of regional low-flow ischemia. ATP content is determined in tissue specimens taken in the vicinity of biopsies for arachidonic acid assessment. *Data* are grouped according to ATP content and divided into cohorts of 3–5 nmol.g^{-1} dry weight. The *figures* near the *median values* refer to the number of observations. *Shaded area* indicates 95% confidence limits of data of all samples from nonischemic myocardium. After Reneman et al. [10]

nic acid content can be observed. A higher myocardial free arachidonic acid content is reached when myocardial ischemia is induced by coronary artery occlusion (Fig. 2; note that the data are presented in nmol.g^{-1} dry weight because myocardial edema can be expected during reperfusion).

After 120 min of low-flow myocardial ischemia, generally no increase in free arachidonic acid content can be observed when blood flow in the area at risk, as assessed by radioactive microspheres, is higher than 0.3 ml.min^{-1}.g^{-1}, irrespective of the layer from which the sample is taken. Samples with a blood flow below this value generally show an increase in free arachidonic acid. Extreme increases in free arachidonic acid are predominantly observed in samples from regions with a blood flow below 0.1 ml.min^{-1}.g^{-1} [10]. The relationship between the content of ATP and free arachidonic acid in all three myocardial layers after 120 min of low-flow ischemia is shown in Fig. 3 (paired data on free arachidonic acid and ATP content in ischemic and nonischemic myocardium are presented). The free arachidonic acid content tends to rise at ATP levels between 7 and 10 nmol.g^{-1} dry weight and increases significantly when ATP values of 4–6 nmol.g^{-1} dry weight are reached.

Origin of Long-Chain Unsaturated NEFAs During Myocardial Ischemia

Free arachidonic acid, accumulating during myocardial ischemia, probably originates from endogenous sources because no significant uptake of this long-chain fatty acid by the ischemic myocardium can be detected [2] and a similar accumulation is observed in Tyrode's solution-perfused (without fatty acids as exogenous substrate), isolated rat hearts subjected to global ischemia (Fig. 4). The most likely source of free arachidonic acid is the group of phospholipids. Firstly, these lipids have a high content of both arachidonic and linoleic acid, which do show the highest relative increase in the regionally ischemic dog heart. Secondly, the time-course of NEFA accumulation [6, 7] resembles the time-course of the

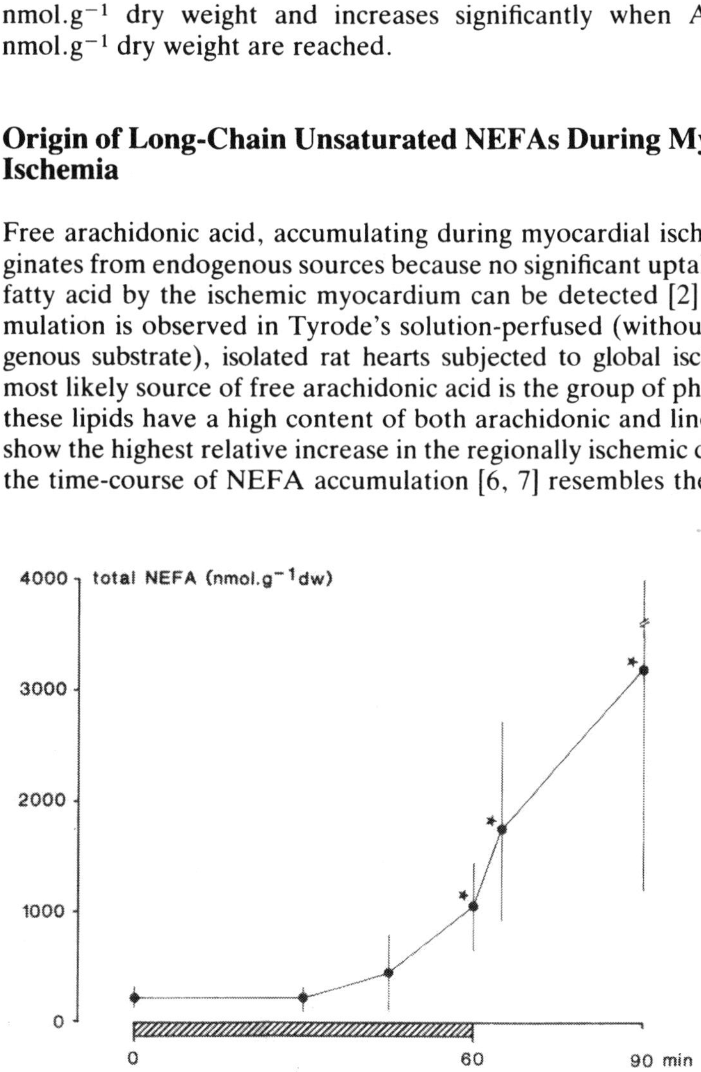

Fig. 4. Nonesterified fatty acid (*NEFA*) content (nmol.g^{-1} dry weight) of rat hearts during normoxia, after 30, 45, and 60 min of ischemia and at various intervals during 30-min reperfusion (means ± SD). The *data* presented are derived from different groups of experiments (n = 7–10/group). The *shaded area* represents the period of ischemia. *Significantly different from the normoxic value ($P < 0.05$). After Van Bilsen et al. [15]

onset of irreversible loss of cell function in ischemic myocardial tissue [11]. Thirdly, the observation by the latter investigators that changes in ultrastructure and membrane function occur when myocardial ATP content is below 5 nmol.g^{-1} dry weight (about 25% of the normoxic ATP level) is in good agreement with the finding that ATP reduction precedes free arachidonic acid accumulation and that this unsaturated fatty acid significantly accumulates when ATP levels of 4–6 nmol.g^{-1} dry weight are reached (Fig. 3). Finally, when ATP levels in cultured myocytes are reduced with the use of specific inhibitors of metabolic activity, arachidonic acid is specifically released from phospholipids when the ATP level drops below 25% of its original value [12].

Mechanism of Accumulation of NEFAs Like Arachidonic Acid and Linoleic Acid

Although the findings described above suggest a causal relationship between a fall in tissue ATP levels and degradation of membrane phospholipids, at present no definite mechanism is available to explain this relationship in full detail. Depletion of ATP will hamper the formation of arachidonyl coenzyme A (CoA), an intermediate required for the incorporation of arachidonic acid into phospholipids. In addition, the accumulation of AMP (due to impaired ATP regeneration under ischemic conditions) will also block the enzymatic process involved in the formation of arachidonyl CoA. Enhanced degradation of phospholipids has to be considered as well (Fig. 5). In this case, a direct relationship between ATP depletion and arachidonic acid release is less evident, since phospholipases are ATP-independent enzymes. The activity of the latter enzymes may be enhanced in the ischemic myocardium by increased intracellular Ca^{2+} levels due to disturbances in ion exchange across cell membranes as a consequence of increased intracellular H^+ concentrations (Fig. 6), impaired ATP-dependent Ca^{2+}-pump activity, reduced binding of Ca^{2+} to membrane-associated proteins [13], or by better contact between the phospholipid substrates and the enzyme proteins due to morphological changes in the cells affected.

Myocardial NEFA Content During Reperfusion

Upon reperfusion, following total coronary artery occlusion (dog; Fig. 2) [14] or global no-flow ischemia (isolated, working rat hearts; Fig. 4), the NEFA content further increases. In the rat experiments, the NEFA levels at the end of 30-min reperfusion following 60 min of ischemia are significantly higher than in hearts freeze-clamped after a period of 90 min of ischemia. Reperfusion after 30 and 45 min of ischemia results in a slight, but significant elevation of tissue NEFA. These findings indicate that reperfusion by itself accelerates hydrolysis of endogenous lipid pools. Concomitantly, a small, but significant increase in myocardial lysophospholipid content can be observed. The less-pronounced quantitative increase in lysophospholipids than in NEFA can possibly be explained by hydrolysis of lysophospholipids by lysophospholipases. The NEFAs accumulating in the reperfused myocardium represent only a small fraction of the fatty

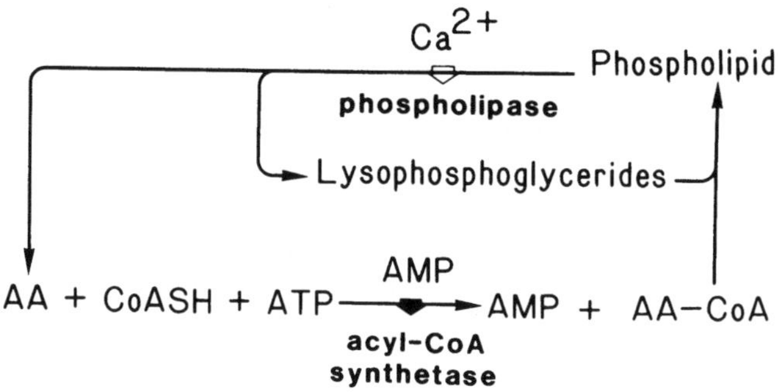

Fig. 5. Schematic representation of phospholipid turnover. In this case arachidonic acid (*AA*) is taken as an example

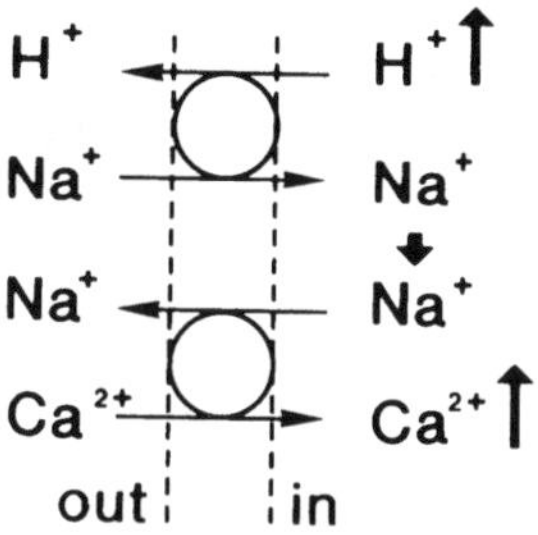

Fig. 6. Schematic representation of the ion-exchange across the cellular membrane in the case of an increased intracellular H^+-ion concentration, as during myocardial ischemia. This increase in H^+ results in an enhanced exchange of this ion with Na^+, leading to elevated Na^+ levels in the myocyte. As a consequence, Ca^{2+} will enter the cell via exchange with Na^+

acids incorporated in the phospholipids. This explains the observation that the total phospholipid content in the tissue does not significantly change during myocardial ischemia [2, 15]. The assay techniques currently available and the intercardiac variations in tissue content of phospholipids do not allow us to detect reliably a decrease in phospholipid content in the order of a few percent.

NEFA Accumulation, Myocardial Function, and Cell Membrane Integrity

Since NEFAs uncouple mitochondrial ATP production from respiratory chain activity [8] and depress Na^+/K^+-ATPase activity [9], a relationship between accumulation of NEFA, myocardial function, and irreversible cell injury has been considered. Moreover, the time-course of NEFA accumulation parallels the time-sequence of loss of essential cellular functions in the absence of oxygen [11]. Experiments on isolated, working rat hearts have shown that recovery of function is adequate after 30 and 45 min of no-flow global ischemia, periods after which the increases in NEFA content are only minor. However, functional recovery is significantly depressed when the ischemic period is extended to 60 min. In hearts freeze-clamped after 60 min of oxygen deprivation, the myocardial NEFA content has been found to be significantly increased [16]. These findings indicate that there is a relation between NEFA accumulation and depression of myocardial function. When these data are regarded on an individual basis, however, after 60 min of ischemia a 75% recovery of stroke volume can be associated with an NEFA content ranging from 1000 to 6000 nmol.g^{-1} dry weight, suggesting that the relation between NEFA accumulation and myocardial function disturbances is not unambiguous. Besides, ventricular fibrillation can be observed at NEFA contents varying between 800 and 8000 nmol.g^{-1} dry weight.

The amount of lactate dehydrogenase (LDH) released from isolated, working rat hearts during 30-min reperfusion, following various periods of no-flow, global ischemia, significantly correlates ($r = 0.79$) with the amount of NEFA accumulated at the end of the reperfusion period (Van Bilsen et al., unpublished results). The amount of LDH released indicates that only about 7% of the cardiac tissue has become irreversibly damaged.

Consequences of Arachidonic Acid Accumulation During Myocardial Ischemia and/or Reperfusion for Eicosanoid Synthesis

Since free arachidonic acid is the common precursor for the formation of leukotrienes, via the lipoxygenase pathway, and prostaglandins, thromboxanes, and prostacyclin, via the cyclooxygenase pathway, one may expect the increase in myocardial free arachidonic acid content during ischemia to lead to the production of eicosanoids. In open-chest dog experiments, in which we studied the arachidonic acid cascade after 2 h of regional low-flow ischemia with and without 2 h of reperfusion, however, the increase in myocardial free arachidonic acid content was not followed by the formation of eicosanoids. Even after 2 h of regional myocardial ischemia, as induced by total coronary artery occlusion, followed by 1 h of reperfusion, when a relatively high tissue content of free arachidonic acid is found (169–431 nmol.g^{-1} dry weight corresponding with 28–67 nmol.g^{-1} wet weight), no eicosanoids can be detected in the jeopardized canine myocardium. Similarly, these products are not released into the local venous blood during the reperfusion period. On the contrary, in Tyrode's solution-perfused, isolated working rat hearts 6-keto PGF 1α, the breakdown product of prostacyclin, is released during reperfusion following a period of 60 min of global no-flow ischemia [15]. The cumulative amount of 6-keto PGF 1α during 30 min of reperfusion, however, is only a fraction (less than 0.5%) of the free arachidonic acid accumulated.

Conclusions

The NEFA content is low in the normoxic myocardium (about 25 nmol.g^{-1} wet weight), but it increases significantly during myocardial ischemia. The NEFA content further increases during reperfusion. Although the content of all NEFAs increases in the dog, the increase in long-chain unsaturated fatty acids, like linoleic acid and arachidonic acid, is relatively most pronouced. These accumulating NEFAs probably originate from phospholipids, major constituents of cell membranes. In low-flow regional myocardial ischemia, the accumulation of nonesterified (free) arachidonic acid is very pronounced in areas with a blood flow lower than 0.1 $ml.min^{-1}.g^{-1}$ and when ATP levels of 4–6 $nmol.g^{-1}$ dry weight are reached. The mechanism responsible for the breakdown of phospholipids during myocardial ischemia is still incompletely understood.

At the present state of knowledge, it is assumed that the accumulation of long-chain unsaturated fatty acids during myocardial ischemia and reperfusion is limited to irreversibly damaged cells. This conclusion is based upon the finding that: (a) the increase in NEFAs represents the breakdown of only a few percent of the phospholipids present in cell membranes, while the amount of LDH released during reperfusion indicates that only 7% of the cardiac cells are irreversiby damaged; (b) there is no unambiguous relation between NEFA accumulation and depression of myocardial function, suggesting that the NEFAs, present in toxic concentrations, do not have access to the contractile machinery of surviving cells; and (c) only very limited amounts of eicosanoids (less than 0.5% of the available arachidonic acid) are produced, indicating that the majority of the substrate arachidonic acid cannot come in contact with enzymes, like lipoxygenase and cyclooxygenase, which are mainly located in endothelial cells. It is possible that the formation of blebs and multilamellar structures, as locally found in membranes during myocardial ischemia and reperfusion [17], is closely related to the accumulation of NEFAs during oxygen deprivation. In particular, Wetzel and Scow [18] recently showed that blebs and lamellar structures are associated with focal sites of lipid hydrolysis.

Acknowledgments. The authors are indebted to Jos Heemskerk and Karin Van Brussel for their help in preparing the manuscript and to Theo Van der Nagel for drawing the figures. This work was supported by grant Nr. 900-516-91 from Medigon/ZWO.

References

1. Opie LH, Owen P, Riemersma RA (1973) Relative rates of oxidation of glucose and free fatty acids by ischaemic and non-ischaemic myocardium after coronary artery ligation in the dog. Eur J Clin Invest 3: 419–435
2. Van der Vusse GJ, Roemen THM, Prinzen FW, Coumans WA, Reneman RS (1982) Uptake and tissue content of fatty acids in dog myocardium under normoxic and ischemic conditions. Circ Res 50: 538–546
3. Van der Vusse GJ, Reneman RS (1984) The myocardial non-esterified fatty acid controversy. J Mol Cell Cardiol 16: 677–682
4. Van der Vusse GJ, Roemen THM, Reneman RS (1985) The content of nonesterified fatty acids in rat myocardial tissue. A comparison between the Dole and Folch extraction procedures. J Mol Cell Cardiol 17: 527–531
5. Weishaar R, Sarma JSM, Maruyama Y, Fischer R, Bing RJ (1977) Regional blood flow, contractility and metabolism in early myocardial infarction. Cardiology 62: 2–20
6. Prinzen FW, Van der Vusse GJ, Arts T, Roemen THM, Coumans WA, Reneman

RS (1984) Accumulation of nonesterified fatty acids in ischemic canine myocardium. Am J Physiol 247: H264-H272
7. Chien KR, Han A, Sen A, Buja LM, Willerson JT (1984) Accumulation of unesterified arachidonic acid in ischemic canine myocardium. Circ Res 54: 313–322
8. Borst P, Loos JA, Christ EJ, Slater EC (1962) Uncoupling activity of long-chain fatty acids. Biochim Biophys Acta 62: 509–518
9. Lamers JMJ, Hulsmann WC (1977) Inhibition of ($Na^+ + K^+$)-stimulated ATPase of heart by fatty acids. J Mol Cell Cardiol 9: 343–346
10. Reneman RS, Prinzen FW, Engels E, Van Bilsen M, Van der Vusse GJ (1987) Arachidonic acid metabolism during myocardial ischemia. Progr Appl Microcirc 12: 152–169
11. Jennings RB, Hawkins JE, Lowe JE, Hill ML, Klotman S, Reimer KA (1978) Relation between high energy phosphate and lethal injury in myocardial ischemia in the dog. Am J Path 92: 187–215
12. Chien KR, Sen A, Reynolds R, Chang A, Kim C, Gunn MD, Buja LM, Willerson JT (1985) Release of arachidonate from membrane phospholipids in cultured neonatal rat myocardial cells during adenosine triphosphate depletion. J Clin Invest 75: 1770–1780
13. Borgers M, Thone F, Xhonneux R, Flameng W (1982) Shifts of calcium in the ischemic myocardium. A structural analysis. In: Wauquier A, et al. (eds) Protection of tissues against hypoxia, Elsevier, Amsterdam, pp 365–375
14. Van der Vusse GJ, Prinzen FW, Reneman RS (1987) Disturbances in myocardial lipid homeostasis during ischemia and reperfusion. In: Sideman S, Beyar R (eds) Activation, metabolism and perfusion of the heart, Nijhoff, Dordrecht, pp 665–682
15. Van Bilsen M, Engels W, Willemsen PHM, Coumans WA, Van der Vusse GJ, Reneman RS (1987) Arachidonic acid accumulation and eicosanoid synthesis during ischemia and reperfusion in isolated rat hearts. Progr Appl Microcirc 12: 236–243
16. Van der Vusse GJ, Van Bilsen M, Reneman RS (in press) Impairment of lipid metabolism in ischemic and reperfused myocardial tissue. In: Sideman S (ed) Analysis and simulation of mechanics, perfusion and electrical performance in ischemic heart disease, CRC Press, Boca Raton
17. Post JA, Leunissen-Bijvelt J, Ruigrok TJC, Verkleij AJ (1985) Ultrastructural changes of sarcolemma and mitochondria in the isolated rabbit heart during ischemia and reperfusion. Biochim Biophys Acta 845: 119–123
18. Wetzel MG, Scow RO (1984) Lipolysis and fatty acid transport in rat heart: electron microscopic study. Am J Physiol 246: C467–C485

Hemodynamic Factors Influencing Regional Ischemia and Infarction of the Myocardium: Difference Between Right and Left Ventricular Myocardial Infarction

Hitonobu Tomoike and Motoomi Nakamura[1]

Introduction

The limitations of myocardial infarct size have been studied both experimentally and clinically [1, 2]. Infarct size depends on the size of the area at risk or the extent of perfusion in the occluded vessel [3, 4]. The infarcted area inside the risk area is modified by collateral blood flow [5, 6], timing of reperfusion [7], and hemodynamic factors which determine the level of myocardial oxygen consumption [8, 9]. Myocardial perfusion through the preexisting collateral channels is often inadequate to the extent that myocardial necrosis is virtually a foregone conclusion [2]. Thus, myocardial necrosis begins approximately 20 min after coronary occlusion and spreads as a "wavefront" from the endocardium to epicardium with increasing duration of ischemia [10]. These concepts were derived from studies on the occlusion of a branch of the left coronary artery in a canine model. The potential applicability of these concepts in the right ventricle was not received full approval.

The pathophysiology of differences in myocardial infarction between the right and left ventricles is not well understood. We have investigated possible topological differences in the development of myocardial necrosis through different transmural layers between the right and left ventricles with reference to the risk areas and regional myocardial blood flow [11].

Distribution of Myocardial Necrosis Inside Area at Risk

Sodium pentobarbital was given intravenously to 51 adult mongrel dogs, and the dogs were ventilated with room air and oxygen as required. A polyvinyl catheter was placed at the ascending aorta through the carotid artery to monitor aortic pressure and for blood sampling. The chest was opened at the left fourth intercostal space and the heart was suspended in a pericardial cradle. The large obtuse marginal branch of the left circumflex coronary artery and the main trunk of the right coronary artery 2–3 cm distal to its orifice were dissected. These

[1] Research Institute of Angiocardiology and Cardiovascular Clinic, Faculty of Medicine, Kyushu University, 1-1, Maidashi 3-chome, Higashi-ku, Fukuoka, 812 Japan

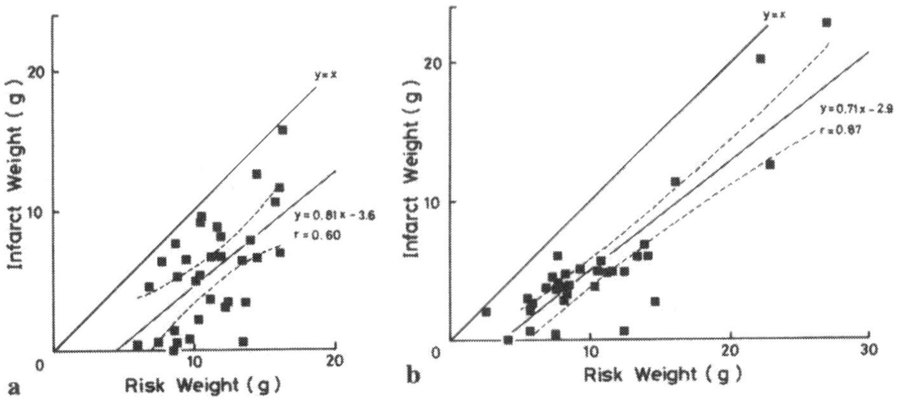

Fig. 1a, b. Relationship between weight of infarcted and risk areas. **a** Right ventricle; **b** left ventricle. The *line* $y = x$ is the line of identity, and the other *line* is the regression line. The standard error of estimate is shown by *broken lines*. Two coronary arteries (obtuse marginal branch and right coronary artery) were ligated at a fairly constant anatomical site. Reproduced from Ohzono et al. [11] with permission

arteries were selected for obstruction because their perfusion areas are remote. The chest was then closed for 24 h. Infarct and risk areas were determined at 24 h of coronary ligation by triphenyl tetrazolium chloride (TTC) staining and postmortem coronary angiograms, respectively.

Of the 51 dogs, 18 died from ventricular fibrillation, three within 5 min, seven between 30 min and 3 h, and eight between 4 and 24 h after the coronary ligation, and the 33 survivors were used for the analysis. The perfusion size was 11.3 ± 0.5 g and 10.5 ± 0.9 g in the right and left ventricles, respectively. The proportion of infarct area to risk area was $47.9\% \pm 5.1\%$ and $46.2\% \pm 3.8\%$ in the right and left ventricles, respectively. Thus, the size of the risk or infarct area was compatible between the right and left ventricles.

There was a linear relationship between the size of the infarct and the risk areas for occlusion of either the right coronary artery or the large obtuse marginal branch of the left circumflex coronary artery (Fig. 1). The infarct area was always located inside the risk area in both the right and left ventricles. Myocardial necrosis in the right ventricle was distributed homogeneously from the subendocardium to the subepicardium. Necrosis was present transmurally in 7 of 33 dogs; in others, there were scattered small islands of necrosis.

The relationship between infarct size and risk area for the subendocardial and subepicardial layers in the right and left ventricles is shown in Fig. 2. In the right ventricle, data from the subepicardial and subendocardial layers were distributed between the x-axis and a line of identity ($y = x$) of an infarct-risk relation. There was no significant difference in variance between these layers. However, in the left ventricle, data from the subendocardial layers were grouped along the line of identity and data from the subepicardial layers were randomly scattered. A marked transmural gradient of infarction was noted in the left ventricle, as previously reported [4], and was negligible in the right ventricle. To elucidate the mechanism of homogeneous and heterogeneous distributions of infarct in

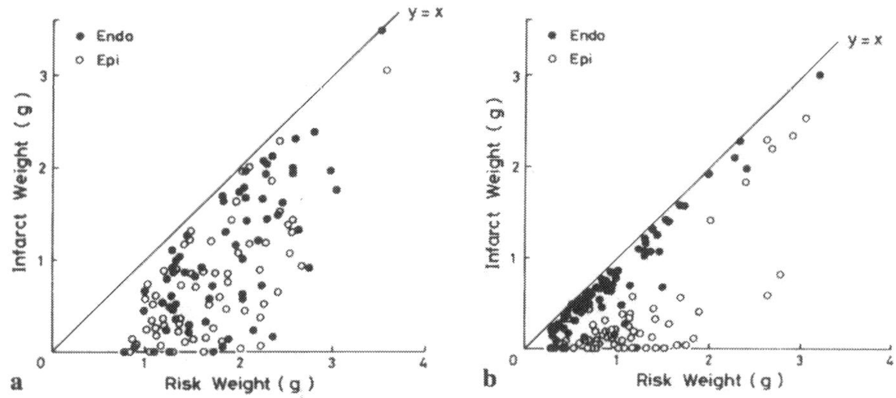

Fig. 2a, b. Relation between weight of infarcted and risk areas at subendocardial (*closed circles*) and subepicardial (*open circles*) layers. **a** Right ventricle; **b** left ventricle. Size of the myocardial infarction was more variable in the right coronary artery occlusion than the obtuse marginal occlusion. Reproduced from Ohzono et al. [11] with permission

the right and left ventricles, respectively, the regional myocardial blood flow was investigated.

Transmural Myocardial Blood Flow and Myocardial Necrosis in Right and Left Ventricles

Regional myocardial blood flow was measured in 11 of the 51 dogs, using tracer microsphere techniques under the following four conditions: control state, 5 min after coronary ligation, 24 h after coronary ligation, and after intravenous administration of dipyridamole (0.5 – 1.0 mg/kg). We used carbonized tracer microspheres, 8–11 μm in diameter, labeled with gamma-emitting nuclides—celium 141, tin 113, scandium 46, strontium 85.

Myocardial samples were obtained from the following regions: (a) normally perfused region—in the left ventricle, the region perfused by the left anterior descending coronary artery, in the right ventricle, the anterior portion of the right ventricular free wall perfused by the left anterior descending coronary artery and/or right coronary artery proximal to the occluded site; (b) inner 5 mm of the risk region from the boundary; (c) outer 5 mm from the boundary of the risk region; and (d) center of the risk region.

Each specimen was subdivided into subendocardial, midwall, and subepicardial layers in the left ventricle and into the subendocardial and subepicardial layers in the right ventricle. Changes in regional myocardial blood flow after dipyridamole were examined at 24 h of coronary occlusion. We noted a marked difference in the amount of incremental flow between the border inside the area of risk and the outer shell just outside the risk area. To minimize further the involvement of the normal tissue, collateral blood flow was defined as the regional blood flow to the center of the risk region [11].

The relation between precentage necrosis of the risk area and transmural col-

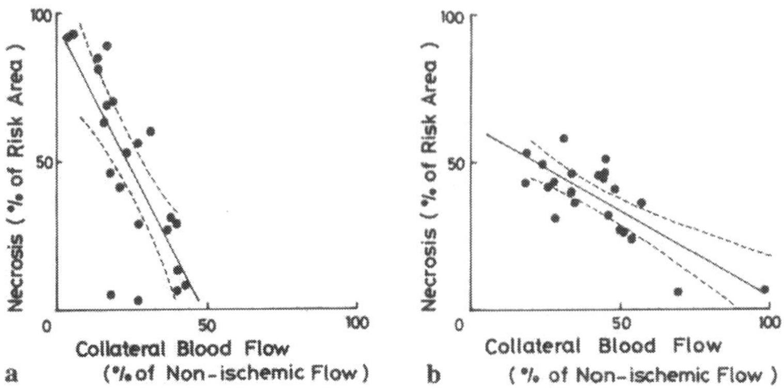

Fig. 3a, b. Relation between percentage necrosis of the risk area and transmural collateral blood flow in percentage of nonischemic flow 24 h after coronary ligation. **a** Right ventricle, $y = -2.1x + 97.8$ ($r = -0.77$). **b** Left ventricle $y = -0.6x + 62.0$ ($r = -0.77$). The standard error of estimate is shown by *broken lines*. Reproduced from Ohzono et al. [11] with permission

lateral blood flow in the percentage of nonischemic flow 24 h after coronary ligation is shown in Fig. 3. The slope of this relationship was steeper in the right than in the left ventricle. The x-axis intercept was lower in the right than in the left ventricle. The correlation coefficients between necrotic area and collateral blood flow remained unchanged between 5 min and 24 h of occlusion in the right ventricle but increased from −0.47 to −0.78 over a period of 24 h in the left ventricle. This observation suggests that a "wavefront" extension of necrotic area inside the risk area was more apparent in the left than in the right ventricle.

The relationship between regional myocardial blood flow in the central risk area 24 h after coronary ligation on the x-axis and the percentage of myocardial necrosis to the risk region on the y-axis in the subendocardial and subepicardial layers is shown in Fig. 4. A slight rightward shift of the relationship was noted in the right ventricle. In the left ventricle, the infarcted area was always larger in the subendocardium than in the subepicardium, along with a markedly reduced slope of this relationship in the subepicardial layer. The transmural gradient of collateral blood flow was evident in the left but not in the right ventricle, as shown in the insets of Fig. 4.

Importance of Hemodynamic Factors in Ischemic Myocardium

Two different types of pump are involved in cardiac output. The left ventricle is a high-pressure chamber and the right is a low-pressure chamber. Inherent differences in the hemodynamics between the right and left ventricles lead to differences in the development of myocardial ischemia and infarction. Comparing the transmural distribution of myocardial necrosis between the right and left ventricles with reference to risk size and collateral flow, we noted several important aspects relating to size of the infarct, as follows.

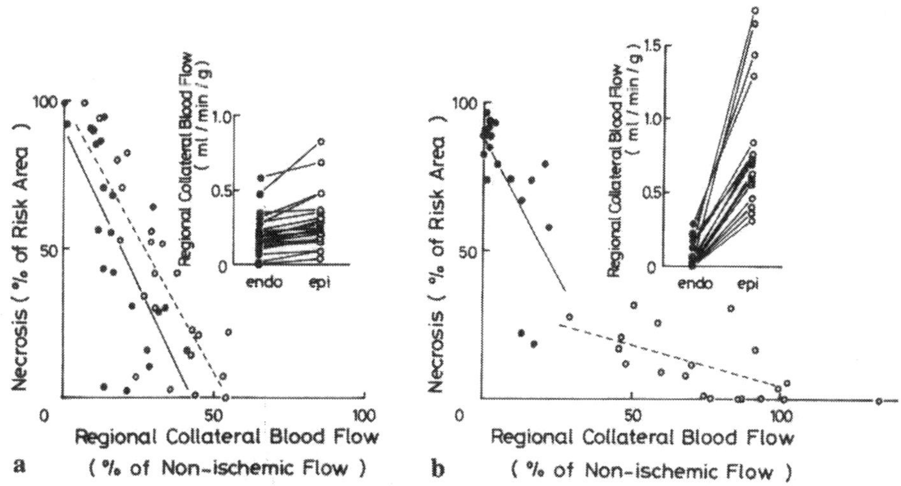

Fig. 4a, b. Relation between collateral blood flow (percentage of control flow at 24 h of coronary ligation) and percent of infarct to risk size in subendocardial (*closed circles*) and subepicardial (open circles) layers in **a** right and **b** left ventricles. Note that the slope of the relationship is steeper for the subendocardium than for the subepicardium in the left but not in the right ventricle. RV subendocardial layer: $y = -2.19x + 93.2$; $r = -0.708$, $n = 20$. RV subepicardial layer: $y = -1.89x + 101.4$; $r = -0.829$, $n = 20$. LV subendocardial layer: $y = -1.92x + 89.4$; $r = -0.668$, $n = 19$. LV subepicardial layer: $y = -0.83x + 32.5$; $r = -0.631$, $n = 19$. *Insets* show regional myocardial blood flow in ml/min/g in the subendocardial (*endo*) and subepicardial (*epi*) layers examined 24 h after coronary ligation. Each *line* in the *insets* represents one slice and shows the transmural distribution of collateral blood flow. Reproduced from Ohzono et al. [11] with permission

Despite similar sizes in risk area and myocardial necrosis between the right and left ventricles, myocardial necrosis was distributed quite homogeneously in the right ventricle and was located subendocardially in the left ventricle. Figure 5 shows a putative mechanism of the difference in the distribution of myocardial necrosis between the right and left ventricles. Transmural distribution of myocardial blood flow depends on the intracavitary pressure and wall thickness, which determine the distribution of myocardial necrosis. For example, subendocardial underperfusion was noted in the case of right ventricular systolic hypertension [12] and right ventricular hypertrophy [13]. Therefore, the greater the similarity in hemodynamic conditions of the right and left ventricles, the greater the necrosis in the subendocardial region of the right ventricle.

The myocardial blood flow required to maintain tissue integrity was 50% of normal flow in the right ventricle, however a small reduction of flow resulted in myocardial necrosis at the subendocardial region in the left ventricle. The lower level of critical coronary flow in the right ventricle may be explained by: (a) a lower level of critical perfusion pressure in the right coronary artery in determining the regional myocardial function [14]; (b) a thinner wall and lower intracavitary pressure in the right ventricle; and (c) a lower level of oxygen consumption [15]. While these are inherent characteristics of the right ventricle, the evidence can be validly extrapolated when attempting to determine the fate of a myocar-

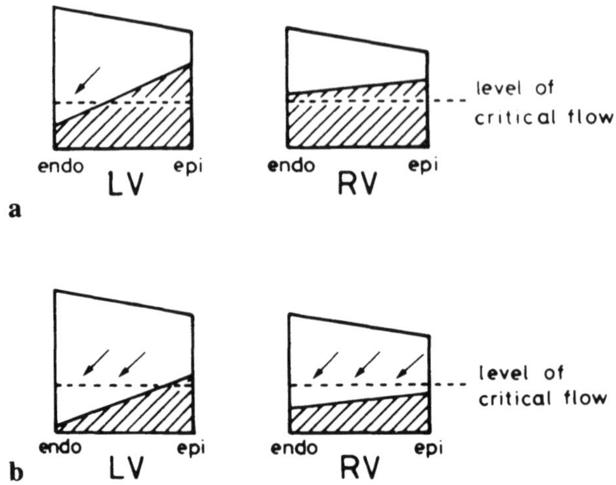

Fig. 5. a Moderate levels of collateral flow and **b** severely reduced level of collateral blood flow. The *broken line* represents the level below which myocardial necrosis appears. In the left ventricle, subendocardial ischemia results in myocardial necrosis largely to the subendocardial zone, however, myocardial necrosis in the right ventricular free wall is distributed homogeneously across the wall

dium which has become ischemic.

A "wavefront" extension of ischemia was evident in the left but not in the right ventricle. This "wavefront" phenomenon is considered to be a tissue-sparing mechanism, i.e., sacrificing the injured myocardium to maintain a viable myocardium in full performance, especially in the left ventricle.

In summary, the extent of the myocardial necrosis after cessation of the forward coronary blood flow can be predicted in terms of collateral blood flow, risk size, and hemodynamics, including wall thickness and intracavitary pressure. In addition to these physical terms, the production of free radicals and lipoxygenase products around the injured myocardium are contributed factors. Alterations in platelet function and coagulability are also responsible for microcirculatory disorders. These parameters are no doubt greatly modified by hemodynamics and the relationship between hemodynamics and the above-mentioned events need to be considered.

Acknowledgments. We are grateful to M. Ohara (Kyushu University) for comments on the manuscript. This work was supported by Scientific Research Grants (60304061, 62570396, 61870037) from the Ministry of Education, Science and Culture, Japan.

References

1. Kloner RA, Braunwald E (1980) Observations on experimental myocardial ischemia. Cardiovasc Res 14: 371–395
2. Becker LC, Ambrosio G (1987) Myocardial consequences of reperfusion. Prog Cardiovasc Disease 30: 23–44

3. Schaper W, Remijsen P, Zhonneux R (1969) The size of myocardial infarction after experimental coronary artery ligation. Z Kreislaufforsch 58: 904–909
4. Sakai K, Tomoike H, Ootsubo H, Kikuchi Y, Nakamura M (1982) Preocclusive perfusion area as a determinant of infarct size in a canine model. Cardiovasc Res 16: 408–416
5. Geary GG, Smith GT, McNamara JJ (1981) Defining the anatomic perfusion bed of an occluded coronary artery and the region at risk to infarction. A comparative study in the baboon, pig and dog. Am J Cardiol 47: 1240–1247
6. Maruoka Y, Tomoike H, Kawachi Y, Noguchi K, Nakamura M (1986) Relations between collateral flow and tissue salvage in the risk area after acute coronary occlusion in dogs; a topological analysis. Br J Exp Pathol 67: 33–42
7. Koren G, Weiss AT, Hasin Y, Appelbaum D, Welber S, Rozenman Y, Lotan C, Mosseri M, Sapoznikov D, Luria MH, Gotsman MS (1985) Prevention of myocardial damage in acute myocardial ischemia by early treatment with intravenous streptokinase. N Engl J Med 313: 1384–1389
8. Shell WE, Sobel BE. (1973) Deleterious effects of increased heart rate on infarct size in the conscious dog. Am J Cardiol 31: 474–479
9. Nienaber CH, Gottwick M, Winkler B, Schaper W (1983) The relationship between the perfusion deficit, infarct size and time after experimental coronary artery occlusion. Basic Res Cardiol 78: 210–226
10. Reimer KA, Lowe JE, Rasmussen MM, Jennings RB (1977) The wavefront phenomenon of ischemic cell death: I. Myocardial infarct size vs. duration of coronary occlusion in dogs. Circulation 56: 786–794
11. Ohzono K, Koyanagi S, Urabe Y, Harasawa Y, Tomoike H, Nakamura M (1986) Transmural distribution of myocardial infarction: Difference between the right and left ventricles in a canine model. Circ Res 59: 63–73
12. Fixler DE, Archie JP, Ullyot DJ, Buckberg GD, Hoffman JIE (1973) Effects of acute right ventricular systolic hypertension on regional myocardial blood flow in anesthetized dogs. Am Heart J 85: 491–500
13. Murray PA, Vatner SF. (1980) Fractional contribution of the right and left coronary arteries to perfusion of normal and hypertrophied right ventricle of conscious dogs. Circ Res 47: 190–200
14. Urabe Y, Tomoike H, Ohzono K, Koyanagi S, Nakamura M. (1985) Role of afterload in determining regional right ventricular performance during coronary underperfusion in dogs. Circ Res 57: 96–104
15. Kusachi S, Nishiyama O, Yasuhara K, Saito D, Haraoka S, Nagashima H (1982) Right and left ventricular oxygen metabolism in open-chest dogs. Am J Physiol 234: H761–H766

Chronic Changes in the Canine Myocardium After Coronary Microembolization

MASATSUGU HORI, YUKIHIRO KORETSUNE, KUNIMITSU IWAI, KOICHI GOTO, HIROSHI SATO, KATSUOMI IWAKURA, AKIRA KITABATAKE, and TAKENOBU KAMADA[1]

Introduction

Recently, there has been interest in acute microcirculatory abnormalities of the coronary arteries, particularly microembolism, as a primary cause of or secondary outcome of the no-reflow phenomenon following recanalization of occluded coronary arteries [1, 2]. It is reported that interruption of the coronary blood flow for more than 30 min produces an incomplete return of blood flow after reperfusion [1], and the area of no-reflow increases with the duration of ischemia [3]. Recanalization of occluded arteries is often observed in the clinical setting either spontaneously or after coronary thrombolytic therapy (PTCR) in patients with acute myocardial infarction. The heart reperfused after a certain time-lag may have regional impairment of coronary perfusion, presumably at the level of the capillaries or feeding arterioles. Several mechanisms for the no-reflow phenomenon have been suggested. Capillary compression by parenchymal cell swelling [2] or interstitial edema [4], obstruction by endothelial cell swelling [5], thrombosis [6], erythrocyte impaction [7], leukocyte plugging [8], and platelet aggregates [9] have been reported as a cause of the perfusion impedance after reperfusion. Although it has been claimed in several studies that plugging of the blood cells in the microvasculature may not be a primary cause of no-reflow [10, 11], entrapment of blood cells secondary to the microcirculatory disturbance could further impede the flow and delay the recovery of ischemia. Prolonged myocardial stunning often observed following reperfusion might be attributed in part to this microcirculatory abnormality. We have previously demonstrated a characteristic hyperemic flow response of coronary blood flow after coronary embolization of microspheres, which mimic blood cell plugging [12]. In this chapter, we shall discuss the chronic changes in coronary blood flow and functional and histological changes in the embolized myocardium.

Coronary Flow Changes After Microembolization

Acute alterations in the coronary blood flow after embolization of coronary arteries have been reported in several studies. Bing et al. reported that the

[1]The First Department of Medicine, Osaka University School of Medicine, 1–50, Fukushima 1-chome, Fukushima-ku, Osaka, 553 Japan

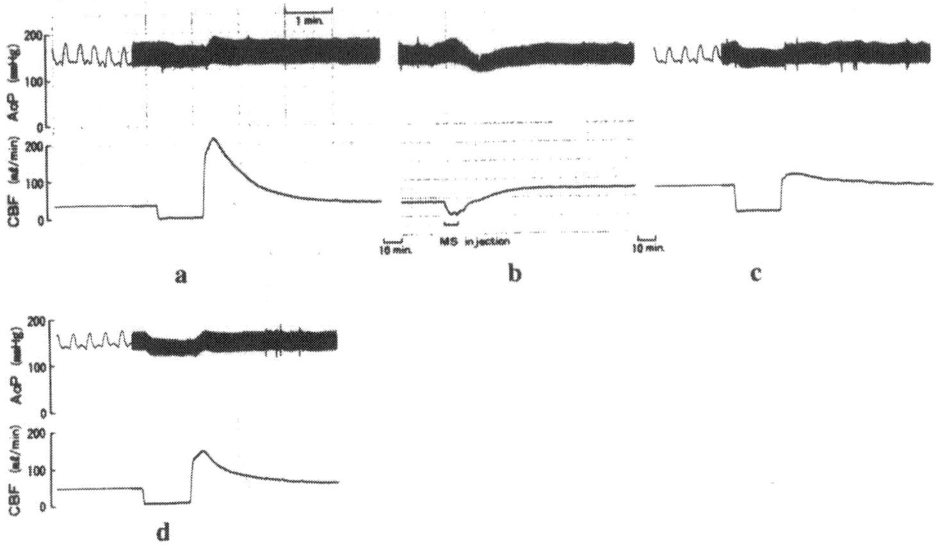

Fig. 1a–d. Representative changes in the resting and reactive hyperemic blood flow in the left circumflex coronary artery after the intracoronary injection of 2.6×10^5/g myocardium of microspheres (15 ± 1 μm in diameter, group I). **a** control; **b** during injection; **c** 10 min after injection; and **d** 2 weeks after injection. *AoP* aortic pressure, *CBF* coronary blood flow, *MS* microsphere. After Hori et al. [15]

coronary vascular resistance decreased following the embolization of plastic spheres suspended in plasma or human albumin, although the coronary flow did not increase because of a marked reduction in blood pressure [13]. They attributed this vasodilation to the neural reflex. The transient increase in coronary blood flow and a decrease in myocardial oxygen uptake after microembolization of canine coronary arteries were also reported by West et al. who attributed the coronary flow change to factors other than the neural reflex since the vasodilation could not be attenuated by the autonomic nerve blockade [14]. Recently, we reported that the hyperemic flow response to coronary microembolization is due to a massive release of adenosine, which dilates the resistance vessels in the nonischemic area surrounding the ischemic foci [12]. It is of interest that the release of adenosine from the ischemic area is sustained for more than several hours and, hence, hyperemic flow is also sustained for a long time. This hyperemic flow had returned to normal 2 weeks after embolization, although the flow reserve was markedly reduced [15]. Figure 1 shows the coronary blood flow in dogs under resting conditions and during the hyperemic response to 1-min occlusion of the coronary artery in controls (before embolization) and 2 weeks after embolization of 15-μm microspheres (2.6×10^5/g.myocardium). The flow reserve is markedly reduced, whereas the resting flow at 2 weeks after embolization is comparable with the control flow. Rapid atrial pacing at the rate of 250/min also provoked myocardial ischemia, as evidenced by the lactate production (Figure. 2). This evidence suggests that the coronary blood flow at rest is well regulated to maintain the oxygen supply to the myocardium even if a micro-

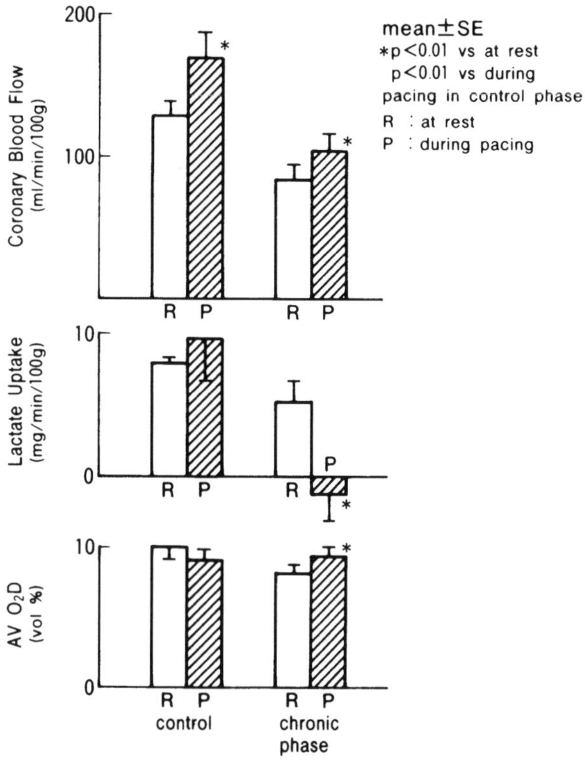

Fig. 2. Coronary blood flow, lactate uptake, and coronary arteriovenous oxygen difference (*AV O_2D*) under resting condtions (*R*) and during rapid atrial pacing (*P*) at 250/min in conscious dogs. Under control conditions (before embolization), pacing stress did not induce ischemia, whereas in chronic phase (2 weeks after embolization of 15-μm microspheres ($5.5 \pm 0.2 \times 10^5$/g myocardium) pacing induced myocardial ischemia, as evidenced by lactate production. After Hori et al. [15]

circulatory abnormality exists. This implies that the chronic microcirculatory abnormality proceeds unnoticed. The electrocardiographic changes also mask the underlying abnormality in the chronic phase. Figure 3 shows electrocardiograms in the standard limb leads and surface mapping 1 h (Fig. 3a) and 2 weeks (Fig. 3b) after microsphere embolization of the left circumflex coronary artery. The QS patterns in leads II, III, and aVF and T-wave inversion observed in the acute phase disappeared in the chronic phase. Since the direct visualization of small coronary arteries in patients is not possible, the detection of the abnormality has to depend on indirect methods, such as the exercise stress test and coronary blood flow measurement during the hyperemic response.

Histological Changes After Microembolization

Sporadic and disseminated myocardial necrosis and/or fibrosis is a characteristic of the histological changes observed in patients with dilated cardiomyopathy.

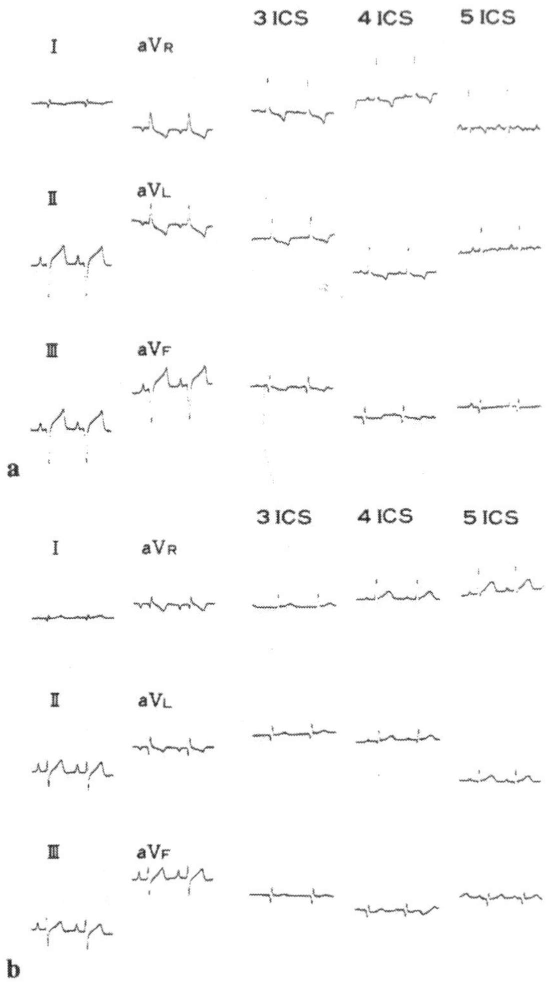

Fig. 3a, b. Representative electrocardiograms obtained **a** 1 h and **b** 2 weeks after embolizaton of 15-μm microspheres (5.4×10^5/g) into the left circumflex artery of the dog. The QS patterns in leads II, III, and aV_F and T-wave inversion in **a** were not seen in **b**, indicating that the transmural ischemia in the acute phase recovered 2 weeks later. *ICS* intercostal space

Coronary embolization with small spheres or emboli mimics the histological changes of this abnormality. Munro et al. embolized styrene divinyl-benzene spheres, 150–600 μm in diameter, in the canine coronary arteries and observed the multiple infarct areas scattered diffusely throughout the myocardium [16]. Smaller microspheres (50 ± 10 μm) also produce smaller infarcts or focal areas of granulation on scar tissue with intercellular edema surrounding the microspheres [17]. Recently, Eng et al. reported that the microinfarct produced by microsphere embolization with 25-μm microspheres could be prevented by prazosin, and without pharmacological intervention they observed infarcts of about

200 × 500 μm in size [18]. In embolization with 15-μm microspheres, however, myocardial necrosis does not occur [15], although the microspheres induce prolonged ischemia as previously described.

One hour after embolization of 15-μm microspheres, microscopic examination demonstrated patchy regions composed of 10–30 myocytes in cross section, which showed a marked intracellular edema. Interstitial edema was also remarkable with dilated capillaries. Electron microscopically, severe intracellular edema and a decrease in glycogen granules were also evident. Five hours after embolization, these changes showed an increase (Fig. 4). However, irreversible changes such as membrane destruction and amorphous dense bodies in the mitochondria were not observed. One day later, demarkation between affected myocytes and intact cells was diffuse and glycogen granules were markedly increased, indicating a decline in ischemic changes. A week later, microscopic inpection showed the absence of necrosis except for a few myocytolytic lesions accompanying the microsphere aggregates (Fig. 5). At this stage, degenerative changes in the mitochondria were prominent, i.e., an increase in the number of small mitochondria or fused mitochondria and sporadically observed giant mitochondria. The rough endoplasmic reticulum was also often observed. These histological changes indicate that the myocardial ischemia elicited by embolization of 15-μm microspheres is sustained but reversible. Whatever the mechanism of the reversibility of ischemia, our results strongly suggest that the blood cell plugging following reperfusion may induce prolonged but reversible myocardial ischemia and, hence, cause the delay of recovery of ischemia after reperfusion.

Cardiac Function After Microembolization

Chronic heart failure in animals is difficult to produce by coronary artery occlusion. Microsphere embolization of the coronary arteries has been done by several investigators to make an animal model of chronic heart failure [17, 19]. Munro et al. observed reduced exercise tolerance in the chronic phase after coronary embolization of relatively large spheres (150–600 μm in diameter [16]. However, the cardiac function in the chronic stage after embolization has not been extensively studied. Smiseth et al. studied the resting hemodynamic and cardiac response to isoproterenol infusion 2 and 4 weeks after coronary embolization of 50 ± 10-μm microspheres [17]. They found moderately elevated left ventricular end-diastolic pressure (LVEDP) in the chronic phase but failed to observe other signs of left ventricular dysfunction. We also observed the recovery of contractile function 1 week after embolization of 15-μm microspheres. Figure 6 depicts the serial changes in left ventriculograms after embolization of 15-μm microspheres into the left main coronary artery. Immediately after embolization, cardiac function was markedly depressed and, thus, left ventricular end-systolic and end-diastolic volumes were increased. Depressed function was still observed 24 h after embolization. One week later, however contractile function of the ventricle returned to normal. However, the time constant (T) of the left ventricular pressure fall during isovolumic relaxation was still prolonged. This impairment of ventricular relaxation was prominent when the afterload was increased by

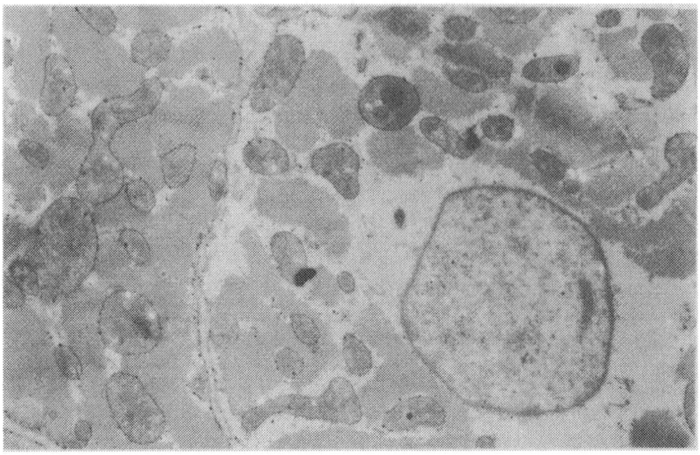

Fig. 4. Electron-microscopic view of the myocardium 5 h after embolization. A marked intracellular edema is observed

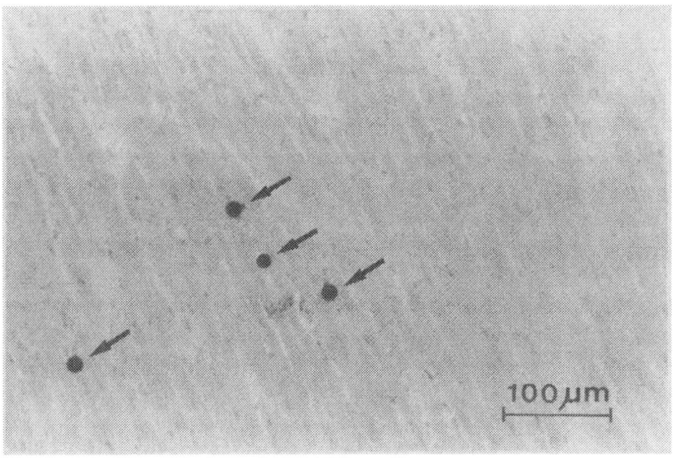

Fig. 5. Microscopic view of the myocardium 24 h after embolization. No necrosis is observed. *Arrows* show the microspheres. H and E

methoxamine infusion. These results indicate that the ventricular relaxation was still impaired when the systolic function (LV dp/dt max) was restored. At this moment, however, it is of interest that the inotropic response to isoproterenol was not significantly impaired, as observed by Smiseth et al. [17] (Fig. 7).

By the radioligand assay of beta-adrenergic receptors of the heart, we found that beta-adrenergic receptors were significantly increased 1 week after embolization (Fig. 8). Therefore, the apparently normal response to isoproterenol may be attributed to the compensatory increase in beta-adrenergic receptor density in this animal model.

The up-regulation of beta-adrenergic receptors has not been observed after

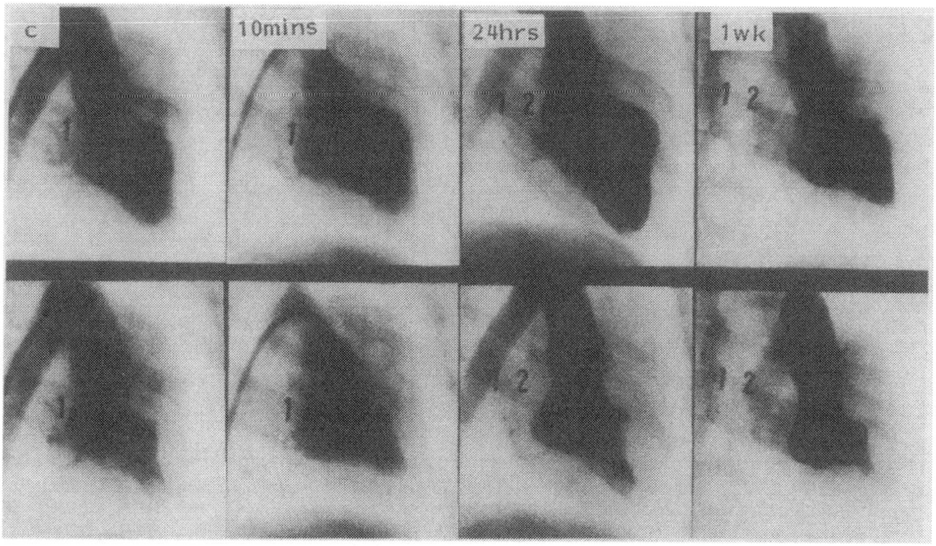

a

b

Fig. 6a, b. Left ventriculograms obtained serially from a dog after the coronary embolization of 15-μm microspheres. **a** Left ventricular end-diastolic volumes; **b** left ventricular end-systolic volumes

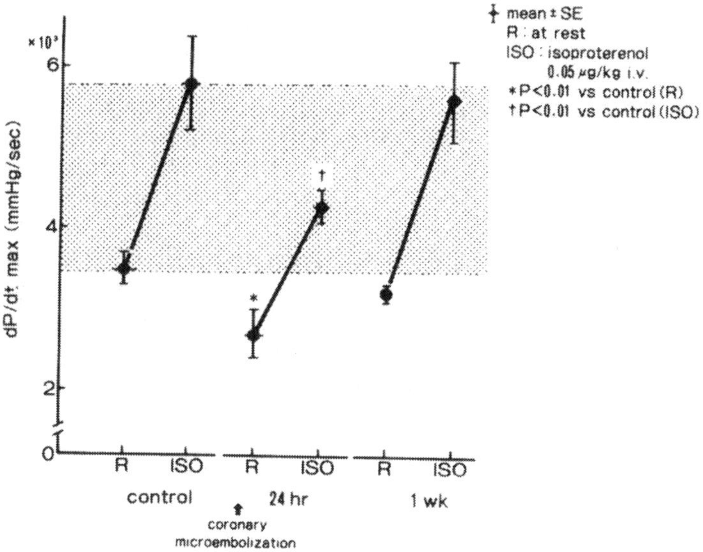

Fig. 7. Inotropic response (LV dp/dt max) to isoproterenol injection (0.05 μm/kg) in dogs before (*control*) and 24 h and 1 week after microembolization of the left main coronary artery. The response almost recovered to normal 1 week after embolization

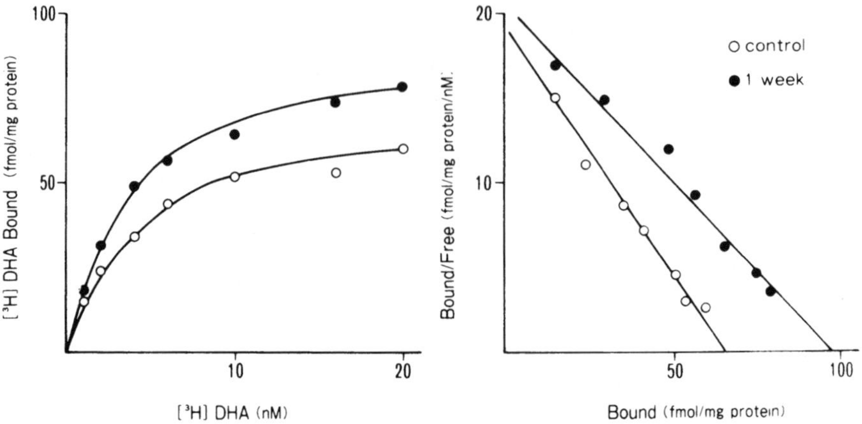

Fig. 8. Saturation curve and Scatchard plots for [^{3}H] dihydroalprenolol (*DHA*) binding to beta-adrenoceptors of embolized canine myocardium. Beta-adrenoceptor density was increased 1 week after embolization

brief ischemia, whereas myocardial ischemia sustained for more than 1 h results in an increase in the beta-adrenoceptor density, which facilitates the intracellular signal transduction [20]. In contrast, a recent study failed to observe the increase in beta-adrenoceptors in experimental myocardial infarction [21]. Our model is different from theirs since the necrotic lesions were very few in our model of microembolization. Although the mechanism by which the beta-adrenoceptors were up-regulated in the previously ischemic myocardium is unknown, the increased beta-adrenoceptors may play an important role in compensation of the contractile function in the damaged myocardium by prolonged ischemia.

Conclusion

Myocardial ischemia produced by the coronary microembolization of 15-μm microspheres is characteristic for its reversibility after prolonged ischemia. The myocardial ischemia was sustained for about 24 h after embolization and it recovers without the occurrence of myocardial necrosis. Cardiac function was markedly depressed at 24 h after embolization, but several days later systolic function recovered, associated with an increase in beta-adrenoceptors. At this time, however, the ventricular relaxation was still impaired, indicating that the subcellular abnormalities still remained. The alterations in the ultrastructure may be compatible with the postischemic dysfunction.

References

1. Krug A, De Rochemont WM, Krob G (1966) Blood supply of the myocardium after temporary coronary occlusion. Circ Res 19: 57
2. Kloner RA, Ganote CE, Jennings RB (1974) The "no-reflow" phenomenon after

temporary coronary occlusion in the dog. J Clin Invest 54: 1496
3. Darsee JR, Kloner RA (1980) The no reflow phenomenon: A time limited factor for reperfusion after coronary occlusion? Am J Cardiol 46: 800
4. Reimer KA, Jennings RB (1979) The changing anatomic reference base of evolving myocardial infarction. Underestimation of myocardial collateral blood flow and overestimation of experimental anatomic infarct size due to tissue edema, hemorrhage and acute inflammation. Circulation 60: 866
5. Armiger LC, Gavin JB (1975) Changes in the microvasculature of ischemic and infarcted myocardium. Lab Invest 33: 51
6. Ruegsegger P, Nydick I, Abarquez F, Cliffton EF, LaDue JS (1960) Effect of fibrinolytic (plasmin) therapy on the physiopathology of myocardial infarction. Am J Cardiol 6: 519
7. Gavin JB, Nevalainen TJ, Seelye RN, Webster V, Thomson RW (1978) An association between the onset of rigor and loss of vascular competence in early myocardial infarcts. Pathology 10: 219
8. Engler RL, Schmid-Schoebein GW, Pavelec RS (1983) Leukocyte capillary plugging in myocardial ischemia and reperfusion in the dog. Am J Pathol 111: 98
9. Schneider MD (1980) Role of the blood platelet in the pathogenesis and complications of experimental myocardial ischemia. Am J Vet Res 45: 451
10. Nevalainen TJ, Gavin JB, Seelye RN, Whitehouse S, Donnell M (1978) The effect of rigor mortis on the passage of erythrocytes and fluid through the myocardium of the isolated dog hearts. Pathology 10: 227
11. Humphrey SM, Gavin JB, Herdson PB (1980) The relationship of ischemic contracture to vascular reperfusion in the isolated rat heart. J Moll Cell Cardiol 12: 1397
12. Hori M, Inoue M, Kitakaze M, Koretsune Y, Iwai K, Tamai J, Ito H, Kitabatake A, Sato T, Kamada T (1986) Role of adenosine in hyperemic response of coronary blood flow in microembolization. Am J Physiol 250: H509-H518
13. Bing RJA, Castellanos E, Grandel C, Luptun C, Siegel A (1956) Experimental myocardial infarction: circulatory, biochemical and pathologic changes. Am J Med Sci 232: 533
14. West JW, Kobayashi T, Anderson FS (1972) Effect of coronary embolization on coronary blood flow and coronary sinus venous blood oxygen saturation in dogs. Circ Res 10: 722
15. Hori M, Koretsune Y, Iwai K, Kitakaze M, Tamai J, Kitabatake A, Inoue M, Kamada T (1987) A possible model of the anginal syndrome with normal coronary arteriograms: Microembolization of canine coronary arteries. Heart Vessels 3: 7
16. Munro G, Balchum OJ, Owens JC, Swan H (1956) Experimental chronic myocardial insufficiency produced by coronary embolization. Surg Forum 6: 204
17. Smiseth OA, Lindal S, Mjos OD, Vik-mo H, Jorgensen L (1983) Progression of myocardial damage following coronary microembolization in dogs. Acta Path Microbiol Immunol Scand Sect A 91: 115
18. Eng C, Cho S, Factor SM, Sonnenblick EH, Kirk ES (1984) Myocardial macronecrosis produced by microsphere embolization: Role of an alpha-adrenergic tonic influence on the coronary microcirculation. Circ Res 54: 74
19. Weber KT, Malinin TI, Dennison BH, Faqua JM, Speaker DM, Hastings FW (1972) Experimental myocardial ischemia and infarction: Production of diffuse myocardial lesions in unanesthetized calves. Am J Cardiol 29: 793
20. Mukherjee A, Bush LR, McCoy KE, Duke RJ, Hagler H, Maxilian Buya L, Willerson JT (1982) Relationship between beta-adrenergic receptor numbers and physioligical responses during experimental canine myocardial ischemia. Circ Res 50: 735
21. Karliner JS, Stevens M, Grattan M, Woloszyn W, Honbo N, Hoffman JIE (1986) Beta-adrenergic receptor properties of canine myocardium: Effect of chronic myocardial infarction. J Am Coll Cardiol 8: 349

Stenosis of Intramyocardial Small Arteries in Hearts with Hypertrophic Cardiomyopathy and Hypertensive Hearts

Hisayoshi Fujiwara, Masaru Tanaka, Tomoya Onodera, Der-Jinn Wu, Mitsuo Matsuda, Yoshihiro Hamashima, and Chuichi Kawai[1]

Introduction

Chest pain is a common symptom of patients with hypertrophic cardiomyopathy (HCM), despite angiographically normal epicardial coronary arteries [1]. Moreover, these patients often demonstrate abnormal myocardial thallium-201 imaging [2] or abnormal lactate metabolism during pacing [3]. Pathologically, these hearts show a greater amount of fibrosis, which is distributed predominantly in the subendocardium rather than in the subepicardium [4].

Intramyocardial small-artery (IMSA) disease has been considered a possible mechanism for myocardial ischemia in HCM and hypertensive heart disease [5]. However, in these studies, stenosis of the IMSA was analyzed only qualitatively. The present study was thus undertaken to evaluate quantitatively stenosis of the IMSA in hearts with HCM [6].

Materials and Methods

Thirty-four autopsied hearts were studied: ten from patients with typical HCM, four from patients with HCM showing features mimicking dilated cardiomyopathy (DCM) in the late stage (DCM-like HCM), ten from hypertensive patients, and ten from normal adults (Table 1). There were no significant differences in age or sex among the four groups, nor in heart weight among the cases of HCM, DCM-like HCM, and hypertensive heart disease. DCM-like HCM was defined as HCM with features mimicking dilated cardiomyopathy in the late stage [7, 8].

The hearts were fixed in 10% formalin and cut transversely from the base to the apex serially at 1-cm intervals. In the hearts with HCM, the slice showing maximal septal hypertrophy was used. In the normal and hypertensive hearts, a slice from the middle third of the heart was used. Each slice was divided into six to eight blocks, which were sectioned at a thickness of 4 μm. These sections were stained with elastica-van Gieson, Masson's trichrome, and hematoxylin-eosin.

---

[1]The Third Division, Department of Internal Medicine and Pathology, Kyoto University, Kawaramachi, Shogoin, Sakyo-ku, Kyoto, 606 Japan

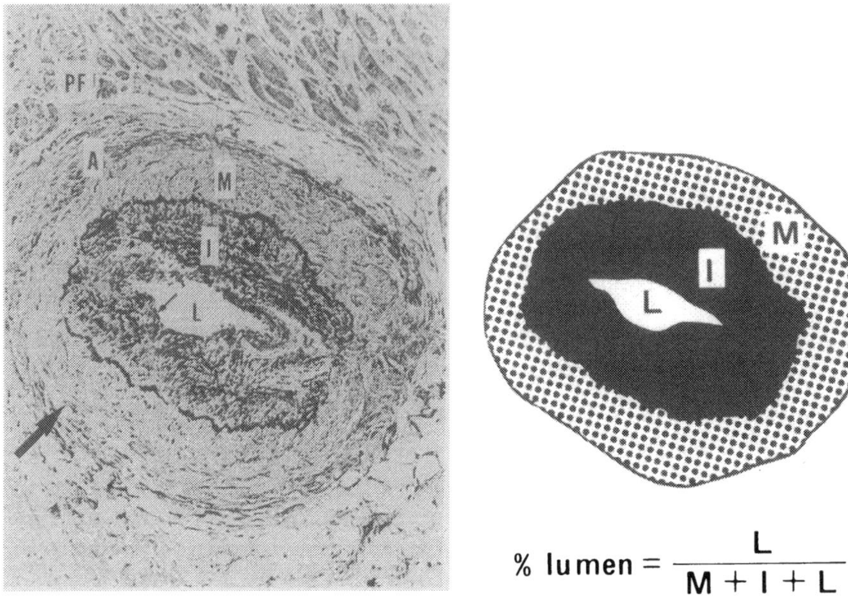

Fig. 1. Method for quantifying stenosis of intramyocardial small arteries [6]. The inner border of the intima (*I*; *short arrow*) and the outer border of the media (*M*; *long arrow*) are traced, and the ratio of the areas encircled by these tracings is calculated as the percentage luminal area; this signifies the percentage of the luminal area (*L*) to the total areas of the media, intima, and lumen. The adventitia (*A*) was excluded, because it was often continuous with perivascular fibrosis (*PF*), which made it difficult to distinguish the border between the two

Quantification of Stenosis of IMSA

Using a multipurpose color image processor (model VIP-21C, Olympus Co.), the 4-μm-thick preparations stained with elastica-van Gieson were enlarged on a high-resolution color television monitor at a $\times 40$–$\times 400$ magnification and stenosis of the IMSA was analyzed. The inner border of the intimal layer and the outer border of the middle layer of the vessel were traced by the light pen, as shown in Fig. 1, and the areas encircled by the tracings were automatically calculated. The ratio of these two areas was defined as the percentage luminal area (%lumen) and used as an index for the degree of luminal stenosis of the IMSA. The external caliber of the IMSA was calculated using the following formula: $1 = 2\sqrt{S/\pi}$, where S is the area within the external border of the middle layer of the IMSA. In this study, the adventitia was excluded because it was often continuos with perivascular fibrosis, which made it difficult to distinguish the border between these two. In quantification, obliquely transected or branching vessels were excluded, and only round vessels were studied. The number of the vessels studied ranged from 85 to 203 (148 ± 22; means ± SD) in each heart. For the regional evaluation of stenosis of the IMSA, the mean %lumen was calculated by averaging all the %lumens of the IMSA in that region. The mean %lumen of

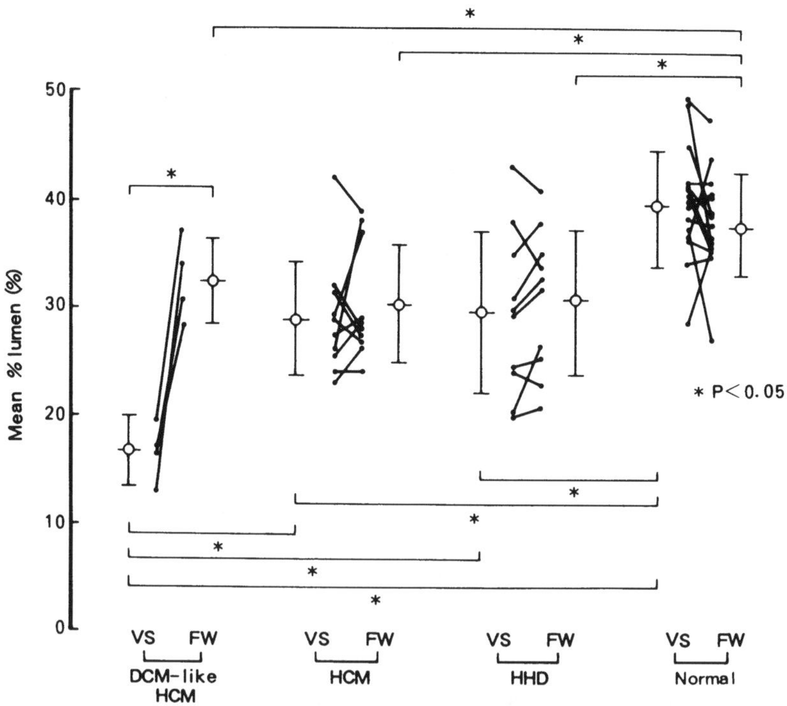

Fig. 2. The mean percentage luminal area (mean *%lumen*) of the intramyocardial small arteries (IMSA) in the ventricular septum (*VS*) and left ventricular free wall (*FW*) of hypertrophic cardiomyopathy showing features mimicking dilated cardiomyopathy (*DCM-like HCM*), hypertrophic cardiomyopathy (*HCM*), hypertensive heart disease (*HHD*), and normal controls [6]. In the VS, the mean %lumen of the IMSA in DCM-like HCM was the lowest of all groups. The mean %lumen of the IMSA was less in HCM and HHD than in the normal controls both in the VS and FW. The mean %lumen of the IMSA was less in the VS than in the FW in DCM-like HCM

the IMSA was calculated separately in the ventricular septum (VS) and left ventricular free wall (LVFW). It was also calculated separately in the right, middle, and left thirds of the VS and in the outer, middle, and inner thirds of the LVFW.

Results

The mean %lumen of the IMSA in the VS was 17% ± 3% in DCM-like HCM, 29% ± 5% in HCM, 30% ± 8% in hypertensive hearts, and 39% ± 6% in normal hearts (Fig. 2). The mean %lumen of the IMSA with an external caliber of more than 60 μm and less than 60 μm was 16% ± 3% and 19% ± 4% in DCM-like HCM, 31% ± 6% and 27% ± 4% in HCM, 31% ± 8%, and 28% ± 9% in hypertensive hearts, and 42% ± 6%, and 36% ± 6% in normal hearts, respectively. Regardless of the size of the IMSA, the mean %lumen of the IMSA in DCM-like HCM was significantly less than in any other group; the mean %lumens of the IMSA in the hearts with HCM and in hypertensive hearts were similar and significantly less than in normal hearts. There was no difference in the mean %lumen of the IMSA among the right, middle, and left thirds of the VS in any group.

The mean %lumen of the IMSA in the LVFW was 33% ± 4% in DCM-like HCM, 31% ± 5% in HCM, 31% ± 7% in hypertensive hearts, and 37% ± 4% in normal hearts (Fig. 2). The mean %lumen of the IMSA with an external caliber of more than and less than 60 μm was 38% ± 6% and 31% ± 4% in DCM-like HCM, 34% ± 5% and 28% ± 4% in HCM, 31% ± 8% and 30% ± 6% in hypertensive hearts, and 40% ± 4% and 36% ± 5% in normal hearts, respectively. Irrespective of the size of the IMSA, the mean %lumen of the IMSA was significantly less in HCM and hypertensive hearts than in normal hearts, but no difference was found between the two disease groups; there was no difference in the mean %lumen of the IMSA between DCM-like HCM and any other group.

The mean % lumen of the IMSA in the inner, middle, and outer thirds of the LVFW was 31% ± 7%, 36% ± 4%, and 34% ± 3% in DCM-like HCM, 28% ± 6%, 31% ± 5%, and 33% ± 6% in HCM, 27% ± 9%, 31% ± 8%, and 35% ± 7% in hypertensive hearts, and 34% ± 4%, 36% ± 6%, and 40% ± 4% in normal hearts. The mean %lumen of the IMSA was less in the subendocardium than in the subepicardium in HCM, hypertensive hearts, and normal hearts.

In DCM-like HCM, the mean %lumen of the IMSA was significantly less in the VS than in the LVFW (Fig. 2). However, no such difference was evident in any other groups.

In the 34 patients examined, the mean %lumen of the IMSA in the left ventricle was inversely correlated with heart weight ($r = -0.51$, $P < 0.01$); the mean %lumen of the IMSA was inversely correlated with the mean size of myocytes both in the VS and the LVFW ($r = -0.60$ and $r = -0.55$, $P < 0.001$, respectively); the mean %lumen of the IMSA was inversely correlated with the extent of fibrosis in the VS ($r = -0.66$, $P < 0.001$; Fig. 3). In HCM, the mean %lumen of the IMSA in the tissue with disarray was compared with that without disarray. The mean %lumen of the IMSA in the tissue with and without disarray was 30% ± 4% and 29% ± 7% in the VS and 30% ± 5% and 30% ± 4% in the LVFW, there being no significant difference between the tissues with and without disarray either in the VS or LVFW.

Discussion

The present study revealed that both in the hearts with HCM and hypertensive hearts, the IMSA did not increase in external caliber and the luminal area was somewhat narrowed despite the marked hypertrophy of the myocytes. The reduction in coronary flow reserve in hypertensive hearts and hearts with HCM and normal epicardial coronary arteries has been reported by many investigators [1, 9]. The coronary reserve has been reported to decrease more in the subendocardium than in the subepicardium [10]. The present study revealed that this was also the case for the mean %lumen of the IMSA. These findings indicate that IMSA disease is a possible pathogenetic mechanism for the reduced coronary reserve both in hearts with HCM and hypertensive hearts.

HCM with features mimicking DCM at a late stage of the diseases has massive

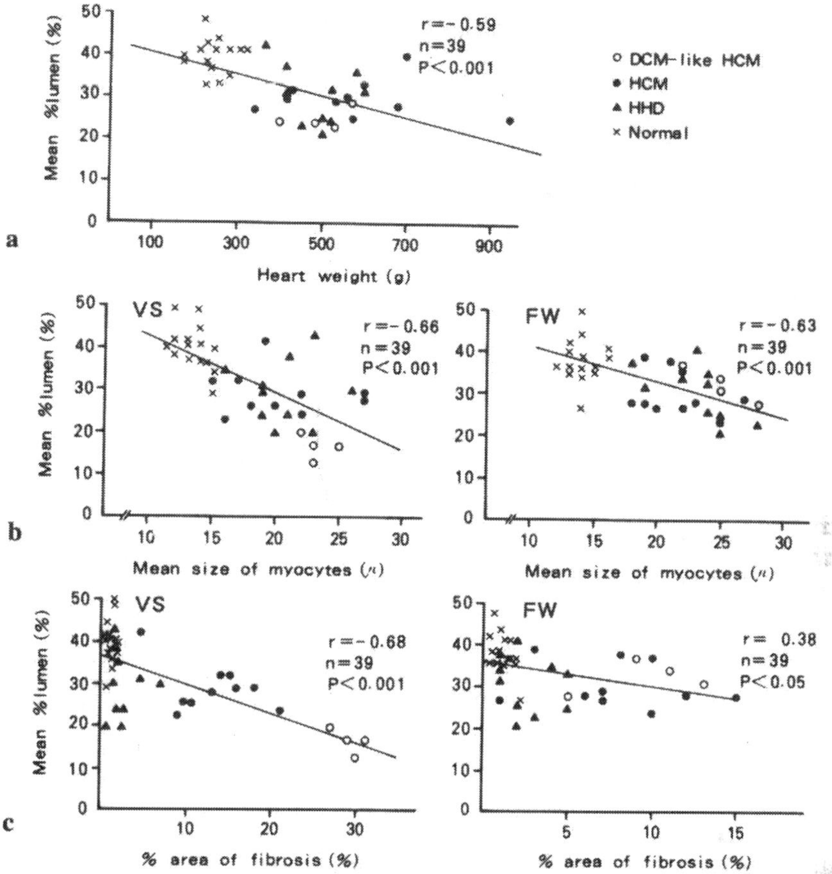

Fig. 3a–c. Relationship of the mean %lumen of the IMSA to **a** heart weight, **b** mean size of myocytes, and **c** percentage fibrotic area [6]. Correlation coefficients and regression lines were obtained from the values of DCM-like HCM (*open circles*), HCM (*closed circles*), HHD (*closed triangles*), and normal controls (*crosses*). Abbreviations are as in Fig. 4

fibrosis, particularly in the VS [6, 7]. Previously, we reported that the extent of fibrosis is greater in hearts with HCM (10.5% ± 4.3%) and hypertensive hearts (2.6% ± 1.5%) than in normal hearts (1.1% ± 0.5%); the extent of fibrosis increases from the epicardial to the endocardial layer of the LVFW [4]. The present study revealed that: the mean %lumen of the IMSA was the least in the VS of DCM-like HCM; the mean %lumen of the IMSA was less in hearts with HCM and hypertensive hearts than in normal hearts; the mean %lumen of the IMSA decreased from the epicardial to the endocardial layer of the LVEW; the mean %lumen of the IMSA was inversely correlated with the extent of fibrosis in the VS. These findings indicate that stenosis of the IMSA is associated with the increased level of fibrosis in hearts with HCM and hypertensive hearts, particularly in the VS of DCM-like HCM. However, the increase of fibrosis in hearts with HCM compared with hypertensive hearts cannot be explained by stenosis of the IMSA, as the mean %lumen of the IMSA was similar in these groups. Other factors such as myocardial fiber disarray are also important in the pathogenesis of extensive fibrosis in hearts with HCM [11, 12].

Our study showed that there was no difference in the mean %lumen of the IMSA between the tissues with and without disarray. This indicates that myocardial fiber disarray is not important in the pathogenesis of stenosis of the IMSA. The mean %lumen of the IMSA was inversely correlated with the heart weight or the mean size of the myocytes. The myocardial fiber diameter has been reported to increase from the epicardial to the endocardial layer of the LVFW [13, 14]. The present study revealed that the mean %lumen of the IMSA decreases. Cardiac hypertrophy is probably one of the pathogenetic factors involved in stenosis of the IMSA in these hearts. However, the pathogenesis of marked stenosis of IMSA in the hearts with DCM-like HCM remains unclear because there was no significant difference in the heart weight or mean size of myocytes between DCM-like HCM and HCM or hypertensive heart disease.

In conclusion, the high prevalence of abnormally stenosed IMSA in patients with HCM, DCM-like HCM in particular, or with hypertension and their association with cardiac hypertrophy and fibrosis indicates that these IMSA alterations are of pathophysiological significance in these patients.

Acknowledgments. We thank Miss M. Jinnai and S. Tomita for assistance in preparing this paper and Mr D. Mrozek for his critical comments on the text. This project was supported in part by a Research Grant for Cardiomyopathy from the Ministry of Health and Welfare of Japan and for project of 60570388, 1985 from the Ministry of Education, Science and Culture of Japan.

References

1. Opherk D, Mall G, Zebe H, Schwarz F, Weihe E, Manthey J, Kubler W (1984) Reduction of coronary reserve: a mechanism for angina pectoris in patients with arterial hypertension and normal coronary arteries. Circulation 69: 1–7
2. Legrand V, Hodgson LM, Bates ER, Aueron FM, Mancinci GBJ, Smith JS, Gross MD, Vogel RA (1985) Abnormal coronary flow reserve and abnormal radionuclide exercise test results in patients with normal coronary angiograms. J Am Coll Cardial 6: 1245–1253
3. Cannon III RO, Rosing DR, Maron BJ, Leon MB, Bonow RO, Watson RM, Epstein SE (1985) Myocardial ischemia patients with hypertrophic cardiomyopathy: contribution of inadequate vasodilator reserve and elevated left ventricular filling pressures. Circulation 71: 234–243
4. Tanaka M, Fujiwara H, Onodera T, Wu DJ, Hamashima Y, Kawai C (1986) Quantitative analysis of myocardial fibrosis in normals, hypertensive hearts and hypertrophic cardiomyopathy. Br Heart J 55: 575–581
5. Maron BJ, Wolfson JK, Epstein SE, Roberts WC (1986) Intamural "small vessel" coronary artery disease in hypertrophic cardiomyopathy: prevalence and potential significance. J Am Coll Cardial 8: 545–557
6. Tanaka M, Fujiwara H, Onodera T, Wu DJ, Matsuda M, Hamashima Y, Kawai C (1987) Quantitative analysis of narrowings of intramyocardial small arteries in normal hearts, hypertensive hearts, and hearts with hypertrophic cardiomyopathy. Circulation 75: 1130–1139

7. Fujiwara H, Onodera T, Tanaka M, Kawai C (1984) Progression from hypertrophic obstructive cardiomyopathy to typical dilated cardiomyopathy like features in the end stage. Jpn Circ J 48: 1210–1214
8. Onodera T, Fujiwara H, Tanaka M, Wu DJ, Hamashima Y, Kawai C (1986) Familial hypertrophic cardiomyopathy mimicing typical dilated cardiomyopathy. Jpn Circ J 50: 614–618
9. Wangler RD, Peters KG, Marcus ML, Tomanek RJ (1982) Effects of duration and severity of arterial hypertension and cardiac hypertrophy on coronary vasodilator reserve. Circ Res 51: 10–18
10. Griggs DM Jr, Nakamura Y (1968) Effects of coronary constriction on myocardial distribution of iodoantipyrine ^{131}I. Am J Physiol 215: 1082–1088
11. Tanaka M, Onodera T, Wu DJ, Fujiwara H, Kawai C (1987) The pathogenesis of myocardial fibrosis in hypertrophic cardiomyopathy with special reference to myocardial fiber disarray. Jpn Circ J 51: 624–630
12. Fujiwara H, Kawai C, Hamashima Y (1979) Myocardial fascicle and fiber disarray in 25μ-thick sections. Circulation 59: 1293–1298
13. Hoshino T, Fujiwara H, Kawai C, Hamashima Y (1983) Myocardial fiber diameter and regional distribution in the ventricular wall of normal adult hearts, hypertensive hearts and hearts with hypertrophic cardiomyopathy. Circulation 67: 1109–1116
14. Fujiwara H, Hoshino T, Yamana K, Fujiwara T, Furuta M, Hamashima Y, Kawai C (1983) Number and size of myocytes and amount of interstitial space in the ventricular septum and in the left ventricular free wall in hypertrophic cardiomyopathy. Am J Cardiol 52: 818–823

Chapter 6
Ischemia of Peripheral Tissues

Microcirculatory Studies on Epidural Spinal Cord Electrical Stimulation in Patients with Severe Lower Limb Ischemia

Michael J.H.M. Jacobs[1], Paul J.G. Jörning[1], Soures R. Joshi[2], Dick W. Slaaf[3], Robert S. Reneman[4]

Introduction

The approach to treatment of patients with chronic occlusive arterial disease of the lower extremities depends on the severity and extent of the obstructive lesions. Arterial reconstructive surgery remains the therapy of choice, but in approximately 20% of patients with ulceration and gangrene, vascular surgery is not effective [1].

Epidural spinal cord electrical stimulation (ESES) is an accepted therapy for the treatment of low back pain, causalgia, and phantom limb pain [2]. Recently, ESES has also been suggested to improve healing of skin ulcers even in patients with limb-threatening occlusive arterial disease, in whom vascular reconstruction is impossible or has failed [3]. It is likely that in these patients ischemic phenomena take place at the level of the microcirculation.

In the present study, we evaluated the effects of ESES on the microcirculation using incident bright-field and fluorescence (dynamic) video capillary microscopy.

Patients and Methods

Patients

ESES was performed on ten patients with severe limb ischemia (Fontaine stage III-IV) due to atherosclerotic or diabetic disease. The mean age of the patients was 77 years. Prior to ESES, patients underwent vascular reconstructive surgery or sympathectomy without satisfactory result. Angiography showed occluded crural arteries that were technically unsuitable for reconstructive surgery. All patients had rest pain and eight of them suffered from nonhealing ulcers. The surgical procedure consisted of a vertical incision parallel to the spinal column; an electrode was introduced into the epidural space at the level of L3–4 and placed in the midline approximately at the level of T10. The lead was then man-

Departments of Surgery[1], Anesthesiology[2], Biophysics[3] and Physiology[4], University of Limburg, P. O. Box 1918, 6201 BX, Maastricht, The Netherlands ipulated until the patients experienced pleasant paresthesia, extending down into both legs. Stimulation was performed with a pulse width of 0.2 ms, a frequency of 120 Hz, and an amplitude varying between 4 and 9 V.

The following macro- and microcirculatory parameters were assessed 1 day before and 1 day after spinal cord stimulation.

Macrocirculation

The systolic ankle/arm pressure index, expressed as a percentage, was measured with a continuous wave Doppler instrument. The systolic toe pressure, expressed in millimeters of mercury, was assessed by photoplethysmography.

Microcirculation

Bright-field microscopy was used to assess capillary diameters and red blood cell (RBC) velocity (flying spot method) in the nailfold [4]. Fluorescence microscopy was used in combination with intravenously injected sodium fluorescence to study capillary density (i.e., number of capillaries/mm^2), sodium fluorescein appearance time (seconds), and distribution in the dorsum of the toe.

Results

After ESES, nine of the ten patients had complete relief of pain and in the other patient the pain was reduced. During the follow-up period, in five of the eight patients with ischemic ulcers, complete healing occurred. In the other three patients, amputation could not be avoided.

Macrocirculation

The mean systolic ankle/arm pressure index was 32 prior to ESES and did not change significantly after stimulation (Table 1). The mean toe pressure increased from 9 to 19 mmHg, which was not a significant difference.

Microcirculation

Morphological investigation of the skin capillaries showed that the number of perfused capillaries increased significantly after ESES (Table 2). Skin capillary diameter did not change after treatment. RBC velocity in capillaries already perfused before ESES increased from 0.054 to 0.762 mm/s ($P < 0.001$) after treatment. The appearance time of sodium fluorescein decreased in all patients ($P < 0.001$).

Discussion

Intravital skin capillary microscopy was shown to be a noninvasive method for evaluating microcirculatory changes induced by ESES. The significant increase in skin capillary density and RBC velocity explains the observed clinical im-

Table 1. Macrocirculatory parameters before and after ESES

	Before	After	Significance[a]
Systolic ankle/arm Pressure index (%)	32 ± 14	37 ± 14	NS
Systolic toe pressure (mmHg)	9 ± 16	19 ± 23	NS

Values are means ± SD
NS not significant
[a] Student's *t*-test

Table 2. Microcirculatory parameters before and after ESES

	Before	After	Significance[a]
Skin capillary diameter (μm)	15.7 ± 1.8	15.5 ± 1.5	NS
Red blood cell velocity (mm/s)	0.054 ± 0.014	0.762 ± 0.205	$P < 0.001$
Sodium fluorescein perfused capillaries (n/mm^2)	20 ± 4	44 ± 5	$P < 0.001$
Sodium-fluorescein appearance time (s)	72 ± 15	45 ± 9	$P < 0.001$

Values are means ± SD
NS not significant
[a] Student's *t*-test

provement and ulcer healing. Although the patients in this study were all in the last phase before amputation, seven patients reported subjective improvement, while in three patients amputation still became necessary. Similar beneficial effects were also reported by Augustinsson and co-workers [5].

The mechanisms by which spinal cord stimulation exerts pain relief are still unclear. Pain is a symptom of tissue damage, caused by stimulation of A-delta and C fibers. Melzack and Wall [6] propose that pain is determined by interaction of stimuli transmission to the cells of the substantia gelatinosa, the dorsal-column fibers, and the first central transmission cells in the dorsal horn. The idea of dorsal root electrical stimulation is based on blockade of pain stimuli. Consequently, pain relief may release the reflex vasoconstriction that is known to occur in response to pain.

Hilton and Marshall [7] described vasodilatation in the cat gastrocnemius muscle following dorsal root stimulation and postulated that this effect is due to antidromic stimulation of small-diameter fibers. They found an interaction with prostaglandines release in muscles.

In conclusion, epidural spinal cord stimulation improved wound healing and caused pain relief in patients with severe limb ischemia, which could be explained by improved skin nutritional blood flow. Further prospective clinical and physiological studies are necessary in order to clarify the indications and investigate the mechanisms involved.

References

1. Gregg RO (1985) Bypass or amputation? Concomitant review of bypass arterial grafting and major amputations. Am J Surg 149: 397–402
2. Long DM (1977) Electrical stimulation for the control of pain. Arch Surg 112: 884–888
3. Cook AW, Oygar A, Baggenstos P, Pacheco S, Kleriga E (1976) Vascular disease of extremities. Electric stimulation of spinal cord and posterior roots. NY St J Med 76: 366–368
4. Jacobs MJHM, Breslau PJ, Slaaf DW, Reneman RS, Lemmens HAJ (1987) Nomenclature of Raynaud's phenomenon. A capillary microscopic and hemorheologic study. Surgery 101 (2): 136–145
5. Augustinsson LE, Holm J, Carlsson CA, Jivegard L (1985) Epidural electrical stimulation in severe limb ischaemia. Evidence of pain relief, increased blood flow and a possible limb-saving effect. Ann Surg 202: 104–111
6. Melzack R, Wall PD (1965) Pain mechanism: a new theory. Science 150: 971–979
7. Hilton SM, Marshall JM (1980) Dorsal root vasodilatation in cat skeletal muscle. J Physiol 299: 277–288

Microcirculation of Canine Hindlimbs in Hemorrhagic Hypotension

Toshio Ozeki, Hiroshi Kumazaki, Y. Kohketsu T. Okada, and S. Hirakawa[1]

Introduction

We have previously studied the changes in the diffusion capacity for ^{22}NaCl and ^{86}RbCl in the hindlimbs of dogs with and without acute hemorrhagic hypotension [1–3]. The diffusion capacity is defined as the product of P and S, where P is the permeability coefficient and S is the surface area. The diffusion capacity is measured by the "indicator diffusion" method. We found that acutely induced hemorrhagic hypotension decreased the diffusion capacity [4].

In separate groups of dogs, we also studied microvascular flow density of the hindlimbs, using low-viscosity silicone rubber, with and without acute hemorrhagic hypotension [5]. We found that the number of patent capillaries per single muscle fiber decreased in response to hemorrhagic hypotension [6].

The decreased diffusion capacity and decreased number of patent capillaries indicate that the microvascular blood flow tends to shift toward the nonexchange vessels, such as thoroughfare channels, resulting either from an increased activity of local sympathetic nerves or from an increased amount of circulating catecholamine. To determine which factor is responsible, we investigated the diffusion capacity after acute hemorrhagic hypotension by pretreating the animal with different interventions, such as acute sciatic denervation, alpha-adrenergic blockade, and beta-adrenergic blockade.

Methods

Measurement of Diffusion Capacity

We anesthetized mongrel dogs with intravenous sodium pentobarbital. The dogs were observed to breathe spontaneously. An extracorporeal circuit made of polyethylene tubing was inserted into the right femoral artery, and to this we applied a constant-flow pump, electromagnetic flow meter, electromanometer; an aperture was made for the injection of indicators, a mixture of ^{86}Rb and

[1]Second Department of Internal Medicine, Gifu University School of Medicine, 40 Tsukasamachi, Gifu, 500 Japan

radioactive ^{131}I serum albumin. We also constructed an extracorporeal circuit in the right femoral vein. By placing an open end to a side branch of the T tube connected to the venous circuit at the level of peripheral venous pressure, we kept the venous pressure constant and collected venous blood. Through a tube inferted into the left carotid artery, we measured systemic blood pressure and depleted the blood to induce acute hemorrhagic hypotensive state as required.

The method of measuring the diffusion capacity (PS) in the baseline state was as follows. We measured the blood flow of the right femoral artery and perfused the hindlimb at the same measured rate of blood flow. Then, we made a bolus injection of a mixture of the indicators—^{86}Rb and ratioactive ^{131}I serum albumin—into the arterial circuit through the aperture. At the same time, we clamped the proximal end of the venous extracorporeal circuit and collected venous blood from the end of the venous side branch at intervals of 3 s for 1 min (a total of 20 samples). During this indicator diffusion study, the rate of venous outflow was maintained constant at the same level as in the control period by adjusting the pump. After completion of sample collection, we turned off the pump and clamped off the venous line.

We produced acute hemorrhagic hypotension by depleting the blood to a carotid artery pressure level of 60 mmHg for 10 min. To determine the PS in acute hemorrhagic hypotension, we repeated the same procedure as in the baseline state.

To evaluate the effect of acute hemorrhagic hypotension on the PS, the fundamental protocol was to determine the PS in the baseline state and again at the end of acute hemorrhagic hypotension for 10 min.

To observe the extent to which local sympathetic nerves affect the response of the PS to acute hemorrhagic hypotension, the PS was studied in acute hemorrhagic hypotension in dogs pretreated with acute sciatic denervation.

To observe the extent to which humoral factors affect the response of the PS to acute hemorrhagic hypotension, we used dogs pretreated with beta blockade (propranolol) and alpha-blockade (phenoxybenzamine).

PS determination. We counted the radioactivity (base 300–450 keV and 1000–1300 keV) per unit gram of each sample for the ^{86}Rb (diffusible indicator) and ^{131}I serum albumin (nondiffusible indicator) with a Packard auto Gamma 500/800 c Counter. These values were divided by the original radioactivity of the fluid injected intra-arterially. Thus, the relative concentration was obtained for ^{86}Rb and ^{131}I serum albumin. Figure 1 shows representative experimental records.

The extraction ratio (E) is defined as follows:

$$E = \frac{C_A - C_V}{C_A} \tag{1}$$

where C_A is the arterial test substance and C_V the venous test substance. The Renkin-Crone equation for the single-capillary model is as follows [7–11]:

$$E = 1 - e^{-(PS/Q)} \tag{2}$$

$$PS = -Q\ln(1 - E) \tag{3}$$

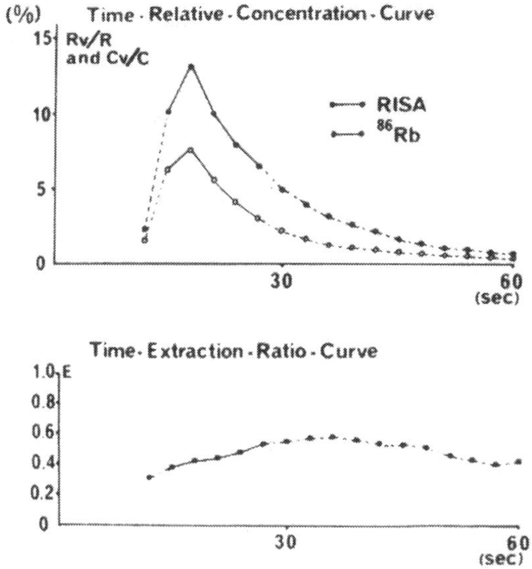

Fig. 1. Typical records of an experiment for the measurement of PS. *Closed circles* indicate radioactivity level of ^{131}I serum albumin (*RISA*), *open circles* radioactivity of ^{86}Rb

where e is the exponential, P the permeability coefficient, S the effective surface area of capillaries, Q the rate of blood flow through the single-capillary model, and ln the natural logarithm.

In our experiments, Q was by definition the femoral venous outflow rate, and this was held constant at two points in the course of an experiment—in the control period and 10 min after the start of hemorrhagic hypotension. We used the following equation to obtain the extraction ratio (E) from relative concentrations, such as Cv/C or Rv/R:

$$1 - E = \frac{Cv/C}{Rv/R} \tag{4}$$

where Cv is the concentration of the test substance, e.g., $^{86}RbCl$, in the venous blood plasma, C is the concentration of the test substance in the injection fluid, Rv is the concentration of the reference substance, e.g., ^{131}I serum albumin, in the venous blood plasma, and R is the concentration of the reference substance in the injection fluid. A single value of E, representing a time-E curve, was obtained as the first point of E where the time-E curves were relatively flat and where the relative concentrations of ^{131}I serum albumin were more than 5%.

Applying the data of the extraction ratio E and the venous blood outflow rate Q into Eq. (3), one obtains the PS.

Measurements of Microvascular Flow Density

Low-viscosity silicone rubber injection studies were performed [12]. An extracorporeal circuit was installed in the right femoral artery. To this circuit, we applied an electromagnetic flowmeter. We installed a reservoir of low-viscosity silicone rubber and a constant-flow pump to a side branch. The low-viscosity silicone rubber (Microfil, Canton Biomedical) has a viscosity of 15–25 cP.

To perfuse the right hindlimb with this silicone rubber, the normal blood circulation of the hindlimb was suddenly switched to perfusion with the silicone rubber. The constant-flow pump was operated such that the volume flow rate of the silicone rubber perfusate was the same as that of the blood circulation observed just before the moment of switching. A side branch was installed to the femoral vein in the same mammer as in the PS studies

Perfusion with low-viscosity silicone rubber continued for 5 min, and then both the inflow and outflow of the hindlimb were closed. We waited 15 min to allow polymerization of the silicone rubber. The dog was then killed. The gastrocunemius muscle was removed, fixed in 10% buffered formalin, and examined under the light microscope without staining. By definition, all blood vessels less than 6.3 μm in diameter are capillary blood vessels. The microvascular flow density was expressed by the capillary/fiber ratio. All variables are given as means ± one standard error of the mean.

Results

Diffusion Capacity

From the average PS for ^{86}RbCl in the control state before hemorrhagic hypotension, i.e., 3.90 ± 0.33 (mean ± SE) ml/min/100 g muscle [4], and an assumed capillary surface area, i.e., 7000 cm^2/100 g skeletal muscle [13], we calculated the capillary permeability coefficient, $P = 0.93 \times 10^{-5}$cm. s^{-1} [4].

Individual percentage changes in PS due to acute hemorrhagic hypotension were −42% ± 8% (mean ± SE) in the control group, −3% ± 6% in pretreatment with alpha blockade, −28% ± 7% in pretreatment with sciatic denervation, and −28% ± 12% in pretreatment with beta blockade. Alpha blockade (phenoxybenzamine) successfully suppressed the reduction of PS that normally occurs following acute hemorrhagic hypotension. On the other hand, neither sciatic denervation nor beta blockade prevented the reduction of PS accompanying the hemorrhagic hypotension.

Microvascular Flow Density

The capillary/fiber (C/F) ratio in the control state was 1.39 ± 0.04 (mean ± SE); after acute hemorrhagic hypotension of 10-min duration, the C:F ratio decreased to 1.14 ± 0.04, which indicates that patent capillaries decrease by 20%. This reduction in the C:F ratio after acute hemorrhagic hypotension was inhibited neither by pretreatment with acute sciatic denervation of 90-min duration (C:F ratio 1.16 ± 0.05) nor by pretreatment with intravenously injected propranolol (beta-blockade; C:F ratio, 1.14 ± 0.08). In contrast, after acute hemorrhagic hypotension by pretreatment with phenoxybenzamine (alpha blockade; C:F ratio 1.34 ± 0.04; mean ± SE), there was no change from the baseline state. This finding implies that the alpha blockade almost completely inhibits the usual decrease in microvascular flow density caused by acute hemorrhagic hypotension.

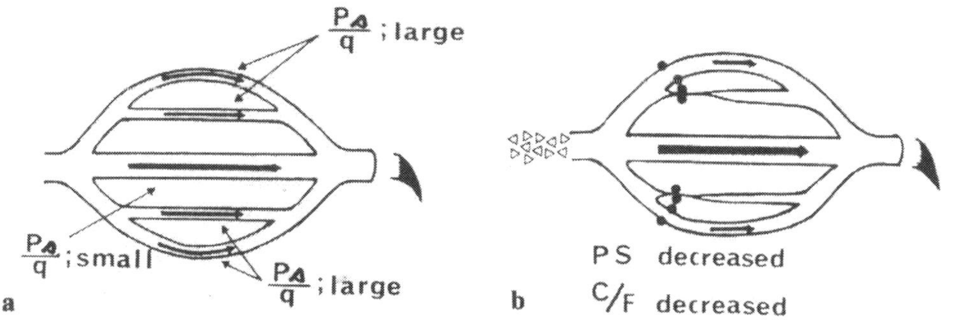

Fig. 2a, b. A model "capillary" bed in the skeletal muscle of the hindlimbs of the dog in **a** the control state and *b* during 10-min hemorrhagic hypotension. The *arrows* express the magnitude of the blood flow volume. During the measurement of PS, femoral venous outflow rate was controlled constant. *P* capillary permeability coefficient, *s* local microvascular surface area, *q* local microvascular blood flow

Discussion

In Fig. 2, we present a speculative model of the microvascular bed in the baseline and experimental states. In the nonexchange vessel, which is shown as a single central large channel, the permeability coefficient is smaller, surface area smaller, and blood flow larger. Therefore, as an index, the rate of PS to blood flow, Ps/q will be small in the nonexchange vessel. In the exchange vessels, which are shown as arched, small channels, the permeability coefficient is larger, surface area larger, and blood flow smaller. Therefore, Ps/q will be large in the exchange vessel.

We found that acute hemorrhagic hypotension decreased PS by 42% and C:F ratio by 20% in the hindlimb. Because the venous blood outflow was maintained constant, as in the baseline state, the blood flow in the microvascular beds is believed to be redistributed from the true exchange vessels to the nonexchange vessels, like a thoroughfare channel. As a result, PS in the hindlimb decreases as a whole.

We further speculate that the catecholamines as shown by triangular particles decrease or block the blood flow into true capillaries, depending on the responsiveness of precapillary sphincters to catecholamines. Since this reduction in diffusion capacity after acute hemorrhagic hypotension was prevented only by the pretreatment with alpha blockade, we conclude that circulating catecholamines, such as adrenaline and noradrenline, exert their effects on alpha receptors on some of the precapillary sphincters, producing: (a) closure of some true capillaries and, (b) redistribution, which tends to be from exchange vessels, true capillaries, to nonexchange vessels.

Summary

We studied diffusion capacity (PS) and capillary/fiber ratio in the striated muscle of intact hindlimbs of the dog in two ways: physiological study of ^{86}Rb for PS, and morphological study using low-viscosity silicone rubber for capillary/fiber ratio.

Both PS and C/F ratio decreased after acute hemorrhagic "shock." This reduction in PS and C/F ratio was completely prevented in dogs with acute hemorrhagic hypotension pretreated with alpha blockade. However, this reduction was not prevented by pretreatment with beta blockade or sciatic denervation.

We, therefore, speculate that microvascular blood flow tends to redistribute toward nonexchange vessels, together with closure of some capillaries during acute hemorrhagic hypotension (60 mmHg, 10 min) by humoral mechanism.

References

1. Imao T (1971) The influence of elevated venous pressure on blood-tissue exchange of ^{22}Na in perfused hindlimbs of dogs. Jpn Circ J 35: 1–20
2. Yoshimura T (1972) Influence of venous congestion on the blood-tissue exchange of ^{22}Na in dog's hindlimbs with special reference to the role of the autonomic nervous system. Jpn Circ J 36: 1047–1055 (in Japanese)
3. Sato E, Kida K, Yokoyamah, Hirakawa S (1983) Redistribution of the blood flow in the microvascular beds of skeletal muscle of dogs during acute venous congestion of a hindlimbs. Acta Scholae Medicinalis Universitatis in Gifu 31: 708–724 (in Japanese)
4. Sato M, Ozeki T, Kumazaki H, Hirakawa S (1986) Effect of acute hemorrhagic hypotension on the blood flow in the microvascular beds of skeletal muscles of dog's hindlimbs. Acta Scholae Medicinalis Universitatis in Gifu 34: 1–14 (in Japanese)
5. Kida K, Sato E, Yokoyama H, Hirakawa S (1980) Quantitative study on the blood flow density in microcirculatory beds of the striated muscle. Acta Scholae Medicinalis Universitatis in Gifu 28: 18–29 (in Japanese)
6. Yokoyama H, Kida K, Sato E, Hirakawa S (1983) The effect of acute hemorrhagic hypotension on blood flow density in cicrocirculatory beds of the striated muscle of dog's hindlimbs. Acta Scholae Medicinalis Universitatis in Gifu 31: 290–303 (in Japanese)
7. Crone C (1970) Capillary permeability-techniques and problems. In: Crone C, Lassen NA (eds) Alfred Benzon symposium II: Capillary permeability. Munksgaard, Copenhagen, pp 15–31
8. Crone C (1963) The permeability of capillaried in various organs as determined by use of the 'indicator diffusion' method. Acta Physiol Scand 58: 292–305
9. Renkin EM (1969) Exchange of substances through capillary walls. In: Wolstenholme GEW, Knight AB (eds) Circulatory and respiratory mass transport, a Ciba foundation symposium. Churchill, London, pp 50–66
10. Renkin EM (1968) Transcapillary exchange in relation to capillary circulation. In: Biological interfaces: flows and exchanges. Little Brown, Boston pp 96–108
11. Renkin EM (1965) Blood flow and transcapillary exchange in skeletal muscle. Federation Proc 24: 1092–1094
12. Plyley MJ, Groom AC (1975) Geometrical disturbance of capillaries in mammalian striated mescle. Am J Physiol 228: 1376–1383
13. Landis EM, Pappenheimer JR (1963) In: Handbook of physiology, sect. 2, vol. 2. Am Physiol Society, Washington pp 961–1034

Impaired Microcirculation in Patients with Peripheral Vascular Disease: Pathophysiological and Therapeutic Aspects

A.M. Ehrly[1]

Introduction

The common causal explanation for ischemic symptoms in chronic occlusive arterial disease, based on arteriosclerosis, is the existence of stenosis and occlusions of the larger arteries like the femoral artery. This almost anatomical and mechanistic way of thinking led to the surgical therapy of "desobliteration" or bypass operations, which is in fact helpful in selected cases. However, only 30% of all patients suffering from intermittent claudication, rest pains, or ischemic ulcers can be operated upon. The remaining 70% with very peripheral occlusions are unsuitable for surgical therapy and must be treated conservatively. Since this is the case, noninterventional types of therapy are needed. These therapies should be based on a more detailed knowledge of the pathophysiology of the disease. This was and is the aim of the scientific work of many groups. The direction of research was outlined in the late 1960s—away from the large arteries and toward the microcirculation. This makes sense, since if the macrocirculatory flow is reduced by stenoses or occlusions, the blood flow in the microcirculation must be impaired and vice versa. What we did not know at that time was that functional vicious circles and mechanisms exist which act in a self-perpetuating way. So far, the logical consequence was to investigate what happens in the ischemic microcirculation in muscle tissue and skin and, if possible, to draw therapeutical consequences from these results.

Here, I shall not speak about the so-called classic microcirculatory disorders of the limbs like diabetic microangiopathy or Raynaud's syndrome, which are very specific vascular disorders and should not be compared with common chronic arteriosclerosis. I shall discuss some microcirculatory aspects of ischemic peripheral arterial disease including the therapeutic consequences.

Microvascular Aspects

Historically, the old rationale of improving blood flow in the microcirculation in order to improve tissue supply was used in the same sense as in former times for

[1] Division of Angiology, Department of Internal Medicine, J.W. Goethe-University Medical School, Theodor-Stern-Kai 7, 6000 Frankfurt am Main 70, Federal Republic of Germany

the macrocirculation. In this connection, I refer to the unsuccessful therapeutic attempts with so-called classic vasodilators like papaverine. Lassen and co-workers [1] created the concept of an increase in systemic blood pressure in order to increase the poststenotic pressure gradients, an approach which really works in ischemic patients in whom the systemic blood pressure values are low. Another therapeutic concept which has become more and more important is the improvement of the flow properties of blood in the macrocirculation as well as in the microcirculation [2, 3]. Again, the main idea was to increase the microcirculatory blood flow, for example, by hemodilution, by reducing the plasma fibrinogen level, reducing the red cell aggregation, or by improving the red cell deformability. The basic rationale for this type of therapy was that in patients with vascular disease the flow properties of blood are impaired, an assumption which may be true from the statistical point of view but must not necessarily be true in the individual patient. Another point of view was that the flow properties of blood would be impaired directly in the ischemic tissue by local acidosis, hyperosmolarity, and other mechanisms. Indeed, it could be shown that, for example, under exercise conditions, the flow properties of blood obtained from the femoral veins of claudicants were worse than in blood obtained from the antecubital veins [4]. This can be explained not only by a local increase in acidosis and osmolarity but also by vicious circles, which may occur in the postocclusive or poststenotic low-pressure areas, particularily in the macrocirculation [3, 5, 6].

All these mechanisms and vicious circles are thought to be responsible for the reduction of blood flow and hence for the decrease in overall perfusion. When we started measurements of the tissue oxygen pressure directly in the ischemic muscle tissue in claudicants and compared these results with plethysmographic or xenon clearance data under resting conditions, we learned that there is a tremendous gap between blood flow values in ischemic tissue and tissue oxygen supply.

The results led us to conclude that the supply of tissue is both a quantitative and a qualitative problem. A therapy which would decrease blood viscosity and break the vicious circles would, hence, lead to an increase in blood flow and to a disapperence of ischemic symptoms. Indeed, some well-known therapeutic concepts have involved this approach, e.g., hemodilution, defibrinogenation, reduction in red cell rigidity.

It has become increasingly obvious that the amount of total blood flow in an ischemic limb, for example, as measured by venous occlusion plethysmography, is not a valid parameter for assessing what really happens in ischemic tissues. Thus, extremely low blood flow and ankle pressure values can be measured in elderly patients with pale, cool skin. In spite of this, they do not exhibit rest pain or even gangrene. On the other hand, in other patients, in particular those with diabetic microangiopathy, high blood flow values and warm feet can be found in spite of the presence of arterial toe ulcers. There is obviously a discrepancy between blood flow and tissue supply.

This can be explained according to Renkin [7] and Schroeder and Rathscheck [8] as a nonhomogenous flow distribution, whereby a large amount of blood is obviously shunted through microvessels—maldistribution [9, 10], whereas in the case of the above-mentioned patients with pale skin and low overall blood flow values the distribution of the remaining small amount of blood flow is homogenous and so a minimal tissue supply can be maintained.

An answer to these open questions can be given since we were able to quantify blood flow and tissue oxygen supply simultaneously in patients with peripheral arterial disease. The technique for measuring tissue oxygen pressure with microplatinum needle electrodes has been published elsewhere [11, 12]. The frequency distribution of the pO_2 values obtained during the withdrawal of the electrode through the ischemic muscle tissue shows a clear difference between normal volunteers and patients with intermittent claudication.

The overall blood flow values as measured by venous occlusion plethysmography as well as by the ^{131}xenon clearance technique, however, did not show any difference between the two groups under resting conditions. This can be explained by the shunting of blood through short, so-called high-flow channels, whereby the longer "nutritive capillaries" [13] remain underperfused. This may happen when a rigid red cell blocks the entrance of a nutritive capillary. The consequence is that the blood flow now tends to utilize shorter "bridging" capillaries in the sense of microshunting, which leads to an impaired oxygen delivery. If the deformability of red cells is improved by a drug like pentoxifylline, the pO_2 values will increase with time and dose [14] and the pO_2 histogram will indicate a more homogenous distribution of the tissue oxygenation, which can be explained by a more homogenous capillary blood flow distribution.

Theoretically, the situation is further complicated when hemodilution is used as a treatment in ischemic disease, since intravenous infusion of so-called plasma substitutes decrease blood viscosity and increase blood flow; however, they also decrease hematocrit and thus the number of oxygen-transporting cells. After hypervolemic hemodilution, though, with 500 ml hydroxyethyl starch (molecular weight 200000), the muscle tissue pO_2 in claudicants increases in spite of a decrease in hematocrit. The pO_2 histograms indicate a shift to the right, which can be explained by a more homogenous capillary distribution in blood flow under these conditions [15].

On the other hand, improvement of the flow properties of blood per se does not necessarily mean an increase in tissue pO_2, as demonstrated by the use of a 5% human albumin solution given intravenously (500 ml within 30 min) in patients with intermittent claudication. In spite of the fact that all hemorheological data are improved (blood and plasma viscosity, red cell aggregation, and red cell filtrability), the tissue pO_2 is decreased during the first 30 min after the end of the infusion. We believe that substances like serotonin may counteract the vasomotor tone, thereby leading to more nonhomogenous flow through short bridging capillaries [16].

Concluding Remarks

According to the hypothesis we presented some years ago—microcirculatory blood maldistribution [9, 10]—blood flow in the microcirculation in ischemic tissues is nonhomogenous due to various mechanisms and hence less effective with respect to tissue supply. This theory enables us to explain the paradox of high flow and insufficient tissue supply and low flow and sufficient supply. Thus, we must be aware of the fact that blood flow or blood perfusion in the microcirculation is both a quantitative and a qualitative problem.

References

1. Lassen NA, Laren OA, Sörensen AW (1968) Conservative treatment of gangrene using mineralocorticoid induced moderate hypertension. Lancet I: 606
2. Ehrly AM (1976) Improvement of the flow properties of blood: A new therapeutical approach in occlusive arterial disease. Angiology 27: 188–196
3. Ehrly AM (1973) Verbesserung der Fließeigenschaften des Blutes: Ein neues Prinzip zur medikamentösen Therapie chronischer peripherer arterieller Durchblutungsstörungen. VASA 2, Suppl. 1
4. Forconi S, Pieragalli D, Acciavatti A, Del Bigo C, Galigani C, Ralli L, Guerrini M, Di Perri T (1984) Positive effect of oral Buflomedil on exercise-induced hemorheological damage and on claudication distance in peripheral obliterative arterial disease patients. J Int Med Res 12: 188–192
5. Ehrly AM (1969) The effect of plasma substitutes on erythrocyte aggregation and blood viscosity. Bibl Heamat 33: 302
6. Ehrly AM, Köhler HJ (1976) Impaired erythrocytes deformability in patients with chronic occlusive arterial disease. In: Seki K, Mishima Y (eds) Proceedings X International Congress of Angiology, Tokyo. p 407
7. Renkin EM (1968) Transcapillary exchanges in relation to capillary circulation. J Gen Physiol 52: 96
8. Schroeder W, Rathscheck W (1973) Investigation of the influence of acetylcholine on the distribution of capillary flow in the skeletal muscle of the guinea pig by recording of the pO_2 in the muscle tissue. Pflügers Arch 345: 335
9. Ehrly AM, Schroeder W (1979) Zur Pathophysiologie der chronischen arteriellen Verschlußerkrankung: I. Mikrozirkulatorische Blutverteilungsstörung in der Skelettmuskulatur. Herz Kreislauf 11: 275
10. Ehrly AM (1980) New pythophysiological concept of ischemic diseases: Microcirculatory blood maldistribution (MBM). Bibl Anat 20: 456
11. Ehrly AM, Köhler HJ, Schroeder W, Müller R (1975) Sauerstoffdruckwerte im ischämischen Muskelgewebe von Patienten mit chronischen peripheren arteriellen Verschlußkrankheten. Klin Wschr 53: 687
12. Ehrly AM, Schroeder W (1977) Oxygen pressure in ischemic muscle tissue of patients with chronic occlusive arterial diseases. Angiology 28: 101
13. Ehrly AM (1983) Verbesserung der nutritiven Durchblutung bei peripheren ischämischen Erkrankungen. VASA 12: [Suppl] 11
14. Ehrly AM, Schroeder W, Dannhof S (1977) The effect of pentoxifylline on the oxygen pressure of ischemic muscle tissue on patients with chronic arterial occlusion. IRCS Med Science 5: 411
15. Ehrly AM, Landgraf H (1984) Effects on muscle tissue oxygen tension in claudicants: infusions of 5% albumine versus 10% hydroxyethylstarch solution (200/0,5) Int J Microcirc 3 (3–4): 521
16. Ehrly, AM, Landgraf, H, Saeger-Lorenz K (1987) Effect of infusion of 500 ml 5% human albumin on the muscle tissue oxygen pressure in patients with intermittent claudication. In: Ehrly AM, Hauss J, Huch R (eds) Clinical oxygen pressure measurement. Springer, Berlin Heidelberg New York Tokyo, pp 104–108

Nailfold Capillary Abnormalities in Patients with Connective Tissue Diseases

Hildegard R. Maricq[1]

Introduction

Pathological changes in the microvasculature are found in many patients with connective tissue diseases and can often be observed in vivo by capillary microscopy. The nailfold capillary bed has been the main site for such observations, although this technique can also be applied to other areas.

A variety of morphological changes have been described in all connective tissue diseases, but the most characteristic and specific patterns of nailfold capillary abnormalities are seen in the scleroderma spectrum disorders (SDS), which include systemic scleroderma (systemic sclerosis) and closely related disorders, such as the calcinosis, Raynaud phenomenon, esophageal dysfunction, sclerodactyly, telangiectasia (CREST) syndrome, dermatomyositis, mixed connective tissue disease (MCTD), overlap syndromes with scleroderma features, and undifferentiated connective tissue disease (UCTD), which includes scleroderma patients in the preclinical stage. A study of the nailfold microvasculature in these disorders is relevant, because the fingers are frequently involved in the pathological process and are often the first site of symptoms noticed by the patient, such as Raynaud's phenomenon, sclerodactyly, or ulcerations.

Several types of techniques can be applied to the nailfold, as follows:

a) In vivo microscopic techniques
   Capillary microscopy and photomicrography
   Cinephotomicrography of nailfold capillary blood flow
   TV microscopy combined with methods to measure RBC velocity
   Fluorescence videomicroscopy
b) Capillary pressure measurements
c) Biopsy of nailfold
   Light and electron microscopy
   Immunofluorescence studies

They include in vivo microscopic techniques to investigate both morphological and functional aspects of this capillary bed and more invasive methods, such as

[1]Department of Medicine, Medical University of South Carolina, Charleston, SC 29425, USA

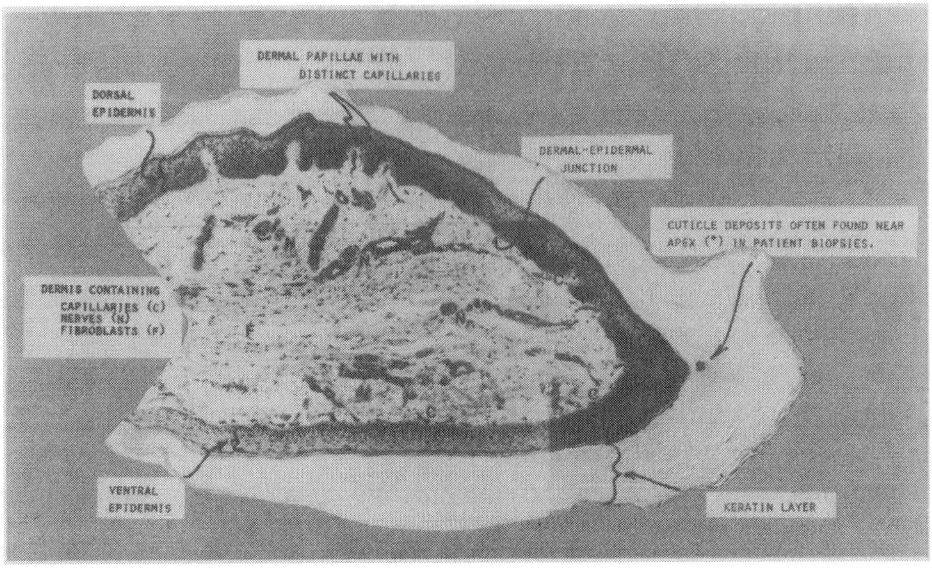

Fig. 1. Periodic acid-Schiff (PAS)-stained sagittal section of a normal nailfold. From Thompson et al. [1]

nailfold biopsy, to analyze both vascular and connective tissue elements. A cross section of the nailfold is shown in Fig. 1 [1] to display the architecture of this particular portion of the skin.

Morphological Abnormalities

The morphological abnormalities seen by means of in vivo microscopic techniques include enlargement and distortion of capillary loops, decrease in capillary density, localized avascular areas, disorganization of the normal pattern of the nailfold capillary bed, neoformation of capillaries, hemorrhagic and thrombotic phenomena, and edema formation [2].

Some of these features are observed more frequently in some scleroderma spectrum disorders than in others, e.g., "bushy" formations are seen more often in dermatomyositis than in scleroderma and are practically never seen in CREST; they seem to be associated with a more active disease process and likely represent capillary neoformation. Extremely large, giant capillaries are often associated with CREST, either in the nailfold or in clusters elsewhere; the latter correspond clinically to the punctate telangiectases characteristic of CREST.

We have shown in prospective [3] and epidemiological [4] studies that this in vivo technique is useful in detecting patients at risk for SDS because typical microvascular abnormalities are often present in the nailfold in the early, preclinical stage.

Evolution of Capillary Abnormalities

Morphological changes in nailfold capillaries are not a static end result. On serial observations, considerable changes in the nailfold capillary morphology can be seen in some SDS patients and these changes appear to parallel the clinical disease activity and severity. In others, there is little change in the nailfold capillary patterns over years of observation, especially in patients with slowly progressing disease. We have defined, therefore, "active" and "slow" patterns of SDS-type capillary abnormalities as follows. Active pattern: avascular areas of more than 2 mm^2/nailfold; bushy formations and disorganization of the nailfold capillary bed; change in number, size, and shape of capillaries on serial observations over weeks or months. Slow pattern: extremely large (giant) capillaries with no avascular areas or, if present, of less than 2 mm^2/nailfold and/or capillary telangiectases elsewhere on the hands; no or minimal change after years.

The sequence of pathological events in the nailfold has been best demonstrated in patients with dermatomyositis by serial observations documented by photography (Fig. 3). In this connective tissue disease, hemorrhagic and thrombotic phenomena and permeability changes occur first and are followed by the destruction of nailfold capillaries. Evidence of neoformation and eventual return toward normalization of the nailfold capillary bed can also be observed, which may in turn be followed by a new cycle of capillary destruction [5].

In scleroderma, observed changes occur over longer periods of time, and the transition from normal to abnormal is rarely seen. A return to normal can also occur, albeit rarely.

Capillary Blood Flow

The red blood cell velocity can be measured by different techniques, e.g., dual-window videodensitometric method [6], flying spot technique [7]. All studies have reported a remarkably slow red blood cell velocity in scleroderma patients, both in comparison with normal controls and with patients with known abnormalities in digital blood flow, such as those with primary Raynaud's phenomenon [8, 9].

The clinically most meaningful observation in scleroderma patients is a complete standstill of capillary flow in response to a cold stimulus at relatively high skin temperature, which can persist for a considerable time after the end of the stimulus [10]. This cessation of capillary blood flow can be documented by observation alone or recorded by a video or movie camera.

There is a close correlation between morphological and functional changes in the nailfold capillaries of scleroderma patients, but neither appears systematically to precede the other during the clinical course [2].

The volume flow in capillary vessels cannot be calculated by the standard in vivo techniques used in humans, because the capillary wall is invisible and only the red blood cell column is recorded. A few authors have recently attempted to estimate the true capillary diameter by injection of fluorescein isothiocyanate (FITC)-tagged albumin [11] or indocyanine green [12].

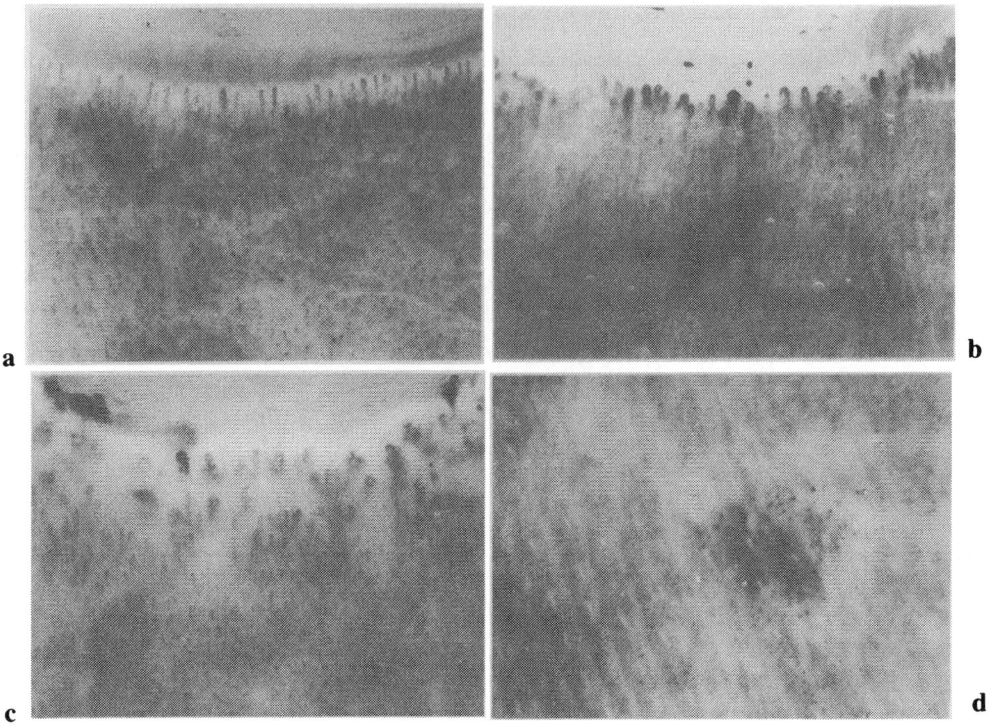

Fig. 2. **a** Example of a normal nailfold. **b** Considerably enlarged nailfold capillaries with little capillary loss in a patient with slowly progressing scleroderma. **c** Enlarged capillaries associated with extensive avascular areas in a patient with undifferentiated connective tissue disease. **d** Telangiectases composed of enlarged capillaries in a patient with CREST

Permeability of Nailfold Capillaries

Permeability changes in capillaries can already be suspected clinically by the observation of edematous fingers in the early stages of scleroderma and in MCTD. Although skin capillaries are normally permeable to sodium fluorescein, the diffusion pattern in scleroderma, both spacially and chronologically, is distinctly different from the one seen in normals and in other diseases, such as diabetes, as shown by Bollinger et al. [13], using fluorescence videomicroscopy.

Nailfold Biopsy

Since in vivo capillary observations in the human skin use reflected light and, therefore, do not allow the visualization of the capillary wall, the question could be raised as to whether the avascular areas listed under morphological in vivo observations are truly avascular or include capillaries that are empty of red blood cells. Our biopsy studies support the hypothesis of a true decrease in capillary density because there is a good correlation between the in vivo capillary counts and those taken from a biopsy specimen obtained on the same day [14].

a b c d

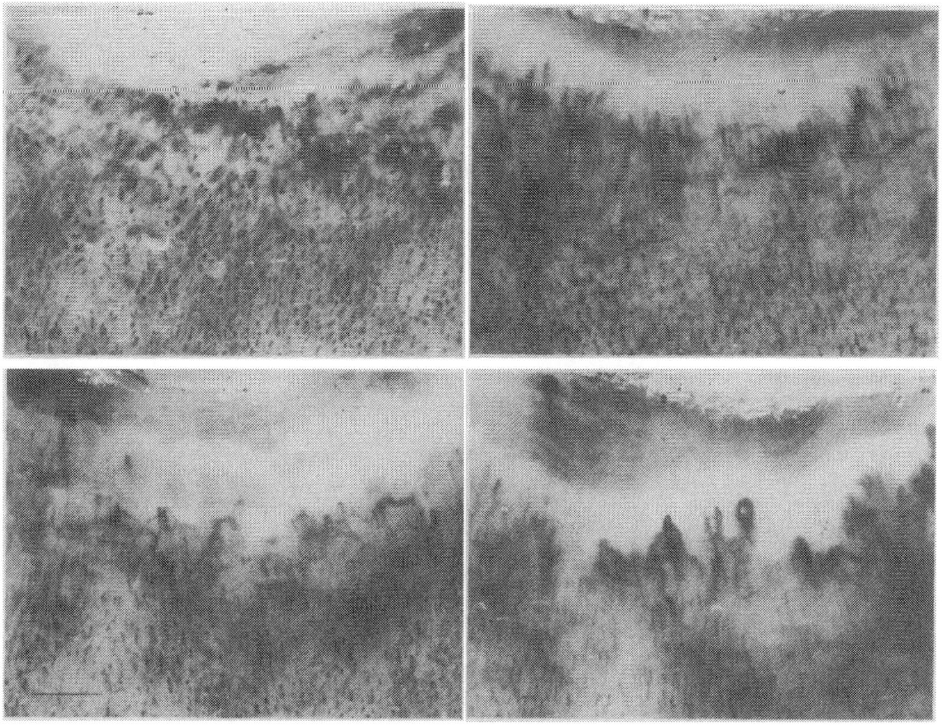

Fig. 3a–d. Evolution of microvascular lesions in dermatomyositis shown on serial photographs of the same nailfold of an 11-year-old patient. **a** Hemorrhagic and thrombotic changes 3 weeks after the first symptoms of dermatomyositis. **b** Disappearance of capillaries along the edge of the nailfold 6 weeks after the onset of illness. **c** Extensive avascular area seen at 9 weeks. **d** Pattern of nailfold capillary abnormalities typical of dermatomyositis, showing giant capillary loops, avascular areas, hemorrhages, and "bushy" formation at 3 months from the onset. *Bar* = 1 mm

A striking finding is the presence of immunoglobulins, fibrinogen C_3, and albumin in the apical portion of the nailfold and in the cuticle [15]. These deposits, seen as amorphous periodic acid-Schiff (PAS)-positive deposits under light microscopy, are correlated with the extent of the avascular areas, i.e., of apparent capillary destruction, seen by in vivo technique [14]. In vivo observations also show a diffuse yellow-orange staining of the cuticle in these patients, often associated with capillary hemorrhages, which are quite different in distribution from those seen in normal subjects or in other types of patients.

These findings suggest considerable permeability changes, both at the capillary level and at the dermoepidermal junction, which may correspond to the observations discussed in the previous section.

Conclusion

The noninvasive character of in vivo microscopic methods, the accessibility of the nailfold, and the early presence of disease manifestations in that area of the skin make nailfold capillary microscopy a useful tool for examining patients with connective tissue diseases, especially those with scleroderma spectrum disorders, for detecting subjects at risk, and for evaluating the severity and evolution of microvascular lesions and their relationship to the clinical course.

Acknowledgment. This work was supported in part by grant AR 31283 from the National Institute of Arthritis and Musculoskeletal and Skin Diseases.

References

1. Thompson RP, Maize JC, Maricq HR (1981) Histology of the nailfold in connective tissue disease. Arthritis Rheum 24: S102
2. Maricq HR (1982) The microcirculation in scleroderma and allied diseases. In: Davis E (ed) Advances in microcirculation. Karger, Basel, pp 17–52
3. Maricq HR, Harper FE, Khan MM, Tan EM, LeRoy EC (1983) Microvascular abnormalities as possible predictors of disease subsets in Raynaud phenomenon and early connective tissue disease. Clin Exp Rheumatol 1: 195–205
4. Maricq HR, McGregor AR, Diat F, Weinrich MC, Keil JE, LeRoy EC (1987) Detection of scleroderma spectrum disorders by capillary microscopy among subjects with Raynaud phenomenon in the general population. Proceedings of the Chinese Academy of Medical Sciences and the Peking Union Medical College 2 (Suppl): 65
5. Maricq HR, Silver RM (1986) Follow-up of microangiopathic lesions in childhood dermatomyositis. Arthritis Rheum 29: S91
6. Intaglietta M, Tompkins WR (1972) On-line microvascular blood cell flow velocity measurement by simplified correlation technique. Microvasc Res 4: 217–220
7. Tyml K, Ellis CG (1982) Evaluation of the flying spot technique as a television method for measuring red cell velocity in microvessels. Int J Microcirc Clin Exp 1: 145–155
8. Jacobs MJHM, Breslau PJ, Slaaf DW, Reneman RS, Lemmens JAJ (1987) Nomenclature of Raynaud's phenomenon: A capillary microscopic and hemorheologic study. Surgery 101: 136–145
9. Diat F, Intaglietta M, Weinrich MC, Maricq HR (1986) Effect of temperature on capillary blood flow in scleroderma spectrum disorders and in Raynaud phenomenon. Int J Microcirc Clin Exp 5: 259
10. Maricq HR, Downey JA, LeRoy EC (1976) Standstill of nailfold capillary blood flow during cooling in scleroderma and Raynaud's syndrome. Blood Vessels 13: 338–349
11. Mahler F, Kneubuhl F (1981) Application of fluorescein-tagged albumin in human nailfold capillaries. 11th European Conference on Microcirculation, Garmisch-Partenkirchen, 1980. Bibl Anat 20: 684–687
12. Moneta G, Brulisauer M, Jager K, Bollinger A (1986) Infrared fluorescence videomicroscopy of skin capillaries with indocyanine green. Int J Microcirc Clin Exp 5: 252
13. Bollinger A, Jager K, Siegenthaler W (1986) Microangiopathy of progressive systemic sclerosis. Evaluation by dynamic fluorescence videomicroscopy. Arch Int Med 146: 1541–1545
14. Thompson RP, Harper FE, Maize JC, Ainsworth SK, LeRoy EC, Maricq HR (1984) Nailfold biopsy in scleroderma and related disorders. Correlation of histologic, capillaroscopic and clinical data. Arthritis Rheum 27: 97–103
15. Chen Z, Dobson RL, Ainsworth SK, Silver RM, Rust PF, Maricq HR (1985) Immunofluorescence in skin specimens from three different biopsy sites in patients with scleroderma. Clin Exp Rheumatol 3: 11–16

The Interaction of Immune Complexes in Microcirculatory Impairment in Patients with Vasculitis

TERENCE J. RYAN[1]

Vasculitis is an inflammatory response as a consequence of injury to small vessels. However, a concept popular during the past decade is that vasculitis is an immunological response, but many factors other than immunological processes are responsible for the final pathology and clinical picture of vasculitis [1, 2]. The injury done to blood vessels produces changes in their perfusion, damage to the endothelium with exhaustion of many of its functions, leakiness so that materials of all kinds can finally escape into the tissues, and during the process of repair, angiogenesis gives rise to abnormal or changed vascular patterns [3].

The functions of the endothelium are now so many that the understanding of its response to injury in vasculitis requires a knowledge of coagulation, fibrinolysis, lipoxygenesis and many enzyme activities responsible for detoxicating pharmacological and biochemical agencies released in the neighbourbood of blood vessels. Many of these account for the localisation of numerous white cells within the lumen or wall of the vessel or in the surrounding tissues. Particularly, those processes leading to complement activation are responsible for neutrophil accumulation. Other less well-studied systems account for lymphocytes accumulating in the area of injury.

In Fig. 1, some of the components of the immunological attack on the vessel are illustrated, such as complexes of antibody, antigen and complement in contact with the endothelium. It illustrates that when there is a complex in which antibody is in excess of antigen, it is soluble, diffuses widely, and is usually harmless since it is phagocytosed by cells and cleared by the lymphatics [4]. When antigen is greatly in excess, a different kind of immune complex develops, which is less soluble, often more damaging, and tends to localise wherever the vasoactive agent encourages permeability of the vessel or where there is contact with macrophages or neutrophils. The more damaging kind of complex arises when there is overwhelming infection, overwelming breakdown of tissues such as the autoimmune processes of lupus erythematosus, or overwhelming breakdown of tumours. The main effect of the agents which cause vasculitis is to activate neutrophils. Besides complement, leucotrienes and fibrin degradation products, ischaemia and reperfusion play some part in the injury that results from immune complexes. Ischaemia and reperfusion will be mentioned later because of the

[1]Department of Dermatology, Slade Hospital, Headington, Oxford, OX3 7JH, England

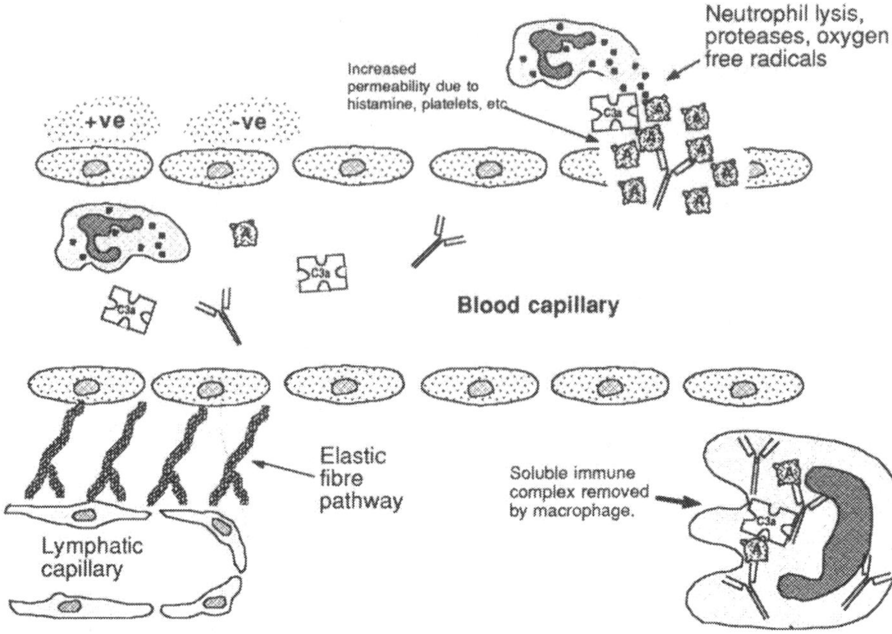

Fig. 1. Principal factors determining damage by immune complexes

role of oxygen free radicals. The combination of impaired perfusion, exhaustion of endothelial cells and leakiness, together with changes in vascular pattern resulting during repair, leads to a vulnerable and exhausted vascular system. This system is then repetitively the site of urticaria, purpura, and ischaemic necrosis. If one imagines a spectrum of activity along a vessel ranging from slight leakiness to typical palpable purpura with white cells and red cells escaping, to a vessel which is completely blocked, due to aggressive injury, then one can explain the spectrum either by the virulence of the immune complex or by gradual exhaustion of the most protective mechanisms in the wall of the blood vessel. Some sites in the body are already exhausted when they meet their first noxious trigger. They include wounds and scars, but they also include, as in Shwartzman's phenomenon, sites which have recently experienced damage from bacteria such as *Escherichia coli* at any time between 12 h and 100 days. They include, as in the "delay phenomenon" known to plastic surgeons, sites which have been recently subjected to ischaemic insult, and over the course of a week have adapted to the ischaemia. There are some tissues of the body, which I have emphasised, are permanently exhausted of protective mechanisms. These include areas such as the lower leg, which experiences gravitational stasis, and the anterior nasal septum, which is a rich, slow-flowing venous system and always slightly hypoxic [5]. In meningococcal septicaemia, a range of injuries from urticaria to ischaemic necrosis can be observed, showing, different clinical patterns due to the localisation of meningococcus at different sites. This range of clinical patterns is explained not so much by the noxiousness of the trigger itself but by the host response. An important feature of the more necrotising and damaging aspects of vasculitis is ischaemic necrosis, and wherever a purpura leads to so much inflammation that the smallest blood vessels are blocked, the blood flow through the incoming artery will also be affected and the purpuric lesion will become necrotic due to ischaemia. Studies of ischaemia have shown that certain cells are more susceptible than others, and in the skin it is the fat lobule and the smooth muscle of the arterial wall which are most susceptible to ischaemia [6]. Only 2 h of poor perfusion can lead to the death of such cells though the epidermis can survive up to 24 h of poor perfusion [1, 3].

It is important to understand the differencs in venules and arteries [3]; venules, which normally have low oxygenation, are vulnerable but not easily injured by hypoxia. Arteries, on the other hand, are not normally leaky, they are not normally exhausted, but they normally exist in an atmosphere of high oxygenation; they have poor resistance to ischaemia. Particularly, the smooth muscle of the arterial wall suffers very rapidly when there is an absence of perfusion. Certain factors in the arterial wall predispose it to additional injury. One of them is high blood pressure and either a hypertensive or hypotensive episode can mean that a vasculitis is more damaging in the region of an artery. Coagulation and platelet thrombi frequently play a part in the determination of injury to the vessel wall, but in fact most commonly the arteries are affected by poor perfusion because distal vessels are blocked by the inflammatory process of vasculitis. The clinical picture of vasculitis can occur from entirely non-immunological processes affecting ischaemic necrosis; an example of this is secondary hyperparathyroidism of renal disease, in which there is blockage of skin vessels by calcium deposits; another example is that of atheromatous emboli from the lower end of the aorta leading to multiple infarcts in the lower legs.

The problem of localisation is of particular interest and has been studied in my department in a number of PhD studies [7], including that of Kanan [5], who showed that the high incidence of vasculitis in the anterior septum of the nose and the high incidence of the localisation of bacteraemia, such as in leprosy or tuberculosis, accounting for a number of diseases of the anterior part of the nose, including vasculitis of Wegener's type, can be explained by the fact that the venules in the anterior septum are already vulnerable. They are vulnerable in respect of being leaky, hypoxic and to some extent, exhausted of many of their protective functions. Kanan showed that any particulate matter injected into the blood stream, provided it is in excess of that which Kupffer's cells of the liver can take up, will find its way to the nose and localise in the venules of the anterior septum. Because vasculitis and some of these bacterial diseases seen to be worse either in pregnant animals or animals exposed to the cold, Kanan studied the effects of castration and the giving of oestrogen in one set of animals and the effect of exposure to cold in others. In both the cases, increased localisation of particulate matter in the venules of the nose could be demonstrated [7].

There have been papers on oxygen free radicals in vasculitis [8], which point out that there are a number of protective enzymes, such as superoxide dismutase and catalase, which are damaged by a process of ischaemia so that when the tissues are reperfused the oxygen cannot be properly used and therefore it damages by inappropriate metabolism of oxygen free radicals. It is thought that this process can occur in the impaired perfusion-reperfusion state of vasculitis. Another new concept is that the tissues have domains where, because of heparan

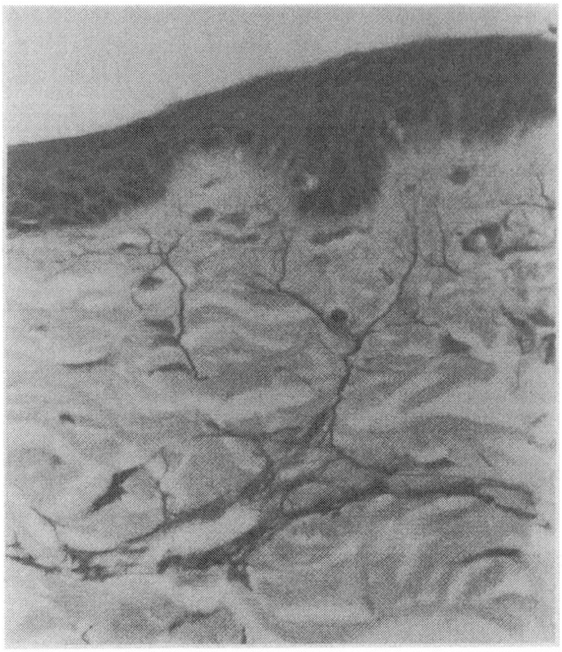

Fig. 2. Elastin and its association with the dermal lymphatics are ideally placed as low-resistance pathways for the passage of macromolecules through the interstitium

sulphate and other materials in the ground substance, cationic proteins tend to localise at so-called anionic sites. This has been studied in the lung and the kidney and, more recently, in the skin [9] and there are certainly sites within the skin where complexes may be localised because they have the appropriate charge

Another concept which has interested me during the last 3 years has been the possibility that damage to the lymphatics also plays a part in vasculitis. It has to be understood that the lymphatics are responsible for the removal, in partnership with macrophages, of all proteins, all immune complexes and all particulate matter, and that none of these agents normally is removed via the blood stream. We have demonstrated that the preferential or low-resistance pathway into the lymphatics may well be along the elastin fibre (Fig. 2), as previously demonstrated by Hauck [10] in the mesentery. As Parish has shown, the elastin fibre is damaged very early on by neutrophil elastases in pathological conditions such as vasculitis [11]. Elastases of membrane bound to monocytes are of significance to granuloma [12]. Elastin fibres are also damaged by bacterial infection, which may explain how bacteria in the skin are not usually cleared by the lymphatics [13].

Some of our studies on the level within the skin at which the lymphatics are most efficient have shown that if one injects macromolecules deeply into the skin, particularly into the fat lobule, almost no clearance takes place [14]. I suspect that this may partially explain the localisation of erythema nodosum in the deep dermis and fat. Following, for instance, a streptococcal sore throat, soluble complexes are leaked out through the tissues quite indiscriminately. But in most tissues, they are quickly removed and cause no damage. In the fat lobule, where leaky vessels are physiological and equipped with receptors to aid the passage of albumin, other macromolecules cannot be immediately removed because there is no satisfactory macrophage or lymphatic system. I believe that more studies need to be done in this respect, if only because none have so far looked at the role of the lymphatics in partnership with the macrophage in the fat in these diseases. Nor in respect to common problems of acne vulgaris or psoriasis have low-resistance pathways for the clearance of macromolecules been thoroughly investigated. Aberrant pathways could account for damage by soluble immune complexes simply because such routes are not as well equipped to deal with them as the lymphatics and lymph nodes.

References

1. Ryan TJ (ed) (1976) Microvascular injury, Major problems in dermatology, vol. 7. Lloyd Luke, London
2. Ryan TJ, Wilkinson DS (1986) Vasculitis and angiitis. In: Rook A, Wilkinson DS, Ebling FJG, Champion RH, Burton JL (eds) Textbook of dermatology, 4th edn. Blackwell, Oxford, pp 1121–1185
3. Ryan TJ (1980) Anatomical features relevant to vasculitis. In: Wolff K, Winkelmann RK (eds) Vasculitis. Major problems in dermatology, vol. 10. Lloyd Luke, London, pp 25–30
4. Ueki H, Masuda T (1982) Immune complex and cutaneous disease. Dermatology (Japan) 9: 255–264
5. Kanan MW, Ryan TJ (1976) Localisation of granulomatous diseases and vasculitis in the nasal mucosa. In: Ryan TJ (ed) Microvascular injury. Major problems in dermatology, vol. 7. Lloyd Luke, London, pp 195–220
6. Willms-Kretschmer K, Majno G (1969) Ischaemia of the skin. Am J Pathol 54: 327–343
7. Kanan MJ (1975) The biological behaviour of the nasal mucosa towards blood borne particulate matter. D. Phil Thesis, Oxford University
8. Miyachi Y, Yanase K, Imamura S, Niwa Y (1982) Increased hydroxyl radical generation by normal polymorphonuclear leukocytes incubated in sera from patients with leukocytoclastic vasculitis. Arch Dermatol Res 274: 65–71
9. Joselow SA, Gown A, Mannik M (1985) Cutaneous deposition of immune complexes in chronic serum sickness of mice induced with cationized or unaltered antigen. J Invest Dermatol 85: 559–563
10. Hauck G (1982) The connective tissue space in view of lymphology. Experientia 38: 1121–1122
11. Parish WE (1985) Cutaneous elastin degradation in ageing and inflammation. J Appl Cosmetol 3: 187–210
12. Hsu PS, Izaki S, Hibino T, Izaki M (1986) Elastase activity in granulomatous inflammation in experimental murine leprosy. Exp Mol Pathol 45: 84–92
13. DeLong TG, Simmons RL (1982) Role of lymphatic vessels in bacterial clearance from early soft-tissue infection. Arch Surg 117: 123–128
14. Ryan TJ, Mortimer PS, Jones RL (1986) Lymphatics of the skin: neglected but important. Int J Dermatol 10: 411–417

Decubital Ulcers of Pads Induced by Hyperlipidemia in the Rabbit

CHIYOJI OHKUBO and MAKISHIGE ASANO[1]

Introduction

There have been many hypotheses concerning the pathogenesis of atherosclerosis and no single one has thus far completely been able to explain it. We have noticed a high incidence of ducubital ulcers of the pads during cholesterol-induced hyperlipdemia in the rabbit [1–3]. In the present study, we tried to elucidate the etiological factors of decubital ulcers of pads induced by experimental hyperlipidemia from hemorheological aspects of the cutaneous microcirculation in the rabbit.

Materials and Methods

Two groups of six male rabbits weighing about 3.0 kg were fed a regular diet (Cont. group) or one supplemented with 1.5% cholesterol (CH group) for 12 weeks. All rabbits had a transparent round table chamber (rabbit ear chamber, REC) [4], in which the microvascular net regenerated and matured completely. The animals were subjected to vital microscopic observation on the microvascular net, biochemical and hematological analyses of the macrocirculatory blood every 3 weeks, and visual inspection of decubital ulcers of the pads weekly.

Results

Development of Decubital Ulcers of Pads

The ulcers developed in the CH group by the 6th week (Table 1), at an incidence of 3/6 according to the number of cases or 7/24 according to the number of ulcerous pads. However, no ulcers were noticed in the Cont. group until the end of the experimental period. The typical appearance of the ulcers is presented in Fig. 1.

[1]Department of Physiological Hygiene, The Institute of Public Health, 6–1, Shirokanedai 4-chome, Minato-ku, Tokyo, 108 Japan

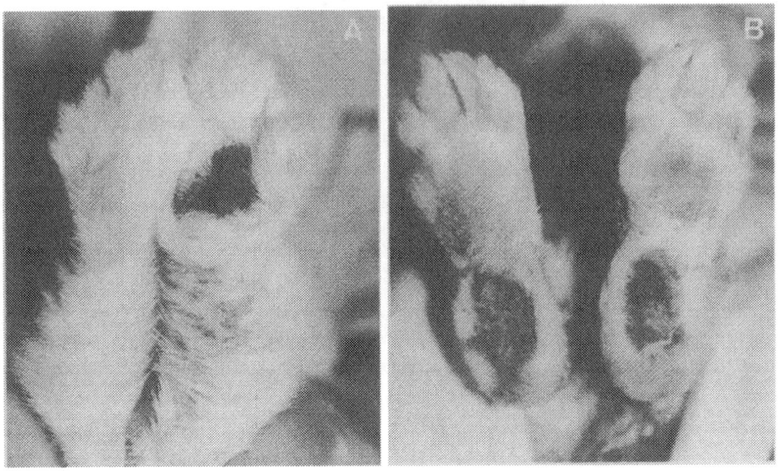

Fig. 1A, B. Typical decubital ulcers of pads of **A** fore- and **B** hindlimbs at the end of the experiment

Changes in Plasma Lipid Levels

Progressive and profound hyperlipidemia (total CH, β-lipoproteins, phospholipds, triglycerides) developed in the CH group, while no appreciable changes were observed in the Cont. group, as shown in Fig. 2.

Changes in Hematological Measurements

Definite macrocirculatory changes such as decreases in red blood cell (RBC) count, hematocrit value, and hemoglobin concentration and increases in white blood cell (WBC) adhesiveness [5] and erythrocyte sedimentation rate (ESR) were developed in the CH group. On the other hand, noticeable changes were not observed in the Cont. group in any parameters, as shown in Fig. 3.

Vital Microscopic Findings of Microcirculation

Although there were no appreciable changes in the cutaneous microcirculation within the REC of the Cont. group throughout the experimental period for 12 weeks, marked and persistent microcirculatory hemorheological changes were developed until the end of the period of CH feeding in the CH group; these changes are chronologically summarized in Table 1.

Six hours after initiation of the CH-supplemented diet, intravascular WBCs became very adhesive to the endothelial surfaces of both venules and capillaries. In addition to increased numbers of the rolling WBCs passing a given venule, some of them adhered singly or in groups to the vascular walls for periods of over 10 min, as shown in Fig. 4; however, they were eventually taken up by circulating WBCs. The masses of adhering WBCs resembled thrombi, but

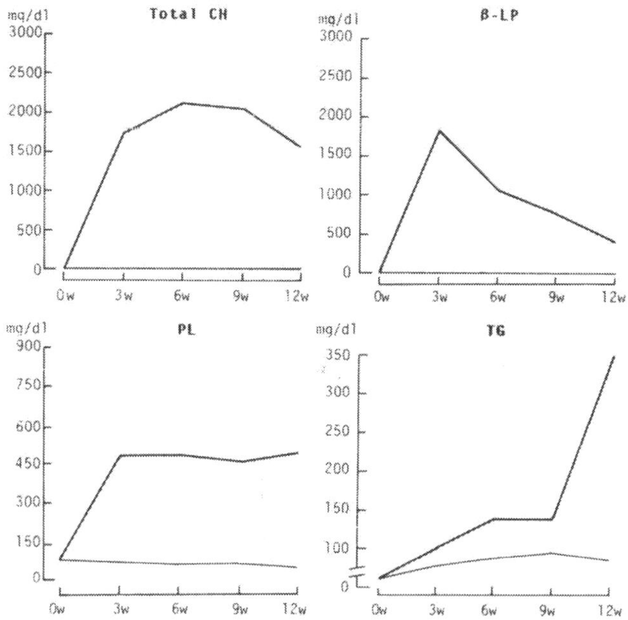

Fig. 2. Chronological changes in plasma lipid levels induced by cholesterol feeding during a period of 12 weeks ($n = 6$). *Thin* and *bold lines* represent mean values for control and cholesterol groups, respectively. *Total CH* total cholesterol, *β-LP* β-lipoprotein, *PL* phospholipid, *TG* triglyceride

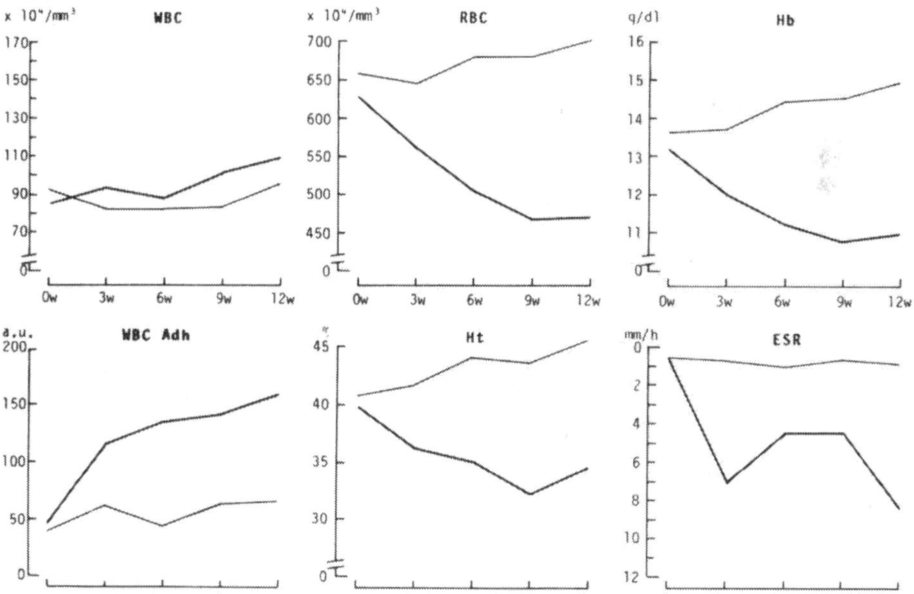

Fig. 3. Chronological changes in hemorheological parameters induced by cholesterol feeding during a period of 12 weeks ($n = 6$). *Thin* and *bold lines* represent mean values for control and cholesterol groups, respectively. *WBC* white blood cell counts, *WBC Adh* white blood cell adhesiveness, *RBC* red blood cell counts, Ht *hematocrit values, Hb* hemoglobin concentrations, *ESR* erythrocyte sedimentation rates

Table 1. Chronological changes in the cutaneous microcirculation induced by cholesterol feeding in male rabbits

	Before	6 h	24 h	1 wk	3 wks	6 wks	9 wks	12 wks
White blood cells								
Increased number	−	++	+++	+++	+++	+++	+++	+++
Lodging	−	++	+++	+++	+++	+++	+++	+++
Plugging	−	++	+++	+++	+++	+++	+++	+++
Thrombus-like structure	−	++	+++	+++	+++	+++	+++	+++
Pavement-like alignment	−	−	+	+	+	+	+	+
Red blood cells								
Rouleau formation	−	−	−	+	++	+++	+++	+++
Sludging	−	−	−	+	++	+++	+++	+++
Bleeding	−	−	−	+	+	+	+	+
Stasis	−	+	+	+	+	+	+	+
Plasma, skimming[a]	−	−	−	+	++	+++	+++	+++
Endothelia, swelling	−	−	−	+	++	++	++	++
Macrophages, amorphous proliferation	−	−	−	+	++	+++	+++	+++
Ulcers of pads, ulceration rate ($n = 6$)	−	−	−	−	−	3/6	3/6	3/6

[a] Refers to abnormal occurrence

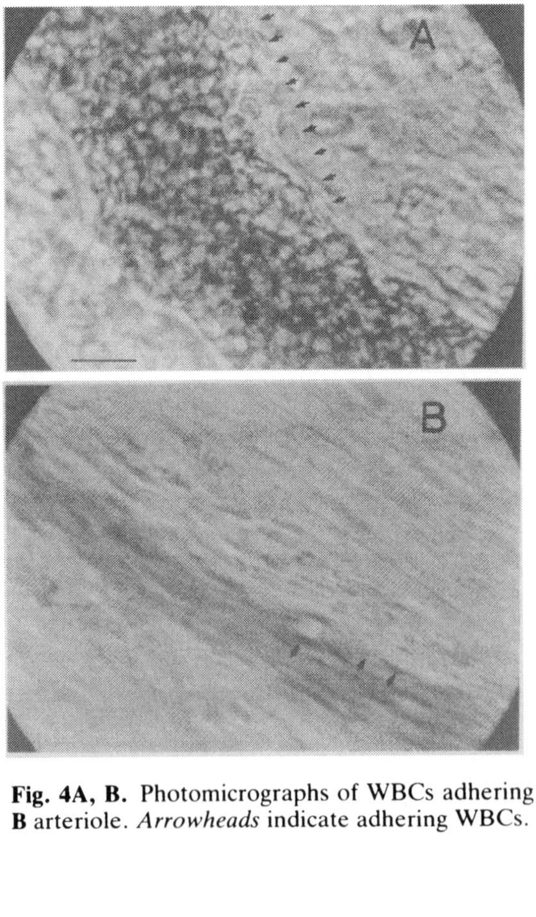

Fig. 4A, B. Photomicrographs of WBCs adhering to the lumenal walls of **A** venule and **B** arteriole. *Arrowheads* indicate adhering WBCs. *Bar* 20 μm

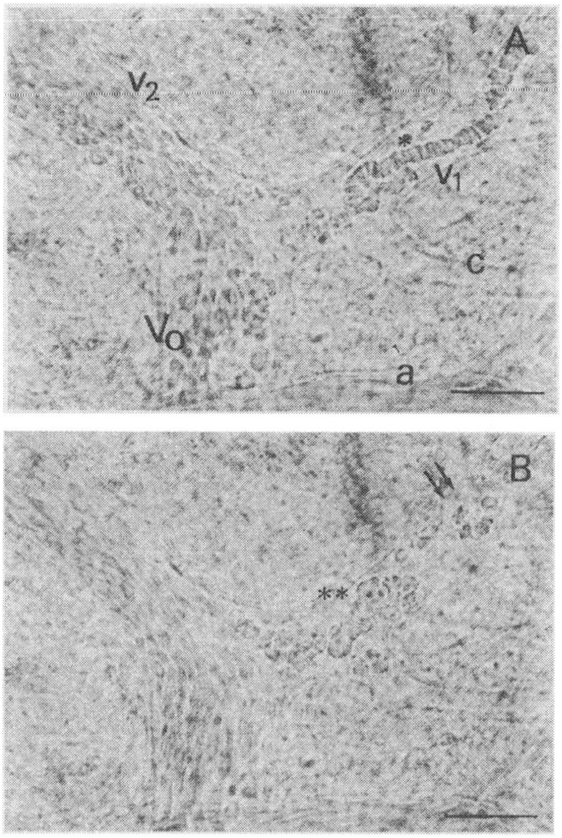

Fig. 5A, B. Photomicrographs of RBCs abnormally aggregating in postcapillary vessels. Between **A** and **B** an interval of 5 min was intercalated. RBCs forming rouleaux and sludges are indicated by *single* and *double asterisks* in the same venule (V_1), respectively. *Double arrow* indicates echinocytes. *Bar* 40 μm. *a* arteriole, V_0, V_1, V_2 venules, *c* capillary

platelets appeared not to participate in forming the thrombus-like structures. Within a week following the initiation of CH feeding, the visible WBCs became much adhesive and adhered even to the walls of arterioles, though they did not form large masses, as shown in Fig. 4.

In addition to the changes in the intramicrovascular behavior of WBCs, the streaming RBCs were apt to make abnormal aggregates, such as heavy rouleaux and sludges, with which many echinocytes mingled, as shown in Fig. 5; endothelial cells of postcapillary vessels began to swell in many places. In addition, within a few days after the initiation of CH feeding, large cells in the interstitial tissue space gathered in large numbers along the outer walls of postcapillary vessels, as shown in Fig. 6. The cells increased in number with time and proliferated into broccoli-like structures even in lymphatic capillaries, as shown in Fig. 7.

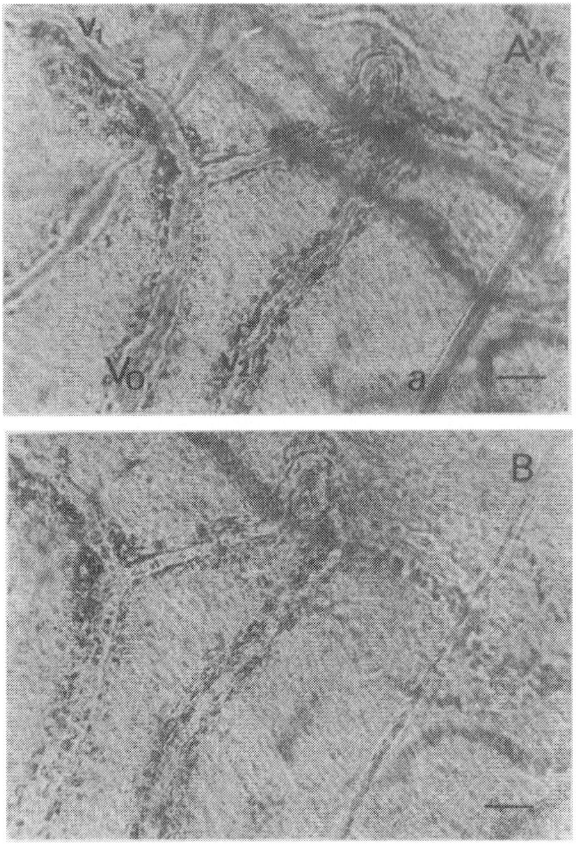

Fig. 6A, B. Photomicrographs of large cells lining the outer walls of postcapillary vessels. **A** and **B** were taken at the dilating and constricting phase of vasomotion, respectively. *a* arteriole, V_0, V_1, V_2 venules. *Bar* 40 μm

Discussion

In the present study, we demonstrated that the decubital ulcers of pads develop at a high incidence in susceptible rabbits fed CH during the development of atherosclerosis due to dietary-induced hyperlipidemias, which caused marked and persistent hemorheological changes in both the macrocirculatory and microcirculatory systems.

Intravital microscopic observation indicated that the immediate behavioral change in blood corpuscles within the REC was increased adhesiveness of WBCs. This phenomenon is well in accordance with the results obtained by an in vitro assay of WBC adhesion [5]. The increased adhesiveness of WBCs to the vessel walls observed as lodging, plugging, and thrombus-like structures may disturb normal behavior of RBCs. The present study indicates that remarkable changes in WBC adhesiveness may help to confer one of the etiological forms of

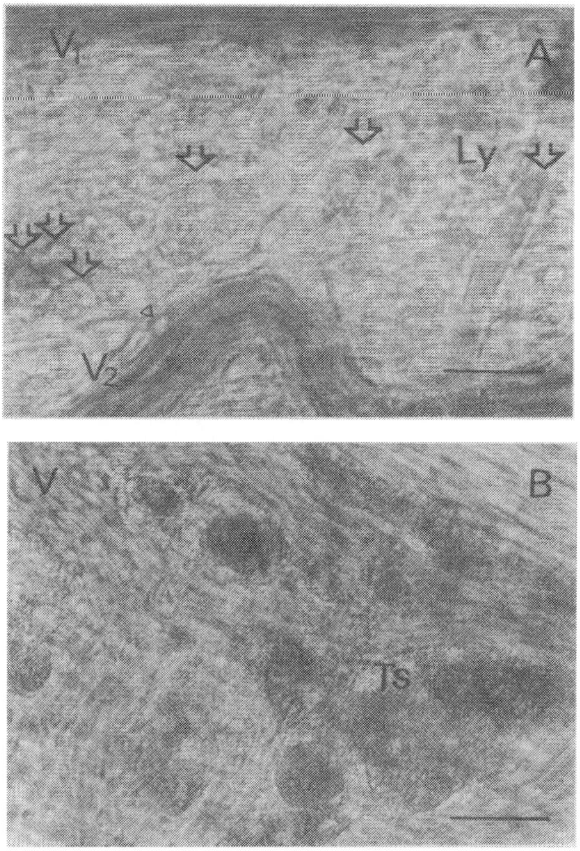

Fig. 7A, B. Photomicrographs of large cells containing numerous droplets in **A** a lymphatic capillary (*Ly*) and **B** interstitial tissue spaces (*Ts*). *Large arrowheads* indicate large cells and *small arrowhead* shows a WBC. *V*, V_1, V_2 venules, *Ly* lymphatic capillary. *Bar* 40 μm

the "response-to-injury hypothesis" [6] in the earliest stage of atherosclerosis. This implies an important role of WBCs in promoting the atherosclerosis without participation of the platelets. Concurrently with the microcirculatory disturbance induced by the increased WBC adhesiveness, increased RBC aggregation observed as heavy rouleaux formation, sludging, and echinocytosis may promote tissue hypoxia. These changes in blood corpuscles may be involved in developing the decubital ulcers in combination with the concomitant systemic anemia and also with the influence of gravity.

As previously reported [3, 7], intravital microscopy at the highest magnification revealed the amorphous proliferation of large cells to include numerous droplets; postmortem histological investigation of the tissues within the REC of CH-fed animals revealed macrophages containing fats, which resembled foam cells surrounding the microvessels. The ulcers of pads were evidenced histologically to be accompanied by underlying xanthomas. Accordingly, the proliferation of macrophages within the REC partly suggests the xanthomatous process of decubital ulcers. The fact that the foam cells isolated from atheromatous lesions of the rabbit aorta exhibit some properties of macrophages [8] is also interesting with respect to the amorphous proliferation of macrophages within the REC.

In conclusion, the microcirculatory hemorheological changes detected by intravital microscopy might be important in developing the atherosclerotic decubital ulcers of pads in combination with the concomitant macrocircultory hemorheological changes and the influence of gravity during CH-induced hyperlipidemia.

Acknowledgments. This work was supported in part by grants of the Ministry of Health and Welfare and the Kanae Fundation of Research for New Medicine.

References

1. Asano M, Hirokawa A, Ohkubo C, Ogawa S, Sawanobori K, Yonekawa K (1981) Hemorheological observations on cutaneous microcirculation in cholesterol-fed rabbits. II. Possible association with systemic hematological changes. Proc Jpn Soc Biorheol 4: 162–165
2. Asano M, Hirokawa A, Ohkubo C, Ogawa S, Sawanobori K, Yonekawa K, Yotsuya T (1983) Hemorheological observations on cutaneous microcirculation in cholesterol-fed rabbits: IV. Relationships between macro- and microcirculatory behaviors of blood cells and decubital ulcers of paws during chronic hyperlipidemia. Proc Jpn Soc Biorheol 6: 147–150
3. Asano M, Ohkubo C, Hirokawa A, Sasaki A, Ogawa S, Sawanobori K (1985) Cutaneous microcirculatory changes during dietary-induced hyperlipidemia in rabbits—Possible roles in development of decubital unlers of pads. In: Tsuchiya M, Asano M, Oda M, Okazaki I (eds) Microcirculation Annual 1985. Excerpta Medica, Amsterdam, pp 338–334
4. Asano M, Yoshida K, Tatai K (1962) On in vivo observation of the behavior of microcirculation by the rabbit ear chamber technique. Seitai No Kagaku 13: 285–294
5. Ohkubo C, Asano M (1985) Changes in the adhesiveness of leukocytes during development of experimental atherosclerosis in the rabbit. In: Tsuchiya M, Asano M, Oda M, Okazaki I (eds) Microcirculation Annual 1985. Excerpta Medica, Amsterdam, pp 56–62
6. Ross R (1986) The pathogenesis of atherosclerosis—an update. N Engl J Med 314: 488–500
7. Asano M, Ohkubo C, Hirokawa A, Sasaki A, Tochihara Y, Sawanobori K, Nagano H, Chiba M, Okeda R (1986) Hemorheological studies on the macro- and microcirculation during development of dietary-induced experimental atherosclerosis. In: Isogai Y (ed) Angiopathy in relation to hemorheology—Fundamental and clinical considerations. Hoechst Japan, Tokyo, pp 19–26
8. Fowler S (1980) Characterization of foam cells in experimental atherosclerosis. Acta Med Scand [Suppl] 642: 151–158

Microangiopathy in Diabetes Mellitus

MUNEKI SAKAKURA[1], MANABU KABA[1], and NOBUKO TSUSHIMA[2]

Many complications of diabetes mellitus are widely known, while the etiology is not as yet clearly understood. It is generally suspected that hemorheological alterations and microhemodynamic changes play major roles in the pathophysiological mechanism of diabetic microangiopathy. In an attempt to clarify the etiology of diabetic microangiopathy, diabetic subjects, boderline subjects, and normal subjects were examined with respect to microhemodynamic changes in the venules on the human bulbar conjunctiva and hemorheological changes in peripheral blood before and after performing a 75 g oral glucose tolerance test (75g-OGTT).

Materials and Methods

As shown in Table 1, five groups were employed in examining the hemodynamics and hemorheology. Group A indicates patients without diabetic retinopathy, group B diabetic patients with simple retinopathy, group C patients with proliferate rentinopathy, group BD borderline subjects, and group N normal subjects.

Retinopathy was diagnosed by an ophthalmologist using the fluorescein occlular fundus angiographic technique. The clinical background of the patients is shown in Table 2. The value of hemoglobin A (HbA) in group C was significantly ($P < 0.01$) higher than that in group A and the value in group B was between that in groups A and C. The duration of illness in group C was the longest of the three groups. Many patients (65%) in group A were treated by diet only, but all patients in group C were treated with insulin or oral drugs. Group C patients suffered the most severe complications of the three groups. Microhemodynamic changes were measured before and after administration of 75 g glucose (per os).

For the observation and recording of the circulation of microvessels in the bulbar conjunctiva, an ophthalmomicroscopy technique developed by Tsushima

[1]Saiseikai-Izuo Hospital, 13–20, Izuo 4-chome, Taisho-ku, Osaka, 551 Japan
[2]National Cardiovascular Center Hospital, 7-1, Fujishirodai 5-chome, Suita, Osaka, 565 Japan

Table 1. Experimental subjects

	Group				
	N	BD	DM		
			A	B	C
n	14	11	23	20	16
M:F	10:4	8:3	19:4	16:4	9:7
Age (yrs)[a]	46 ± 3.9	50 ± 3.8	53 ± 1.9	52 ± 2.6	53 ± 1.9

N normal subjects, *BD* borderline subjects, *DM* diabetes mellitus, *A* without retinopathy, *B* with retinopathy (simple type), *C* with retinopathy (proliferate type)
[a] Means ± SD

Table 2. Clinical background

	Group			
	A	B	C	BD
n	23	20	16	11
HbA_1	6.5 ± 0.1	6.9 ± 0.2	9.6 ± 0.8	6.2 ± 0.2
Ht	42 ± 1.3	4.2 ± 1.2	41 ± 1.2	42 ± 1.3
Duration of disease (yrs)	2.0 ± 0.2	4.6 ± 0.5	8.1 ± 0.9	
Therapy				
Diet only	15/23 (65%)	3/20 (15%)	0/16 (0%)	11/11 (100%)
Oral drug	8/23 (35%)	10/20 (50%)	2/16 (12%)	0/11 (0%)
Insulin	0/23 (0%)	7/20 (35%)	14/16 (88%)	0/11 (0%)
Complications				
Neuropathy	6	6	12	0
Retinopathy	0	20	16	0
Nephropathy	0	4	10	0
Hypertension	3	8	8	4
Heart disease	4	6	7	2
Cerebral disease	0	3	5	2
ASO	0	0	2	0

HbA_I hemoglobin A, *Ht* hematocrit, *ASO* arteriosclerosis obliterans
$^{*}P<0.05$, $^{**}P<0.01$, $^{***}P<0.001$

et al. [1] and Tsushima and Nakayama [2] was used (Fig. 1). With this system, a microscope with an object lens (× 5) and a halogen lamp light source (6 V, 30 W) is connected to a video recorder system, which displays × 280 magnifications on its 20-in. screen. The internal diameters of the venules and blood flow velocities were measured on the screen. Blood flow velocities were measured using the distance meter method [1, 2], which involved an apparatus linked to a distance meter and a stop watch. Erythrocytes were followed in microvessels with a distance meter; the distance millimeters they advanced and the time (seconds) re-

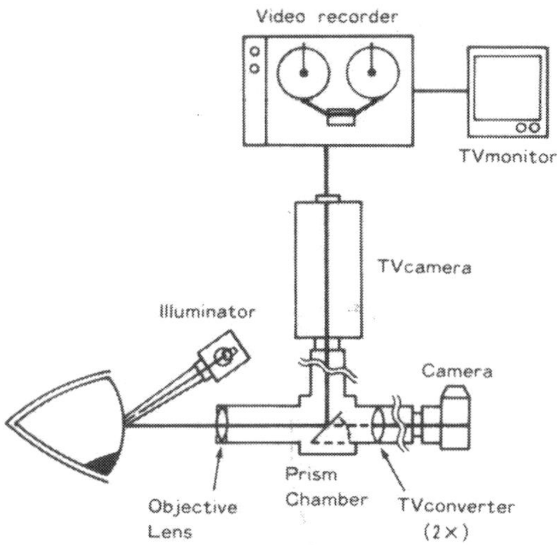

Fig. 1. System of ophthalmo-microscopy—Intra-vital-video microscopic system (IVVMS)

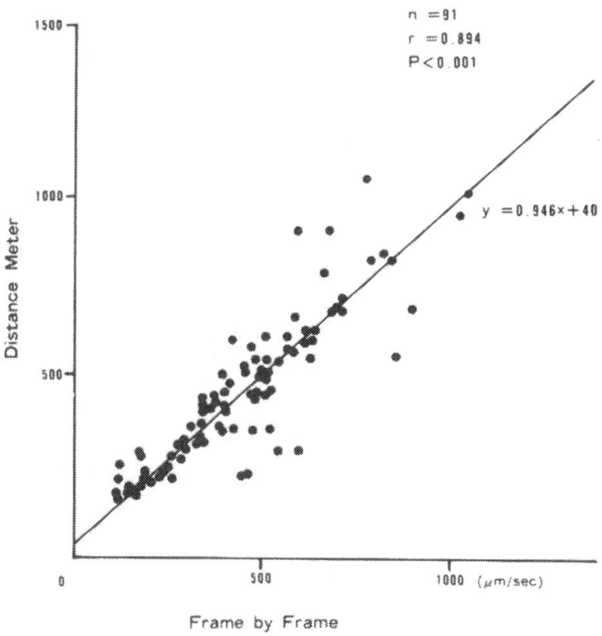

Fig. 2. Correlation between frame-by-frame and distance meter methods

quired for the advance were shown on the distance meter. There is a significant correlation between the conventional frame-by-frame method [2] and distance meter method, as shown in Fig. 2. The diameters of the erythrocyte column were used as the internal diameters of blood vessels, excluding the plasma sheath. Blood flow volume was calculated by multiplying cross-sectional area and average blood flow velocity on the assumption that the vessel cross section was circular. The microcirculation was observed and measured at the same part of the same blood vessel before and after glucose administration.

Increases in internal diameter, blood flow velocity, and blood flow volume are expressed as percentages, taking the preadministration level as 100% and the increments are represented by:

$$\text{Increment (\%)} = \frac{\text{Mean X after administration}}{\text{Mean X before administration}} \times 100 - 100$$

where mean X signifies the mean value of the diameters, velocities, and volumes. The diameters of the venules used for these examinations were about $47.7 \pm 3.4\ \mu m$.

The viscosities of whole blood were measured at high shear rate ($94.5\ s^{-1}$) and low shear rate ($0.375\ s^{-1}$) by Contraves Low Shear-30. In order to determine the deformability of erythrocytes [3], the passage times of 40% red cell suspensions through the micropore filter membrane ($5\ \mu m$) under $-10\ cmH_2O$ pressure were measured. Factors of hemocoagulation and fibrinolysis were also measured (fibrinogen, a_2-plasmin inhibitor, a_2-macroglobulin, antithrombin-III, and plasminogen). Blood samples were withdrawn from the cubital vein at 0, 30, 60, 90 and 120 min after glucose administration.

All calculated results were expressed as means ± SE. The significance was assessed using Student's *t*-test.

Results

Increments of internal diameters of the venules of the conjunctiva of diabetic patients, borderline subjects, and normal subjects after 75g-OGTT are shown in Fig. 3. The maximal increments were observed at 60 min after glucose administration in normal and borderline subjects and 90 min in diabetic subjects. In

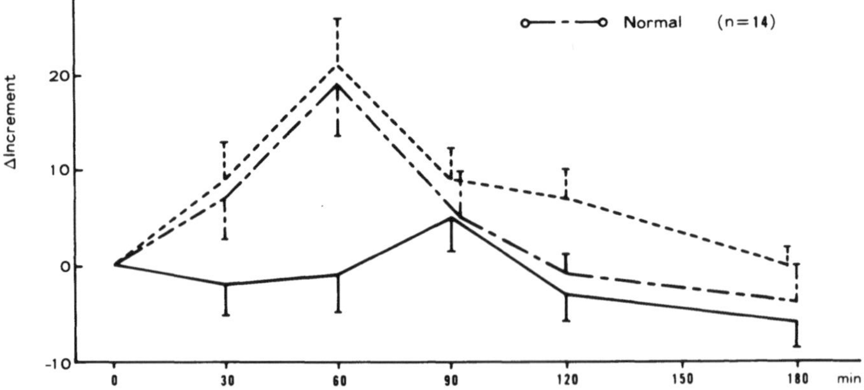

Fig. 3. Increment of internal diameter after 75g-OGTT (means ± SE)

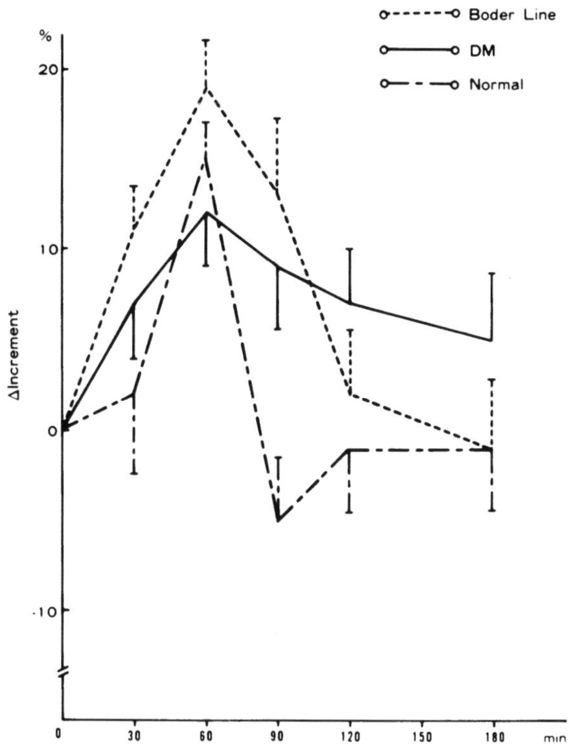

Fig. 4. Increment of blood flow velocities (means ± SE)

Fig. 4, the maximal values of flow velocities appeared 60 min after the test began. Increments of flow volumes in three groups are illustrated in Fig. 5; the maximal increments were observed 60 min after 75g-OGTT in all the groups. The largest increment was measured in the borderline group and the smallest in diabetic subjects.

From the data recorded above, the diabetic patients were divided into three subgroups—A, B, and C—and the increments of internal diameter, flow velocity, and flow volume were measured 60 min after glucose administration in groups A, B, C, BD, and N. Internal diameters of groups B and C after the test were decreased significantly ($P<0.05$) compared with groups N, BD, and A, as shown in Fig. 6, but flow velocities of group C only showed a tendency to decrease when compared with another group, as illustrated in Fig. 7.

Flow volumes of groups B and C were decreased significantly ($P<0.05$) compared with groups N, A, and BD. On the other hand, flow volume was increased significantly ($P<0.05$) compared with groups N (Fig. 8).

Viscosities of whole blood at high shear rate ($94.5\ s^{-1}$) and low shear rate ($0.376\ s^{-1}$) of group C decreased significantly ($P<0.05$) compared with groups A and BD but did not show a marked decrease compared with group N, as shown in Fig. 9. Plasma viscosities did not show significant changes after glucose administration.

The passage time of 40% erythrocyte suspensions are presented in Fig. 10 and the value of group C was increased significantly compared with groups N and A.

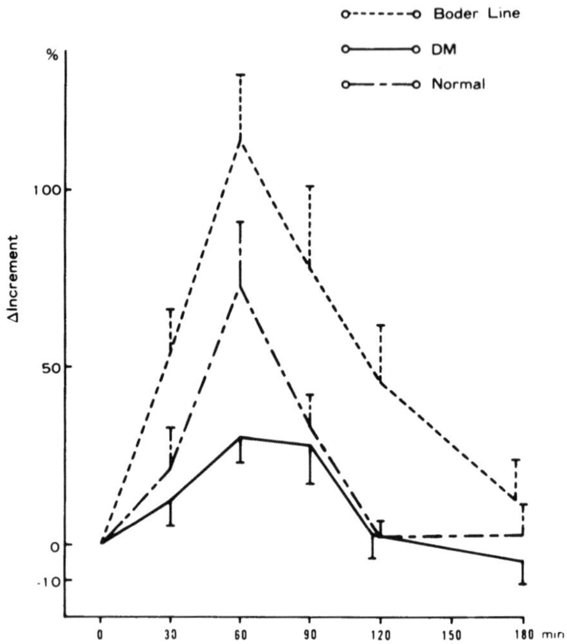

Fig. 5. Increment of blood flow volume (mean ± SE)

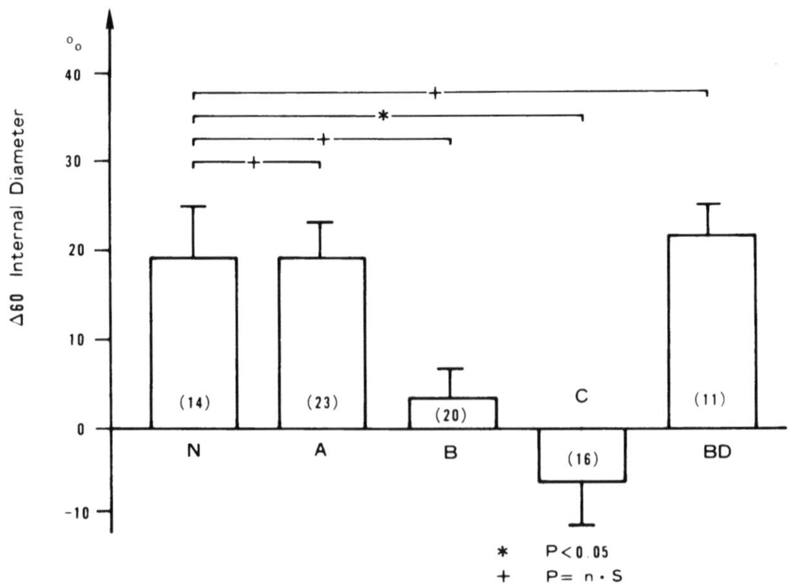

Fig. 6. Increments of internal diameter 60 min after 75g-OGTT in groups N, A, B, C, and BD. The figures in the *columns* indicate the number of experimental subjects

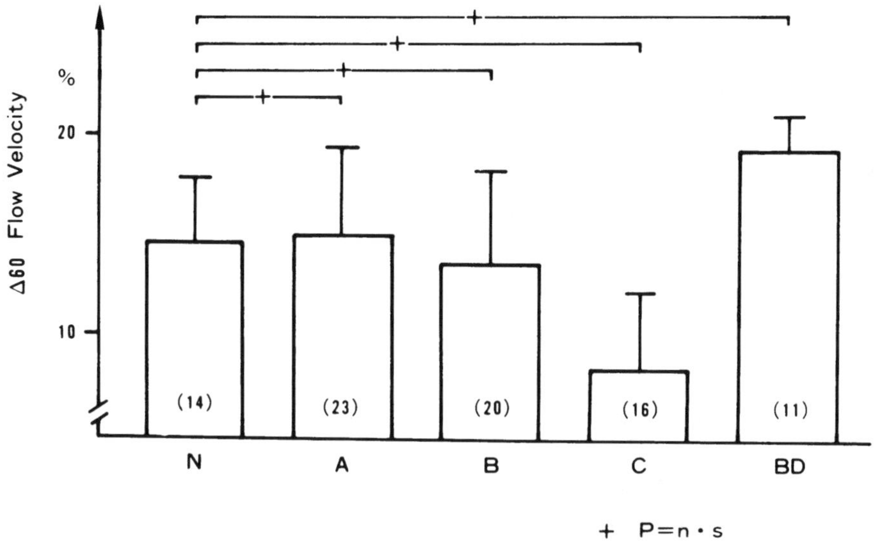

Fig. 7. Increments of blood flow velocity 60 min after 75g-OGTT

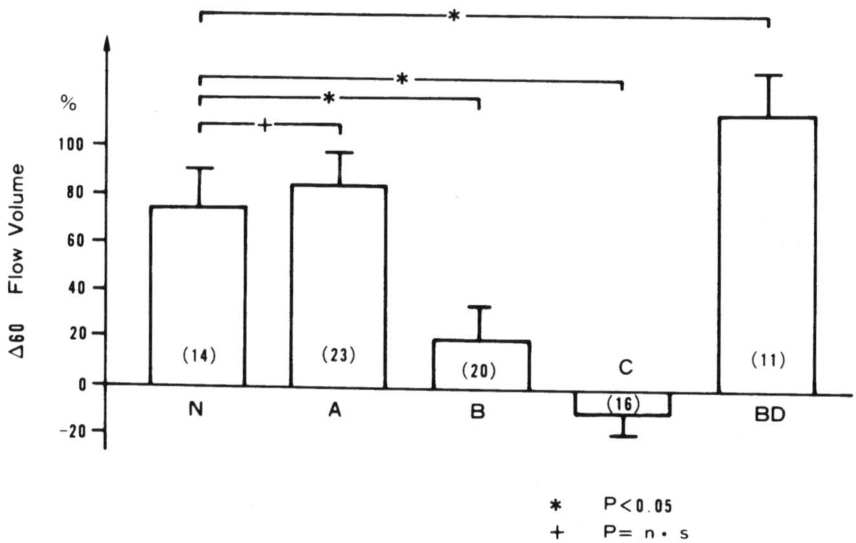

Fig. 8. Increments of blood flow volume 60 min after 75g-OGTT (mean ± SE)

The passage time of group A was significantly slower than that of group N.

Fibrinogen and a_2-macroglobulin of group C were significantly increased compared with groups A, BD, and N. On the other hand, a_2-plasmin inhibitor was significantly decreased in group C, as whown in Fig. 11.

Antithrombin-III of group C was also markedly decreased compared with groups A, BD, and N (Fig. 12).

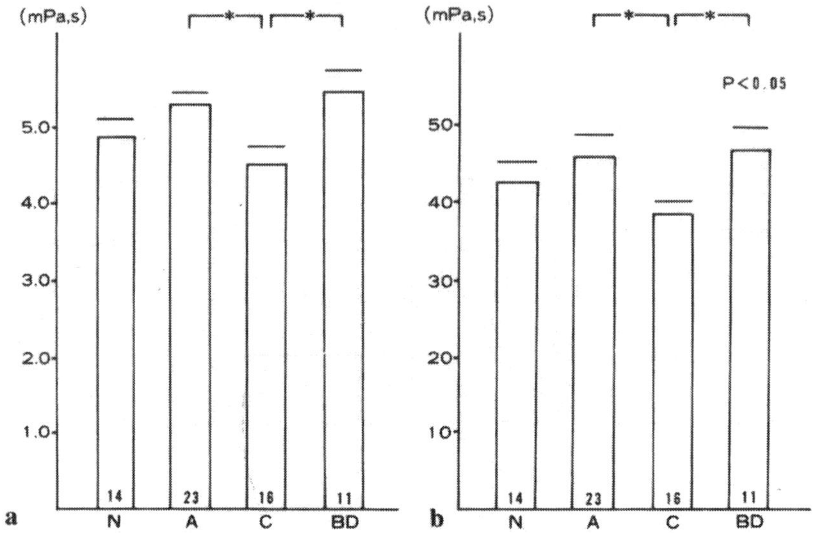

Fig. 9. Whole blood viscosity at **a** high shear rate (94.5 s) and **b** low shear rate (0.376 s)

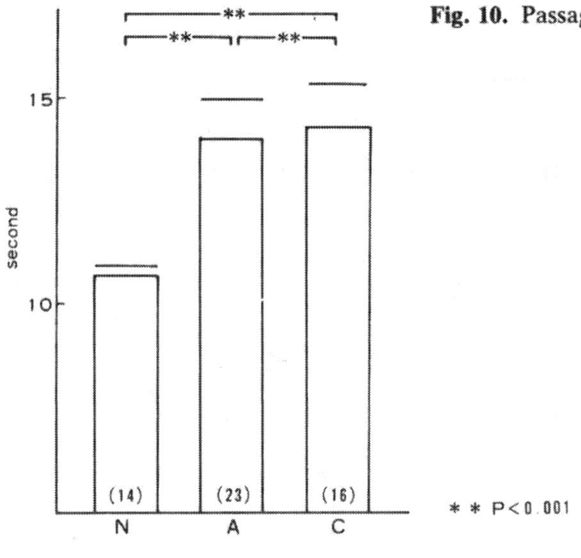

Fig. 10. Passage time of 40% RBC suspensions

Discussion

Diabetes mellitus is common, but its etiology is not as yet clearly understood. Pyke and Tattersall [4] and Leslie et al. [5] proposed that hereditary factors may play a major role in the develop the disease. On the other hand, Stout [6, 7] reported that the development of diabetes mellitus may be caused by metabolic disturbance in the peripheral organs on account of the lack of insulin action.

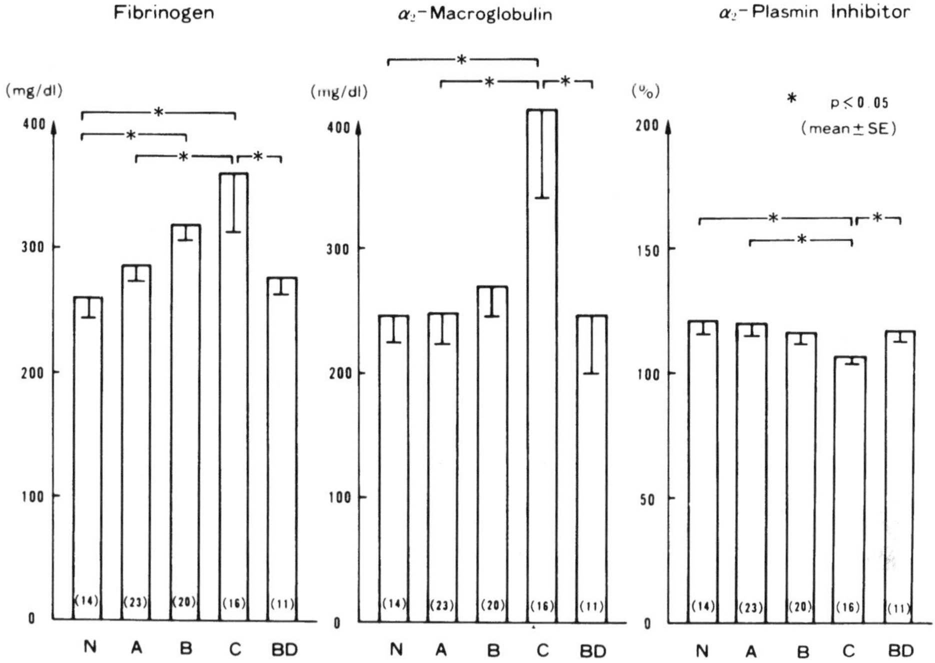

Fig. 11. Coagulation factors

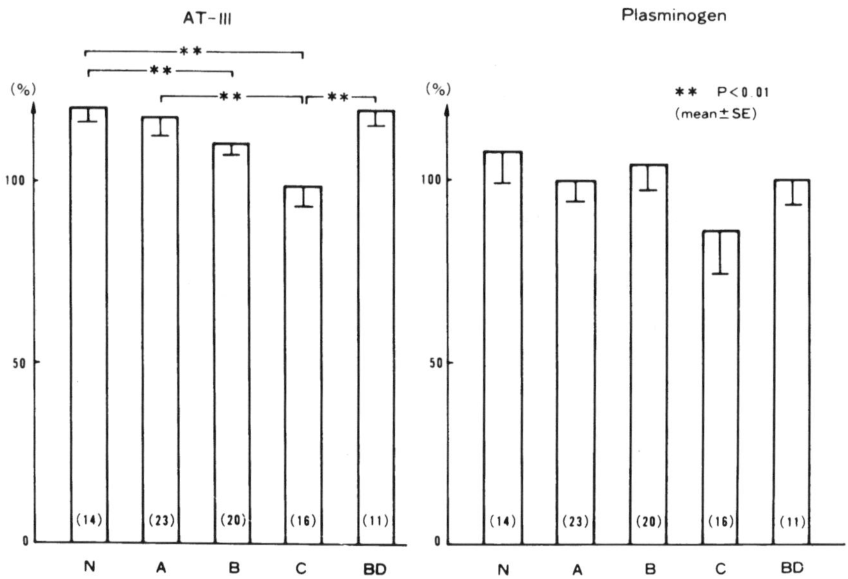

Fig. 12. Fibrinolytic factors

From our experiments, the following results were obtained. In group BD, blood flow volume increased markedly and whole blood viscosity also showed a tendency to increase compared with group N. In diabetic subjects with slignt microangiopathic changes, the deformabielity of erythrocytes was worse and whole blood viscosity and blood coagulability increased. Blood flow volume was similar to that in normal subjects. In advanced diabetes mellitus, on the other hand, the deformability of erythrocytes became more severely worse and the blood coagulability increased, but the whole blood viscosity decreased. Conversely, a fibrinolytic state existed and blood flow volume decreased.

These facts suggest that diabetes mellitus may be caused by a hereditary factor and advanced by a microangiopathic disorder. However, the causes of the microangiopathic changes in the vessels are not known. Possible explanations are: (a) Hypoxia in peripheral tissue may cause microangiopathic changes; (b) aldose reductase in the basement membrane of microvessels may be increased congenitally; and (c) hypoglycemia in cells may cause microangiopathic changes.

More data are required concerning these points to clarify the etiology.

Conclusions

Microhemodynamic disorders were observed in diabetic patients. A hypercoagulable state existed in diabetic patients with proliferate retinopathy. A borderline group showed a hyperresponse to glucose in the microhemodynamics. Whole blood viscosity of diabetic patients with proliferative retinopathy showed a significant ($P < 0.05$) decrement at both shear rates (94.5 and 0.376 s^{-1}). Deformability of erythrocytes in group C was decreased compared with groups N and A.

References

1. Tsushima N, Satoh T, Koyama T (1981) Human microcirculation (MC) by intra-vital microsopic system (IVVMS). Bibltheca Anat 20: 716–719
2. Tsushima N, Nakayama R (1983) Microcirculation of bulbar conjunctiva. Excepta Medica ICS 625: 15–28
3. Kikuchi Y, Arai T, Koyama T (1983) Improvement filtration method for red cell deformability measurement. Med Biol Eng Comput 21: 270–276
4. Pyke DA, Tattersall RB (1973) Diabetic retinopathy in identical twins. Diabetes 22: 613–618
5. Leslie RBG, Barnett AH, Pyke DA (1979) Chlorpropamide alcohol flushing and diabetic retinopathy. Lancet 1: 997–999
6. Stout RW (1979) Diabetes and atherosclerosis—The role of insulin. Diabetologica 16: 141–150
7. Stout RW (1968) Insulin stimulated lipogenesis in arterial tissue in relation to diabetes and atheroma. Lancet 2: 702–703

Microcirculation in Diabetic Gangrene

Yukihide Isogai, Nobuhiko Saito, Takao Shimada, Sanae Tanaka, and Hidetoshi Ito[1]

One of the major complications of diabetes mellitus is diabetic gangrene, which has been increasingly observed in recent years. It is very specific in its features in that: (a) the peripheral pulsation remains intact, (b) the skin temperature is high, (c) the gangrene is wet, and (d) sensory nerve disturbance is present. It is often caused by friction from shoes or by thermal wounds and has a tendency to relapse. The many reports on this complication indicate that the probable etiology of the gangrene is diabetic microangiopathy (though there are reports that the degree of microangiopathy makes no difference in the presence of the gangrene [1]) and diabetic neuropathy, causing sensory nerve disturbance (as happens in the cases where shoes and thermal injuries are involved) and autonomic nerve disturbance [2]. The latter results in the inability to control vascular tone in the peripheral circulation. However, there has been insufficient explanation as to why this type of gangrene relapses so often.

From the results of our investigations over the years, which we summarize here, we have come to the conclusion that the most important underlying factor in the development of diabetic gangrene is diabetic autonomic nerve disturbance. This is the starting point of the chain of events ending in the development of diabetic gangrene, which will also be discussed in this report.

Methods

The first of our investigations was done on the distribution of blood flow in the lower extremities of diabetics. The ^{99m}Tc-microsphere albumin (MA) intra-arterial injection method [3, 4] was used to evaluate 82 diabetics. MA is an almost spherical albumin particle, 7–25 μm in diameter, labeled with ^{99m}Tc. It was injected into both femoral arteries, and distribution pictures were taken by a gamma camera (Fig. 1a). The injected MA was distributed by the blood flow and trapped as microthrombi in peripheral vessels smaller than the MA; other MA particles passed through open arteriovenous anastomoses (AVAs) and were eventually trapped in the pulmonary capillaries (Fig. 1b). The shunt rate was

[1] 3rd Department of Internal Medicine, Jikei University School of Medicine, 25–8, Nishi-Shinbashi 3-chome, Minato-ku, Tokyo, 105 Japan

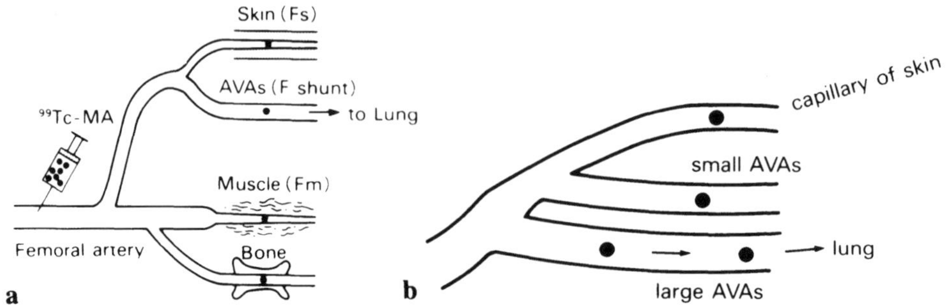

Fig. 1. a Method of ^{99m}Tc-microsphere albumin (*MA*) intra-arterial injection to observe the distribution rate of MA in muscle and skin, respectively. **b** Model of arteriovenous anastomoses (AVAs). The injected MA was trapped in a capillary smaller than the MA, other MA particles passed through open AVAs and became trapped in the pulmonary capillary network

calculated from the ratio of radioactivity in the lung and the whole body, i.e., shunt rate (%) = pulmonary radioactivity/whole body radioactivity × 100. This method is an effective way of observing the distribution of the blood flow, but, unfortunately, the actual amount of blood flow cannot be calculated. We, therefore, attempted to calculate the effective skin and muscle blood flow by the ^{133}Xe-clearance method [5]. We applied this method further to check whether the regulation of AVAs by the sympathetic nerves was intact in the diabetics as compared with healthy subjects. The effective blood flow of the calf was measured by ^{133}Xe-clearance, the total blood flow by admittance plethysmography [6, 7], and the shunt flow was then calculated from the results of the two (Fig. 2). The condition of sympathomimetic regulation was investigated by observing the changes in shunt flow by the core heating method [8]. Finally, the skin perfusion pressure of the diabetic patients was determined by application of ^{133}Xe-clearance, measuring the pressure necessary to stop local blood flow by a cuff (Fig. 3).

Results

Figure 4 shows the results obtained from the MA method. The actual configuration of the distribution is shown in Fig. 4. Two distinct types of distribution were observed: (a) the muscular (M) type—almost equivalent to the distribution in healthy subject, with the blood flow distributed mainly in the muscles; (b) the dermal (D) type—the majority of the blood flow distributed in the skin and subcutaneous tissues together with distribution into the lungs, resulting in a high-shunt ratio as well. The actual numerical values are shown in Table 1, confirming the visual findings. Since all the patients with diabetic gangrene were classified as type D, it can be assumed that this type of blood flow distribution is closely related to the pathogenesis of the gangrene.

Figure 5a indicates the results of ^{133}Xe-clearance. Though the apparent skin blood flow in the MA type D group is increased, the results of this method show the effective skin blood flow to be actually greater in type M.

Figure 5b indicates the result of a comparison of the effective and total blood

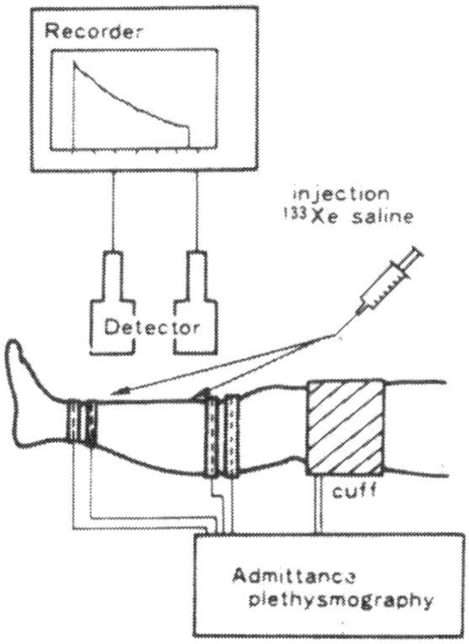

Fig. 2. Method of ^{133}Xe-clearance and admittance plethysmography following ^{99m}Tc-microsphere albumin intra-arterial injection

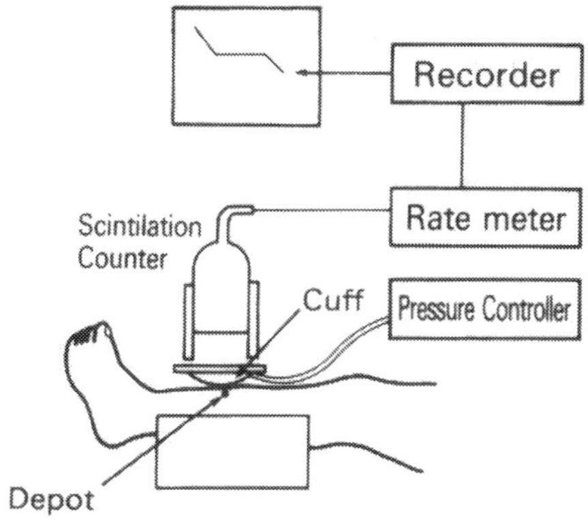

Fig. 3. Measurement of skin perfusion pressure

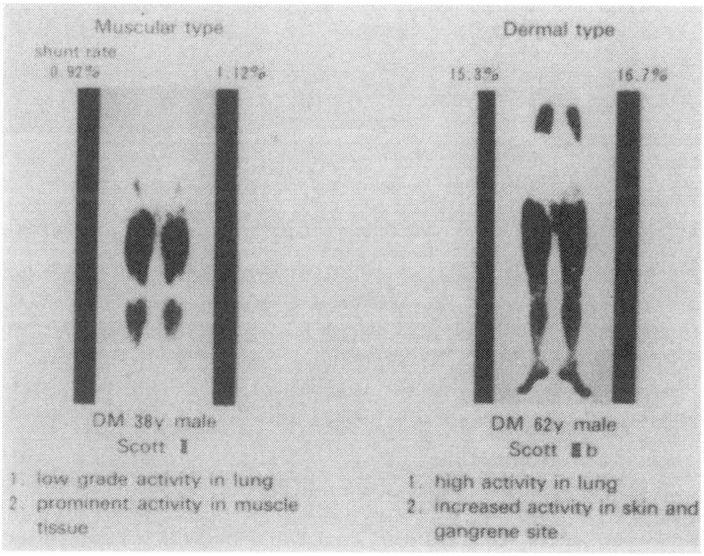

Fig. 4. Result of ^{99m}Tc-microsphere albumin intra-arterial injection

Table 1. Muscular and dermal types of distribution of ^{99m}Tc-microsphere albumin

	M type	D type
Number of cases	43/82 (52%)	39/82 (48%)
Gangrene without ASO	0/18 (0%)	18/18 (100%)
Shunt rate	1.74% ± 0.66%	7.94% ± 3.75%

M muscular, *D* dermal, *ASO* arteriosclerosis obliterance

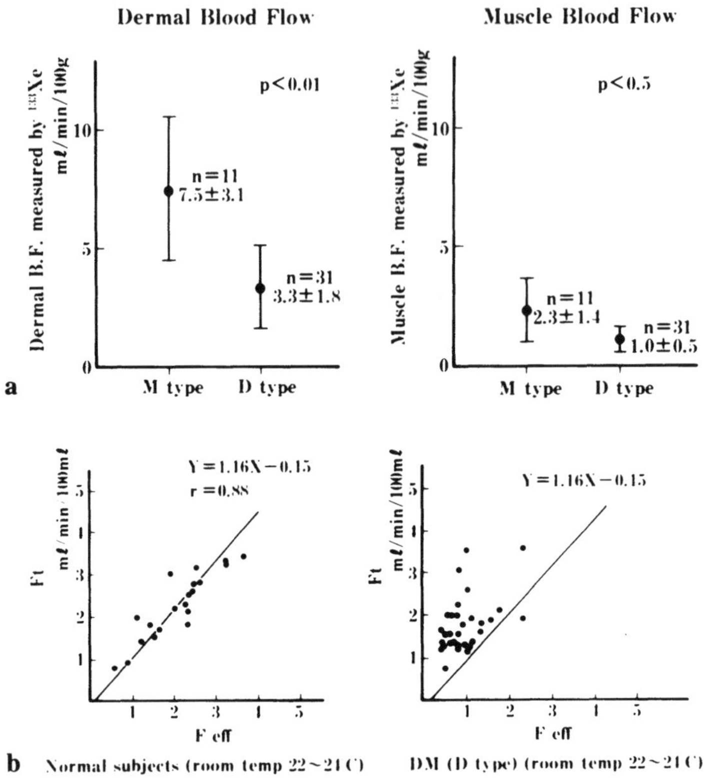

Fig. 5a, b. Results of **a** ^{133}Xe-clearance and **b** admittance plethysmography. *F eff* effective blood flow, *Ft* total blood flow

flow of the calves. At rest, healthy subjects (on the left), show a good correlation between effective and total blood flow, with the regression line at approximately 45°, while in the type D group the results are varied and no correlation can be observed.

The results of the effect of core heating on skin, muscle, and total blood flow are indicated in Fig. 6a. Figure 6b shows the change in shunt flow due to thermal stress. While the healthy subjects react well to thermal stress, the type D patients do not.

Figure 7 shows the results of skin perfusion pressure and it can be seen that it is significantly low in type D diabetics as compared with healthy subjects.

Discussion and Conclusion

From the results of the MA studies, two distinct groups of blood flow distribution were recognized and accordingly classifed as types M and D. The visualized blood flow distribution in the skin of type D patients was apparently increased. However, from the results of ^{133}Xe-clearance, it was in type M patients that the actual blood flow was greater. These apparently contradictory results imply that

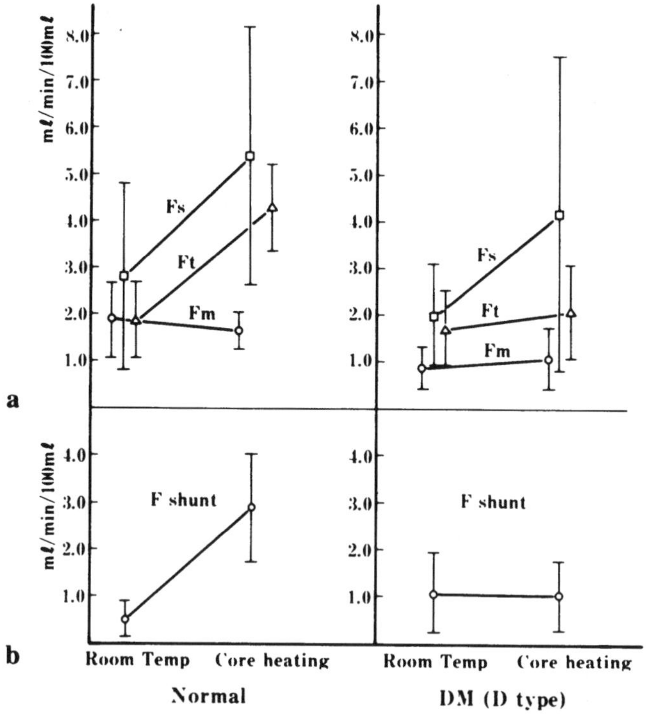

Fig. 6a, b. Result of core heating. **a** Changes in total, muscle, and skin blood flow after core heating. **b** Changes in calculated shunt flow after core heating. In normal subjects shunt flow is low at room temperature and increases markedly after core heating. No remarkable change is observed in type D diabetics (*DM*)

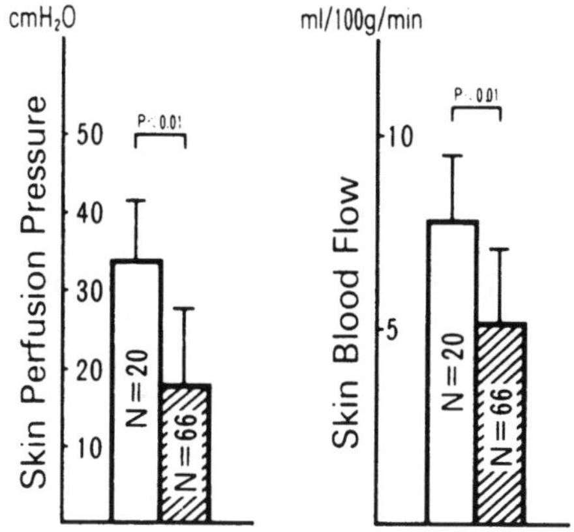

Fig. 7. Result of skin perfusion pressure measurement in normal subjects (*unshaded columns*) and diabetics (*shaded columns*)

the increased skin blood flow in MA imaging was actually a false image. We reasoned from these results that there were various sizes of AVA, and because of this, as the MA particles flowed into the AVAs, the MA smaller than the diameter of the AVA passed through and went on to be finally trapped in the pulmonary capillary bed, while those larger than the AVA were trapped at the particular location. In consequence, the increase in skin distribution of MA observed in type D patients indicated only increased shunt blood flow through the smaller AVAs. These AVAs are, in healthy subjects, regulated by the sympathetic nerves, and are opened dramatically by thermal stress [8–10]. Comparison of the reaction of effective and total blood flow and shunt rate to core heating between healthy and type D subjects showed the reaction in the type D group to be almost nonexistent, indicating that in the patients classed as type D, sympathomimetic regulation of the peripheral vasculature was impaired. These results seem to indicate that the decrease of effective skin blood flow was due to the steal phenomenon while the AVAs were opened. It can also be assumed that the decreased skin perfusion pressure in the diabetics is consistent with and supportive of this hypothesis.

In summary, we have made the following conclusions concerning the development of diabetic gangrene. First, diabetic autonomic nerve disturbance sets in. This results in the dilatation of the AVAs followed by an increase in shunted blood flow. This, in turn, brings about the steal phenomenon in the skin blood flow. This reduction in skin blood flow is also evidenced by the fact that in such subjects, reduction in skin perfusion pressure is observed. It is this continual decrease in skin blood flow that finally results in diabetic gangrene and its protraction.

References

1. Strandness DE, Pruest RE, Gibbons GE (1964) Combined clinical and pathologic study of diabetic and nondiabetic peripheral arterial disease. Diabetes 13: 366–372
2. Grover-Johnson NM, Baumann FG, Imparato AM, Kim GE, Thomas PK (1981) Abnormal innervation of lower limb epineurial arterioles. Diabetologia 20: 31–38
3. Rhodes BA, Greyson ND, Siegel ME, Giargiana FA (1973) The distribution of radioactive microspheres in patients with peripheral vascular disease. Am J Roentgenol Radiother Nucl Med 118: 820–826
4. Spence RJ, Rhocles BA, Wagner HN (1972) Regulation of arteriovenous anastomotic and capillary blood flow in the dog leg. Am J Physiol 222: 326–332
5. Lassen NA, Lindjerg IF, Munck O (1964) Measurement of blood through skeletal muscle by intramuscular injection of xenon-133. Lancet I: 686–689
6. Yamakoski K, Shimazu H, Togawa T, Ito H (1978) Admittance plethysmography for accurate measurement of human limb blood flow. Am J Physiol 235: 821–829
7. Kawakami K, Katuyama N, Mori Y, Shimada T, Tamura T, Togawa T, Shimazu H, Yamakoshi K, Fukuoka M, Ito H, Fujisaki N (1981) A combined study of admittance plethysmography and radionuclide methods for measurement of peripheral circulation. In: Proceedings of the ICEBI, Tokyo 1981. Japanese Society of Medical Electronics and Biological Engineering, Tokyo, pp 333–336
8. Zanick DC, Delaney JP (1973) Temperature influences on arteriovenous anastomoses. Proc Soc Exp Biol Med 144: 616–620
9. Hales JRS, Iriki M (1975) Integrated changes in regional circulatory activity evoked spinal cord and peripheral thermoreceptor stimulation. Brain Res. 87: 267–279
10. Deleaney J, Scarpino J (1973) Limb arteriovenous shunting following sympathetic denervation. Surgery 73: 202–206

Chapter 7
Methodology for Microvascular Disorders

Regulation of Plasma Membrane Ca-Pump ATPase of Vascular Smooth Muscle by cGMP

Ken-Ichi Furukawa, Yuko Tawada, Hiroshi Nakamura, and Munekazu Shigekawa[1]

Introduction

Relaxation of vascular smooth muscle can be induced by several agents, such as nitrovasodilators, natriuretic factor, and endothelium-derived relaxant factor (EDRF), which increase the cyclic guanosine monophosphate (cGMP) level within vascular smooth muscle cells (VSMCs; Fig. 1) [1, for review]. There is a good parallel between the cGMP accumulation and reduction of vascular tone [1, 2]. cGMP-dependent protein kinase (G-PK) phosphorylates several proteins in VSMCs [3]. However, the function of these proteins and their relevance to vasodilation remain unclear. The Ca-pump ATPase in the plasma membrane of VSMCs presumably plays an important role in the relaxation of VSMCs through its ATP- and calmodulin-dependent Ca^{2+} extrusion. Therefore, we examined whether the plasma membrane Ca pump is a target for G-PK-dependent regulation.

Experimental Procedures

The preparation of bovine aortic microsomes and purification of the Ca-pump ATPase by calmodulin-affinity chromatography were performed as described by Furukawa and Nakamura [4]. G-PK was purified from the bovine lung by the method of Lincoln [5]. The purified Ca-pump ATPase was incorporated into soybean phospholipid liposomes according to the method of Niggli et al. [6]. For assaying of cGMP-dependent phosphorylation, reconstituted proteoliposomes were phosphorylated with 100 μM [$\gamma-{}^{32}P$]ATP at 37°C in a medium containing 0.13 M KCl, 10 mM $MgCl_2$, 0.5 mM EDTA, and 20 mM Hepes-Tris (pH 7.4), with or without 1 μM cGMP and 0.03 μg G-PK. The phosphorylation was stopped by adding 6% trichloroacetic acid (TCA), and then hydroxylaminolysis was carried out, as described previously, to remove acylphosphoprotein [4]. Formation of the acylphosphoenzyme intermediate of the Ca-pump ATPase was measured as described previously [4]. Sodium dodecyl sulfate (SDS) polyacrylamide

[1]Department of Molecular Physiology, National Cardiovascular Center Research Institute, 7-1, Fujishirodai 5-chome, Suita, Osaka, 565 Japan

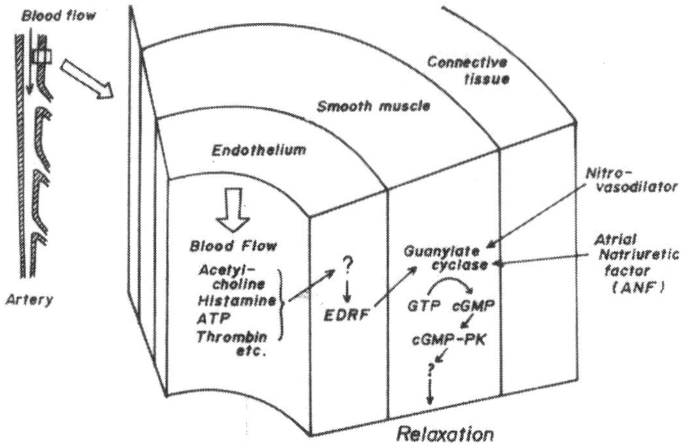

Fig. 1. cGMP-dependent relaxation of vascular smooth muscle

gel electrophoresis of the [^{32}P]-phosphoprotein was performed at 2°C using a slab gel (7.5% acrylamide) and the Laemmli buffer system [7]. Following the electrophoresis, the gel was stained with Coomassie Brilliant Blue R-250 in 10% acetic acid/45% ethanol at 2°C. The gel was then dried and exposed to Kodak XAR-5 film for 24 h. ^{45}Ca uptake was measured at 37°C in Ca-uptake medium containing 5 μg/ml calmodulin, 0.13 *M* KCl, 20 m*M* Hepes-Tris (pH 7.4), 1 m*M* $MgCl_2$, 1 m*M* ATP, 0.2 m*M* $^{45}CaCl_2$, and 0.18–0.29 m*M* EGTA, and otherwise as described previously [4]. Free Ca^{2+} concentration was calculated as described previously [4].

Results and Discussion

Proteoliposomes containing 1 μg purified Ca-pump ATPase were phosphorylated in 0.13 *M* KCl, 20 m*M* Hepes-Tris (pH 7.4), and 10 m*M* $MgCl_2$ in the presence (lanes A and B, Fig. 2) or absence (lane C) of 0.3 μM free Ca^{2+}. cGMP-dependent phosphorylation of the proteoliposomes was carried out at 37°C for 10 min in the presence (lanes D and E) or absence (lane F) of 1 μM cGMP plus 0.03 μg pyruvate kinase (PK). Further incubation did not increase the amount of phosphoprotein. Lanes B and E were treated with 0.4 *M* hydroxylamine for 10 min at pH 5.3 and 37°C.

When the phospholipid liposomes containing the purified Ca-pump ATPase (Molecular weight 135000) were phosphorylated with [γ-^{32}P]ATP (Fig. 2), only the 135-kilodalton protein was phosphorylated in the presence of either Ca^{2+} (lane A) or cGMP plus G-PK (lane D). In the former case, all the ^{32}P label incorporated into this protein was released on hydroxylamine treatment (lane B), indicating that the phosphoprotein formed was of the acylphosphate type. On the other hand, the ^{32}P label incorporated in the latter case was found to be resistant to hydroxylaminolysis (lane E). These results, therefore, suggest that it was the Ca-pump ATPase that was phosphorylated by G-PK. The maximum

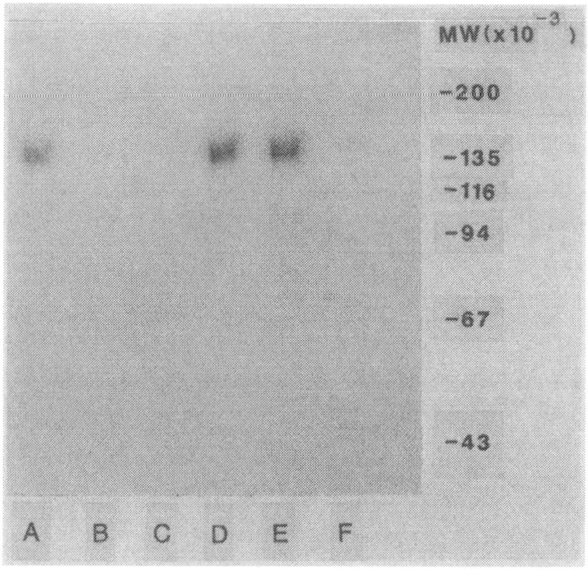

Fig. 2. Autoradiographic characterization of phosphoproteins formed in reconstituted proteoliposomes. After Furukawa and Nakamura [8]

observed level of cGMP-dependent ^{32}P label incorporation was 0.4 mol/mol 135-kilodalton protein. This value may indicate that 80% of the ATPase molecules, whose phosphorylation sites were accessible from the outside, were phosphorylated by [γ-^{32}P]ATP, because orientation of the ATPase molecules may well have been random in the reconstituted proteoliposomes.

Proteoliposomes containing 2.0 μg ATPase were phosphorylated with G-PK (0.04 μg) plus cGMP (1 μmol/L) in the presence of 100 μM ATP at 37°C for 10 min. Ca^{2+} uptake was assayed at 37°C for 1 min in the presence of various concentrations of Ca^{2+}. The Ca^{2+} uptake proceeded linearly for the initial 3 min.

Figure 3 shows the effect of the cGMP-dependent phosphorylation on the Ca^{2+} dependence of the Ca^{2+}-uptake rate of the reconstituted proteoliposomes. Nonphosphorylated proteoliposomes showed a K_m value of 0.3 μmol/L for Ca^{2+} and a maximum velocity, Vmax, of 2.1 μmol/min/mg protein. When the proteoliposomes were phosphorylated with cGMP plus G-PK up to a level of 0.4 mol of ^{32}P/mol 135-kilodalton protein, the K_m value decreased to 0.1 μmol/L, while the Vmax value increased to 2.6 μmol/min/mg protein.

Cyclic GMP-dependent phosphorylation was carried out with [γ-^{32}P] ATP and proteoliposomes containing 5.0 μg ATPase in the presence of G-PK (0.1 μg) plus cGMP (1 μmol/L) for 0, 3, and 10 min and was terminated by adding 6% TCA. For assaying ^{45}Ca uptake, cGMP-dependent phosphorylation was performed with nonradioactive ATP and otherwise as described above; it was terminated by diluting the phosphorylation medium ten fold with the Ca^{2+}-uptake medium. Then, ^{45}Ca uptake was measured for 1 min at 37°C with 0.3 μM free Ca^{2+}. During this 1-min period, the cGMP-dependent phosphorylation did not

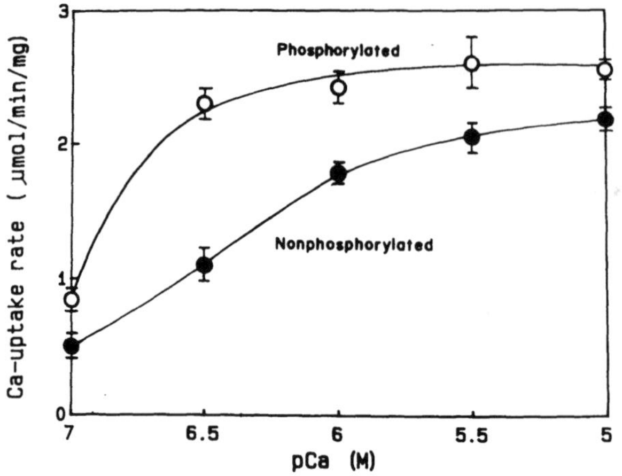

Fig. 3. Ca^{2+} dependence of the rates of ^{45}Ca uptake by phosphorylated and nonphosphorylated reconstituted proteoliposomes. The data are means ± SD ($n = 3$). After Furukawa and Nakamura [8]

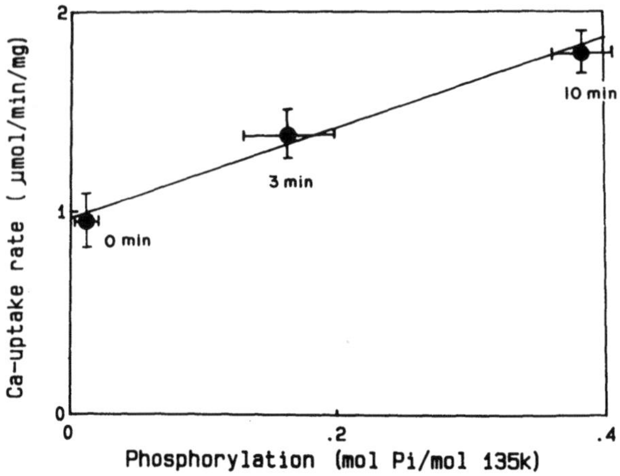

Fig. 4. Correlation between the extent of cGMP-dependent phosphorylation and stimulation of the Ca^{2+}-uptake rates. The data are means ± SD for three determinations for the phosphorylation and Ca^{2+} uptake rate. After Furukawa and Nakamura [8]

increase significantly because of the dilution and the use of a low Mg^{2+} (1 mmol/L) concentration.

Figure 4 shows the relationship between the cGMP-dependent phosphorylation and the observed rate of Ca uptake by the phosphorylated proteoliposomes. In this experiment, the free Ca^{2+} concentration was fixed at 0.3 µmol/L to observe the maximum effect of phosphorylation (Fig. 3). As shown in Fig. 4, there was a good parallel between the Ca^{2+}-uptake rate and the extent of phosphorylation. These results, therefore, suggest that the activity of the plasma membrane Ca pump of vascular smooth muscle is regulated by cGMP-dependent phosphorylation of the ATPase protein. The results strongly support the view that cGMP stimulation of the plasma membrane Ca pump activity is one of the mechanisms for the cGMP-induced relaxation of smooth muscle.

References

1. Murad F (1986) Cyclic guanosine monophosphate as a mediator of vasodilation. J Clin Invest 78: 1–5
2. Gruetter CA, Gruetter DY, Lyon JE, Kadowitz PJ, Ignarro LJ (1981) Relationship between cyclic guanosine 3'.5'-monophosphate formation and relaxation of coronary arterial smooth muscle by glyceryl trinitrate, nitroprusside, nitrite and nitric oxide. J Pharmacol Exp Ther 219: 181–186
3. Casnellie JE, Ives HE, Jamieson JD, Greengard P (1980) Cyclic GMP-dependent protein phosphorylation in intact medial tissue and isolated cells from vascular smooth muscle. J Biol Chem 255: 3770–3776
4. Furukawa K-I, Nakamura H (1984) Characterization of the (Ca^{2+}-Mg^{2+}) ATPase purified by calmodulin-affinity chromatography from bovine aortic smooth muscle. J Biochem 96: 1343–1350
5. Lincoln TM (1983) cGMP-dependent protein kinase. In: Colowick SP, Kaplan NO (eds) Methods in enzymology, vol. 99. Academic, New York, pp 62–71
6. Niggli V, Adunyah ES, Penniston JT, Carafoli E (1981) Purified (Ca^{2+}-Mg^{2+}) ATPase of the erythrocyte membrane. J Biol Chem 256: 395–401
7. Laemmli UK (1970) Cleavage of structural proteins during the assembly of the head of bacteriophage T4. Nature 277: 680–685
8. Furukawa K-I, Nakamura H (1987) Cyclic GMP regulation of the plasma membrane (Ca^{2+}-Mg^{2+}) ATPase in vascular smooth muscle. J Biochem 101: 287–290

Molecular Regulation of Calcium, Calmodulin-Dependent Myosin Phosphorylation

Toshio Tanaka, Tomohiko Ishikawa, Satoshi Matsushima, and Hiroyoshi Hidaka[1]

Introduction

The calcium ion plays a critical role in vascular smooth muscle contraction and platelet activation as a second messenger [1]. Increase in the intracellular calcium ion concentration induced by various agonists is due to the release from intracellular calcium stores and/or influx of extracellular calcium ions (Fig. 1). It is generally accepted that intracellular calcium ion function in smooth muscle and nonmuscle cells is mostly regulated through calcium, calmodulin-dependent protein kinases and ultimate modulation of the extent of protein phosphorylation [2]. To investigate the molecular mechanisms involved in the calcium-regulated system in smooth muscle cells and platelets, we developed selective inhibitors of each process of the calcium, calmodulin-dependent protein phosphorylation system [3]. The major mechanism for calcium activation of contractile proteins in vertebrate skeletal and cardiac muscle is a system consisting of calcium regulation of thin filaments by troponin-tropomyosin [4]. However, contractile activity in smooth muscle and nonmuscle cells is thought to be primarily regulated by calcium, calmodulin-dependent myosin light-chain phosphorylation (Fig. 1) [5]. The biochemical processes of the calcium, calmodulin-dependent regulatory system in the microcirculation have though proved difficult to study. Here, we provide data on two selective inhibitors of myosin light-chain phosphorylation, which have different sites of action and are potent vasorelaxants and platelet inhibitors. These compounds are N-(6-aminohexyl)-5-chloro-1-naphthalenesulfonamide (W-7) and 1-(5-chloronaphthalenesulfonyl)-1H-hexahydro-1, 4-diazepine (ML-9; Fig. 2).

Selective Inhibition of Myosin Light-Chain Phosphorylation

Myosin light-chain kinases of smooth muscle and platelets are calcium, calmodulin-dependent protein kinases and catalyze the transfer of the γ-phosphate from ATP to the myosin light chain (Fig. 3). This reaction is necessary for the

[1]Department of Molecular and Cellular Pharmacology, Mie University School of Medicine, 174 Edobashi 2-chome, Tsu, Mie, 514 Japan

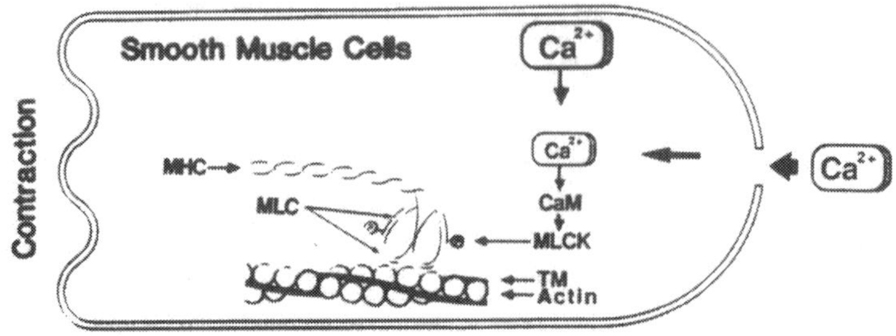

Fig. 1. Biochemical regulation of calcium, calmodulin-dependent myosin light-chain phosphorylation in smooth muscle and nonmuscle cells. *MHC* myosin heavy chain, *MLC* myosin light chain, *CaM* calmodulin, *MLCK* myosin light-chain kinase, *TM* tropomyosin

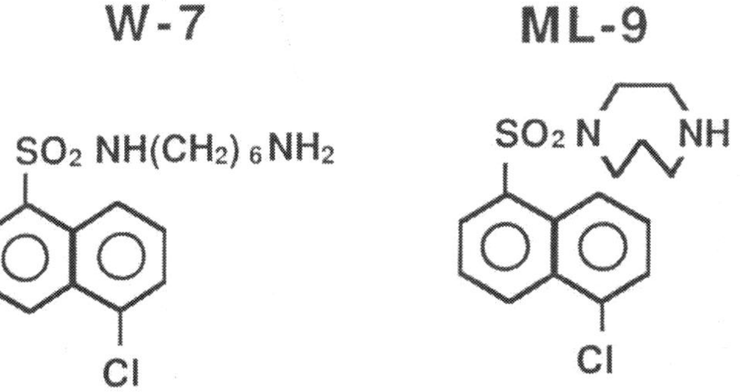

Fig. 2. Chemical structure of N-(6-aminohexyl)-5-chloro-1-naphthalenesulfonamide (*W-7*) and 1-(5-chloronaphthalenesulfonyl)-1H-hexahydro-1, 4-diazepine (*ML-9*)

stimulation of actin-activated, myosin ATPase in smooth muscle and nonmuscle cells and is a prerequisite for tension development of smooth muscle and platelet activation [5]. We investigated the effects of these compounds on myosin light-chain kinase from smooth muscle [6] and platelets [7]. We have demonstrated previously that myosin light-chain kinase is alternatively activated in an irreversible manner by trypsin treatment [8]. The catalytically active fragment produced by this treatment was entirely independent of the calcium-calmodulin complex. Kinetic analysis of the W-7-induced inhibition of myosin light-chain kinase revealed that W-7 inhibited the activity in competitive fashion with calmodulin, with a Ki value of 12 μmol/l (Table 1). W-7 was found to be less potent in inhibiting trypsin-treated myosin light-chain kinase, protein kinase C, and cAMP-dependent protein kinase. These results suggest that W-7 selectively inhibits calmodulin-induced activation of the enzyme. On the other hand, the Ki values of ML-9 for calcium, calmodulin-dependent and trypsin-treated myosin light-chain kinase from smooth muscle were 3.8 μmol/l and 4.0 μmol/l, respectively [9]. The Ki values of ML-9 for the myosin kinase from human platelets and rabbit skeletal muscle were 3.8 μmol/l and 49 μmol/l, respectively. These data suggest that ML-9 has excellent selectivity toward smooth muscle and non-

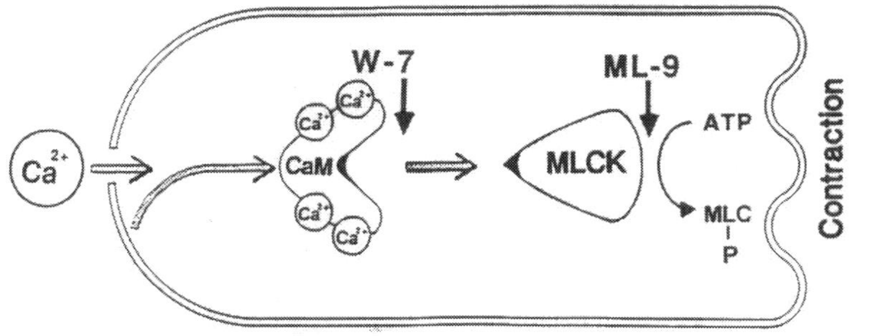

Fig. 3. Selective inhibitors of calcium, calmodulin-dependent myosin light-chain phosphorylation

Table 1. Effect of W-7 and ML-9 on protein kinases. After Tanak et al. [6] and Saitoh et al. [9]

Enzyme	Ki (μmol/L)	
	W-7	ML-9
MLC kinase + Ca^{2+} −CaM	12	3.8
Trypsin treated + EGTA	110	4.0
Protein kinase C + Ca^{2+} −PS	110	54
Trypsin treated + EGTA	340	56
cAMP-dependent protein kinase	170	32

MLC myosin light-chain, *CAM* calmodulin, *PS* phosphatidylserine

muscle myosin light-chain kinase and the inhibitory effects of ML-9 may be due to direct action on the catalytic site of the protein kinase and not to effects on the enzyme activation process. The mode of interaction of ML-9 with myosin light-chain kinase was investigated by Lineweaver-Burk plots and it was revealed that this compound was a competitive inhibitor with ATP and a noncompetitive inhibitor with the phosphate acceptor, myosin light chain. ML-9 is a selective inhibitor of myosin light-chain kinase from smooth muscle and nonmuscle cells and less potent in inhibiting other calcium, calmodulin-dependent enzymes, such as calcium-dependent cyclic nucleotide phosphodiesterase. On the other hand, a calmodulin antagonist, W-7 inhibits all calmodulin-dependent enzymes studied, such as myosin light-chain kinase, calcium-dependent cyclic nucleotide phosphodiesterase, and Ca^{2+}, Mg^{2+}-ATPase of human erythrocytes to a similar extent. Therefore, it is difficult to evaluate which calmodulin-dependent enzyme is dominantly responsible for the calcium-dependent regulatory system in smooth muscle and nonmuscle cells using the calmodulin antagonist W-7 [10].

Myosin Light-Chain Phosphorylation in Cell Physiology

We have established that ML-9 is a selective myosin light-chain kinase inhibitor of smooth muscle and nonmuscle cells and W-7 is a calmodulin antagonist.

We studied the physiological role of calcium, calmodulin-dependent myosin light-chain phosphorylation in smooth muscle and platelets, using these ML-9 and W-7. We found that W-7 and ML-9 produced relaxation of isolated vascular strips contracted by various agonists such as norepinephrine, serotonin, histamine, and angiotensin II to the same degree [11]. These compounds inhibited the maximun contractile response of intact and skinned muscles by calcium ions. The results indicate that W-7 and ML-9 have an affect on the common intracellular pathway in the regulation system of smooth muscle contraction, which may be calcium, calmodulin-dependent myosin light-chain phosphorylation [12].

To elucidate the physiological significance of calcium, calmodulin-dependent myosin light-chain phosphorylation in human platelet secretion, the effects of W-7 and ML-7 on the release reaction and protein phosphorylation of washed human platelets preincubated with ^{14}C-serotonin or ^{32}P-orthophosphate were investigated. These compounds inhibited myosin light-chain phosphorylation and secretion of human platelets. These observations suggest that myosin light-chain phosphorylation catalyzed by myosin light-chain kinase may play a critical role in platelet activation [13]

Conclusion

Diverse calcium-dependent cellular processes, such as vascular smooth muscle contraction and platelet secretion of biologically active substances, are thought to be involved in regulation of the microcirculation. The data described in this paper clearly indicate the physiological significance of calcium, calmodulin-dependent myosin light-chain phosphorylation in smooth muscle and nonmuscle cells, and these selective inhibitors may be useful tools in elucidating the physiological functions of myosin phosphorylation in the microcirculation.

Acknowledgments. This study was supported in part by Grants from the Ministry of Education, Science and Culture and the Ministry of Health and Welfare of Japan.

References

1. Campbell AK (1983) Intracellular calcium; its universal role as regulator. Wiley, New York
2. Means AR, Tash JS, Chafouleas JG (1982) Physiological implications of the presence, distribution, and regulation calmodulin in eukaryotic cells. Physiol Rev 62: 1–39
3. Hidaka K, Tanaka T (1987) Transmembrane Ca^{2+} signaling and a new class of inhibitors. Methods Enzymol 139: 570–582
4. Ebashi S (1983) Regulation of contractility. In: Stracher A (ed) Muscle and nonmuscle motility, vol. 1. Academic, New York. pp 217–232
5. Adelstein RS, de Lanerolle P, Sellers JR, Pato MD, Conti Ma (1982) Calmodulin and intracellular Ca^{2+}-receptors. In: Kakiuchi S, Hidaka H, Means AR (eds) Calmodulin and intracellular Ca^{++} receptors. Plenum , New York, pp 313–331
6. Tanaka T, Ohmura T, Yamakado T, Hidaka H (1982) Two types of calcium-dependent protein phosphorylation modulated by calmodulin antagonists: naphthalenesulfonamide derivatives. Mol Pharmacol 22: 408–412

7. Nishikawa M, Tanaka T, Hidaka H (1980) Ca^{+}-calmodulin dependent phosphorylation and platelet secretion. Nature 287: 863–865
8. Tanaka T, Naka M, Hidaka H (1980) Activation of myosin light chain kinase by trypsin. Biochem Biophys Res Commun 90: 694–699
9. Saitoh M, Naka M, Hidaka H (1986) the modulatory role of myosin light chain phosphorylation in human platelet activation. Biodem Biophys Res commun 140: 280–287
10. Hidaka H, Tanaka T, (1983) Naphthalenesulfonamides as calmodulin antagonists. Methods Enzymol 102: 185–194
11. Hidaka H, Hartshorne DJ (eds) (1985) Calmodulin antagonists and cellular physiology. Academic, New York
12. Tanaka T, Kanamori M, Hidaka H (1983) N-(6-aminohexyl)-5-chloro-1-naphthalenesulfonamide (W-7): a novel smooth muscle relaxant and intracellular calcium blocking agent. In: Bevan JA, Maxwell RA, Fujiwara M, Shibata S, Toda N, Mori K (eds) Vascular neuroeffector mechanism. Raven, New York, pp 315–218
13. Tanaka T, Saitoh M, Naka M, Inagaki M, Hidaka H (1987) Calcium-dependent protein phosphorylation in platelet activation and the selective inhibitior. In: Yamazaki H, Mustard JF (ed) Platelet activation. Academic, New York, pp 17–26

Erythrocyte Aggregation Induced by Immunoglobulin G and Related Macromolecules Studied with Rheoscope-Image Analyzer-Computer System

Nobuji Maeda, Masahiko Seike, Kazuhiko Imaizumi, Kazunori Kon, and Takeshi Shiga[1]

Erythrocyte aggregation is induced in blood flowing at low shear rates, especially in the stasis of blood, by macromolecular bridging between adjacent erythrocytes [1]. The process of erythrocyte aggregation is reversible; aggregates disintegrate at high shear rates. Since the facilitation of erythrocyte aggregation reduces the blood flow, the kinetic analysis of erythrocyte aggregation is very important for understanding the control of blood flow, rheologically. This paper describes a method for measuring the velocity of erythrocyte aggregation and the effect of immunoglobulin G and related macromolecules on the velocity.

Materials and Methods

Erythrocytes and Plasma

Fresh heparinized blood from healthy adult males was centrifuged at $1200 \times g$ for 5 min at 4°C. Plasma was used after recentrifugation at $15\,000 \times g$ for 20 min at 4°C to remove platelets. Erythrocytes were washed twice with 20 volumes of isotonic phosphate-buffered saline (50 m*M* Na phosphate, 90 m*M* NaCl, 5 m*M* KCl, 5.6 m*M* D-glucose, pH 7.4, 285 mosmol) at 4°C and were used within 5 h after blood-collecting.

Macromolecules

Immunoglobulin G (IgG; human) was purchased from Miles Lab. (Naperville, IL, USA): The red cell type-specific agglutinins were removed by adsorption to erythrocytes [2, 3]. IgM, IgA, and IgG fragments [$F(ab')_2$, Fc, and Fab] were purchased from Green Cross Corp. (Osaka, Japan). Commercial immunoglobulin preparations (polyethyleneglycol-treated, sulfonated, pepsin-treated, and plasmin-treated) for therapeutic purposes were used (Table 1). Human serum albumin (fatty acid free, fraction V) was purphased from Miles Lab. Inc. (Naperville, IL, USA).

[1] Department of Physiology, School of Medicine, Ehime University, Shigenobu, Onsen-gun, Ehime, 791–02 Japan

Table 1. Erythrocyte aggregation by commercial immunoglobulin preparations

Preparation	Composition[f]	[C] at $v/v_o = 2$[h]			
		A^+	B^+	AB^+	O^+
Polyethyleneglycol-treated[a]	IgG (84%)[g]	0.6	0.6	0.6	0.6
Sulfonated[b]	H_2L_2 (92%)[g]	0.7	0.7	0.7	0.7
Pepsin-treated-1[c]	$F(ab')_2$ (77%) IgG (12%) C_H3 (11%)	0.3	0.3	0.3	1.2
Pepsin-treated-2[d]	$F(ab')_2$ (89%) IgG (11%)	0.8	0.8	0.8	>2
Plasmin-treated[e]	Fc + Fab (45%) IgG (55%)	0.6	0.6	1.1	>2

[a] Globulin-N, from Yamanouchi Pharmaceutical Co., Tokyo
[b] Venilon, from Fujisawa Pharmaceutical Co., Osaka
[c] Gamma-Venin, from Boehringwerke, Hoechst
[d] Glovenin, from Takeda Pharmaceutical Co., Osaka
[e] Venoglobulin, from Green Cross Corporation, Osaka
[f] Determined by sedimentation analysis and polyacrylamide gel electrophoresis [2]
[g] Others are aggregates of IgG
[h] Erythrocyte aggregation of red cell type, A^+, B^+, AB^+, and O^+ was measured in presence (v) and absence (v_o) of immunoglobulin preparations in 60% autologous plasma + 40% isotonic phosphate-buffered saline (pH 7.4); [C] is concentration of immunoglobulin preparation (g/dl) at $v/v_o = 2$

Measurement of Velocity of Erythrocyte Aggregation

The rheoscope [4] (composed of a transparent 0.8° cone-plate viscometer and an inverted microscope) was combined with a video-camera (Sony, AVC 1150, Tokyo, Japan), an image analyzer (Luzex 450, Toyo Ink Co., Tokyo, Japan), and a computer (Hewlett Packard, HP-85, Palo Alto, CA, USA) for the measurement of the velocity of erythrocyte aggregation [5] (Fig. 1).

Erythrocytes suspended in various media were poured into the gap between the cone and the plate of the rheoscope. The measurements were carried out at a final hematocrit of 0.26%, shear rate of 7.5 s^{-1}, and temperature of 25°C (in this condition, the sensitivity and reproducibility were satisfactory) [5]. The particles count, i.e., the total number of single erythrocytes, one-dimensional aggregates (rouleaux), or three-dimensional aggregates, and the total projected area of the particles in the video frame ($200 \times 150\ \mu m^2$) were consecutively encoded by the analyzer at an interval of ca. 1.3 s, and transferred to the computer. The velocity of erythrocyte aggregation was expressed by the increasing rate of area/count (v, μm^2/min).

Results and Discussion

Erythrocyte Aggregation by IgG and Related Macromolecules

With increasing concentration of IgM, IgA, $F(ab')_2$, and IgG, added in 60% autologous plasma, the velocity of erythrocyte aggregation increased (Fig. 2).

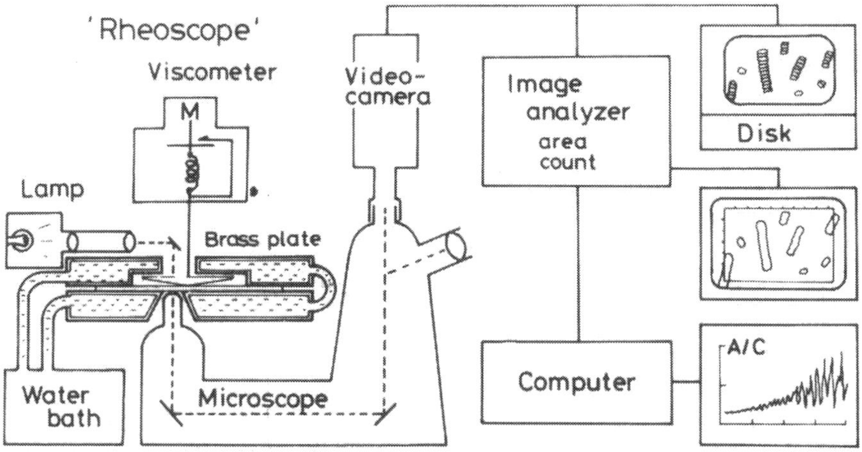

Fig. 1. Apparatus for measuring the velocity of erythrocyte aggregation

The facilitating effect was in the order—IgM > IgA ≈ $F(ab')_2$ > IgG. However, the addition of Fc and Fab did not alter the velocity of erythrocyte aggregation (Fig. 2).

Generally, with increasing molecular weight, the bridging force of the macromolecules increases, since: (a) the number of attaching sites on the erythrocyte surface increases due to the increased molecular size, and (b) the repulsive force between negatively charged erythrocytes is reduced due to the increased distance between cells [1]. The stronger facilitating effect of $F(ab')_2$ (92 kilodaltons) than IgG (150 kilodaltons) [3] may be due to: (a) the flexible structure at the hinge region [6], and (b) the more positive charge at the Fab region in comparison with the Fc region of IgG [2, 7]. Fc (50 kilodaltons) and Fab (45 kilodaltons) may be too small to bridge between adjacent cells, though they can attach to the erythrocyte surface [3] (also, see below).

Inhibition of IgG-Induced Erythrocyte Aggregation by Albumin

As the concentration of IgG in isotonic phosphate-buffered saline (pH 7.4) was increased, the velocity increased in various concentrations of albumin. Contrarily, the velocity of erythrocyte aggregation induced by IgG was inhibited with increasing albumin concentration. An empirical equation between the velocity (v) and the concentrations of IgG and albumin was obtained [8]:

$$v = \alpha\,[\text{IgG}]^{1.8} / [\text{albumin}],$$

where α is constant.

The inhibition of IgG-induced erythrocyte aggregation by albumin may be interpreted by the molecular size of these macromolecules and the number of bound molecules on the erythrocyte surface [8], i.e., the bridging by IgG is prevented by albumin occupying the erythrocyte surface.

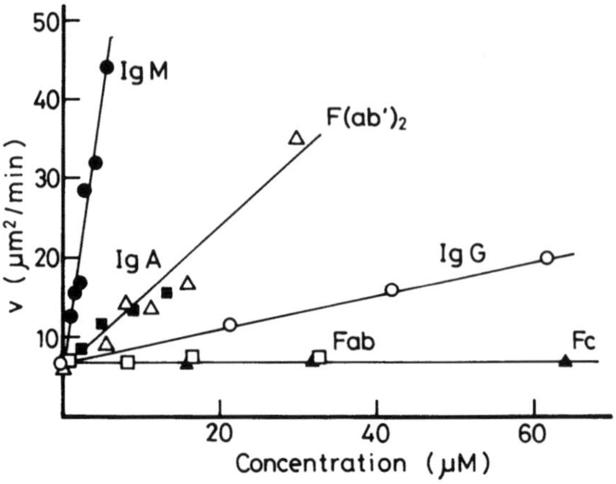

Fig. 2. Effect of immunoglobulins and the fragments on the velocity of erythrocyte aggregation. Immunoglobulins and the fragments were added in 60% autologuous plasma + 40% isotonic phosphate-buffers saline (pH 7.4), and the velocity was measured at 7.5 s^{-1} at 25°C. IgM (●), IgA (■), IgG (○), F $(ab')_2$ (△), Fc (▲), Fab (□)

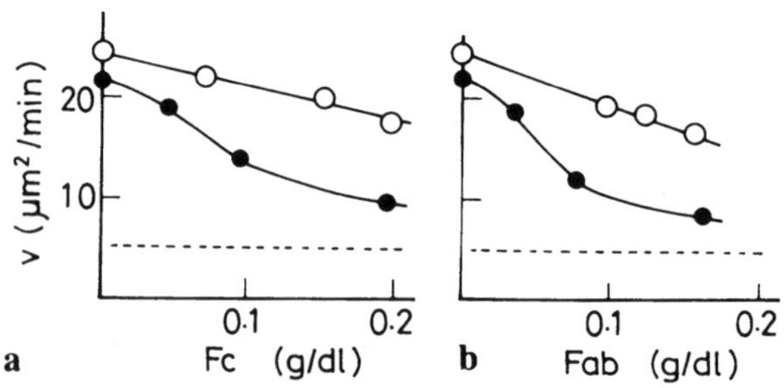

Fig. 3a, b. Inhibitory effect of **a** Fc and **b** Fab for IgG- and $F(ab')_2$-induced erythrocyte aggregation. Measured in 50% autologous plasma + 50% isotonic phosphate-buffered saline (pH 7.4) at 7.5 s^{-1} at 25°C. *Dotted line* velocity level in 50% autologous plasma. ○ 0.97g/dl IgG added to 50% autologous plasma; ● 0.28 g/dl F $(ab')_2$ added to 50% autologous plasma

Inhibition of IgG- and $F(ab')_2$-Induced Erythrocyte Aggregation by Fc and Fab

Fc and Fab inhibited the erythrocyte aggregation facilitated by IgG and $F(ab')_2$ in 50% autologous plasma (Fig. 3). The inhibitory effect was larger for $F(ab')_2$-induced than for IgG-induced aggregation, and Fab was more effective than Fc for the inhibition.

Fc and Fab prevent the bridging of IgG and $F(ab')_2$ between the erythrocyte surfaces, probably by competing for binding sites with IgG and $F(ab')_2$ [9]. The more positively charged Fab is more effective for the interaction with negatively charged erythrocytes than the less positively charged Fc.

Erythrocyte Aggregation by Commercial Immunoglobulin Preparations

All immunoglobulin preparations were contaminated by red cell type-specific agglutinins. After the removal of these agglutinins, the facilitating effect of immunoglobulin preparations on the erythrocyte aggregation was compared in 60% autologous plasma (Table 1). The degree of facilitation was evaluated by the concentration of each preparation to produce a twofold increase in the relative velocity of erythrocyte aggregation: v/v_o, where v and v_o are the velocities in the presence and absence of the immunoglobulin preparation, respectively.

The facilitating effect of some preparations (pepsin- and plasmin-treated) depended on the red cell type, while that of others (polyethyleneglycol-treated and sulfonated) did not. On the whole, the facilitating effect was weaker for O^+-erythrocytes than for A^+-, B^+-, and AB^+-erythrocytes.

The erythrocyte aggregation by immunoglobulin preparation greatly depends on the molecular composition and may be interpreted by: (a) the molecular weight, (b) the conformation, (c) the electric charge, (d) the competitive binding of bridging and nonbridging molecules on the erythrocyte surface [2, 10].

Summary

An apparatus for measuring the velocity of erythrocyte aggregation at constant shear rate and temperature was constructed by combining the rheoscope with a video camera, an image analyzer, and a computer. The accelerating effect of IgG and the related macromolecules on the velocity of erythrocyte aggregation was examined. The effect was in the order $IgM > IgA \approx F(ab')_2 > IgG$. Albumin inhibited IgG-induced erythrocyte aggregation. Fc and Fab did not induce the erythrocyte aggregation but inhibited the IgG- and $F(ab')_2$-induced erythrocyte aggregation. The effect of commercial immunoglobulin preparations for therapeutic purposes on the erythrocyte aggregation (for different blood groups) was examined.

Acknowledgments. The work was supported in part by grants from the Ministry of Education, Culture and Science of Japan and from the Ehime Medical Foundation.

References

1. Chien S, Jan K-M (1973) Ultrastructural basis of the mechanism of rouleau formation. Microvasc Res 5: 155–166
2. Maeda N, Sekiya M, Kameda K, Shiga T (1986) Effect of immunoglobulin preparations on the aggregation of human erythrocytes. Eur J Clin Invest 16: 184–191
3. Imaizumi K, Shiga T (1983) Effect of immunoglobulins and IgG-fragments on the human erythrocyte aggregation, studied by a rheoscope combined with image analyzer. Biorheology 20: 569–577
4. Schmid-Schönbein H, Wells R, Schildkraut R (1969) Microscopy and viscometry of blood flowing under uniform shear rate (rheoscope). J Appl Physiol 26: 674–678
5. Shiga T, Imaizumi K, Harada N, Sekiya M (1983) Kinetics of rouleaux formation using TV-image analyzer: I. Human erythrocytes. Am J Physiol 245: H252–H258

6. Valentine RC, Green NM (1967) Electron microscopy of an antibody-hapten complex. J Mol Biol 27: 615–617
7. Edelman GM, Heremans JF, Heremans M-T, Kunkel HG (1960) Immunological studies of human γ-globulin. Relation of the precipitin lines of whole γ-globulin to those of the fragments produced by papain. J Exp Med 112: 203–223
8. Maeda N, Shiga T (1986) Opposite Effect of albumin on the erythrocyte aggregation induced by immunoglobulin G and fibrinogen. Biochim Biophys Acta 855: 127–135
9. Imaizumi K, Imai A, Maruyama T, Shiga T (1984) Inhibition of IgG-, $F(ab')_2$- and myeloma protein-induced erythrocyte aggregation, by small Ig G-fragments. Clin Hemorheol 4: 431–439
10. Maeda N, Shiga T (1985) Inhibition and acceleration of erythrocyte aggregation induced by small macromolecules. Biochim Biophys Acta 843: 128–136

Blood Pressure in Mesenteric Microvessels of Normotensive and Hypertensive Rats: Application of a Servo-Nulling Micropressure System

Sotaro Hanai[1], Hideyuki Niimi[1], Yasuyuki Nishio[2], and Takuji Suzaki[2]

Introduction

It is of physiological importance to measure directly the pressure in in vivo microvessels since this may reflect the hemodynamic nature in the microvascular network. A number of techniques have been proposed for the direct measurement of microvascular pressure, but a servo-nulling technique [1] has been commonly used because it can provide accurate information about the microhemodynamics. In fact, this method has made it possible to measure blood pressure at a particular point in the microvascular network and to measure unsteady micropressure because of its high-frequency response capability. According to various reports, the response frequency ranges from 0 to 20–60 Hz [1–4]. In this paper, applications of the servo-nulling method to the microvasculature of normotensive and hypertensive rats are investigated.

The frequency response of the micropressure system may be greatly influenced by characteristics of the glass micropipette used as a pressure sensor. We tested our servo-controlled device and glass micropipettes in a plastic chamber. After the in vitro test, we measured blood pressure distributions in the mesentery of normotensive and spontaneously hypertensive rats using the micropressure system.

Methods

Micropressure System

A servo-controlled device (W–P Instruments, New Haven, USA) was used in combination with two kinds of glass micropipette. The micropipettes were made from cleaned glass tubes using a pipette puller with a two-step traction feature (Narishige PP–83, Tokyo, Japan). The shape of the tip was observed using a scanning electron microscope (SEM).

After the micropipette was filled with 99.5% ethanol under reduced pressure,

[1]Department of Vascular Physiology, National Cardiovascular Center Research Institute, 7-1, Fujishirodai 5-chome, Suita, Osaka, 565 Japan
[2]Tateisi Institute of Life Sciences, 3 Nakamikado-cho, Hanazono, Ukyo-ku, Kyoto, 616 Japan

the contents were replaced by 1–2 *M* NaCl solution; the ethanol and NaCl solution were filtered through a Millipore filter (0.2-μm pore). To examine the passive properties of the micropressure system, we immersed it in normal saline and measured its electrical resistance under various trans-tip pressure gradients.

We determined the active characteristics of the micropressure system by measuring responses to the pressure applied to a closed plastic chamber filled with normal saline. The linearity and stability of the system were calibrated against a reference pressure transducer (Statham P23D, Hato Rey, Puerto Rico). The frequency response of the system was estimated based on the response to transient pressure.

In Vivo Measurement

Fourteen male Wistar rats (WR; 163 ± 47 g body weight) and ten male spontaneously hypertensive rats (SHR; 180 ± 29 g) were used. The animals were anesthetized with sodium pentobarbital (40 mg/kg i.p.) and the respiration was maintained spontaneously through a tracheal cannula. The mesentery was exposed through an abdominal median incision and loosely draped over a plastic organ bath. The preparation was mounted on a mechanically positioning stage (Nikon 9VA-J1, Tokyo, Japan, 1-μm accuracy) and the mesentery was monitored using a TV-microscope system (Nikon UM-3, Hamamatsu Photonics C-2400, Hamamatsu, Japan). Microvessels in the mesentery were randomly selected for the present pressure measurement. A micropipette was held on the micromanipulator, which allowed three-dimensional linear movement, rotating, and tilting. The ECG of the rats was recorded simultaneously with pressure.

When we measured pressure in the microvessels, we examined the pulsation in pressure to judge whether the vessel was penetrated or not. When the pulse pressure was synchronized with the cardiac rhythm, we judged the vessel to be penetrated.

We measured the vessel diameter at the pressure-measuring site using the vessel image on the TV monitor. By moving the mechanical stage, we successively superimposed each side of the vessel wall on a fixed cursor and then measured the amount of stage displacement during this operation.

Results and Discussion

Characteristics of Servo-Nulling System with Micropipette

Two kinds of micropipette were manufactured from thick and thin glass tubes (1.5- and 1.0-mm outer diameter). Figure 1 shows SEM images of their tips. The thick pipette has a larger outer diameter, larger bore, and thinner wall than the thin one. The hydraulic and electrical resistance of the thick pipette was relatively low compared with the thin one. The thick pipette was convenient for the servo-nulling operation but not so effective for puncturing the vessels, especially small vessels. It is quite difficult to control the tip shape of pipettes suitable for each object. For this reason, we routinely used thick pipettes in in vitro and in vivo measurements.

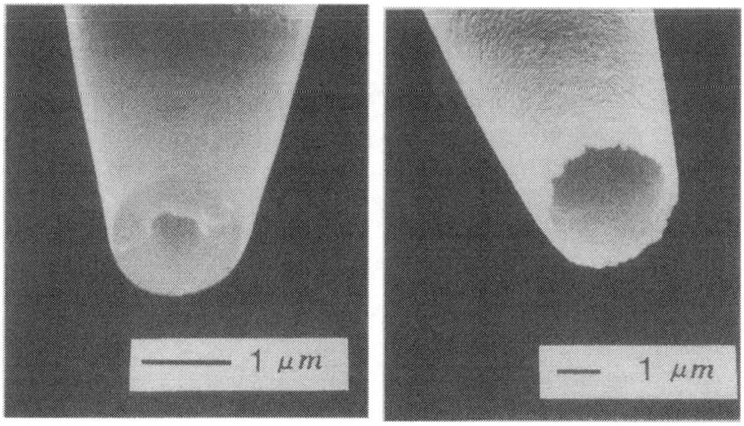

a b

Fig. 1a, b. Scanning electron micrographs showing tip shapes of micropipettes. These are made from glass tubes of **a** 1-mm and **b** 1.5 mm outer diameter

The micropipette (3-μm outer diameter and filled with 2 *M* NaCl) was changed in electrical resistance from 300 kohm to 2.2 Mohm, associated with a change in the hydrostatic pressure gradient between the pipette and chamber (Fig. 2a). The resistance change fell within the recommended range of operation for the servo-controlled device. In general, the resistance of the micropipette was determined by both the dimension of its tip and the electrical conductivity of the filling solution [2]. For example, when the tip is completely filled with the internal pipette fluid (2 *M* NaCl), the resistance may reach minimum value. If influx of the external fluid (saline) generates a fluid interface in the tip, on the other hand, the resistance may gradually increase with the inward movement of the interface. When the effective part of the tip is entirely filled with the external fluid, the resistance will decline [2].

A transient change in the pipette resistance was caused by the stepwise application of pressure to the chamber (Fig. 2b). The magnitude and duration of the response were varied among the pipettes, but in most cases the pipette resistance could attain a stationary level within 10 min; the levels were higher than the original values after the pressure restoration. This hysteresis may be caused by lowered electrolyte concentration in the internal fluid around the pipette tip. A relatively large amount of the external fluid entered the pipette at an early stage of the transient phase.

When a pipette is installed in a servo-system, the passive characteristics of the pipette may be eliminated because the fluid cannot move through the pipette tip after servo-operation has been established. Considering this tendency, we evaluated the active characteristics of the entire servo-system. The present calibration against a reference pressure showed that the system was linear within 0.5% of the full scale (100 mmHg) and that the long-term drift of the baseline was less than 0.5 mmHg/h. The frequency response of the system can be evaluated from the step response (Fig. 3) as follows. According to the circuit theory, the rise time (ts) and the frequency band width (BW) in a given system are practically

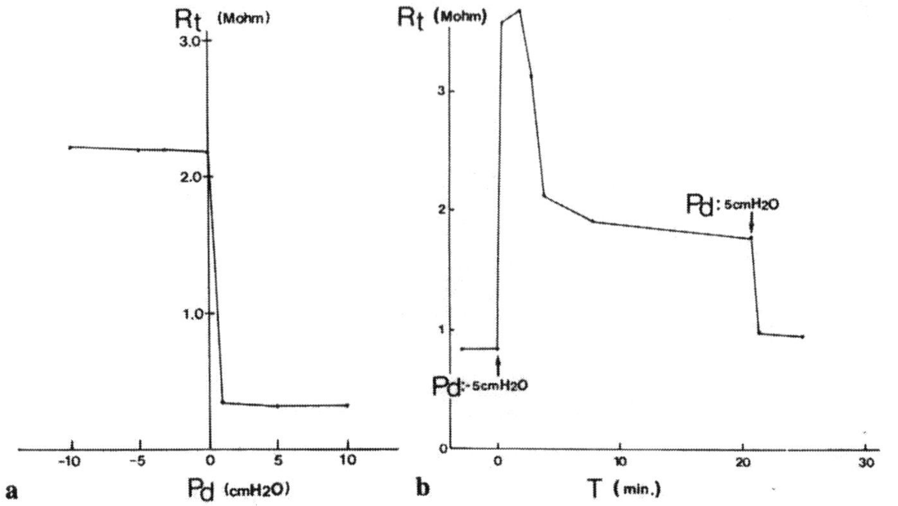

Fig. 2. **a** Static and **b** hysteretic characteristics between electrical resistance and pressure for a relatively large pipette. *Pd* pressure differences between pipette and chamber. Positive values of Pd mean that internal pressure of pipette is higher than external pressure. To obtain hysteretic response, small opposite pressures are applied at the moments indicated by *arrows*

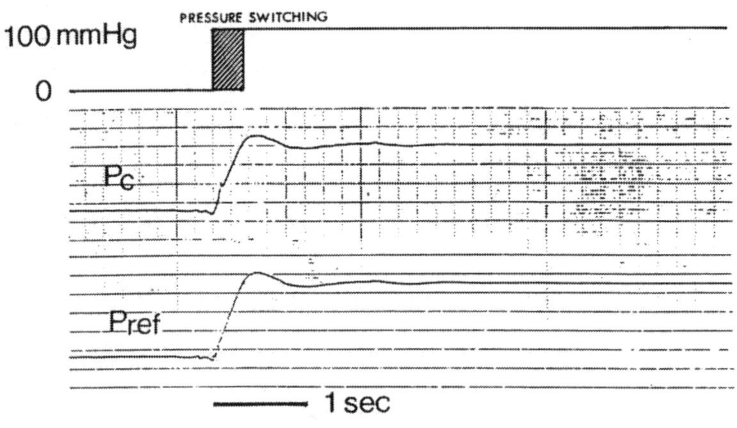

Fig. 3. Transient response for a large pipette. *Pc* counter pressure generated by the servo-controlled system, *Pref* pressure within a chamber measured with a reference pressure probe

expressed in terms of two rise times, t_o, t_i, of the output and input signal, respectively, as:

$$t_s^2 = t_o^2 - t_i^2, \; BW = 0.35/t_s$$

Then, ts and BW in the present system are estimated to be 11 ms and 30 Hz, respectively. These frequency capabilities are similar to those reported previously.

In Vivo Measurements

The pressure pulsation was observed in venules as well as in arterioles. Figure 4 shows two typical recordings of the micropressure measured in mesenteric arteriole and venules. The mean pulse pressure in arterioles was 25.7% ± 11.3% of the mean pressure; no significant difference was found between SHR and WR. The pulse pressure was greatly damped in venules, but it was often detectable.

Figure 5 shows the mean pressure plotted against the vessel diameters. SHR have a higher mean pressure than WR in arterioles larger than 25 μm in diameter. The gradient of the pressure distribution of arterioles in SHR was twice that in WR at the same level in the smallest vessels. The venular pressure in SHR appeared to be somewhat higher than in WR; this was not significant. The pressure in SHR agrees well in distribution pattern with other results reported for the microvasculature of the intestine [5] and skeletal muscle [6]. Furthermore, the pressure recorded here from the smallest arterioles to large venules is similar in absolute value to that in the intestinal mucosa [5] and skeletal muscle [6], except for the intestinal muscle layer [5].

There is some discrepancy in the capillary pressure measured in hypertensive and normotensive rats. Some experimental studies have reported that the capillary pressure is higher in SHR than in normotensive rats. Other studies have stated that the capillary pressure in SHR is the same as in normotensive rats. We did not measure the capillary pressure directly, but the present experimental results strongly suggest a possible similarity in capillary pressure between SHR and WR.

As mentioned above, the blood pressure may vary even in a small extent of the microvasculature, associated with the diameter and branching order of vessels. Moreover, the micropressure is likely to be disturbed under some pathological conditions. The micropressure system based on a servo-nulling technique can provide accurate information for analysis of the hemodynamic behavior in the microvasculature under both physiological and pathological conditions.

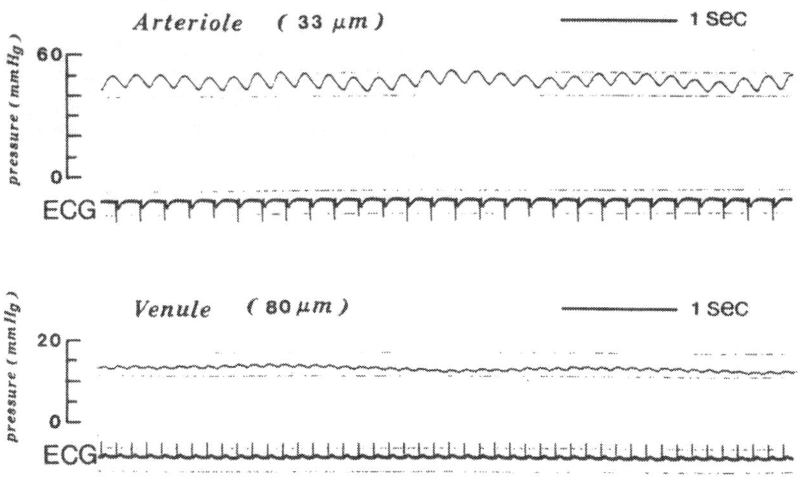

Fig. 4. Characteristic pressure patterns in the arteriole and venule

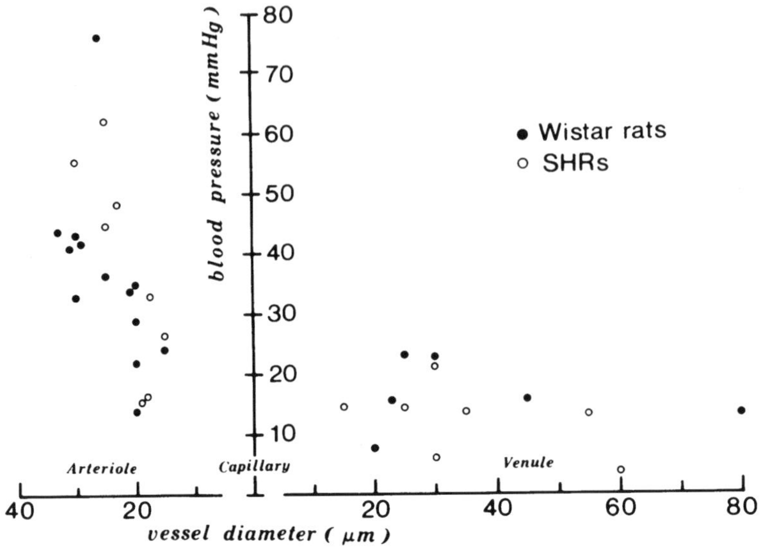

Fig. 5. Microvascular pressures in Wistar rats and spontaneously hypertensive rats (*SHRs*)

References

1. Wiederhielm CA, Woodbury JW, Kirk S, Rushmer RF (1963) Pulsatile pressures in the microcirculation of frog's mesentery. Am J Physiol 207: H173–H176
2. Fox JR, Wiederhielm CA (1973) Characteristics of the servo-controlled micropipet pressure system. Microvasc Res 5: 324–335
3. Fein H (1972) Microdimensional pressure measurements in electrolytes. J Appl Physiol 32: 560–564
4. Intaglietta M, Pawula RF, Tompkins WR (1970) Pressure measurements in the mammalian microvasculature. Microvasc Res 2: 212–220
5. Bohlen HG (1983) Intestinal microvascular adaptation during maturation of spontaneous hypertensive rats. Hypertension 5: 739–745
6. Zweifach BW, Kovalcheck S, De Lano F, Chen P (1981) Micropressure-flow relationships in a skeletal muscle of spontaneously hypertensive rats. Hypertension 3: 601–614

Analysis of Diameter and Flow Velocity Changes in Small Pulmonary Vessels During Regional Alveolar Hypercapnia

Mikiyasu Shirai, Kouji Sada, and Ishio Ninomiya[1]

Introduction

Effects of alveolar hypercapnia on the pulmonary vessels have been studied chiefly by measuring the pressure-flow relationship [1–3]. Some of the results have suggested an increase in the vascular resistance to blood flow in the hypercapnic lung area [1, 2], whereas others have not [3]. However, we consider that for detecting the local pulmonary vasomotion during alveolar hypercapnia, it is necessary to measure directly the internal diameter (ID) of small pulmonary vessels with rich smooth muscle layers. In this study, using a new X-ray TV system developed in our laboratory [4], we quantitatively analyzed the changes in ID of the small pulmonary arteries and veins (100–600 μm ID) in unilobar alveolar hypercapnia. Simultaneously, flow velocity and volume flow in the small arteries were analyzed.

Methods

Experimental Procedure and Angiography

The scheme of our system and the experimental setup are shown in Fig. 1. The system consists of three major parts, (a) a specially designed X-ray apparatus, (b) an X-ray-sensitive 1-in. Vidicon camera, and (c) a digital image processor. The picture element is about 20 μm in size, and the time required for one frame is 1/30 s.

The experiments were carried out on 15 cats anesthetized with pentobarbital sodium (35 mg/kg i.p.). Each cat was intubated and artificially ventilated. After the rib cage was partially excised and 4–5 cmH_2O end-expiratory pressure was added to the tracheal tube, the outer half of the left or right lower lung was exposed. It was arranged such that the exposed lung automatically contacted the plate just above the X-ray-sensitive vidicon camera. While ventilation was stopped at end expiration, the contrast medium (60% Urografin) was injected

[1] Department of Cardiac Physiology, National Cardiovascular Center Research Institute, 7–1, Fujishirodai 5-chome, Suita, Osaka, 565 Japan

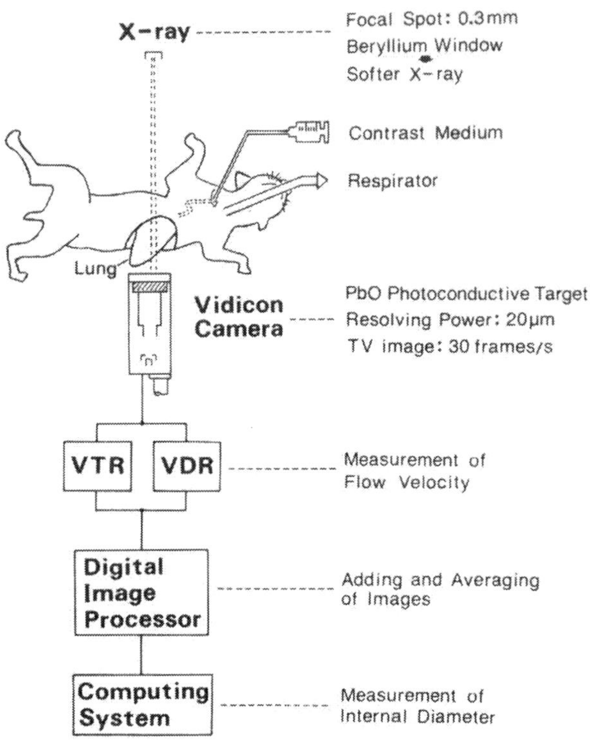

Fig. 1. System and experimental setup

into the main pulmonary artery at a constant speed. Under the exposure of softer X-rays, the passage of the contrast medium through the pulmonary vascular bed was serially recorded on a videodisk recorder and videotape recorder.

Measurement of ID and Flow Velocity

The recorded data were transferred to the digital image processor, and a digital image at a selected phase was obtained. This image was clearly reproduced on paper by image forming. The ID of the small pulmonary vessels on the copy was measured manually using a digitizer coupled with a minicomputer. Flow velocity (V) in the small arteries was estimated from the distance that the leading edge of the contrast medium moved in 0.1 s. Volume flow (F) in the small arteries was calculated from the V and the cross-sectional area (S) of the small arteries: $F = S \times V$. The measurement method of ID, S, V, and F has been reported in detail previously [4].

Experimental Protocol

Studies were made in two groups. In both groups, using a dual concentric tracheal tube system (Fig. 2), hypercapnic gas was administered selectively to the left lower lung (LLL) for a period of 6–8 min. In group 1 ($n = 11$), the

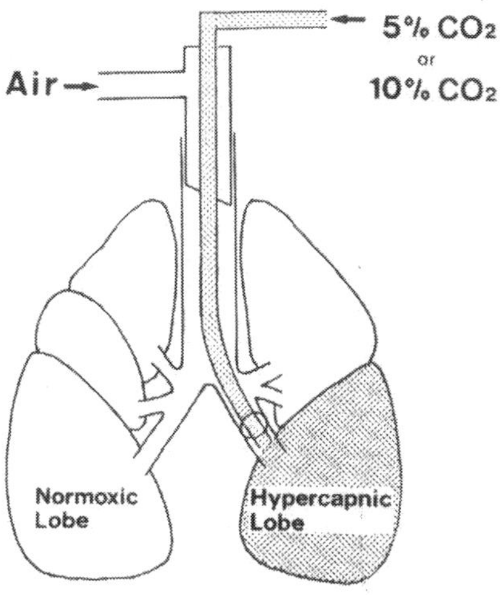

Fig. 2. Dual concentric tracheal tube system for ventilating left lower lobe (LLL) independently of the rest of the lung. The LLL was ventilated with 5% CO_2 or 10% CO_2 through the center tube, while the rest of the lung was ventilated with room air

angiograms before and during unilobar hypercapnia were made in the LLL; in group 2 ($n = 4$), they were made in the contralateral normoxic lobe (right lower lung).

Results

Typical Angiograms with Hypercapnia

Figure 3 shows typical arteriograms and venograms of the LLL before and during the ventilation of the lobe with 5% CO_2. In the arteries, apparent ID constrictions, shown by solid arrows, occurred chiefly in two main branches on the order of 200–300 μm in ID; on the other hand, the larger artery and the smaller branches showed only slight ID constrictions. In the veins, the ID constricted slightly. These findings indicated that in the small pulmonary vessels, the magnitudes of ID responses to alveolar hypercapnia varied depending on the control ID size. Therefore, it was necessary to measure the ID changes at different levels in the pulmonary vascular tree.

Relationship Between Vessel Size and Magnitude of Vasoconstriction

The ID constrictions in the LLL during the ventilation of the lobe with 5% CO_2 and 10% CO_2 are shown in each of the five groups with different ID size (Fig. 4). In both arteries and veins, the ID constricted significantly in proportion to the degree of hypercapnia. The ID constriction was larger in the arteries than in the veins. In the arteries, the ID constricted nonuniformly in the series-arranged vessels, whereas in the veins uniform ID constriction occurred. The ID constriction was maximal in the arteries of 200–300 μm ID, where it was 28% and 36% with 5% CO_2 and 10% CO_2, respectively. In the contralateral normoxic lobe, no significant ID changes were seen.

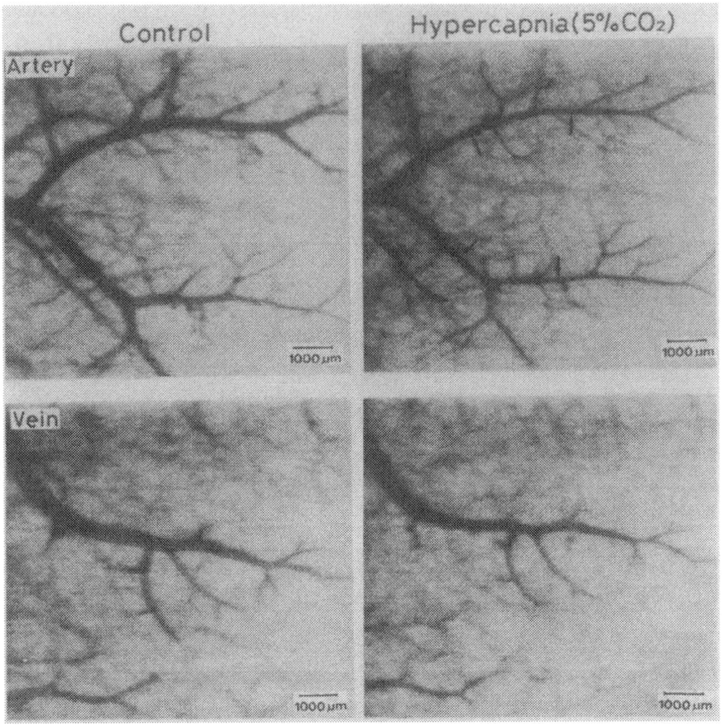

Fig. 3. Typical arteriograms and venograms of left lower lung under control and hypercapnic conditions in the same cat. *Arrows* indicate apparent vasoconstrictions

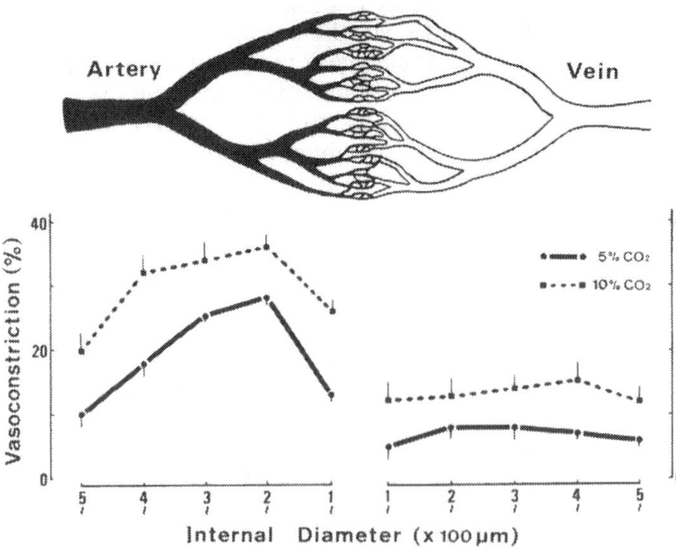

Fig. 4. Vasoconstrictions in arteries and veins to 5% CO_2 and 10% CO_2 inhalations. Values are means ± SE

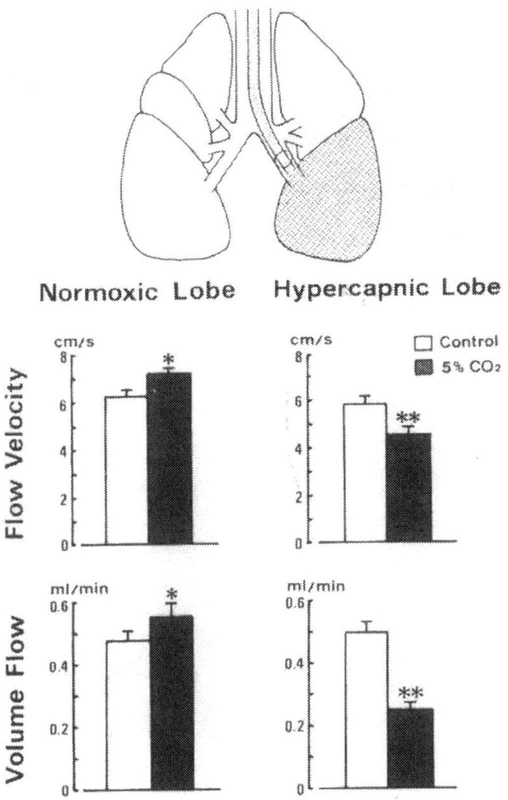

Fig. 5. Effects of regional alveolar hypercapnia on flow velocity and volume flow of small pulmonary arteries. Significant difference from control: * $P<0.05$, ** $P<0.01$

Changes in Flow Velocity and Volume Flow in Response to Alveolar Hypercapnia

Changes in the mean flow velocity and volume flow in the hypercapnic and the normoxic lobes are summarized in Fig. 5. In the hypercapnic lobe, the flow velocity decreased, with 5% CO_2, by 23%. The volume flow further decreased by 50%, because the vasoconstriction occurred in the hypercapnic lobe. On the other hand, in the normoxic lobe, the flow velocity increased by 14%. The volume flow showed almost the same degree of increase as the flow velocity, because no significant vasomotion occurred in the normoxic lobe.

Conclusions

We conclude that regional alveolar hypercapnia induced a nonuniform vasoconstriction in the small pulmonary arteries. The maximum constriction occurred in the arteries of 200–300 μm ID. Such local vasoconstriction diverted blood flow from the hypercapnic lung region to the normoxic one.

References

1. Hyman AL, Kadowitz PJ (1975) Effects of alveolar and perfusion hypoxia and hypercapnia on pulmonary vascular resistance in the lamb. Am J Physiol 228: 397–403
2. Manfredi F, Sieker HO (1960) The effect of carbon dioxide on the pulmonary circulation. J Clin Invest 39: 295–301
3. Peters RM (1957) Effect of unilateral carbon dioxide breathing on pulmonary blood flow. Am J Physiol 191: 399–403
4. Sada K, Shirai M, Ninomiya I (1985) X-ray TV system for measuring microcirculation in small pulmonary vessels. J Appl Physiol 59: 1013–1018

Measuring the Dimensions of a Thin Cylindrical Vessel by Processing Ultrasonic Reflections with an MEM Cepstrum

MOTOMU MINAMIYAMA[1] and SHIN-ICHI YAGI[2]

Introduction

Many different methods have been developed for the measurement of blood vessel dimensions, such as diameter and wall thickness. Especially for microvessels, optical and electronic techniques have been widely used [1–4]. With such techniques, the vessel must be observed under a transparent light source during the invasive operation. In contrast, for noninvasive evaluation of living tissue dimensions, ultrasonic echography is commonly used [5]. The diameter and wall thickness of the artery are visually observed from an echo signal chart [6] or by the ultrasonic echo-tracking method with a phased locked loop [7]. However, the conventional pulse-echo method has only a limited range of resolution, inversely proportional to the frequency bandwidth of the measurement system.

For exactly measuring the wall thickness of a human carotid artery, a computer algorithm for time-delay extraction from a composite echo signal has been developed [8]. It is fundamentally the Cepstrum method, but it has attained sufficient accuracy for this evaluation by combination with Burg's maximum entropy method (MEM). The purpose of this study is to measure exactly the diameter and wall thickness of a small vessel using this ultrasonic MEM Cepstrum method.

Method

Data Acquisition

For acquisition of ultrasonic echo signals from a small vessel, the cylindrical wall of the vessel was attached to a bath filled with physiological solution maintained at 37°C and pH 7.35 (Fig. 1). An ultrasonic beam was aligned perpendicularly

[1]Department of Vascular Physiology, National Cardiovascular Center Research Institute, 7–1, Fujishirodai 5-chome, Suita, Osaka, 565 Japan
[2]Department of Electrical and Electronics Engineering, Sophia University, 1 Kioi-cho 7-chome, Chiyoda-ku, Tokyo, 102 Japan

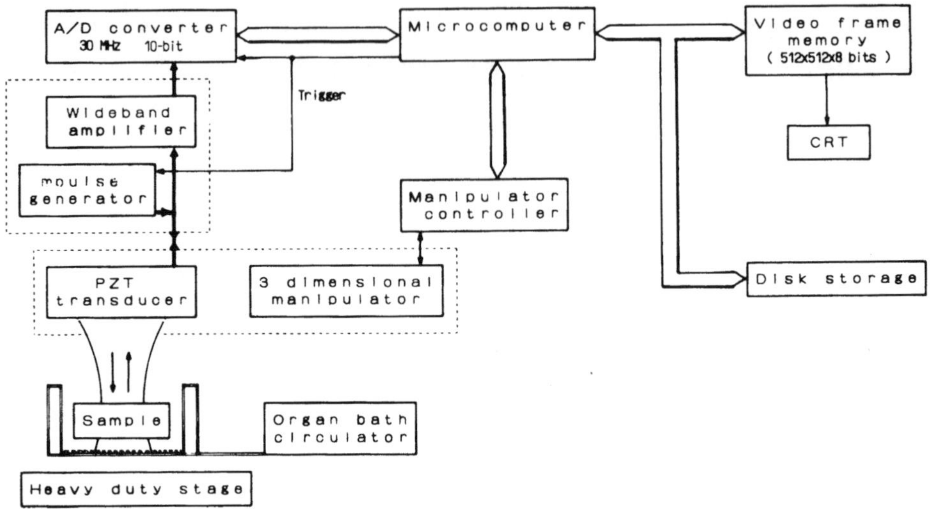

Fig. 1. Block diagram of data acquisition and processing system

to the cylindrical wall using a microcomputer-controlled three-dimensional manipulator (KOGAKU HD-8).

The r-f echo signal from a nominal 10-MHz, 6-mm diameter, middle internal focus PZT transducer (KB-AEROTEC BST10BS) was then digitized into a time series at a 30-MHz sampling rate with 10-bit resolution with an auto-digitizer (AUTONICS S-121). The digitized data was transferred into mass storage by a microcomputer (NEC PC-9801). In order to verify the alignment of the ultrasonic beam against the wall surfaces, an ultrasonic tomogram of the vessel was made using a video frame memory unit (HAMAMATSU C-1900) and the microcomputer (Fig. 1).

Signal Processing

To estimate exactly the dimension and wall thickness of a small vessel, we developed a computer algorithm, which contains the following steps.

Windowing ultrasonic echo signal. An r-f echo signal from a small vessel (about 0.8 mm in outer diameter) is shown in Fig. 2a. In order to truncate the measuring site on the echo signal, the digitized echo signal was windowed by a raised cosine gate (Fig. 2b).

Normalization of echo spectrum. For normalization of the echo spectrum from the vessel (Fig. 2c), the response function of the measurement system could be obtained experimentally as a Fourier transform of the echo signal from a spherical steel target in a certain range from the transducer (Fig. 3). Thereafter, the normalized log spectrum of the echo signal of the vessel was truncated by the effective bandwidth of the response function (Fig. 4a, b). Thus, we obtained input data as a limited frequency series for the MEM Cepstrum method.

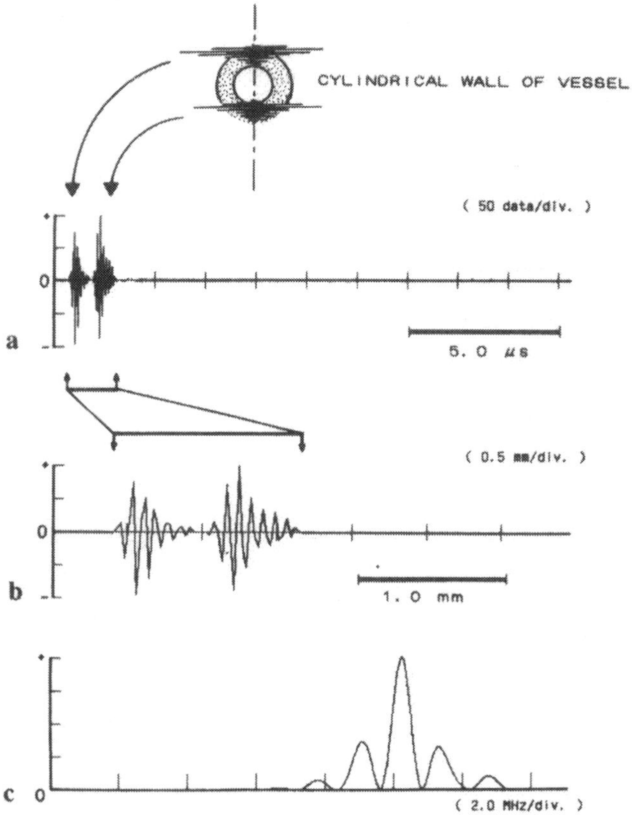

Fig. 2. **a** Ultrasonic r-f echo signal from a small vessel. **b** Data of the echo signal truncated by a raised cosine type gate. **c** Power spectrum of an ultrasonic r-f echo signal from a small vessel

Estimation of time delay carrier. The time delay carrier of the frequency series was estimated by the MEM Cepstrum method. These carriers are shown as peaks in Fig. 4c, d. Thus, since the velocity fluctuation is very small in soft tissues, the time delay could be directly translated into the distance separating the reflection surfaces. The distance between the reflection surfaces indicated the diameter and wall thickness of the small vessel (Fig. 4c, d).

Performance Characteristics

We examined the accuracy of this ultrasonic method by measuring the dimension of some cylindrical ployethylene tubes. These tubes were between 0.77 and 3.51 mm in outer diameter and the polyethylene sound velocity was taken as 1950 m/s. An exactly linear relation was found between the outer diameters estimated by the ultrasound method and those directly measured with a scale and a microscope (Fig. 5).

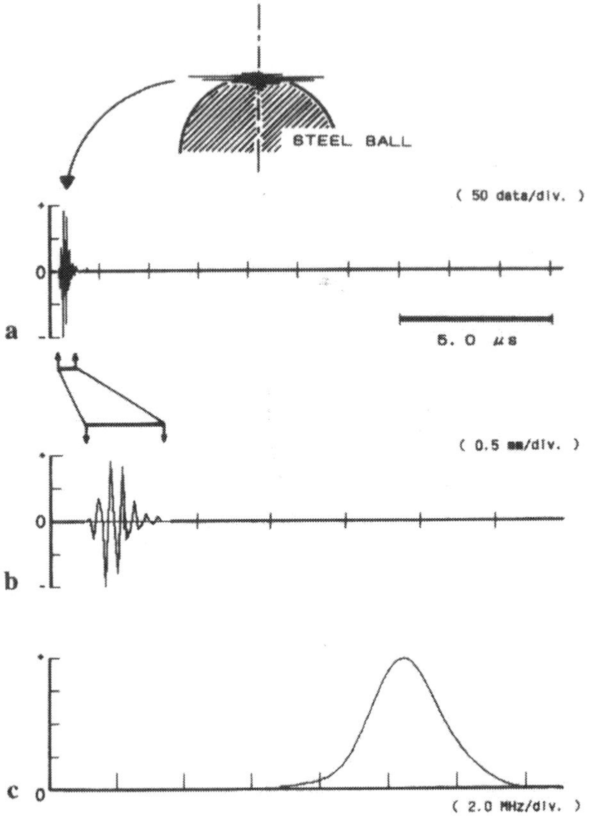

Fig. 3. **a** Ultrasonic r-f echo signal from a standard reflector. **b** Data of the echo signal truncated by a raised cosine type gate. **c** Power spectrum of an ultrasonic r-echo signal from a standard reflector

Discussion and Conclusion

The MEM Cepstrum method we have developed allows measurements to be made of the diameter and wall thickness of a small vessel with an outer diameter greater than 100 μm. The resolution is limited by the effective bandwidth of the measurement system due especially to the transducer and the sampling rate of A/D conversion. The frequency response depends only on the sampling time for A/D conversion and the time taken to transfer the digitized data into the mass storage, since the actual digital computing to estimate the dimensions is done offline. The estimated values by the MEM Cepstrum method agreed fairly well with the actual dimensions (Fig. 5). In conclusion, this ultrasonic method of measuring the diameter and wall thickness of small vessels may be useful for studying the function of small vessels in a parenchymal organ.

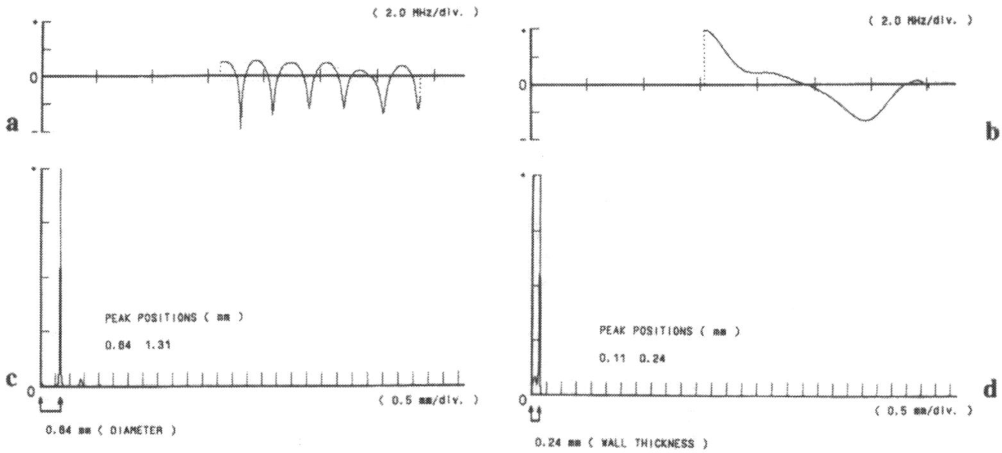

Fig. 4. **a** Log compression of normalized echo spectrum of a small vessel. This tracing is a truncated frequency series including the echo signal from both the forward and rear wall along the ultrasonic beam. **b** Log compression of normalized spectrum of small vessel. This *tracing* is a truncated frequency series including the echo signal from the forward wall. **c** Cepstrum output of truncated frequency series by MEM. A *peak* shows the distance between reflection surfaces, which indicates the diameter of the vessel. **d** Cepstrum output of truncated frequency series by MEM. A *peak* shows the distance between reflection surfaces, which indicates the thickness of the wall of the vessel

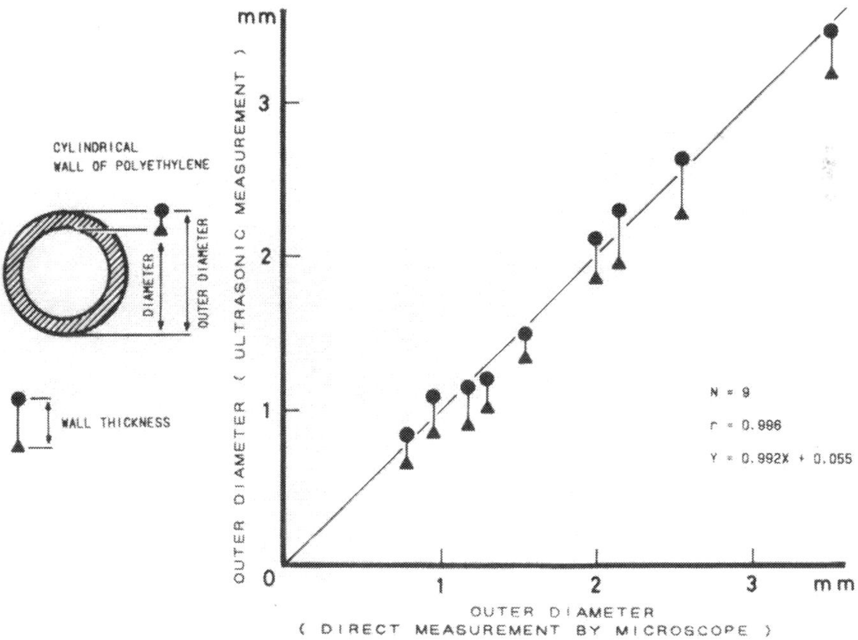

Fig. 5. Relation between ultrasonic measurement by the MEM Cepstrum method and direct measurement with a microscope. The outer diameter, measured directly by a microscope, is the sum of the thinkness of the wall and the diameter which the ultrasonic MEM cepstrum method measured separately

References

1. Asano M, Yoshida K, Tatai K (1965) Microphotoelectric plethysmograph using a rabbit ear chamber. J Appl Physiol 20: 1056–1062
2. Baez S (1966) Recording of microvascular dimensions with an image splitter television microscope. J Appl Physiol 21: 299–301
3. Intaglietta M, Tompkins WR (1973) Microvascular measurements by video image shearing and splitting. Microvasc Res 5: 309–312
4. Sakaguti M, Ohhashi T, Azuma T (1976) A photoelectric diameter gauge utilizing the image sensor. Pflug Arch 378: 263–268
5. Hill CR (1986) Pulse-echo imaing and measurement. In Hill CR (ed) Physical principles of medical ultrasonics. Ellis Horwood, New York, pp 278–304
6. Orson RM (1974) Human carotid artery wall thickness, diameter and blood flow by a non-invasive technique. J Appl Physiol 37: 955–960
7. Furuhata H, Kitsukawa K, Yoshimura S (1982) Non-invasive measurement of wall thickness of artery by ultrasound and derivation of incremental modulus. Proc Jap Soc Biorheol 5: 57–60 (in Japanese)
8. Yagi S, Nakayama K (1983) Analysis of MEM Cepstrum algorithm for ultrasonic dynamical measurements of living arterial wall thickness. Proc Jap Soc Biorheol 6: 139–142 (in Japanese)

Alterations in Membrane Fluidity of Hypertension Determined by an Electron Spin Resonance Method

Kazushi Tsuda[1], Seiko Tsuda[2], Yohsuke Minatogawa[3], Hideo Iwahashi[3], Hiroki Shima[1], Masanori Hamada[1], Hiroyuki Yoshikawa[1], Masako Ura[1], Jiro Takeda[1], Ichiro Nishio[1], Ryo Kido[3], and Yoshiaki Masuyama[1]

Introduction

It has been proposed that essential hypertension and genetic hypertension may be associated with various functional or structural abnormalities of cell membranes [1–3]. The data of these studies support the concept that changes in electrolyte handling or physiochemical properties of membrances may be a key etiological factor in hypertension. Recently, electron spin resonance (ESR) and a spin-label technique have been widely used to elucidate the composition, structure, and behavior of biomembranes and perturbations of the membranes by external agents [4–6].

To obtain further information about the membrane abnormalities of hypertension, we examined alterations in fluidity of cell membranes from spontaneously hypertensive rats (SHR) and patients with essential hypertension by means of an ESR method. Further, Ca-related changes of ESR spectra of hypertension were also investigated.

Materials and Methods

Male SHR (Okamoto and Aoki strain) and WKY rats were studied at the ages of 4 and 10–13 weeks. Forty-five patients with essential hypertension (males 26, females 19, age 47 ± 2 years, blood pressure 160.0 ± 3.1/97.9 ± 2.0 mmHg) were examined and compared with normotensive subjects (males seven, females five, age 43 ± 2 years, blood pressure 128.4 ± 2.8/77.2 ± 3.0 mmHg). For secondary hypertension, patients with primary aldosteronism (male one, female one), pheochromocytoma (female one), and renovascular hypertension (females two; age 41 ± 6 years, blood pressure 195.6 ± 11.3/109.2 ± 5.9 mmHg) were examined.

All hypertensive patients were in stage I or II of the WHO classification of hypertension and had no medication for at least 2 weeks before the study.

Division of Cardiology, Department of Medicine[1], Third Division of Department of Medicine[2], and Department of Biochemistry[3], Wakayama Medical College, 1, 7-Bancho, Wakayama, 640 Japan

The rats were anesthetized under pentobarbital anesthesia (40 mg/kg, intraperitoneal injection) and the abdominal cavity was opened. Heparinized blood was obtained from the inferior vena cava in each animal. In human subjects, blood sampling was performed by venipuncture after at least 30-min bed rest. After plasma and buffy coat were carefully removed by centrifugation, erythrocytes were washed three times in physiological saline. The cells were resuspended in isotonic buffer (140 m*M* sodium chloride, 20 m*M* Tris-HCl, pH 7.4) at a hematocrit of 50%.

Cultured vascular smooth muscles were obtained from the thoracic aortae of 10- to 13-week-old SHR and WKY rats according to the method described by Campbell et al. [7]. Morphological examination revealed the characteristics of vascular smooth muscle cells with crisscross patterns, undulations, and nodular structures in confluent cultures with phase-contrast microscopy. Cells at passage levels four to five were used for the experiments.

Spin Label of Erythrocytes and Cultured Vascular Smooth Muscle Cells

Erythrocyte or cultured vascular smooth muscle cell suspensions were preincubated for 30 min and then spin-labeling was performed [8].

A fatty acid spin-label agent, 5-nitroxy stearate (5-NS), was purchased from Syva Associates Palo Alto, USA) and kept at a stock solution of 0.01 mol/l in 100% ethanol. The agent was diluted in NaCl-Tris buffer before the experiment (5×10^{-5} mol/l). Two hundred microliters of the spin-label-containing solution was added to 400 μl erythrocytes or cultured vascular smooth muscle cells (about 5 mg of protein), and then the solution was incubated for 2 h at 37°C with gentle shaking.

ESR measurements were carried out using an ESR spectrometer (JES-FE2XG, Nihon Denshi Co., Ltd., Japan) with a microwave control unit (ES-SCXA, Nihon Denshi Co., Ltd.). The temperature was controlled by ES-DVT1 control unit (Nihon Denshi), and its accuracy was within ± 0.5°C.

Erythrocytes, or vascular smooth muscle cells, after washing in isotonic NaCl-Tris buffer, were packed in a quartz ESR flat cell (ES-LC11, Nihon Denshi Co., Ltd.). The microwave power was 5 mW, and the modulation frequency was 100 kHz with an amplitude of 2.0 G. The recorder scan width was 3280 ± 50 G, and the sweep time was 8 min. The receiver gain was $4.0 \times 10^3 - 7.9 \times 10^3$ with a response time of 1.0 s.

Ca-Related Changes of ESR Spectra

Washed erythrocytes were preincubated in NaCl-Tris buffer with or without Ca-ionophore A23187 (0.9 μmol/l, Hoechst, USA) and 1.0 m*M* of $CaCl_2$ (at a hematocrit of 50%, 37°C, 30 min). Then, spin-label containing NaCl-Tris buffer (200 μl) was added to 400 μl erythrocytes. After incubation at 37°C for 2 h, the ESR spectra were obtained by the same procedures as described above.

All values were expressed as means ± SEM. Statistical significances were determined by paired or unpaired Student's *t*-test. A value of $P < 0.05$ was considered significant.

Results

The values of outer and inner hyperfine splitting ($2T'_{//}$, $2T'_{\perp}$ in gauss) were evaluated in each ESR spectrum, and order parameter (S) was calculated from $2T'_{//}$ and $2T'_{\perp}$ [9]. The greater values of $2T'_{//}$ and S are associated with the lesser freedom of motion of the spin-label in the biomembrane bilayers, indicating the decreased membrane fluidity.

The values of $2T'_{//}$ and S were significantly higher in erythrocytes from SHR than those from WKY both at 4 and 10–13 weeks of ages ($2T'_{//}$ at 30°C: 4-week-old SHR 57.22 ± 0.40 G, $n = 6$, WKY 55.00 ± 0.16 G, $n = 6$, $P < 0.01$; 10- to 13-week-old SHR 57.11 ± 0.25 G, $n = 9$, WKY 53.88 ± 0.40 G, $n = 4$, $P < 0.01$; Fig. 1).

The fluidity of cultured vascular smooth muscle cell membranes may also be decreased in SHR compared with WKY ($2T'_{//}$ at 30°C: SHR 57.57 ± 0.39 G, $n = 4$, WKY 53.95 ± 0.05 G, $n = 4$, $P < 0.05$; Fig. 1).

Similarly, the ESR spectrum parameters in patients with essential hypertension (EH) were increased compared with those in normotensive (NT) subjects ($2T'_{//}$ at 30°C: EH 58.58 ± 0.25 G, $n = 45$, NT 56.33 ± 0.24 G, $n = 10$, $P < 0.01$; S: EH 0.742 ± 0.004, $n = 45$, NT 0.695 ± 0.004, $n = 10$, $P < 0.01$; Fig. 2). However, the ESR values of secondary hypertension were not changed compared with those of NT subjects. These findings indicate that the membrane fluidity of erythrocytes may be decreased in SHR and EH.

When calcium was loaded to erythrocytes with Ca-ionophore A23187, the parameters of ESR spectra showed a greater increase (membrane fluidity was decreased) in SHR and patients with essential hypertension than that in the normotensive controls. These Ca-induced changes in membrane fluidity were not definitely observed in secondary hypertension (Fig. 3).

Discussion

In the present study, we showed that the cell membranes of SHR and EH patients could permit different spin motions from those of NT controls, suggesting that the cell membranes in hypertension may be stiffer and less fluid. Additionally, the decreased membrane fluidity was observed in erythrocytes from SHR at the prehypertensive stage (4 weeks old) and in vascular smooth muscle cells from SHR. These data support the concept that alteration in cellular physical properties may be a genetically determined and generalized abnormality of hereditary hypertension.

It is well known that membrane fluidity is a function related to the microviscosity of the membrane, lipid component, water content, and divalent cation content [9]. The intracellular Ca level seems to regulate the size, shape, and some physical properties of erythrocytes [10]. On the basis of these previous findings, we investigated the Ca-induced changes in membrane fluidity of erythrocytes in hypertension. Treatment of erythrocytes with the Ca-ionophore A23187 and Ca caused a decrease in membane fluidity (the S value in ESR spectra was increased), and this change was more prominent in SHR and EH

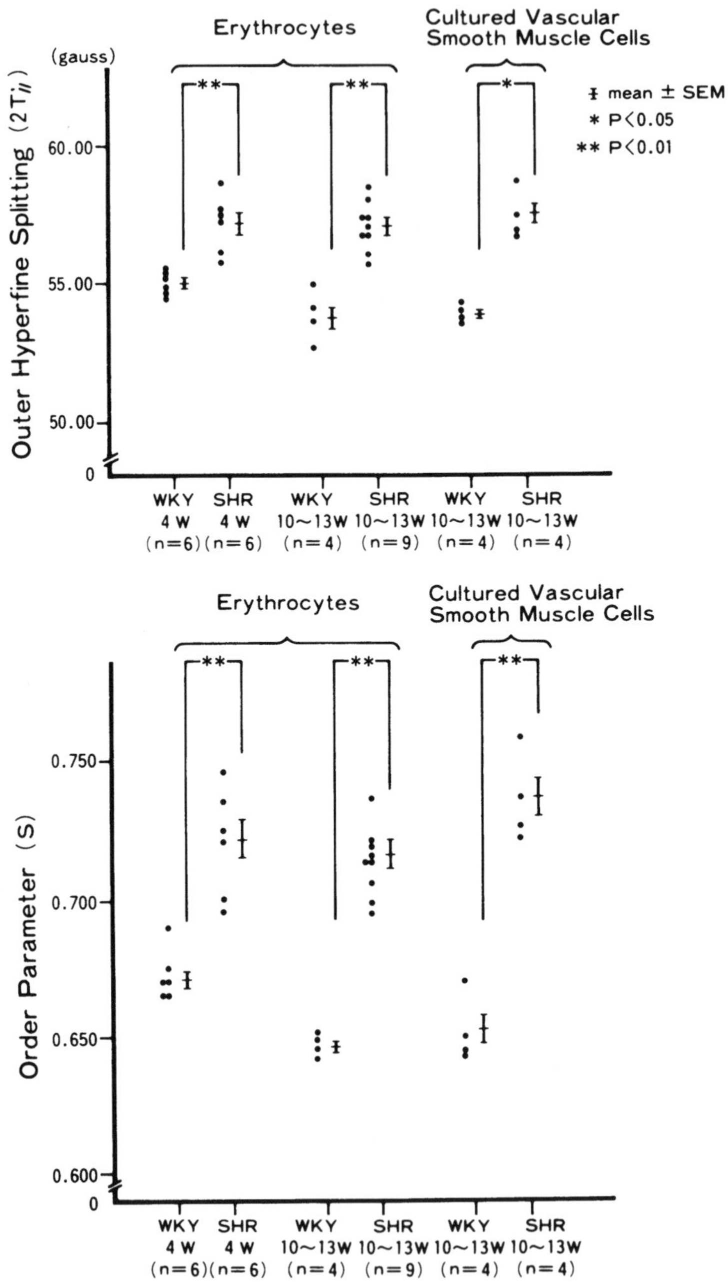

Fig. 1. Comparison of outer hyperfine splitting (2T'//) and order parameter (S) of *electron spin resonance* spectra in erythrocytes and cultured vascular smooth muscle cells between spontaneously hypertensive rats (*SHR*) and WKY rats at 30°C. The higher values of 2T'// and S are associated with lower membrane fluidity

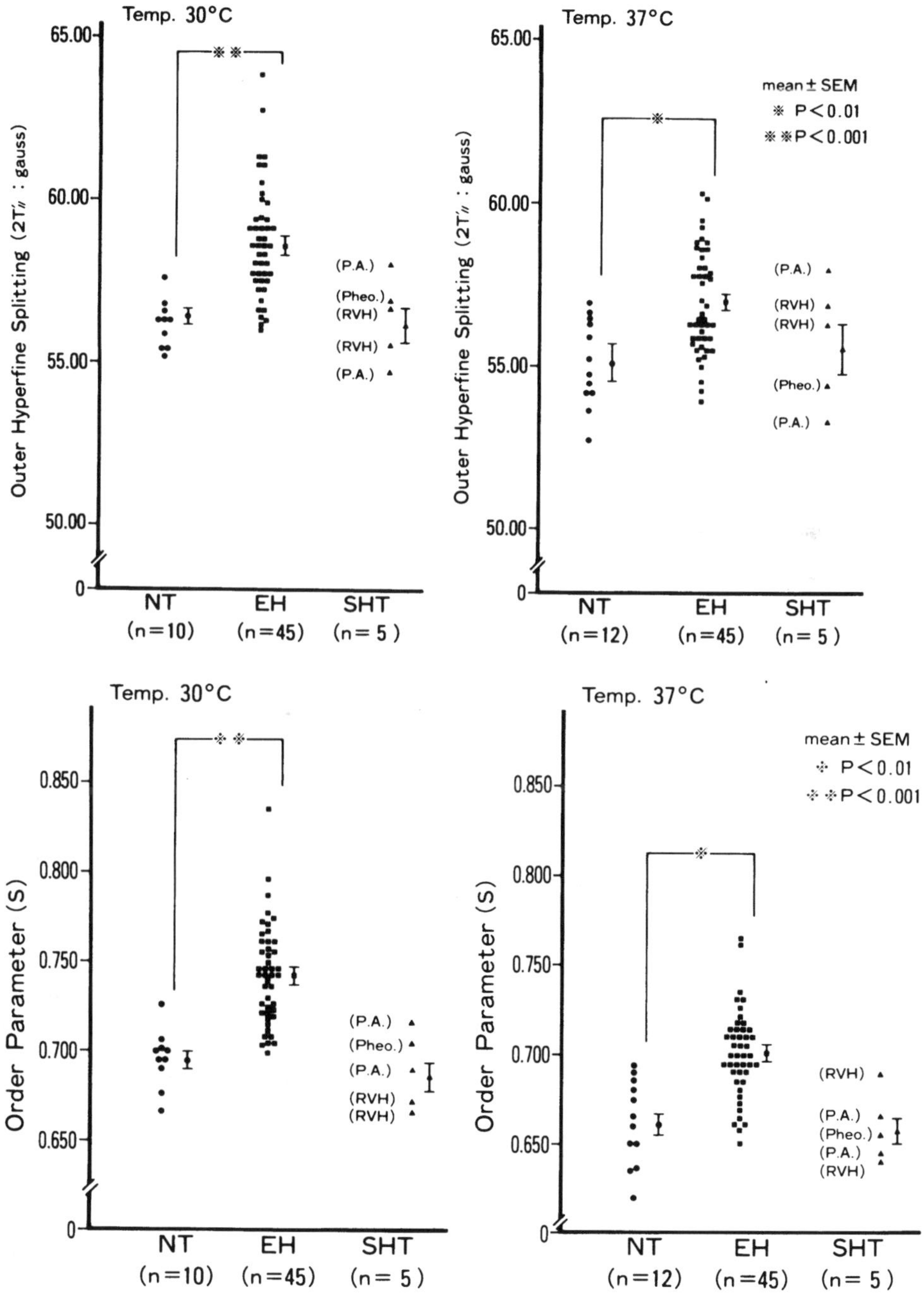

Fig. 2. Values of $2T'_{//}$ and S of ESR spectra in normotensive subjects (*NT*), patients with essential hypertension (*EH*), and patients with secondary hypertension (*SHT*). *PA* primary aldosteronism, *Pheo* pheochromocytoma, *RVH* renovascular hypertension

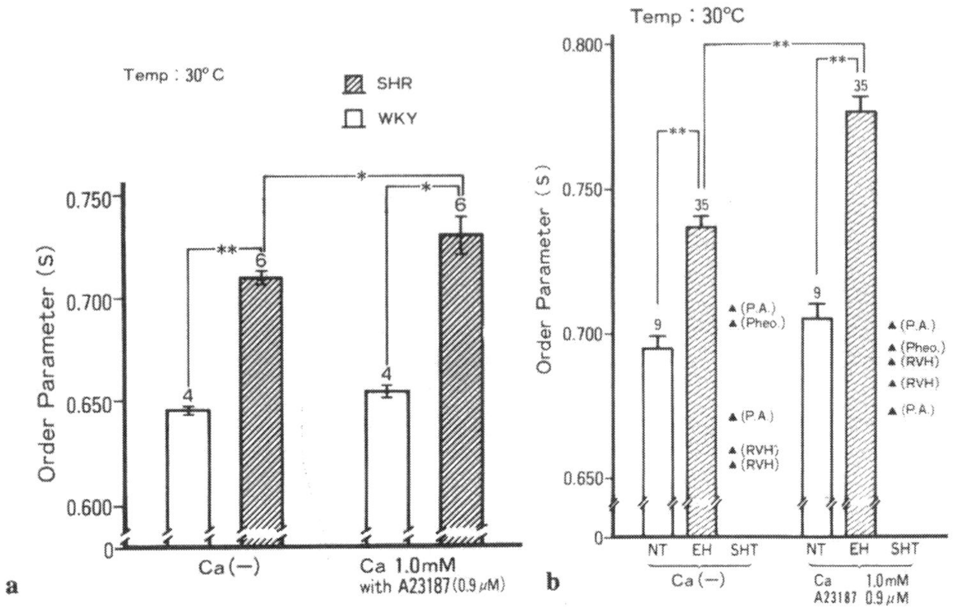

Fig. 3a, b. Effects of Ca loading on membrane fluidity of erythrocytes in **a** SHR and **b** essential hypertension. Ca loading to erythrocytes was performed with Ca ionophore A23187 (0.9 μmol/L) and $CaCl_2$ (1.0 mmol/L) in vitro. The *figures* above each *column* are the numbers in each experiment

patients than in NT controls. Our previous report showed that A23187 and Ca reduced the osmotic fragility of erythrocytes, implying an increase in membrane rigidity. In addition, the Ca-induced change in osmotic fragility was greater in EH patients than in NT subjects [11]. Therefore, our results indicate that Ca influx across the membranes or interactions of Ca with erythrocyte membranes could be enhanced in SHR and EH patients.

Details about the role of membrane fluidity in hypertension are still unknown. However, decreased fluidity could induce an increase in the vascular resistance since the membrane fluidity appears to be inversely correlated with the membrane stiffness.

In conclusion, ESR studies with a fatty acid and spin-label agent indicated that the cell membranes of SHR and EH patients could tolerate different spin motions than those of NT controls, suggesting that the membrane fluidity is decreased in these genetic forms of hypertension.

The marked reduction of the membrane fluidity in SHR and EH patients when Ca was loaded to erythrocytes supports the hypothesis that an abnormality of Ca handling at cellular levels could affect physical properties of the biomembranes in hereditary hypertension.

Summary

In this study, we examined alterations in membrane fluidity of hypertension by means of an electron-spin resonance (ESR) and spin-labeling method.

Washed erythrocytes from spontaneously hypertensive rats (SHR; Okamoto and Aoki strains, 4 and 10–13 weeks of age) and patients with essential hypertension, and cultured vascular smooth muscle cells from SHR were investigated and compared with those from normotensive controls.

ESR spectra were obtained for a fatty acid spin-label agent (5-nitroxy stearate) into the membranes. The values of outer hyperfine splitting and order parameters of the spectra were significantly higher in erythrocytes from SHR and essential hypertensives than in their normotensive controls. Similar results were obtained in cultured vascular smooth muscle cells of SHR. These findings indicate that the membrane fluidity is decreased in SHR and essential hypertensives.

When calcium was loaded to erythrocytes with the Ca ionophore A23187, the fluidity was decreased. This Ca-induced change was more marked in SHR and essential hypertensives.

These results suggest that decreased membrane fluidity in SHR and essential hypertensives is a genetically determined abnormality of hypertension, which could be more prominent in the presence of calcium.

Acknowledgments. This study was supported partly by Grants-in-Aids for Scientific Research (60570404, 60440049, 62304041) from the Ministry of the Education, Science and Culture of Japan, and by Nanki Scholarship Fund.

References

1. Postnov YV, Orlov SN, Gulak P, Shevchenko A (1976) Evidence of altered permeability of the erythrocyte membrane for sodium and potassium ions in spontaneously hypertensive rats. Clin Sci Mol Med 51: 169s–172s
2. Canessa M, Adragna N, Solomon HS, Tosteson DC (1980) Increased sodium-lithium countertransport in red cells of patients with essential hypertension. N Engl J Med 302: 772–776
3. Devynck MA, Pernollet MG, Nunez AM, Meyer P (1981) Analysis of calcium handling in erythrocyte membranes of genetically hypertensive rats. Hypertension 3: 397–403
4. Tanaka K, Ohnishi S (1976) Heterogeneity in the fluidity of intact erythrocyte membrane and its homogenization upon hemolysis. Biochim Biophys Acta 426: 218–231
5. Butterfield DA, Chesnut DB, Appel SH, Roses AD (1976) Spin label study of erythrocyte membrane fluidity in myotonic and Duchenne muscular dystrophy and congenital myotonia. Nature 263: 159–161
6. Hubbel WL. McConnell HM (1971) Molecular motion in spin labeled phospholipid and membranes. J Am Chem Soc 93: 314–326
7. Campbell JC, Campbell GR, Ross R (1979) The smooth muscle cell in culture. Physiol Rev 59: 1–61
8. Simon I (1979) Differences in membrane unsaturated fatty acids and electron spin resonance in different types of myeloid leukemia cells. Biochim Biophys Acta 556: 408–422

9. Cooper RA (1977) Abnormalities of cell-membrane fluidity in the pathogenesis of disease. N Engl J Med 297: 371–377
10. Lake W, Rasmussen H, Goodman DBP (1977) Effect of ionophore A23187 upon membrane function and ion movement in human and toad erythrocytes. J Membrane Biol 32: 93–113
11. Tsuda K, Minatogawa Y, Furuya S, Ueda E, Shima H, Tamaki T, Nishio I, Kido R, Masuyama Y (1986) Enhanced calcium-sensitivity of erythrocytes in hypertension—Calcium-induced changes of erythrocyte osmotic fragility in essential hypertension Jpn Circ J 50: 1158–1164

Assessment of Systemic and Regional Blood Flows with the Radioactive Microsphere-Reference Sample Method in Rats

JIN YAMAMOTO and MASATSUGU NAKAI[1]

Introduction

The radioactive microsphere-reference sample (RMRS) method has become applied to hemodynamic studies even in small animals such as rats [1, 2]. The assumptions and prerequisites of this method in determining systemic and regional blood flows have been described previously [1–3]. Cardiac output and regional blood flow can be obtained by determining the amount of the radioactivity injected and that of the reference sample withdrawn at a known rate and then by comparing them with the radioactivity entrapped by regional organs. The accuracy and precision of this technique are influenced by many factors, including the number of microspheres injected, the site of injection, the rate of reference blood withdrawal, and the kind of suspension agents [1–7]; however, appropriate experimental conditions seem to be now established in rats [2, 6, 7]. In comparison with an independent method, Ishise et al. demonstrated that cardiac output determined by the RMRS method correlated excellently with that determined simultaneously by electromagnetic flowmetry in rats [2].

We report here our study with the RMRS technique in the assessment of systemic and regional blood flows in rats.

Methods

The rats were anesthetized with ether [2, 8–10]. Polyethylene catheters were positioned in the femoral artery and vein and left ventricle. These catheters were brought out at the nape. After a 16- to 18-h recovery period, each rat was placed in a small nonconfining cage. Hemodynamic parameters were determined on a recorder by connecting the catheters to transducers and a polygraph. Reference blood samples were withdrawn from the arterial catheter at a constant rate (0.8–1.2 ml/min) using a Harvard pump over a 50-s period. Beginning 10 s after the start of sampling, approximately 40 000–100 000 radioactive microspheres (15

[1] Department of Cardiovascular Dynamics and Function, National Cardiovascular Center Research Institute, 7-1, Fujishirodai 5-chome, Suita, Osaka, 565 Japan

μm in average diameter, suspended in 0.05 ml 0.9% saline containing 0.01% Tween 80, vigorously preagitated; 3M, St. Paul or NEN, Boston, USA) were injected into the left ventricle and flushed with fresh donor blood over a 20 period. Blood loss was replaced immediately by blood infusion. After the rats were killed, the organs were removed and weighed. Reference samples and organs were counted in a computerized scintillation counter (LKB, Stockholm, Sweden).

Cardiac output (CO) and regional blood flow were calculated as follows:

$$\text{CO (ml/min)} = \frac{\text{sampling rate (ml/min)} \times \text{injected isotope counts (cpm)}}{\text{reference sample counts (cpm)}}$$

$$\text{Organ blood flow (ml/min)} = \text{CO} \times \text{organ fractional distribution of CO.}$$

CO and regional flows were normalized for body and organ weights. Total peripheral and regional vascular resistance was obtained by dividing the mean arterial pressure by normalized systemic and regional blood flows. The adequacy of mixing was assessed by comparing blood flows between the right and left hemispheres of the brain and between the right and left kidneys.

Results and Discussion

In the first set of experiments, 0.9% saline, norepinephrine, angiotensin II, or sodium nitroprusside was infused into conscious rats through the femoral venous catheter using a Harvard pump. The doses in the drug-infused rats were selected so as to make their mean arterial pressure (MAP) approximately 20% higher or lower than that of the saline-infused control rats. Cardiac output and regional blood flow were determined with the RMRS method 15–20 min after the initiation of infusion, during which period a steady hemodynamic state was reached. Analysis of variance followed by the Bonferroni procedure was employed for statistical analysis in all the studies described below. MAP was 115 ± 3 (mean $\pm$ SE) mmHg in the saline group ($n = 10$), 137 ± 3 mmHg in the norepinephrine group ($n = 10$), 139 ± 3 mmHg in the angiotensin II group ($n = 11$), and 94 ± 2 mmHg in the sodium nitroprusside group ($n = 10$). The cardiac index was 306 ± 15 ml/min/kg with saline, 304 ± 14 ml/min/kg with norepinephrine, 274 ± 7 ml/min/kg with angiotensin II, and 360 ± 11 ml/min/kg with sodium nitroprusside; the cardiac index was significantly ($P < 0.05$) greater in the sodium nitroprusside group than in the saline group. The heart rate was 371 ± 8 beats/min in the saline group, 345 ± 8 beats/min in the norepinephrine group, 356 ± 8 beats/min in the angiotensin II group, and 431 ± 9 beats/min in the sodium nitroprusside group. Accordingly, increased cardiac index observed with sodium nitroprusside may be related in part to reflex tachycardia in this group of rats.

Figure 1 shows regional blood flow data in various organs and tissues. The data are given in terms of percentage of change of each value compared with the mean values of the saline-infused group. Regional blood flows were not significantly altered by nonrepinephrine infusion. Blood flow to the viscera (splanchnic blood flow—gastrointestinal tract, spleen, and pancreas) and kidneys were significantly decreased with angiotensin II. On the other hand, blood flow

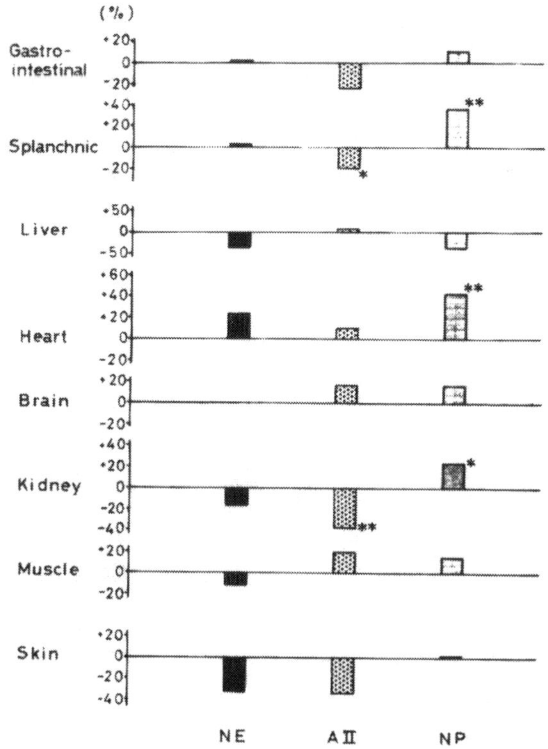

Fig. 1. Regional blood flow data during infusion of norepinephrine (*NE*), angiotensin II (*A II*), and sodium nitroprusside (*NP*). Data during drug infusion are expressed as percentage of change of values during 0.9% saline infusion. Only means of values are given. * $P<0.05$, ** $P<0.01$ vs. 0%

to these two vascular beds was increased with sodium nitroprusside. Blood flow to the heart tended to be increased during infusion of norepinephrine and angiotensin II, and significantly increased heart blood flow occurred during sodium nitroprusside infusion. Notably, there was no change in cerebral blood flow with any of the drugs. The majority of effects of these vasoactive drugs with known actions were as anticipated. With the doses used, the most responsive was the splanchnic vascular bed, and the second most responsive was the renal vasculature. The finding of unaltered cerebral blood flow is consistent with the well-established concept of autoregulation of cerebral circulation. The results of these experiments indicate, therefore, that the reference sample method can be used to evaluate drug-induced specific changes in systemic and regional blood flow in rats.

Systemic and regional hemodynamics were then studied in conscious rats with deoxycorticosterone acetate (DOCA)-salt hypertension, an experimental model of mineralocorticoid excess hypertension, at 8 weeks of treatment [8, 9]. The rats were made hypertensive by weekly injections of 30 mg DOCA and the provision of 1% saline as a drinking solution. Placebo-treated rats were used as controls. Compared with the controls, DOCA-salt rats showed strikingly increased MAP (186 ± 4 mmHg vs. 122 ± 3 mmHg), which was associated with increased total peripheral resistance index and increased cardiac index (291 ± 8 ml/min/kg vs. 257 ± 12 ml/min/kg). As illustrated in Fig. 2, the percentage of the fraction of cardiac output per gram of organ (% CO/g) and blood flow to the

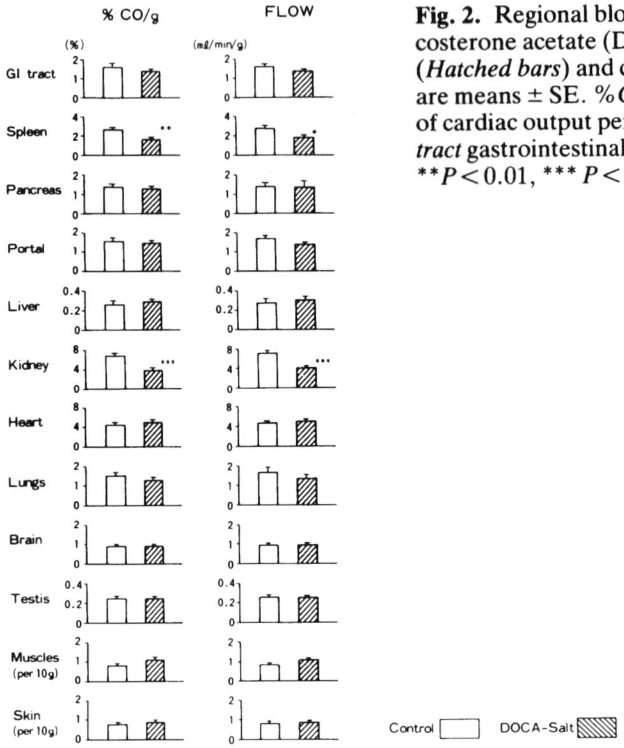

Fig. 2. Regional blood flow data in deoxycorticosterone acetate (DOCA)-salt hypertensive (*Hatched bars*) and control (*open bars*) rats. Data are means ± SE. *%CO/g* percentage of fraction of cardiac output per gram of organ weight, *GI tract* gastrointestinal tract. * $P<0.05$, ** $P<0.01$, *** $P<0.001$ vs. control rats

organs were similar in the hypertensive and control rats, for the most part. Noticeably, these parameters were significantly decreased in the spleen and kidneys. In addition, portal (gastrointestinal tract, spleen, and pancreas) blood flow tended to be decreased in the hypertensive rats ($0.05<P<0.10$). The RMRS method was thus able to detect significant hemodynamic changes in DOCA-salt hypertensive rats.

Systemic and regional hemodynamics were also investigated in spontaneously hypertensive rats (SHR), an experimental model of genetic hypertension, and the control strain of Wistar-Kyoto rats (WKY) [10]. Measurements were made in conscious rats over a wide range of ages, i.e., at 8, 24, 48, and 96 weeks. In SHR, MAP was already increased (average 142 mmHg) at 8 weeks of age, reached a near plateau level of 160 mmHg at 24 weeks, and remained at this level thereafter. MAP was 120–130 mmHg in all WKY groups. The cardiac index was similar in SHR and WKY at 8–96 weeks of age. Accordingly, increased MAP was maintained by increased total peripheral resistance index in SHR, compared with WKY, at all ages studied. Regional blood flows were not different in SHR and WKY at most ages tested. Notably, in SHR, there was a tendency toward decrease in renal blood flow at 8–48 weeks of age, and significantly decreased renal blood flow was observed at 96 weeks (SHR 499 ml/min/100 g vs. WKY 664 ml/min/100 g; $P<0.05$). Splanchnic blood flow was significantly decreased in SHR vs. WKY, when comparison was made between both strains as a whole; however, no significant difference was noted in splanchnic blood flow when comparison was made at each individual age.

These data indicate that the characteristic feature of systemic hemodynamics in SHR hypertension was an increased total peripheral resistance, a finding identical to that seen in human essential hypertension [11]. Our observations of the regional hemodynamic pattern, consisting of almost unaltered blood flow to most organs except for reduced renal blood flow in the oldest age-group of SHR, also agree with findings in human essential hypertension. Reviewing the literature revealed that some controversy exists as to cardiac output in very early and advanced stages of SHR hypertension [10, 11]. We showed that the cardiac index was unaltered in young-through-old SHR when the RMRS method was used under conscious, quiescent conditions [10].

SHR hypertension develops slowly according to a genetically programmed mode [10, 11], whereas DOCA-salt hypertension develops rapidly with artificial DOCA-salt treatment [8, 9]. Nonetheless, considering our results with DOCA-salt rats and SHR together, we believe that the most vulnerable among the peripheral vascular beds was the renal circulation in experimental models of hypertensive disease. Thus, hypertension-specific circulatory alterations were successfully detected with the RMRS method.

Collectively, the RMRS method permits reliable, simultaneous assessment of cardiac output and regional blood flows in rats. This method is useful for evaluation of circulatory alterations in disease models and also of those provoked by chemical and other agents [12–14].

Acknowledgment. This work was supported in part by a grant-in-aid (C-62570408) for Scientific Research by the Ministry of Education, Science and Culture.

References

1. Malik AB, Kaplan JE, Saba TM (1976) Reference sample method for cardiac output and regional blood flow determinations in the rat. J Appl Physiol 40: 472–475
2. Ishise S, Pegram BL, Yamamoto J, Kitamura Y, Frohlich ED (1980) Reference sample microsphere method: cardiac output and blood flows in conscious rat. Am J Physiol 239: H443–H449
3. Buckberg GD, Luck JC, Payne DB, Hoffman JIE, Archie JP, Fixler DE (1971) Some sources of errors in measuring regional blood flow with radioactive microspheres. J Appl Physiol 31: 598–604
4. Tsuchiya M, Ferrone RA, Walsh GM, Frohlich ED (1977) Systemic hemodynamic effects of microspheres in conscious rats. Am J Physiol 233: H617–H621
5. Flaim SF, Morris ZQ, Kennedy TJ (1978) Dextran as a radioactive microsphere suspending agent: severe hypotensive effects in rat. Am J Physiol 235: H587–H591
6. Stanek KA, Smith TL, Murphy WR, Coleman TG (1983) Hemodynamic disturbances in the rat as a function of the number of microspheres injected. Am J Physiol 245: H920–H923
7. Tuma RF, Vasthare US, Irion GL, Wiedeman MP (1986) Consideration in use of microspheres for flow measurements in anesthetized rats. Am J Physiol 250: H137–143
8. Yamamoto J, Goto Y, Nakai M, Ogino K, Ikeda M (1983) Circulatory pressure-volume relationship and cardiac output in DOCA-salt rats. Hypertension 5: 507–513
9. Yamamoto J, Yamane Y, Umeda Y, Yoshioka T, Nakai M, Ikeda M (1984) Cardiovascular hemodynamics and vasopressin blockade in DOCA-salt hypertensive

rats. Hypertension 6: 397–407
10. Yamamoto J, Nakai M, Natsume T (1987) Cardiovascular responses to acute stress in young-to-old spontaneously hypertensive rats. Hypertension 9: 362–370
11. Trippodo NC, Frohlich ED (1981) Similarity of genetic (spontaneous) hypertension: man and rat. Circ Res 47: 922–933
12. Yamamoto J, Akabane S, Yoshimi H, Nakai M, Ikeda M (1985) Effects of taurine on stress-evoked hemodynamic and plasma catecholamine changes in spontaneously hypertensive rats. Hypertension 7: 913–922
13. Nakai M, Matsui Y, Yamamoto J (1986) Systemic and regional hemodynamic effects of E614 (tripamide) as studied in conscious SHR. Arch Int Pharmacodyn Ther 279: 291–303
14. Nakai M, Yamamoto J, Matsui M (1986) Acute systemic and regional hemodynamic effects of alphal-adrenoceptor blockade in conscious spontaneously hypertensive rats. Clin Exp Hypertension A8 (6): 981–996

Angiotensin Converting Enzyme Activity in Brain Microvessels of Rats

Satoko Itoh, Yoshiharu Kanayama, Hiromi Inariba, Mikio Okamura, Kazuo Takaori, Takatoshi Inoue, and Tadanao Takeda[1]

Introduction

Angiotensin converting enzyme (ACE) is a carboxyl terminal dipeptidyl dipeptidase, which is known to convert angiotensin I to angiotensin II (Ang II) and to hydrolyze bradykinin and enkephalin. In the brain, ACE is located in endothelial cells of capillaries throughout the brain, in the subfornical organ, and in the brush border of choroidal epithelial cells in contact with cerebrospinal fluid [1]. Administration of Ang II into the brain ventricles induces thirst [2], a rise in arterial blood pressure, and secretion of vasopressin [3]. Recently, the specific binding of Ang II to the membrane fraction of canine brain microvessels was detected, suggesting the role of Ang II in regulation of the brain microcirculation and transport across the blood-brain barrier [4]. Since ACE in the brain microvessels might affect the brain microcirculation by modulating the local production of Ang II, we measured ACE activity in brain microvessels obtained from 13-week-old spontaneously hypertensive rats (SHR), Wistar-Kyoto rats, and SHR of the same age under antihypertensive therapy to clarify the effect of hypertension on the brain microvessels.

Materials and Methods

Male 13-week-old SHR and Wistar-Kyoto rats (WKY) were used. Male 4-week-old SHR were treated with hydralazine (5 mg/kg, p.o.) for 9 weeks (HD-SHR). Systolic blood pressure was measured by the tail-cuff method in conscious rats. Brain microvessels were isolated according to the method of Goldstein et al. [5]. The rats were killed by decapitation. The gray matter of the cortices was minced and homogenized in oxygen-saturated Ringer's solution (pH 7.4). The homogenate was passed through the three nylon meshes (900,200, and 100 μm) and centrifuged. The pellet was resuspended in the same buffer containing 30% bovine serum albumin and centrifuged. The pellet was resuspended in the original buffer and applied to a column of glass beads (0.2 mm diameter). The

[1]First Department of Internal Medicine, Osaka City University Medical School, 5–7, Asahimachi 1-chome, Abeno-ku, Osaka, 545 Japan

microvessels attached to the glass beads were removed by gentle agitation and centrifuged. The purity of isolation of the brain microvessels was determined by phase-contrast micrography.

Brain microvessels were homogenized in Tris-HCl buffer (pH 8.3) containing 0.5% Nonidet P-40 and centrifuged to obtain the enzyme solution. ACE activity was measured by the production rate of hyppuric acid from Hip-His-Leu using high-performance liquid chromatography [6]. γ-Glutamyl transpeptidase (γ-GTP) activity, a marker enzyme of brain microvessels, was measured according to the method of Orlowsky and Meister [7].

Results

The systolic blood pressure of SHR (172.9 ± 8.7 mmHg) was higher than that of WKY (128.9 ± 2.5 mmHg; $P < 0.01$) and HD-SHR (156.3 ± 4.8 mmHg; $P < 0.01$; Fig. 1.). In the phase-contrast micrograph of brain microvessels, the preparation was composed mainly of capillaries and appeared free of neuronal and glial elements. The purity of isolation of brain microvessels was also confirmed by measurement of γ-GTP activity. γ-GTP activity in brain homogenates was 16.9 ± 8.6 in WKY, 17.1 ± 3.0 in SHR, and 18.2 ± 3.7 nmol/min/mg protein in HD-SHR. γ-GTP activity in brain microvessels was 127.8 ± 25.1 in WKY,

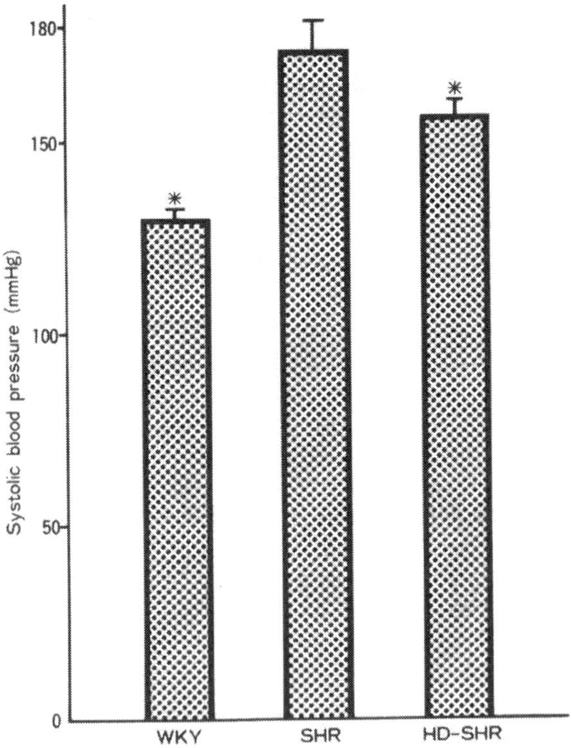

Fig. 1. Systolic blood pressures of WKY ($n = 16$), SHR ($n = 16$), and HD-SHR ($n = 10$). Values are means ± SD. * $P < 0.01$ vs. SHR

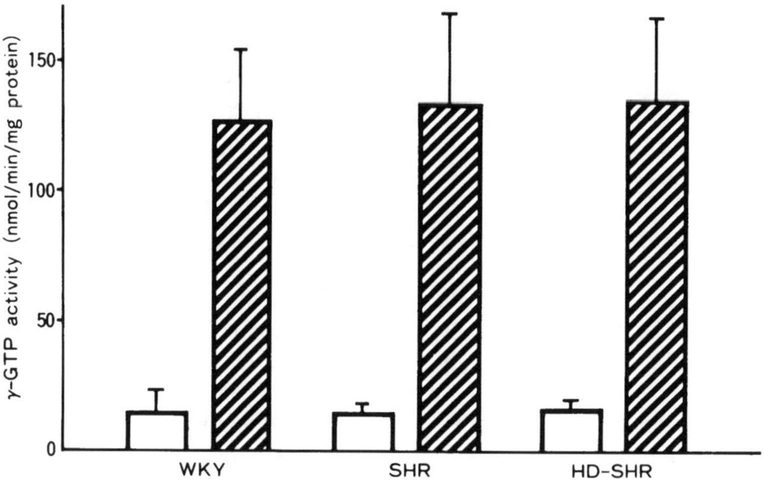

Fig. 2. γ-Glutamyl transpeptidase activity in brain homogenate (*open bars*) and brain microvessles (*hatched bars*) of rats. Values are means ± SD

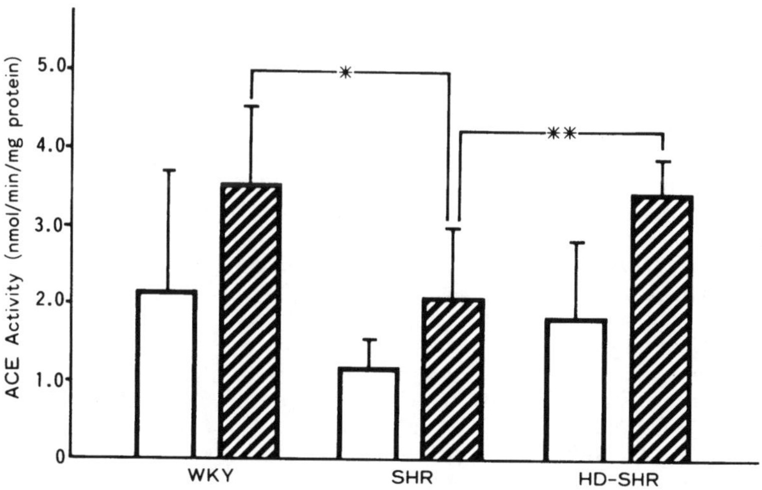

Fig. 3. ACE activity in brain homogenate (*open bars*) and brain microvessels (*hatched bars*) of rats. Values are means ± SD. $*P<0.01$, $**P<0.05$

130.8 ± 35.2 in SHR, and 132.8 ± 30.7 nmol/min/mg protein in HD-SHR. There was no significant difference among the three groups (Fig. 2.).

ACE activity in brain microvessels of SHR (2.11 ± 0.92 nmol/min/mg protein) was lower than that of WKY (3.55 ± 1.06; $P<0.01$) and HD-SHR (3.44 ± 0.45; $P<0.05$; Fig. 3.), but there was no significant difference in the ACE activity of brain homogenates among the three groups.

Discussion

The development of methods for the isolation of brain microvessels has made it possible to measure the activity of enzymes such as ACE in the brain microvessels [8]. In this study, the ACE activity in brain microvessels of SHR was lower than that of WKY. However, the ACE activity in brain microvessels of hydralazine-treated SHR was higher than that of SHR. These results suggest that the ACE activity of brain microvessels is modulated by high blood pressure in rats.

Examination of ACE activity in cultured endothelial cells revealed a decrease in the specific activity of the enzyme as the population-doubling level of the cultures increased [9]. The activity of histidine decarboxylase, which may alter the permeability of endothelial cells, was extremely sensitive to shearing stress [10]. These reports indicated that the enzyme activity in endothelial cells is altered by increased turnover of the cell cycle or by shear stress [11].

The low activity of ACE in the brain microvessels of hypertensive rats may contribute to the regulation of the blood flow or permeability of the brain microcirculation.

References

1. Brownfield MS, Reid IA, Ganten D, Ganong WF (1982) Differential distribution of immunoreactive angiotensin and angiotensin-converting enzyme in rat brain. Neuroscience 7: 1759–1769
2. Epstein AN, Fitzsimons JT, Rolls BJ (1969) Drinking induced by injection of angiotensin into the brain of the rat. J Physiol (London) 210: 457–474
3. Severs WB, Daniels-Severs AE (1973) Effects of angiotensin on the central nervous system. Pharmacol Rev 25: 415–440
4. Speth RC, Haric SI (1985) Angiotensin II receptor binding sites in brain microvessels. Proc Natl Acad Sci USA 82: 6340–6343
5. Goldstein GW, Wolinsky JS, Csejtey J, Diamond I (1975) Isolation of metabolically active capillaries from rat brain. J Neurochem 25: 715–717
6. Horiuchi M, Fujimura K, Terashima T, Iso T (1982) Method for determination of angiotensin-converting enzyme activity in blood and tissue by high-performance liquid chromatography. J Chromatog 233: 123–130
7. Orlowsky M, Meister A (1965) Isolation of γ-glutamyltranspeptidase from hog kidney. J Biol Chem 240: 338–347
8. Brecher P, Tercyac A, Gavras H, Chobanian AV (1978) Peptidyl dipeptidase in rabbit brain microvessels. Biochim Biophys Acta 526: 537–546
9. Del Vecchio PJ, Smith JR (1982) Aging of endothelium in culture: Decrease in angiotensin-converting enzyme activity. Cell Biol Int Reports 6: 379–384
10. Rosen LA, Hollis TM, Sharma MG (1974) Alterations in bovine endothelial histidine decarboxylase activity following exposure to shearing stresses. Exp Mol Pathol 20: 329–343
11. Shepro D, D'Amore PA (1984) Handbook of physiology. The cardiovascular system: IV. American Physiological Society, Bethesda, Maryland, pp 103–164

Assessment of the Adequacy of Mucosal Oxygenation in Patients with Intraluminally Located Silicone Tonomitors

Richard G. Fiddian-Green[1]

An indirect method for measuring the pH in the gastrointestinal mucosa has been applied to the monitoring and evaluation of patients who are critically ill. The method depends upon the knowledge that tissues are highly permeable to CO_2 and that the PCO_2 of fluid instilled into the lumen of a hollow organ will equilibrate with the PCO_2 of tissue fluid and cells in the superficial layers of the wall of the hollow organ [1–4]. This is true for all parts of the gut including the stomach, for the PCO_2 of fluid instilled into the lumen of this hollow organ rises and falls in parallel with changes in PCO_2 in arterial blood [1]. The measurement of pH depends also upon the assumption that the $[HCO_3^-]$ in the wall of the organ is the same as that being belivered to it in arterial blood and upon the assumption that the pH in the tissue fluid is the same as that in plasma. The pH is calculated by substituting the measurements of PCO_2 in luminal fluid and the $[HCO_3^-]$ in arterial blood in the Henderson-Hasselbalch equation.

The measurement of PCO_2 in luminal fluid is facilitated by using a Tonomitor (Tonometrics Inc, Bethesda, MD, USA). In its commercial form, the Tonomitor consists of a sillicone balloon that is freely permeable to CO_2 and a sampling tube that is impermeable to CO_2. The Tonomitor permits fluid to be placed in any segment of the gut long enough for the CO_2 in the fluid to equilibrate with the PCO_2 in the superficial layers of the mucosa with which it is in contact. The volume capacity of the Tonomitor buffers local variations in PCO_2, occurring from the buffering of gastric acid by duodenal bicarbonate and regional differences in metabolic activity. The PCO_2 of fluid in the Tonomitor provides an indirect measure of the mean ambient PCO_2 in superficial layers of the mucosa with which it is in contact.

Alterations in pH of luminal fluid do not influence the equilibrium PCO_2 in the Tonomitor. The indirect measurements of pH in the mucosa vary independently of variations in the pH of luminal fluid [2] and the reproducibility of measurements of intramucosal pH in the stomach is of the same order as that in the other parts of the gut [1]. The independence of the equilibrium PCO_2 in the Tonomitor from variations in the pH in luminal fluid was confirmed in a simple in vitro experiment. In this experiment, a Tonomitor was inserted into each of

[1] Department of Surgery, University of Massachusetts Medical Center, 55 Lake Avenue North, Worcester, MA 01605, USA

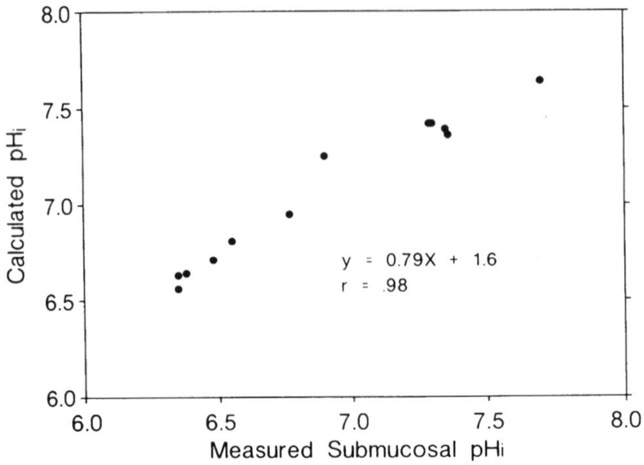

Fig. 1. Correlation between the indirect measurements of intramucosal pH calculated from the PCO_2 in a Tonomitor and the $[HCO_3^-]$ in arterial blood and measurements in the submucsosal space of the intestine of an anesthetized dog made directly with a pH probe. The measurements were made before and at 20-min intervals after occluding the blood supply to the gut

nine silicone bags (permeable to CO_2) filled with nine solutions of different pH, ranging from pH 1 to 9. All nine bags were then immersed into the same container of saline being bubbled with CO_2. The PCO_2 of saline introduced into each of the nine Tonomitors equilibrated with the PCO_2 in the container independently of the pH in the silicone bags into which they had been immersed.

The assumption that the $[HCO_3^-]$ in the mucosa is the same as that in arterial blood is valid for an adequately perfused organ but invalid for an ischemic organ that is generating lactic acid. Despite this source of error, the indirect measurements of pH in gut mucosa correlate remarkably well with measurements of pH made directly with a microprobe (Fig. 1). Thus, even though the indirect measurement of pH might not be an accurate reflection of the actual pH within the mucosa, it does reflect the direction and magnitude of the fall in tissue pH from control values that occur in ischemia.

The assumption that the $[HCO_3^-]$ in the body of the stomach is the same as that in arterial blood is invalid during the stimulation of acid secretion, when an alkaline tide is generated in the gastric tissues. This potential source of error may be avoided by inhibiting the secretion of acid with an H_2 receptor antagonist. The long-term and compulsive administration of antacids to prevent stress ulceration may also induce a local tissue alkalosis and could mask a fall in pH occurring in ischemia [2].

Intramucosal pH, Mucosal Oxygenation, and Ischemia in Animals

The indirect measurement of pH in the gut mucosa provides a metabolic measure of the adequacy of mucosal oxygenation [3], the first part of the gut to be affected in ischemia [5]. The pH in the mucosa remains constant in the face of a progressive decrease in oxygen delivery until a critical point is reached at which oxygen delivery becomes equal to the oxygen requirements of the tissue (Fig. 2). Below this point, which varies depending upon the manner in which oxygen delivery is reduced, the pH in the mucosa falls in parallel with further decreases in oxygen delivery and the corresponding fall in oxygen consumption by the gut. That the indirect measurement of intramucosal pH reflects the adequacy of mucosal oxygenation is confirmed by the maintenance of the intramucosal pH at control levels and the prevention of mucosal disruption during total arterial occlusion achieved by the intraluminal infusion of oxygenated saline (Fig. 3). Thus, a deviation in intramucosal pH below the statistical limits of normality provides an indication of the presence of anerobic metabolism and, hence, of mucosal ischemia.

The pH in the mucosa remains constant under stable conditions but falls below the statistical limits of normality within minutes of total arterial occlusion (Fig. 3). A fall in intramucosal pH to abnormally low levels for 2 h followed by reperfusion is sufficient to cause complete mucosal infarction. Thus, a fall in intramucosal pH to abnormally low levels for 2 h is indicative of mucosal hypoxia severe enough to cause complete mucosal infarction. It takes about 8 h of total ischemia to cause transmural infarction [5].

There are regional differences in the measurements of intramucosal pH (pHi), which must be taken into account when using the pHi to assess the adequacy of mucosal oxygenation. The pHi in gastric mucosa is slightly higher than the pH in arterial blood (pHa). The pHi in small intestinal mucosa is about the same as the pHa and the pHi in colonic mucosa slightly lower than the pHa [1, 4].

Diagnosis of Mucosal Ischemia in Patients

The indirect measurement of intramucosal pH is a sensitive and specific diagnostic test for mucosal ischemia in patients. In the sigmoid colon, the lowest intramucosal pH encountered on the day of operation in patients having abdominal aortic operations correlates very well with the endoscopic appearance of the sigmoid mucosa [6] and the symptoms [7] of ischemic mucosal colitis developing several days after surgery. A fall in intramucosal pH in the sigmoid colon below the lower limit of normality on the day of operation distinguishes all patients who die from ischemic mucosal colitis from all those who have an uncomplicated postopertive course with a sensitivity of 100% and a specificity of 87% [6]. An abnormally low pH in the stomach distinguished all measurements made in six symptomatic patients with chronic gastrointestinal ischemia from all those made after their symptoms had been relieved by revascularization, with a sensitivity and specificity of 100% [8].

Gastric Mucosal Ischemia in Cardiac Surgery

More than 50% of patients having cardiac operations develop a transient episode of gastric mucosal ischemia during the operation or within the first few hours

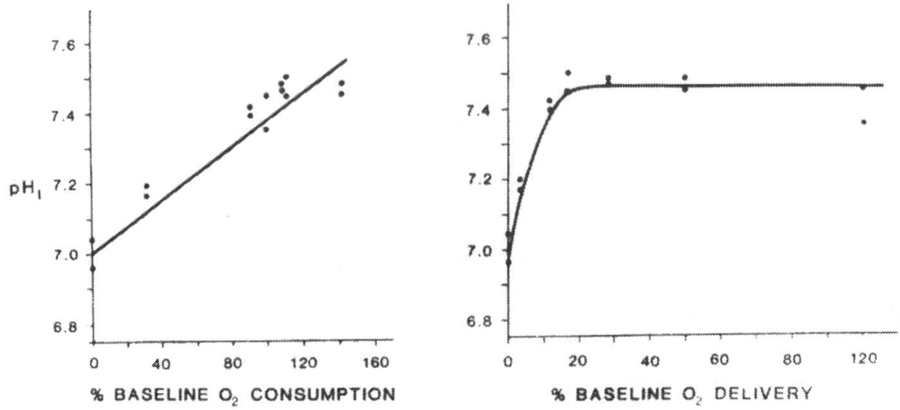

Fig. 2. The relationship between the indirect measurements of pH in the mucosa (pH_I) made with Tomomitors and oxygen delivery to the gut in the small intestine of an anesthetized dog. After Grum et al. [3]

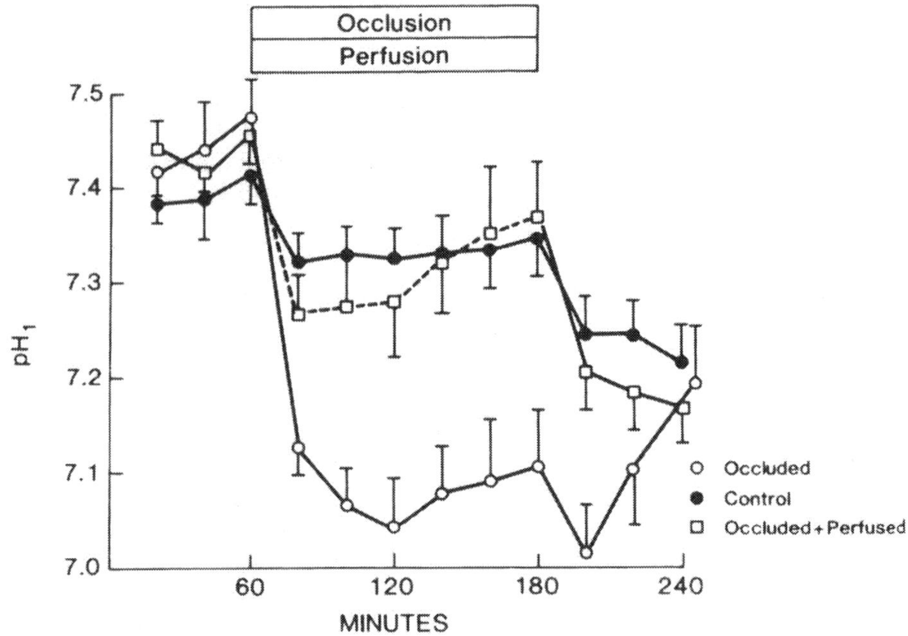

Fig. 3. Indirect measurements of intramucosal pH (pH_I) in three discontinuous segments of the small intestine in the same 12 anesthetized dogs, showing the effects of vascular occlusion and reperfusion in two of the segments. The intramucosal pH in one of the ischemic segments was maintained at control levels and histological evidence of mucosal infarction was prevented by the intraluminal infusion of oxygenated saline during the period of vascular occlusion. The fall in pHi in the control segment of the gut, observed upon occlusion and reperfusion of the two other segments, did not occur in control experiments in other dogs

after the operation, as evident from a fall in intramucosal pH below the lower statistical limit of normality in the stomach derived from 47 elderly patients [9]. Most episodes lasted about 1 h.

The presence of gastric mucosal ischemia and especially the duration of gastric mucosal ischemia on the day of operation was highly predictive for the development of life-threatening complications within 72 h of surgery [9], for death from all causes, and for death from low cardiac output syndrome occurring within 30 days of cardiac surgery [10].

The mucosal ischemia that develops in patients having cardiac surgery is an early indication of impaired core tissue perfusion. The time-course of events and the predictive ability of the transient episodes of gastric mucosal ischemia for outcome are consistent with the hypothesis [5] that the transient episodes of mucosal ischemia are causally related to low-cardic output syndrome, the primary cause of death in our patients.

Gastric Mucosal Ischemia and Stress Ulceration in ICU Patients

Gastric mucosal ischemia, or acidosis, is a common finding in intensive care unit (ICU) patients, occurring in 80% of those with multiple organ failure [11]. The probability of massive bleeding from stress ulceration is very low, even in patients with multiple organ failure, unless the pH in gastric mucosa falls to abnormally low levels [2]. The fall in intramucosal pH in these patients is accompanied by a fall in intramucosal PO_2 and is almost certainly a manifestation of gastric mucosal ischemia [2, 12].

Sigmoid Mucosal Ischemia in Abdominal Aortic Surgery

Acidosis in the sigmoid colonic mucosa occurred on the day of operation in 25% of patients having an abdominal aortic operation [6, 7]. The acidosis, which was highly predictive for the development of endoscopic and clinical evidence of severe ischemic colitis, tended to occur in the elderly and in patients with a significant stenosis of the superior mesenteric artery. The probability of developing ischemic colitis was not influenced by the status of the inferior mesenteric artery, as reported in other studies. Although pH in the sigmoid mucosa fell after application of the aortic clamp [6], it fell more profoundly after the aortic clamp had been removed, and in some instances only after the patient had been transferred to the ICU. As in the patients having cardiac operations, the episodes of ischemia were usually transient and lasted less than 2 h.

The duration of sigmoid mucosal ischemia on the day of operation was highly predictive for the development of sepsis from enteric organisms [13], multiple organ failure, death from all causes, and death from multiple organ failure [6, 7, 10]. These data are consistent with the hypothesis that mucosal disruption in the sigmoid colon is causally related to the development of sepsis from enteric organisms and to the development of multiple organ failure [5].

Monitoring in the Critically Ill

Gastric mucosal ichemia is one of the earliest manifestations of impaired core tissue perfusion in the critically ill. The sensitivity of gastric mucosal ischemia, detected on the day of surgery, as a predictor of impending complications following cardiac surgery is 100% [9]. In some patients who die in the ICU, gastric mucosal ischemia may precede all other evidence of impaired core tissue perfusion by several days [11]. The sensitivity of oliguria, and indicator of impaired tissue perfusion in another regional tissue bed, is only 12.5%. Oliguria was only seen in one of our patients, on the day of surgery, and then only some hours after the onset of the gastric mucosal ischemia, shortly before he died from low cardiac output syndrome. Hypotension and arterial acidosis are also poorly sensitive as predictors of impending complications. Oliguria, hypotension, and arterial acidosis are all later manifestations in deteriorating patients and invariably preterminal events [9].

The specificity of gastric mucosal ischemia as a predictor of impending complications following cardiac surgery is 55% and increases exponentially as the degree and duration of the ischemia increase. The appearance of oliguria was 100% specific for impending complications. Hypotension and arterial acidosis were also highly specific as predictors when the data collected during bypass were excluded from the analysis.

Stepwise logistic regression analysis of all the measurements made on the day of surgery in patients having cardiac operation shows that inclusion of the indirect measurements of pH on the day of surgery improves significantly the prediction of life-threatening complications achieved by conventional forms of monitoring [14]. The best predictive model for impending complications was derived from measurements of intramucosal pH in the stomach, a measure of the adequacy of core tissue perfusion, and the systolic blood pressure, a measure of perfusion pressure. The predictive ability of this model was not improved by inclusion of any other measurement recorded, including the urine output and all the measurements of myocardial performance made with pulmonary artery catheters.

Conclusion

"The detection of microvascular dysfunction in key organ systems early in disease is one of our highest priorities" (See Chap. 1) The indirect method of measuring the intramucosal pH fulfills this need. The method provides clinicians with a safe, simple, and effective means of evaluating the adequacy of gut oxygenation and establishing the diagnosis of mucosal ischemia in patients. Measurements of intramucosal pH in gastric mucosa improve the efficacy of monitoring in the critically ill. Measurements of pH in other parts of the splanchnic circulation may improve further the accuracy of the predictions. The mearements of pH enable minor disturbances in splanchnic tissue perfusion to be dectected hours or days before any impairment of core tissue perfusion can be detected by conventional means. Transient episodes of mucosal ischemia, indicative of an impairment of splanchnic perfusion from low flow and/or vasospasm, are extremely common in the critically ill. The episodes are highly predictive for impending complications, sepsis, and death from low cardiac output syndrome and from multiple organ failure. The predictive ability of these episodes of mucosal ischemia for outcome and the time-course of events are consistent with the hypothesis that transient episodes of splanchnic ischemia are causally related to low cardiac output syndrome, sepsis, and multiple organ failure, Further clinical studies are necessary to determine the best ways of preventing or limiting the degree and duration of these transient episodes of mucosal ischemia to establish whether splanchnic ischemia is indeed causally related to these events.

References

1. Fiddian-Green RG, Pittenger G, Whitehouse WM Jr (1982) Back-diffusion of CO_2 and its influence on the intramural pH in gastric mucosa. J Surg Res 33: 39–48
2. Fiddian-Green RG, McGough E, Pittenger G, Rothman ED (1983) Predictive value of intramural pH and other risk factors for massive bleeding from stress ulceration. Gastroenterology 85: 613–20
3. Grum CM, Fiddian-Green RG, Pittenger GL, Grant BJB, Rothman ED, Dantzker DR (1984) Adequacy of tissue oxygenation in intact dog intestine. J Appl Physiol 56: 1065–69
4. Poole JW, Sammartano RJ, Boley SJ (1987) Hemodynamic basis of the pain in chronic mesenteric ischemia. Am J Surg 153: 171–76
5. Marston A (1986) Laboratory studies of intestinal ischaemia. In: Marston A (ed) Vascular diseases of the gut. Arnold, Melbourne, pp 30–51
6. Shiedler MG, Cutler BS, Fiddian-Green RG (1987) Sigmoid intramurial pH for prediction of ischemic colitis during aortic surgery. Arch Surg 122: 881–6
7. Fiddian-Green RG, Amelin PM, Herrmann JB, Arous E, Cutler BS, Schiedler M, Wheeler HB, Baker S (1986) Prediction of the development of sigmoid ischemia on the day of aortic operations. Arch Surg 121: 654–60
8. Fiddian-Green RG, Stanley J, Nostrant T, Phillips D (1987) Chronic gastric ischemia: a cause of chronic abdominal pain identified from the presence of acidosis in the wall of the stomach. In: Microcirculation—an update, vol 2. Elsevier, Amsterdam, pp 275–276
9. Fiddian-Green RG, Baker S (1987) The predictive value of measurements of pH in the wall of the stomach for complications after cardiac surgery: a comparison with other forms of monitoring. Crit Care Med 15: 153–56
10. Fiddian-Green Amelin P, Baker S (1987) Predictive value of transient episodes of gut ischemia for death after cardiac and aortic operations. In: Microcirculation—an update, vol 2. Elsevier, Amsterdam, pp 447–448
11. Fiddian-Green RG (1987) Hypotension, splanchnic hypoxia and arterial acidosis in ICU patients. Circ Shock 21: 326
12. Kamada T, Sato N, Kawano S, Fusamoto H, Abe H (1982) Gastric mucosal hemodynamics after thermal or head injury. A clinical application of reflectance spectrometry. Gastroenterology 83: 535–40
13. Fiddian-Green RG, Gantz NM (1987) Transient episodes of sigmoid ischemia and their relation to infection from intestinal organisms after abdominal aortic operations. Crit Care Med 15: 835–839
14. Fiddian-Green RG, Baker S (1987) The value of measurements used to monitor patients having cardiac operations. In: Microcirculation—an update, vol 2. Elsevier, Amsterdam, pp 187–188

Comparative Studies on Microcirculation of the Pancreas in Anesthetized and Conscious Dogs

Kazutomo Inoue[1], Tamotsu Kawano[1], Ryo Hosotani[1], Masafumi Kogire[1], Shoichiro Sumi[1], Ryuichiro Doi[1], Mitsutoshi Yun[1], Takashi Suzuki[2], Haruaki Yajima[3], and Takayoshi Tobe[1]

The physiology of pancreatic blood flow has been poorly understood because of the difficulty in measuring it since there is an abundance of anastomoses between the branches of the vessels supplying blood flow to the pancreas. Furthermore, very little information is available regarding the physiology of pancreatic blood flow in the conscious state.

In this study, two methods were used—the hydrogen gas clearance method [1] and the thermoelectric method [2–6]. The former procedure makes it possible to measure quantitatively the basal tissue blood flow, and the latter enables us to measure continuously the changes in tissue blood flow.

Vasoactive intestinal peptide (VIP) is known to have a wide range of biological activities [5, 6]. The present study was conducted to compare the microcirculation of the pancreas and pancreatic blood flow response to VIP in the conscious state with that observed under anesthesia.

Materials and Methods

Mongrel dogs of both sexes, weighing from 8 to 15 kg, were used. Rearing of these dogs and the experiments were carried out at the Institute of Laboratory Animals, Faculty of Medicine, Kyoto University. Each dog was deprived of food for 18 h with free access to water before each experiment.

Basal pancreatic blood flow in the conscious state and following intravenous pentobarbital injection (25 mg/kg body weight) was measured in six dogs by the hydrogen gas clearance method [1] with a platinum electrode, 0.2 mm in diameter (Medical System wire-type element), implanted into the pancreatic tissue.

Changes in pancreatic blood flow in response to synthetic VIP [7] (0.01, 0.1, 0.5, 1.0 μg/kg) in the conscious state (three dogs) and under pentobarbital anesthesia (25 mg/kg body weight, seven dogs) were compared by the thermoelectric

[1] First Department of Surgery, Faculty of Medicine, Kyoto University, 54 Kawara-cho, Shogoin, Sakyo-ku, Kyoto, 606 Japan
[2] Second Department of Surgery, Faculty of Medicine, Yamaguchi University, 1144 Ogushi, Nishi-ku, Ube, Yamaguchi, 755 Japan
[3] Pharmaceutical Sciences, Kyoto University, Yoshida, Sakyo-ku, Kyoto, 606 Japan

method [2–6] with a thin thermocouple, 0.1 mm in diameter (Medical System wire-type element W552) implanted into the pancreatic tissue.

In each experiment under pentobarbital anesthesia, a femoral artery was cannulated for continuous monitoring of intra-arterial pressure; a catheter was attached to a pressure transducer (Nihon Koden Type MPU OSA) and connected to a Medical-Corder (Nihon Koden Type PMP 3004). The blood flow rate in ml/min/100 g pancreatic tissue weight was measured by the hydrogen gas clearance method. A convenient and widely used method of calculating blood flow rate in tissues is by plotting the desaturation curve semilogarithmically according to the formula: $F = 100\ (0.693/t\frac{1}{2})$ ml/min/100 g, where $t\frac{1}{2}$ is the time in minutes for tissue hydrogen concentration to be reduced to half of its numerical value. In this study, however, the slope of the desaturation curve was determined by computer (Facom M 200). The data were expressed as means ± SEM. Student's paired or unpaired *t*-test was used to analyze the data. Changes associated with P values less than 0.05 were considered statistically significant.

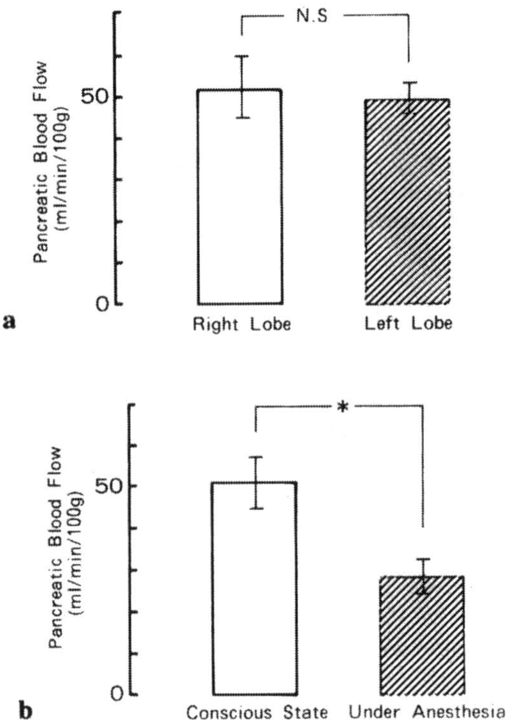

Fig. 1. **a** Comparative studies on the pancreatic blood flow in the right and left lobes of the pancreas in six conscious dogs. Blood flow measurement was performed by the hydrogen gas clearance method. *NS* not significant. **b** Comparative studies on the pancreatic blood flow in the conscious state and after intravenous pentobarbital injection in six dogs. Blood flow measurement was performed by the hydrogen gas clearance method. *Asterisk* represents significant difference between conscious state and under anesthesia

Results

Basal Pancreatic Blood Flow

Pancreatic tissue blood flow in the conscious state was compared between the right and left lobes of the pancreas by performing simultaneous measurement of each lobe of the pancreas (Fig. 1a). No significant difference was detected between the basal blood flow rate in the right (51.6 ± 7.9 ml/min/100 g) and left (49.1 ± 4.7 ml/min/100 g) lobes of the pancreas.

After measurement of pancreatic blood flow in the conscious state, intravenous pentobarbital (25 mg/kg) was given to the same dogs. Pentobarbital injection significantly reduced pancreatic blood to 28.4 ± 4.0 ml/min/100 g (Fig. 1b). Pancreatic blood flow rate was not significantly changed during pentobarbital anesthesia with positive pressure ventilation applied by a respirator through an endotracheal tube.

Pancreatic Blood Flow Response to VIP

Graded doses of synthetic VIP induced graded increases in both conscious and anesthetized dogs (Table 1). Figure 2 illustrates a typical pattern of the pancreatic blood flow response to VIP under pentobarbital anesthesia, measured by the thermoelectric method. VIP induces prominent increases in pancreatic blood flow with simultaneous reduction in the systemic arterial pressure.

Comparative studies on the blood flow response to VIP in the conscious state and under anesthesia revealed that the increased blood flow response of the pancreas in the conscious state is significantly greater than that observed under anesthesia (Table 1).

Discussion

In order to elucidate the physiology of pancreatic blood flow, observation of the microcirculation of the pancreas is indispensable, since there are anatomical complications of blood supply to the pancreas. For that reason, the hydrogen gas clearance method [1, 5] and thermoelectric method [2–6], both of which enable direct measurement of the tissue blood flow of the pancreas, were used in this study.

The hydrogen gas clearance method, which was first introduced by Aukland and colleagues [1], permits the quantitative determination of local blood flow. The weak point of this method is that it does not allow a continuous recording of blood flow changes. On the other hand, the thermoelectric method, which was first introduced by Gibbs [2] and later improved by Grayson [3] and modified by Hensel and Ruef [4], is very useful for measuring continuous changes of the pancreatic tissue blood flow for long periods of time. The disadvantage of this method is that measurement is not quantitative but only qualitative. Therefore, in the present study, we used both methods to measure basal pancreatic blood flow by the hydrogen gas clearance method and pancreatic blood flow response to VIP by the thermoelectric method.

Table 1. Increase in pancreatic blood flow induced by synthetic VIP

VIP (μg/kg)	Increase in pancreatic blood flow (%)	
	Conscious	Anesthesia
0.01	21.5 ± 4.9*	10.5 ± 4.2*[a]
0.1	39.2 ± 6.5*	20.1 ± 7.4*[a]
0.5	43.1 ± 8.1*	34.1 ± 8.9*[a]
1.0	49.0 ± 7.0*	45.3 ± 6.9*

* Significant increase from basal level
[a] Significant difference between conscious ($n = 3$) and anesthetized ($n = 7$) dogs

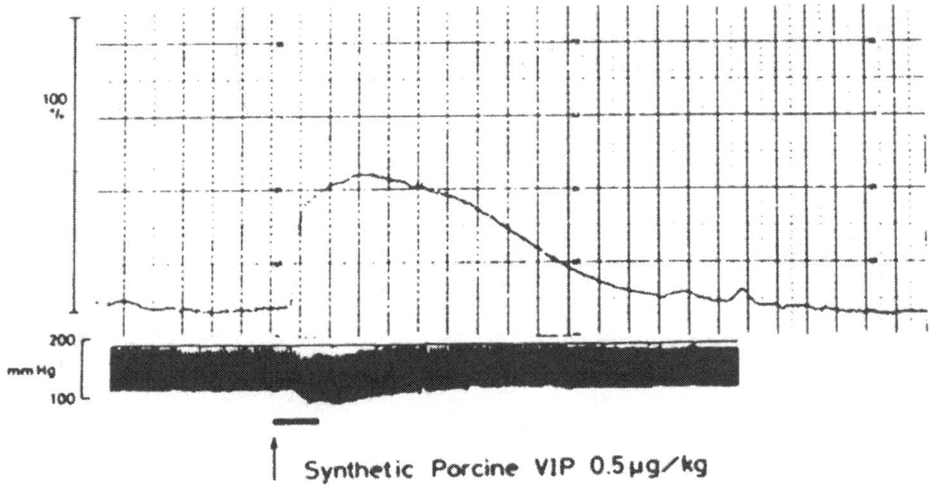

Fig. 2. Continuous recording of changes in pancreatic blood flow in response to 0.5 μg/kg synthetic VIP under pentobarbital anesthesia. Blood flow measurement was carried out by the thermoelectric method

The physiology of the microcirculation of the pancreas in the conscious state has not yet been elucidated. The present study has clarified that basal pancreatic blood flow was significantly greater than that found under anesthesia, suggesting that it is preferable to carry out studies on pancreatic blood flow in the conscious state from the physiological point of view. We have also demonstrated that pancreatic blood flow response to VIP was significantly greater in the conscious dog than in the anesthetized dog, indicating the increased sensitivity of the pancreatic vasculature in the conscious state. Stimulatory action of VIP on pancreatic blood flow has been suggested to be due to the direct effect of VIP on the pancreatic vasculature [5, 6]. It is well known that VIP acts as a neurotransmitter. Prominently increased response of pancreatic blood flow to VIP in the conscious state may be partly attributed to the action of VIP as a neurotransmitter, since the neural pathway is supposedly well maintained in the conscious state.

In conclusion, the present study indicates that the basal pancreatic blood flow in the conscious state is significantly greater than under anesthesia. Pancreatic blood flow response to VIP is significantly greater in the conscious state than under anesthesia, suggesting increased sensitivity of the pancreatic vasculature in the conscious state.

Acknowledgment. This work was supported in part by a grant from the Ministry of Education of Japan (#A 61440060).

References

1. Aukland K, Bower BF, Berliner RW (1964) Measurement of local blood flow with hydrogen gas. Circ Res 14: 164–187
2. Gibbs FA (1933) Thermoelectric blood flow recorder in form of a needle. Proc Soc Exp Biol Med 31: 141–146
3. Grayson J (1952) Internal calorimetry in the determination of thermal conductivity and blood flow. J Physiol 118: 54–72
4. Hensel H, Ruef J (1954) Fortlaufende Registrierung der Muskel-Durchblutung an Menschen mit einer Calorimetersonde. Plfügers Arch 259: 267–280
5. Inoue K, Kawano T, Shima K, Kim T, Suzuki T, Tobe T, Yajima H (1981) Relationship between development of fibrosis and hemodynamic changes of the pancreas in dogs. Gastroenterology 81: 37–47
6. Inoue K, Kawano T, Shima K, Kim T, Suzuki T, Tobe T, Takeyama M, Yajima H (1983) Effect of synthetic chicken vasoactive intestinal peptide on pancreatic blood flow and on exocrine and endocrine secretions of the pancreas in dogs. Dig Dis Sci 28: 724–734
7. Yajima H, Takeyama M, Koyama K, Tobe T, Inoue K, Kawano T, Adachi H (1980) Synthesis of an octacosapeptide amide corresponding to the entire amino acid sequence of chicken vasoactive intestinal polypeptide (VIP). Int J Peptide Protein Res 16: 33–47

Cerebral Microvascular Reserve for Hyperemia

Norio Tanahashi[1]

It is well known that a temporary stoppage of circulation may result in reactive hyperemia in cerebral tissue as in other organs. However, little is yet known about the quantitative characteristics of reactive hyperemia in the cerebral circulation, especially in short periods of ischemia.

Hyperemia is thought to be a condition with an increased blood flow above control level. However, hyperemia is, in the strict sense, an excess of blood in the tissue produced by vascular dilatation and expansion of the vascular bed, which cannot be determined by flow studies alone. Recently, we developed a photoelectric method [1] capable of rapid measurement of the cerebral blood volume together with frequent determinations of cerebral blood flow. By this method, we demonstrated the paradoxical appearance of hyperemia in the ischemic area of the feline brain and termed the phenomenon "low perfusion hyperemia" [2].

In the present study, an attempt was made to clarify the cerebral microvascular reserve for hyperemia by determining the critical duration of middle cerebral artery occlusion for the production of reactive hyperemia in feline cerebral tissue.

Methods

A photoelectric method was used in 21 cats under anesthesia with alpha chloralose and urethane for continuous recording of cerebral blood volume (CBV) and frequent determination of the mean transit time of blood ($\bar{t}$). The measurements were performed in the sylvian area supplied by the middle cerebral artery. From the values of $\bar{t}$ and CBV, the CBF was calculated using the Stewart-Hamilton equation.

Transorbital occlusion of the middle cerebral artery (MCA) at its origin was effected microscopically with a miniature Mayfield clip during continuous recording of the the focal CBV from the core area (sylvian opercula) of the ischemic region and simultaneously from the corresponding area in the opposite

[1]Department of Neurology, Ashikaga Red Cross Hospital, 3-2100 Honjyo, Ashikaga, Tochigi, 326 Japan

hemisphere. CBV values were expressed as changes (CBV vol%) compared with the preocclusive value.

Within 7 min after the MCA occlusion, clips were removed from the MCA to restore the cerebral circulation. All cats were divided into three groups according to the duration of ischemia: (group 1, 0–60 s; group 2, 60–120 s; group 3, 180–420 s). CBV, $\bar{t}$, and CBF values were analyzed to determine the critical duration of MCA occlusion for the appearance of reactive hyperemia in the feline cerebral tissue.

Results

Transorbital clipping of the left MCA at its origin produced a rapid decrease in CBV and a disappearance of the hemodilution curves. The calculated CBF decreased to almost zero. In unclipping, CBV overshot the control level (reactive hyperemia) in group 2 (+0.8 vol%; $P<0.01$) and group 3 (+1.4 vol%; $P<0.005$). The $\bar{t}$ values just after reopening of the MCA were significantly shorter than the preocclusive values only in group 3 ($P<0.001$) and did not show any significant changes in groups 1 and 2. Calculated CBF immediately after reopening of the MCA was significantly greater than the control value in groups 2 ($P<0.05$) and 3 ($P<0.05$) but did not show any significant change in group 1. The CBF increments during reopening was significantly different between groups 2 and 3 ($P<0.05$). Mean arterial blood pressure did not show any significant change by occlusion and reopening of the MCA. CBV, $\bar{t}$, and CBF in the contralateral hemisphere did not show any significant changes after occlusion and reopening of the MCA in all cats.

Discussion

Many studies have been made on the effects of recirculation after major cerebral artery occlusion of the ischemic brain [3–5]. Most work along these lines, however, has been carried out from the viewpoint of changes in CBF, morphology, and clinical signs. The present investigation appears to be the first to perform quantitative estimation of the CBV changes following cerebral ischemia and recirculation.

The data obtained indicate that reactive hyperemia did not appear in the feline cerebral tissue unless the duration of MCA occlusion exceeded 1 min. Such a time lag in the vascular reaction to flow cessation could be accounted for either by a pool of substrates in the tissue or temporary preservation of the autoregulatory mechanism. The latter would mean that the decrease in vascular tone which occurred within 1 min was somehow compensated for by the autoregulatory mechanism upon the sudden recovery of intraluminal pressure.

References

1. Tomita M, Gotoh F, Amano T, Tanahashi N, Tanaka K, Yamamoto M (1978) Photoelectric method for estimating hemodynamic changes in regional cerebral tissue. Am J

Physiol 235: H56–H63
2. Tomita M, Gotoh F, Amamo T, Tanahashi N, Tanaka K (1980) "Low perfusion hyperemia" following middle cerebral arterial occlusion in cats of different age groups. Stroke 11: 629–636
3. Randall JE, Harvath SM (1953) Relationship between duration of ischemia in a single vessel. Am J Physiol 172: 391–398
4. Ishikawa S, Handa J, Meyer JS (1965) Haemodynamics of the circle of Willis and the leptomeningeal anastomoses: An electomagnetic flowmeter study of intracranial arterial occlusion in the monkey. J Neurol Neurosurg Psychiat 28: 124–136
5. Symon L, Ganz JC, Dorsch NWC (1972) Experimental studies of hyperemic phenomena in the cerebral circulation of primates. Brain 95: 265–278

Correlation of Conjunctival Oxygen Tension with Carotid Artery Blood Flow During Hemorrhagic Hypotension

YOSHINORI KIKUTA[1], OTOWA MORITSUNE[1], HIROAKI KAWABATA[1], SHINKICHI TEZUKA[1], KAZUO OKADA[1], and ATSUO FUKUNAGA[2]

Introduction

The palpebral conjunctiva is a very special tissue. The mucous membrane epithelium overlying the conjunctival capillaries is only two to four cell layers thick with minimum oxygen consumption, and this presents a unique opportunity to measure tissue oxygen tension atraumatically [1]. The transconjunctival oxygen monitor measures tissue oxygen tension, which reflects both the oxygen content of the arterial blood and the regional blood flow. If arterial oxygen content remains constant, then any change in tissue oxygen tension should be secondary to a change in the blood flow to that tissue. The purpose of this study was to examine the relationship between the conjunctival PO_2 ($PcjO_2$, in millimeters of mercury) and carotid artery blood flow (CaBF, in millimeters per minute) in the dog during hemorrhagic hypotension.

Method

Six adult dogs weighing 15.8 ± 1.5 (SEM) kg were induced with intravenous thiopental (20 mg/kg), and the trachea was intubated and mechanically ventilated with a constant-volume ventilator to maintain normocapnia. Anesthesia was maintained on enflurane (1.0%) in nitrous oxide (3 l)—oxygen (2 l) and paralysis was caused by pancuronium bromide. An arterial catheter and pulmonary thermodilution catheter were inserted via a femoral cut-down. A polarographic oxygen electrode was mounted on a scleral conformer, a device which conforms to the shape of the eye (Fig. 1). A miniature conjunctival PO_2 sensor (Biomedical Sensors Inc.) was applied noninvasively in the right eye (Fig. 2). The ipsilateral neck was dissected and an ultrasonic blood flowmeter probe (Transonic System Inc.) was placed on the right common carotid artery to measure continuous CaBF. Hemorrhagic hypotension was produced by bleeding from a femoral artery to a reservoir bottle with a constant rate over 30 min until

[1] Department of Anesthesiology, Teikyo University School of Medicine, 11–1, Kaga 2-chome, Itabashi-ku, Tokyo, 173 Japan
[2] Department of Anesthesiology, Harbor-UCLA Medical Center, Torrance, CA 90509, USA

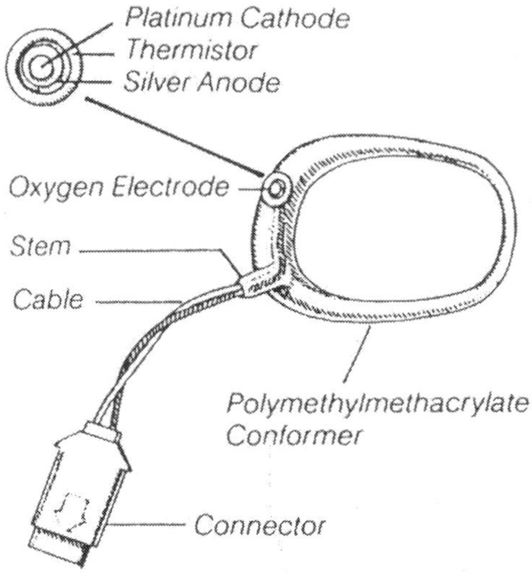

Fig. 1. Polarographic oxygen electrode and scleral conformer

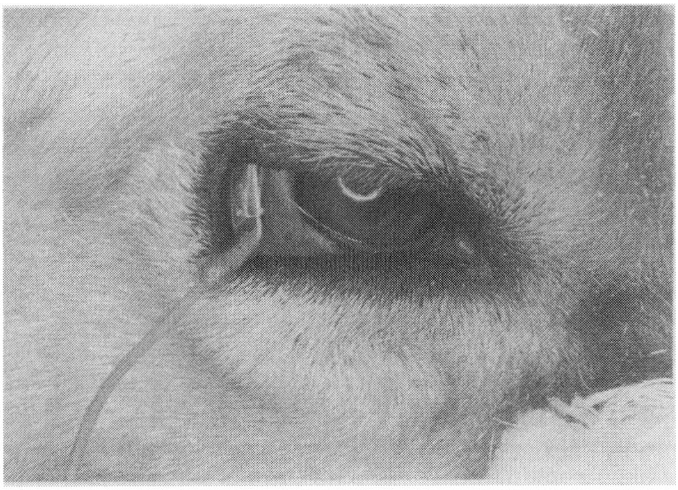

Fig. 2. Application of conjunctival PO_2 sensor to right eye

mean arterial pressure (MAP) reached 50 mmHg, and the MAP was maintained for 180 min by adjusting the height of the reservoir. The data were collected every 5 min and analyzed statistically using linear regression analysis and the paired Student's *t*-test, where applicable, and $P < 0.05$ was considered significant.

Results

MAP decreased from a control value of 119 ± 7 (SEM) mmHg to 90 ± 4 mmHg in 10 min, 66 ± 6 mmHg in 20 min, and attained close to 50 mmHg after 30 min of arterial hemorrhage; it was maintained at this lower level for 180 min. Cardiac

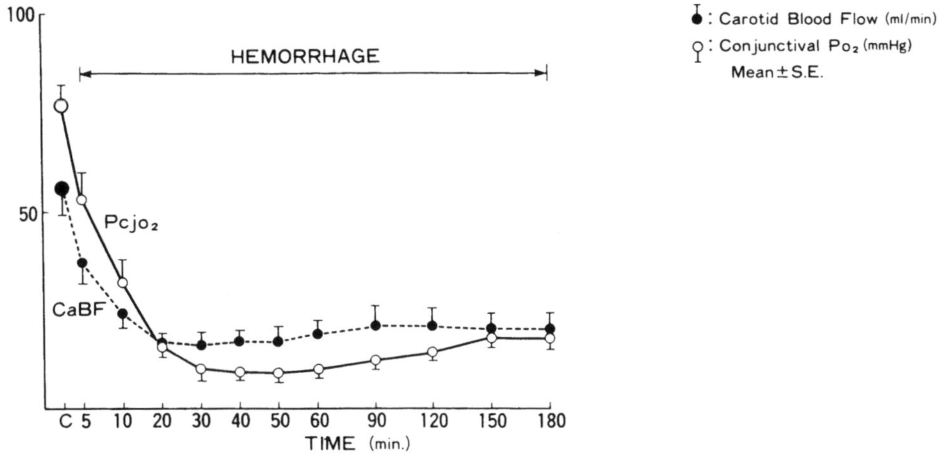

Fig. 3. Changes in carotid blood flow and conjunctival PO_2

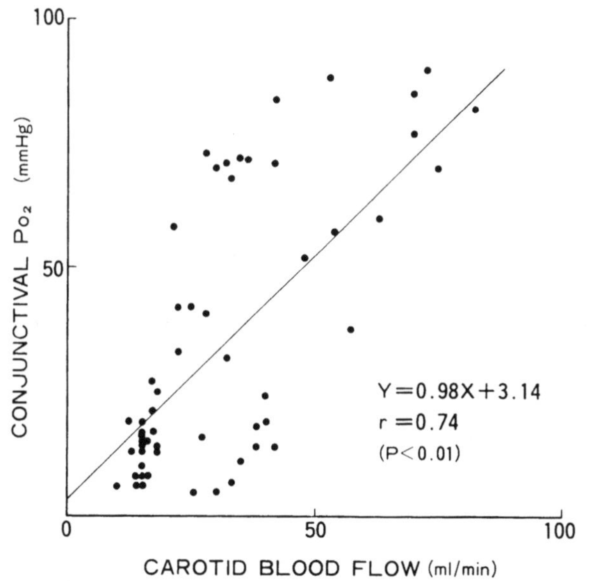

Fig. 4. Correlation between carotid blood flow and conjunctival PO_2

output decreased significantly (0.6 l/min) after 10 min of bleeding from the control value of 2.8 ± 0.3 l/min. Immediately after the beginning of bleeding, $PcjO_2$ fell significantly, concomitant with the significantly decreased CaBF during active hemorrhage; it remained at a lower value during the entire course of hypotension for 180 min (Fig. 3). There was a positively significant ($P<0.01$) correlation ($y = 0.98\,x + 3.14$, $r = 0.74$) between CaBF and $PcjO_2$, as shown in Fig. 4. Figure 5 shows the changes in arterial oxygen tension (PaO_2) and pH during hemorrhagic hypotension. PaO_2 remained unchanged, but pH decreased significantly after 90 min of hypotension.

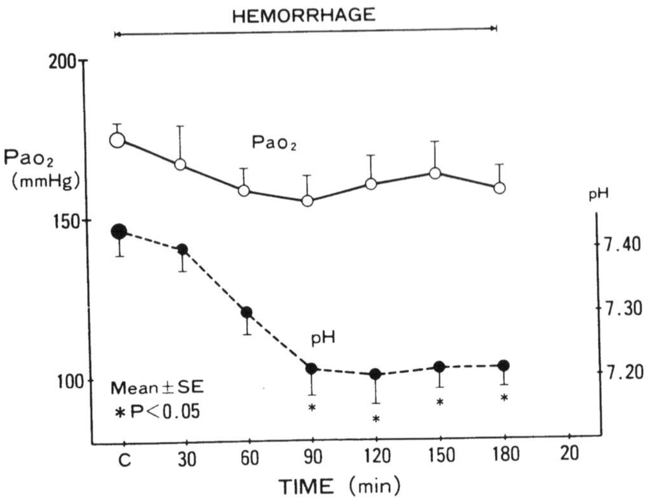

Fig. 5. Changes in arterial oxygen tension and pH

Discussion and Conclusion

Unlike cerebral perfusion [2, 3], the conjunctival tissue did not reveal any sign of an autoregulatory mechanism during hemorrhagic hypotension. $PcjO_2$ decreased significantly and in a dose-related manner during hypotension, despite PaO_2 being maintained. The decrease in $PcjO_2$ was directly related to the lowered blood pressure, cardiac output, and CaBF. Thus, it may be concluded that the conjunctival tissue responded differently to the cerebral organ tissues in spite of the anatomical similarity and proximity of their blood supply.

Acknowledgment. This work was supported by a grant-in-aid for scientific research (no. 62771150) from the Ministry of Education, Japan.

References

1. Kwan M, Fatt I (1971) A noninvasive method of continuous arterial oxygen tension estimation from measured palpebral conjunctival oxygen tension. Anesthesiology 35: 309–314
2. van der Zee HT, Faithfull NS, Kypers MH Dhasmana KM, Erdman W (1985) On-line conjunctival oxygen tension as a guide to cerebral oxygenation. Anesth Analg 64: 63–67
3. Gibson BE, McMichan JC, Cucchiara RF (1986) Lack of correlation between trans-conjunctival O_2 and cerebral blood flow during carotid artery occlusion. Anesthesiology 64: 277–279

Changes in Cerebral Regional Blood Flow and Tissue Oxygen Tension During Hemorrhagic Shock and Post-Cerebral Circulatory Arrest

KAZUO OKADA, OTOWA MORITSUNE, YOSHIMORI KIKUTA, KENZO KAJIYAMA, HIROAKI KAWABATA, and SHINKICHI TEZUKA[1]

Introduction

Tissue PO_2 may be defined as an indicator of the changes in regional blood flow and tissue metabolic rate for oxygen. In metabolically stable tissue, tissue PO_2 (PtO_2) is primarily determined by the local tissue blood flow. It is well recognized that in the brain, the blood flow is maintained by an autoregulatory mechanism, even during hypotension. With the progression of shock, this mechanism may deteriorate.

However, precise investigations have not been carried out into the question of when and from where the disruption of this autoregulatory mechanism occurs in the brain.

The increase of cerebral blood flow becomes manifest suddenly after occlusion ischemia—a phenomenon called the hyperemic response.

The present study was designed to measure PtO_2 and regional blood flow in hemorrhagic shock and the postocclusion period and to differentiate the regional changes in PtO_2 and regional blood flow.

Materials and Methods

Mongrel dogs weighing 10–17 kg were used. Anesthesia was maintained with O_2-enflurane under controlled ventilation. Catheters were inserted into the femoral arteries and veins for both monitoring blood pressure and exsanguination. After craniotomy, the dura was opened at the frontooccipital region. The incision was 10 mm in diameter.

Regional blood flow was measured with the thermal gradient method (Bio-Medical Co. Ltd, Japan); the polarographic method was applied to determine PtO_2 (Mitsubishi Rayon Co. Ltd, Japan). The diameters of both sensors were sufficiently fine to be inserted without damaging the surrounding tissue.

One PtO_2 sensor and a regional blood flow sensor were inserted into the subcortical white matter. Other pairs of these sensors were placed on the cortex.

[1]Department of Anesthesiology, Teikyo University School of Medicine, 11-1, Kaga 2-chome, Itabashi-ku, Tokyo, 173 Japan

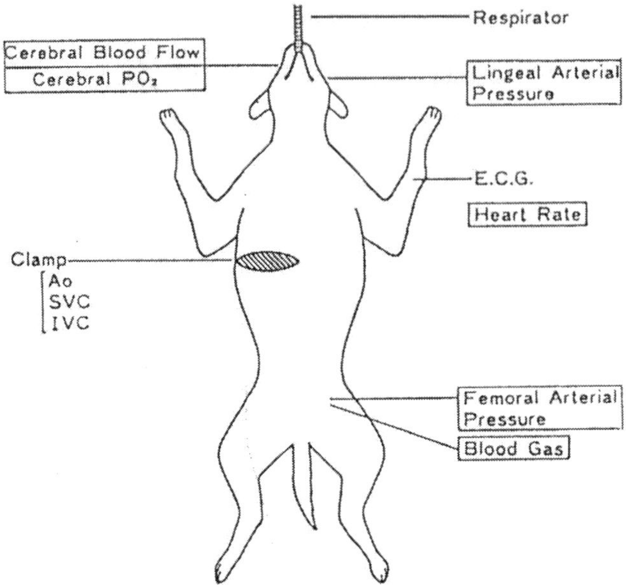

Fig. 1. Experimental procedure. *Ao* aortic artery, *SVC* superior vena cava, *IVC* inferior vena cava, *E.C.G.* electrocardiogram

PtO_2 and regional blood flow in the brain were measured continuously during the whole course of the experiment.

$PaCO_2$ was kept constant during the study period using a Harvard ventilator. The experimental procedure was divided into two parts: part 1—the period of hemorrhagic shock, and part 2—postocclusion ischemia (Fig. 1).

Part 1. Hemorrhagic Hypotension

Hemorrhagic hypotension was induced by exsanguinating from a femoral artery to a reservoir bottle with a constant rate over 30 min until mean arterial pressure (MAP) reached 50 mmHg, and the MAP was maintained for about 3 h by adjusting the height of the reservoir. Then 3 h later, exsanguinated blood was transfused.

Part 2. Total Brain Ischemia

The dogs were thoracotomized and umblical tape occluders were placed around the ascending aorta, inferior vena cava, and superior vena cava to stop both inflow to and outflow from the heart simultaneously (Fig. 2). When this maneuver was accomplished, no blood flowed out from the heart except for the coronary circulation, while the heart did not stop beating. Complete cerebral tissue ischemia was verified quantitatively with lingual arterial pressure monitoring. The ischemic period was arbitrarily decided by the change in this clamping period.

When the occlusion was released, total systemic circulation was reestablished to control level. From the beginning of the stable state until this postischemic

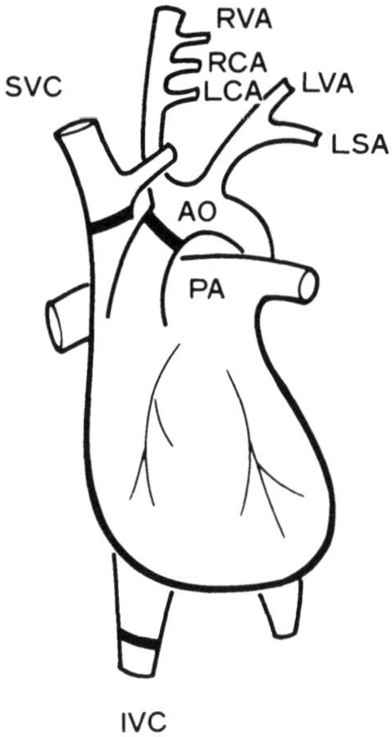

Fig. 2. Schema of total clamping of aorta (*AO*), inferior (*IVC*) and superior (*SVC*) vena cava. *RVA* right vertebral artery, *LVA* left vertebral artery, *RCA* right carotid artery, *LCA* left carotid artery, *LSA* left subclavian artery, *PA* pulmonary artery

period, PtO_2 and regional blood flow were measured continuously together with other hemodynamic parameters. Total occlusion time was decided arbitrarily as follows in different groups—3, 5, 10, and 15 min. The data were statistically evaluated by student's paired *t*-test. Differences were considered significant at $P<0.05$.

Results and Discussion

Hemorrhage resulted in a dose-related decrease in MAP. After attaining 50 mmHg MAP, the MAP level was kept constant during the course of the experiment by Lamson's method. Even though MAP was kept at 50 mmHg, cerebral regional blood flow and PtO_2 began to decrease progressively. Both PtO_2 and cerebral blood flow showed a much greater decrease in the white matter than in the cortex. In each region, the discrepancy ocurrred in the magnitude of the PtO_2 and the regional blood flow changes (Figs. 3, 4). However, this discrepancy could not be explained definitely from these data, and further experiments are required.

It has been noted that autoregulatory mechanism plays a role in trying to maintain the cerebral blood flow in hemorrhagic shock [1]. Using a microsphere technique, we demonstrated the changes in fractional distribution of cardiac output in shock [2]. Blood flow was fairly well maintained in cerebral and coronary regions, with a severe decrease in the distribution to visceral or muscular regions. The change in regional blood flow or PtO_2 in the brain was separately measured by Kovach et al. in hemorrhagic shock [3, 4]. From the results reported here, it was shown more clearly that the autoregulatory mechanism was disrupted after 3 h of shock, but the degree of disruption was not the same in two

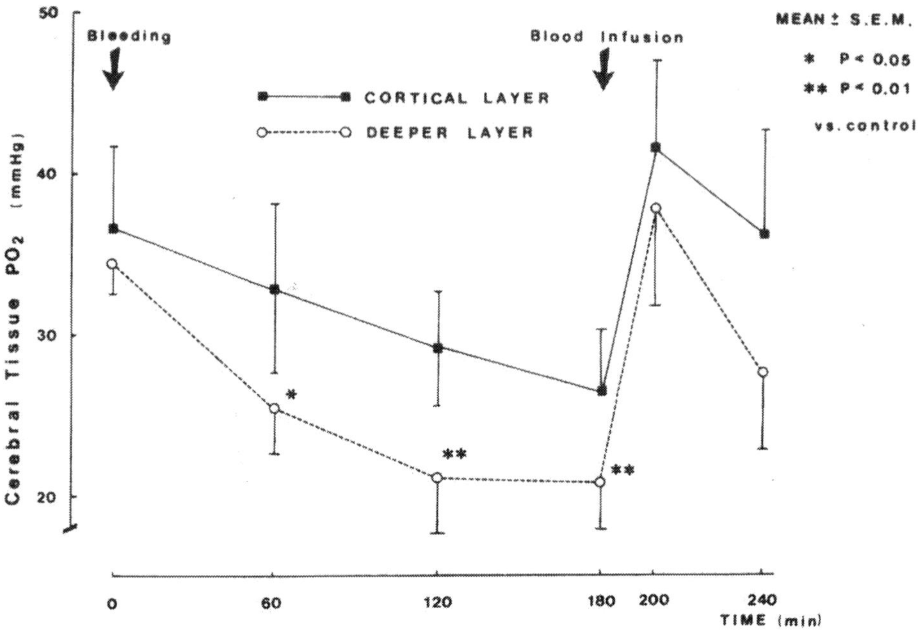

Fig. 3. Tissue PO_2 change in brain tissue during hemorrhagic shock

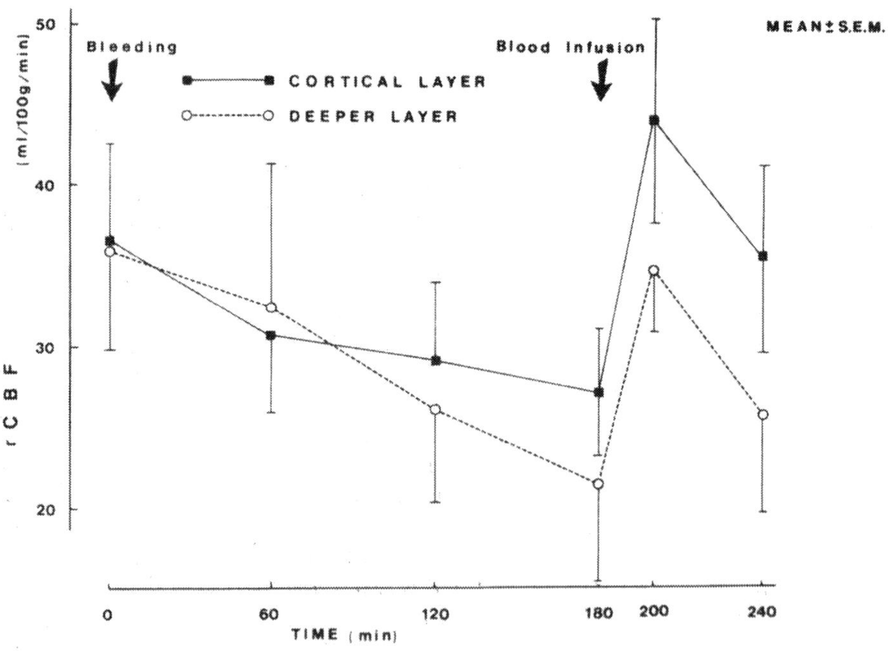

Fig. 4. Regional blood flow change in brain tissue during hemorrhagic shock

regions of the brain; this is clarified by the fact that the magnitude of PtO_2 and blood flow changes was not the same between the two regions of the brain.

Postischemic hypermia has been reported to play the major role in neurological recovery after ischemia [5–7]. In our ischemic model, a rapid decrease in both the cerebral regional blood flow and PtO_2 was found. When the blood flow was reestablished, both the cerebral regional blood flow and PtO_2 were observed to show a rapid recovery, and their values transiently exceeded the control values.

As the duration of the ischemia state was prolonged, the curves showing the transient increase in the cerebral regional blood flow and PtO_2 after the blood flow was reestablished became more gradual, and the time required to reach the peak tended to become prolonged (Figs 5, 6). In addition, the different sites in the brain were observed to show differences in the rate of recovery, with the white matter tending to be slower to recover the blood flow and PtO_2 than the cortex after the reestablishment of blood flow.

Both during the period of total cerebral ischemia and after the reestablishment of cerebral blood flow, the distribution of blood flow within the brain and PtO_2 showed a variation with the site in the brain. In all series of the experiment, the transient increase in the cerebral regional blood flow and PtO_2 was more dominant in the cortex than in the white matter.

The duration of the ischemia also influenced the recovery of cerebral blood flow and PtO_2. The increase in cerebral regional blood flow was more significant in 3-min ischemia than in that of 5, 10, or 15 min.

Increase of both parameters was diminished as the duration of ischemia was prolonged. PtO_2 did not show a completely parallel change with regional blood flow. In contrast to cerebral blood flow, PtO_2 reached higher values after 5- or 10-min ischemia than after 3-min ischemia.

It may be speculated that the decrease of oxygen consumption accompanied by irreversible metabolic change would counteract the decrease of PtO_2. Further studies are required to clarify the autoregulatory mechanism in cerebral circulation.

Conclusion

PtO_2 and cerebral regional blood flow were measured continuously in hemorrhagic shock or occlusion ischemia in dogs. PtO_2 sensors and regional blood flow sensors were inserted simultaneously into both the cortex and white matter. Hemorrhage caused the preferential decrease of PtO_2 and cerebral regional blood flow in white matter.

Autoregulation may be disrupted regionally in the cerebral circulation. After ischemia, an abrupt increase of PtO_2 and cerebral regional tissue blood flow occurred. When blood flow recovered after complete ischemia, the abrupt increase of PtO_2 and cerebral regional blood flow was followed by a gradual decrease of both parameters. A regional difference was found in PtO_2 and cerebral regional blood flow changes. PtO_2 and blood flow in the cortex showed much greater recovery than in the white matter. A disturbance of the regional cerebral circulation was discussed in pathophysiological conditions such as shock or ischemia.

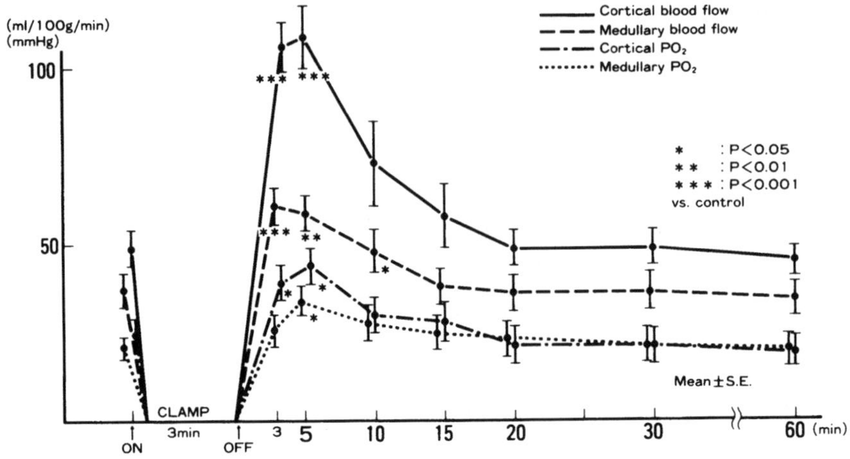

Fig. 5. Blood flow and PO_2 change in brain tissue after 3-min total cerebral ischemia

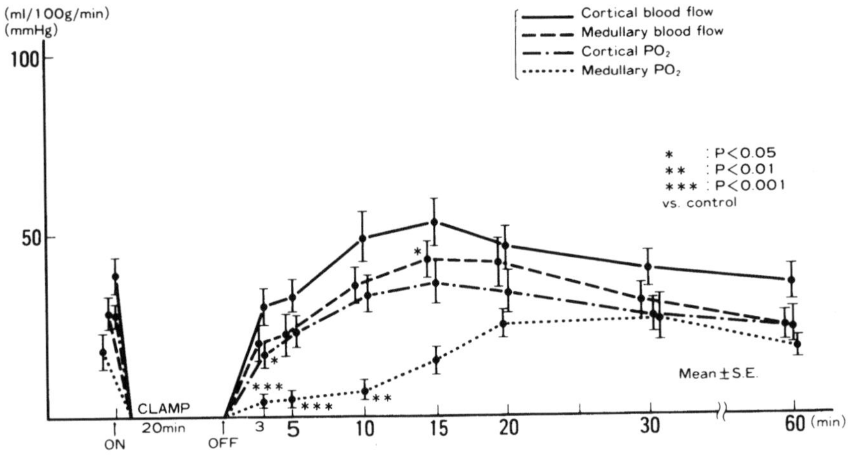

Fig. 6. Blood flow and PO_2 change in brain tissue after 20-min total cerebral ischemia

Acknowledgment. This work was supported by a grant-in-aid for scientific research (no. 60480351) from the Ministry of Education of Japan.

References

1. Maekawa T, McDowall DG, Okuda Y (1979) Brain surface oxygen tension and cerebral cortical blood flow during hemorrhagic and drug-induced hypotension in the cat. Anesthsiology 51: 313–320
2. Okada K, Kosugi I, Kitagaki T, Yamaguchi Y, Yoshikawa H, Kawashima Y, Kawaka-

mi S, Senoh Y (1977) Pathophysiology of shock. Jpn Circ J 41: 346–361
3. Kovach AGB, Dora E, Eke A, Gyulai L (1975) Correlation between the redox state, electrical activity and blood flow in cat brain cortex during hemorrhagic shock. In: Grote J, Reneau D, Thews G (eds) Oxygen transport to tissue: II. Plenum, New York, pp 289–297
4. Kovach AGB, Dora E (1978) Intracellular oxygen tension and energy metabolism in the cat brain cortex during hemorrhagic shock. Acta Physiological Acad Scient Hungaricae 54: 333–346
5. Hossman KA, Kleihues P (1973) Reversibility of ischemic brain damage. Arch Neurol 29: 375–384
6. Hossmann KA, Gruter HL, Hossmann V (1973) The role of cerebral blood flow for the recovery of the brain after prolonged ischemia. Z Neurol 204: 281–299
7. Ishihara N, Noritomi H, Meyer JS, Dodson RF, Deshmukh VD (1978) Differences in the time course of regional cerebral hemodynamics of gray and white matter during experimental hypertension. JN Sciences 38: 97–111

A Combined Method for Immunohistochemistry and Autoradiographic Measurement of Focal Cerebral Blood Flow in Investigation of Pathophysiological Roles of Microcirculation in Cerebral Ischemia

MASAYASU MATSUMOTO[1, 2], TAKAO HATAKEYAMA[1], SHOTARO YONEDA[2], KAZUFUMI KIMURA[2], TAKENOBU KAMADA[2], and TAKEHIKO YANAGIHARA[1]

Introduction

Measurement of focal cerebral blood flow (CBF) using quantitative autoradiography has provided valuable information in the investigation of cerebral ischemia [1]. However, the measurement of CBF alone has not been very successful for elucidation of the pathophysiological mechanism of cerebral ischemia and the selective tissue vulnerability, partly because of the lack of a sensitive morphological method for visualization of early ischemic damage. Since immunohistochemical techniques can detect early ischemic damage [2, 3], we aimed, in the present study, to establish a combined autoradiographic and immunohistochemical method for exact measurement of focal CBF in the area of an early immunohistochemical ischemic lesion. A more detailed description of the present work appears elsewhere [4].

Materials and Methods

Each Mongolian gerbil, weighing 60–80 g, was anesthetized with intraperitoneal ketamine hydrochloride (100 mg/kg) and the tail artery and right saphenous vein were cannulated with a PE-10 polyethylene catheter, as described previously [5]. After recovery from anesthesia at least 3 h later, each animal was lightly anesthetized by ether inhalation and the right common carotid artery was occluded. The gerbils showing onset of ischemic signs within 10 min were reanesthetized with intraperitoneal ketamine hydrochloride (50 mg/kg); seven gerbils with severe, moderate, and mild ischemic signs were selected for the present study. After measurement of arterial blood pressure and collection of the arterial blood sample (100 μl) from the tail artery for blood gas analysis, 30 μCi of 4-iodo[N-methyl-^{14}C]antipyrine dissolved in normal saline (0.8 ml) was infused through the right saphenous vein and serial arterial blood samples were collected according to the method of Sakurada et al. [6]. After infusion for 1 min, the gerbils

[1] Department of Neurology, Mayo Clinic, Rochester, MN 55905, USA
[2] First Department of Internal Medicine, Osaka University Medical School, 1–50, Fukushima 1-chome, Fukushima-ku, Osaka, 553 Japan

were decapitated, and the brains quickly removed and frozen in chilled isopentane (−50°C).

For autoradiographic measurement of focal CBF, brain sections (20 μm) were prepared in a cryostat and processed according to the method of Sakurada et al. (6). For immunohistochemical demonstration of the brain structure, each brain section (10 μm) was taken onto a gelatin-coated glass slide without thawing, immersed in chilled acetone (−20°C) for 10 min, and air-dried. Each section for immunohistochemical investigation was sandwiched between the adjacent two sections for autoradiography. In the immunohistochemical reaction for tubulin, the peroxidase-antiperoxidase light-microscopic method was used, as described previously [2]. Based on the findings from our previous investigations [2, 3], 34 anatomical sites were selected as representative of the vulnerable and nonvulnerable areas for measurement of focal CBF and detection of immunohistochemical ischemic damage. The sections corresponding to the stereotaxic section [7], 0.1–0.3 mm rostral to the bregma and 1.4–1.6 mm caudal to the bregma, were chosen for quantitation of autoradiography. The immunohistochemical and autoradiographic sections were superimposed under microscopic manipulation, and microdensitometric measurement was carried out with a 0.2-mm aperture regardless of the presence or absence of the immunohistochemical lesion. Precise and reproducible manipulation of the autoradiographic film was accomplished by mechanical shift to the x- and y-axis with the aid of a vernier, which we constructed and attached to the densitometer. Focal CBF values were computed according to the method of Sakurada et al. [6].

Results

The immunohistochemical reaction for tubulin using frozen sections visualized neuronal perikarya, dendrites, and the neuropil. After ischemia for 15 min, loss of the immunohistochemical reaction in the neuropil, dendrites, and neuronal perikarya was observed in the subiculum CA1 and CA2 regions of the hippocampus, layer III/IV of the frontoparietal cortex (Fig. 1), and the ventral nucleus of the thalamus on the occluded side, as observed previously [3], while no abnormality was observed on the nonoccluded side.

There was a clear correlation between the severity of the clinical manifestations and the immunohistochemical ischemic lesions. Two gerbils with mild signs did not have any ischemic lesions, while two gerbils with moderately severe signs showed immunohistochemical lesions in the subiculum CA1 and CA2 regions of the hippocampus. Two gerbils with severe clinical signs, including torsion of the neck and seizure, showed ischemic lesions in larger areas of the hippocampus, cerebral cortex, and thalamus (Fig. 1); the third gerbil with a slightly delayed onset of severe clinical signs had ischemic lesions in the hippocampus and cerebral cortex.

Physiological parameters, including mean arterial pressure, PaO_2, $PaCO_2$, arterial pH, and hematocrit values, did not deviate from the normal ranges. A clear correlation was observed again between the abnormality of the autoradiographic pattern and the neurological status. In gerbils with severe clinical signs, focal CBFs in the right hemisphere were extremely and diffusely low except for

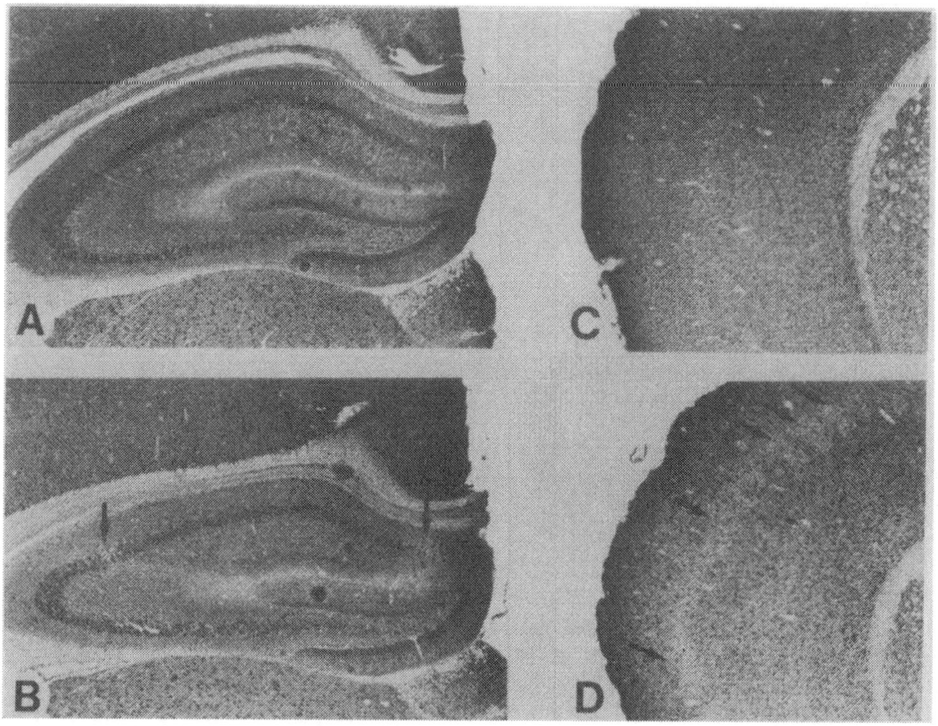

Fig. 1A–D. The immunohistochemical reaction for tubulin in **A, B** the hippocampus and **C, D** frontoparietal cortex on the nonoccluded side (**A, C**) and on the occluded side (**B, D**) after ischemia for 15 min. The ischemic lesions with loss of the immunohistochemical reaction are shown with *arrows* in the subiculum CA1 and CA2 regions of the hippocampus (**B**) and the columnar lesions in layer III/IV of the frontoparietal cortex (**D**) on the occluded side. *Photographs* **A** and **C** are reversed for better comparison. Original magnification × 20

those close to the midline such as the subiculum, the cingulate cortex, the habenular nucleus, and the midline structure of the thalamus (Fig. 2A, B). However, the autoradiogram of a gerbil with a slightly delayed onset of severe clinical signs showed a heterogeneous pattern and perpendicular columns with relatively high and low flow were observed in the right cerebral cortex (Fig. 2C, D). In the moderately affected gerbils, a less widespread decrease of focal CBF was observed in the hippocampus. The mildly affected gerbils showed an even milder degree of decrease of focal CBF in the hippocampus.

Part of an autoradiogram and an immunohistochemical section which were superimposed for measurement of focal CBF at the designated anatomical sites are shown in Fig. 3. In the severely affected gerbil (Fig. 3A–C), the regional CBF in the hippocampus was markedly and diffusely reduced, and the immunohistochemical lesions were clearly seen in the subiculum CA1 and CA2 regions. On the other hand, the moderately affected gerbil (Fig. 3D–F) showed residual focal CBF even in some areas within the hippocampus, and the immunohistochemical

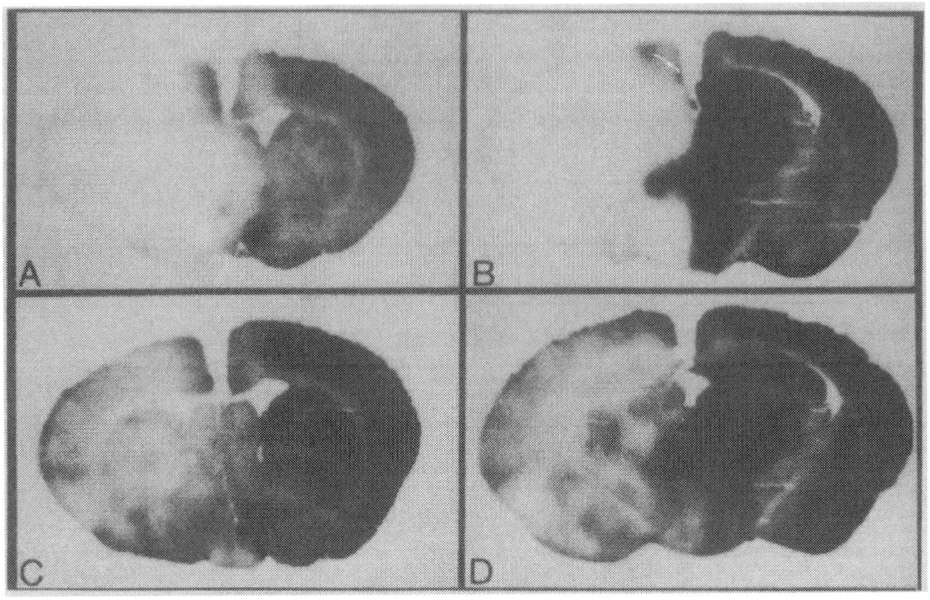

Fig. 2A–D. Representative autoradiographs showing focal CBF patterns in the coronal planes, including **A, C** the frontoparietal cerebral cortex and caudoputamen and **B, D** parietal cortex, hippocampus and thalamus. The gerbil in **A, B** had severe clinical manifestations; the gerbil in **C, D** also had severe clinical manifestations but with a slightly slower onset. Microheterogeneity of the reduction of focal CBF is shown in the hippocampus and thalamus (**D**) and alternating dark and light columns are seen in the cerebral cortex (**C, D**)

lesions were less distinct. Among 34 anatomical sites studied, focal CBF at sites with immunohistochemical lesions over 0.2 mm in diameter was consistently below 8 ml/100 g/min, and where the diameter was less than 0.2 mm the focal CBF was below 15 ml/100 g/min. In the hippocampus, the immunohistochemical lesions in the subiculum CA1 and CA2 regions coincided with the transitional zone between the area with extremely low CBF and the adjacent area with substantial residual CBF (Fig. 3). In the cerebral cortex, however, the immunohistochemical lesions were detected only in layer III/IV even though focal CBF was widely reduced.

Discussion

In the present study, we were able to demonstrate the feasibility of combining autoradiographic and immunohistochemical methods for exact measurement of focal CBF in the area defined by the presence or absence of immunohistochemical lesions. The presence of regional heterogeneity in focal CBF was noted even within the hippocampus, cerebral cortex, and thalamus in the early ischemic period after the occlusion of the common carotid artery. In the cerebral

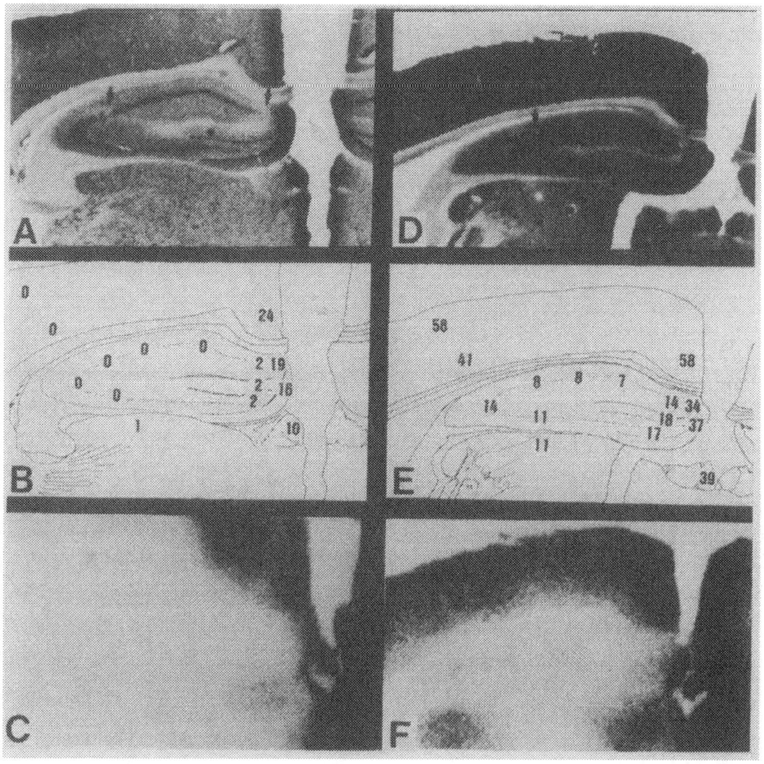

Fig. 3. A, D The immunohistochemical reaction patterns, **B, E** schematic drawings with focal CBF values (ml/100 g/min), and **C, F** corresponding autoradiographic patterns showing the hippocampus and overlying parietal cortex in a gerbil with severe clinical manifestations (**A, B, C**) and another with moderate clinical manifestations (**D, E, F**). In the severely affected gerbil, discrete immunohistochemical lesions were observed in the subiculum CA1 and CA2 regions as shown by *arrows* (**A**) and CBF was almost homogeneously reduced in the hippocampus except for the subiculum and dentate gyrus close to the midline (**B, C**). In the moderately affected gerbil, the immunohistochemical lesions in the subiculum CA1 and CA2 regions were present as shown by *arrows* but less obvious (*D*), and the reduction of CBF was heterogeneous in the hippocampus (**E, F**). Note that the lesion in the subiculum CA1 region occurred at the border between the area with marked reduction of blood flow and the adjacent area with considerable residual blood flow in each instance

cortex, we observed a columnar pattern (alternating light and dark bands) in the autoradiogram (Fig. 2) and the corresponding pattern with the immunohistochemical method (Fig. 1). The dark bands likely correspond to the location of the cortical penetrating arteries, which are known to have residual blood perfusion after carotid occlusion [2]. The present investigation also demonstrated that the anatomical sites where the immunohistochemical lesions develop early [2, 3]—namely the junction between the medial CA1 region and subiculum and the CA2 region of the hippocampus—showed a sharp focal CBF gradient between the site with relatively high residual flow and the site with markedly reduced flow. This "blood flow cliff" (sudden drop in blood flow) may promote severe ischemic damage by detrimental factors such as free radical formation, tissue acidosis, influx of calcium ions, and release of excitatory neurotransmitters. However, the "blood flow cliff" was not present in the vulnerable region of the cerebral cortex (layer III/IV).

The present investigation demonstrated the potential usefulness of a combined method of quantitative autoradiography for measurement of focal CBF and immunohistochemical technique for detection of early ischemic damage.

Summary

A combined autoradiographic and immunohistochemical method was established for exact measurement of focal cerebral blood flow (CBF) in the area of an immunohistochemical ischemic lesion and was applied to the brains of symptomatic gerbils 15 min after occlusion of the right common carotid artery. It was found that the reduction of focal CBF can be heterogeneous at an early ischemic period and that the residual focal CBF was below 8.0 ml/100 g/min in some areas with ischemic lesions, but other areas were tolerant of severe hypoperfusion. This method will be useful for investigation of the pathophysiological roles of microcirculatory changes in cerebral ischemia.

References

1. Mies G, Kloiber O, Drewes LR, Hossmann KA (1984) Cerebral blood flow and regional potassium distribution during focal ischemia of gerbil brain. Ann Neurol 16: 232–237
2. Yanagihara T, Yoshimine T, Morimoto K, Yamamoto K, Homburger HA (1985) Immunohistochemical investigation of cerebral ischemia in gerbils. J Neuropath Exp Neurol 44: 204–215
3. Matsumoto M, Yamamoto K, Homburger HA, Yanagihara T (1987) Early detection of cerebral ischemic damage and repair process in the gerbil by use of an immunohistochemical technique. Mayo Clin Proc 62: 460–472
4. Matsumoto M, Hatakeyama T, Yamamoto K, Yanagihara T (1987) A combined method for measurement of cerebral blood flow and immunohistochemistry for investigation of cerebral ischemia. Brain Res 424: 231–238
5. Matsumoto M, Kimura K, Fujisawa A, Matsuyama T, Asai T, Uyama O, Yoneda S, Abe H (1982) Regional blood flows measured in Mongolian gerbil by a modified microsphere method. Am J Physiol 242: H990–H995
6. Sakurada O, Kennedy C, Jehle J, Brown JD, Carbin GL, Sokoloff L (1978) Measurement of local cerebral blood flow with iodo[^{14}C]antipyrine. Am J Physiol 234: H59–H66
7. Loskota WJ, Lomax P, Verty MA (1974) A stereotaxic atlas of the Mongolian gerbil brain (*Meriones unguiculatus*). Ann Arbor Science Publishers, Ann Arbor

Evaluation of the Behavior of Cerebral Blood Flow and Hemorheological Parameters with Infusions of Hydroxyethyl Starch and Low Molecular Weight Dextran in Normal Baboons

YOSHIYASU TSUDA[1,2], ALEXANDER HARTMANN[1], JÜRGEN WEIAND[1], LASZLO SOLYMOSI[1], and HIROHIDE MATSUO[2]

Introduction

The efficacy of hemodilution with an infusion of oncotic plasma substitutes in cerebral ischemia is still controversial [1], although it is widely performed [2–5]. In general, the infusion with such substances, for example, hydroxyethyl starch (HES) and low molecular weight dextran (LMWD), is known to influence the flow properties of blood markedly by inducing volumetric expansion, i.e., it reduces the flow resistance by decreasing the erythrocyte mass per unit volume and increases the cerebral blood flow (CBF). However, an objective assessment of the rheological behavior associated with changes in CBF over a time-course during and after the infusion of such oncotic substances appears to be necessary to evaluate the efficacy of hemodilution.

LMWD is the most commonly used plasma substitute in therapeutic hemodilution. However, an increase in plasma viscosity due to the infusion of LMWD has often been reported [6, 7]. This may be unfavorable from the hemorheological point of view, although an increase in CBF due to the infusion of LMWD has been reported in patients with cerebral ischemia [2, 4].

In contrast, HES has been reported not to increase the plasma viscosity despite its relatively high molecular weight as a result of the hydrophilic properties of the starch molecules [6]. HES is rapidly degraded to smaller molecules, which are rheologically active and may increase CBF.

In this study, we evaluated the specific effects of hemodilution with infusions of HES and LMWD, as compared with an infusion of 0.9% sodium chloride solution, on the flow properties of hemorheological parameters and CBF under physiological conditions in normal baboons.

Materials and Methods

Twelve adult baboons (*Papio cynocephalus*) of both sexes were used. They were aged between 2 and 4 years, with an average weight of 11.2 ± 1.7 kg. After an

[1]Neurological and Neuroradiological University Clinic of Bonn, 5300 Bonn 1, Federal Republic of Germany
[2]Second Department of Internal Medicine, Kagawa Medical University, 1750-1, Ikenobe, Miki-cho, Kagawa, 761-07 Japan

initial intraperitoneal injection of pentobarbital sodium (20–25 mg/kg), the animals were artificially ventilated with a gas mixture of 75% N_2O and 25% O_2. The stroke volume and ventilation rate were adjusted and controlled by regular measurements of arterial blood gases to achieve a steady state level of $PaCO_2$ of 36–42 mmHg. Immobilization was achieved with repeated injections of pancuronium bromide (0.04 mg/kg). The arterial and central venous blood pressures were continuously recorded by transducers connected to catheters inserted into a femoral artery and vein. The central venous pressure was kept at +2 to +5 mmHg.

Measurements of regional CBF (rCBF) were made using an intraarterial xenon-133 injection technique, according to the method previously reported [8]. The left lingual artery was exposed and a thin polyethylene catheter was introduced into the lingual artery with its tip at the orifice. All arteries of the upper half of the common carotid artery, except for the internal carotid artery, were temporary ligated. This guaranteed that all xenon-133 injected through the catheter entered only the internal carotid artery. The baboon was fixed in the prone position into a stereotaxic frame, which had a lead shield for collimations. The desaturation curves of xenon-133 were recorded by eight NaI crystal detectors, with a collimation of 14 mm, positioned in the lead shield covering the left hemisphere (Fig. 1). For measuring the rCBF, 1–2 mCi xenon-133 in 1 ml saline was injected through the catheter in the lingual artery. The curves were recorded by a multichannel analyzer (Wenzel, Munich, Federal Republic of Germany) for 8.5 min following desaturation, stored on-line, and calculated thereafter for regional flow in ml/100 g/min by stochastic analysis [9]. The correction of the xenon-133 partition coefficient lambda during and after the course of infusion was done according to regularly estimated hemoglobin concentrations [10], and the rCBF values during the protocol were corrected for a standard arterial CO_2 tension of 40 mmHg by individual estimations of CO_2 reactivity with hypercapnia. The rCBF changes in each of the eight detectors were identical before, during, and after infusions. Therefore, hemispheric mean rCBF values were used for evaluations. The hemispheric mean rCBF values were calculated from each of the eight rCBF values being combined and averaged.

The hemorheological variables were also estimated for each rCBF study, and the following variables were evaluated, i.e., the hematocrit (percentage), erythrocyte flow (a product of the mean rCBF and hematocrit—ml/100 g/min), plasma viscosity (mPas), and erythrocyte aggregation index. The plasma viscosity was measured with a capillary tube plasma viscometer, which was fully automated with disposable polyurethane capillary tubes. The erythrocyte aggregation index was determined photometrically in a transparent plate-cone chamber, measured as an increase of the light intensity transmitted through the chamber. The change in intensity as a function of time determines the standardized erythrocyte aggregation index at a constant hematocrit level of 35%.

Of the 12 baboons investigated, six were treated with an infusion of 10% HES (molecular weight 200000) solution at 0.33 ml/kg/min for 60 min (20 ml/kg), while the other six received an infusion of 0.9% NaCl solution at 0.5 ml/kg/min for 60 min (30 ml/kg) and thereafter, 3 h after the end of NaCl infusion, received an infusion of 10% LMWD (molecular weight 20000) solution, at 0.33 ml/kg/min for 60 min (20 ml/kg)

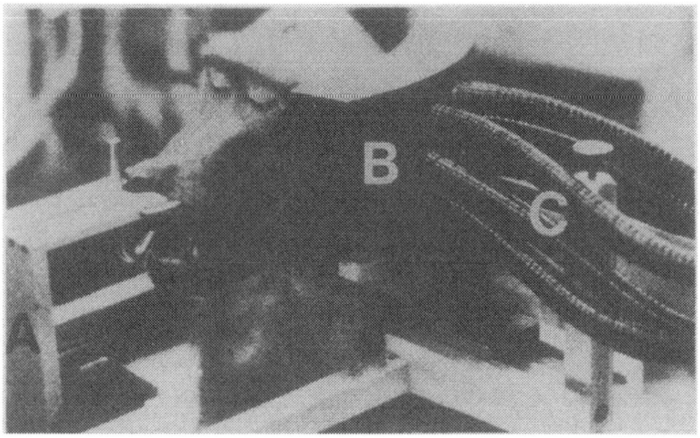

Fig. 1. Apparatus for measuring regional cerebral blood flow (rCBF) in baboons. *A* Stereotaxic frame, *B* lead shield covering left hemisphere of the brain, *C* eight NaI crystal detectors with 14-mm collimations

The CBF runs pre- and postinfusion of 10% HES solution were subjected to six measurements, i.e., steady state, 30 min, 60 min, 3 h, 5 h, and 7 h aftr the beginning of infusion.

The CBF runs pre- and postinfusion of 0.9% NaCl solution and 10% LMWD solution were subjected to 11 measurements, i.e., steady state, 30 min, 60 min, 2 h, 3 h, and 4 h after the beginning of an infusion of 0.9% NaCl solution, and 30 min, 60 min, 3 h, 5 h, and 7 h after the beginning of an infusion of 10% LMWD solution.

The first study of the rCBF was started at least 6 h after a single injection of barbiturate. The mean arterial blood pressure was quite stable during the protocol, ranging from 105 to 115 mmHg, and was not different between the groups of baboons.

Results

The results of the effects of hemodilution on CBF and hemorheological parameters with infusions of HES, LMWD, and NaCl are shown in Table 1. With an infusion of HES, the mean rCBF increased 21% at 30 min and reached a maximal increase of up to 48% 60 min after the beginning of infusion. The significant increase continued for 5 h after the beginning of infusion from the steady state level. With an infusion of LMWD, the mean rCBF values showed a maximal increase of up to 9.6% at 60 min and continued for 3 h after the beginning of infusion from the steady state level. Between the groups with infusions of HES and LMWD, the mean rCBF values showed significant differences at 60 min, 3 h, and 5 h after the beginning of infusion.

The serum hematocrit values significantly decreased during the infusions of HES, NaCl, and LMWD from the steady state levels. After the infusions were ended, the decreased values of hematocrit gradually rose, and no significant

Table 1. Effect of hemodilution on cerebral blood flow and hemorheological parameters with infusions of HES, LMWD, and NaCl

	SS	30 min	60 min	2 h	3 h	4 h	5 h	7 h
Mean rCBF (ml/100 g/min)								
HES	41.5 ± 2.0	50.7 ± 3.6	61.5 ± 3.8****		58.6 ± 2.7****		51.2 ± 3.8*	46.9 ± 3.8
LMWD	38.7 ± 1.5	40.6 ± 1.0	42.4 ± 1.5**		42.3 ± 2.2*		41.0 ± 2.0	41.1 ± 1.9
	NS	NS	$P < 0.001$		$P < 0.001$		$P < 0.05$	NS
NaCl	38.7 ± 1.5	39.2 ± 1.8	40.9 ± 1.5	39.5 ± 1.2	39.2 ± 1.4	40.0 ± 2.0		
Hematocrit (%)								
HES	41.3 ± 1.1	38.2 ± 1.1***	35.7 ± 0.9****		39.0 ± 0.7***		41.2 ± 0.9	41.5 ± 1.0
LMWD	38.7 ± 2.3	33.7 ± 3.1***	30.3 ± 2.7****		33.0 ± 2.8****		33.8 ± 2.9***	35.8 ± 3.0**
	NS	NS	NS		NS		$P < 0.05$	NS
NaCl	39.7 ± 2.3	38.0 ± 2.4****	36.7 ± 2.5****	38.5 ± 2.7	39.2 ± 2.7	38.5 ± 2.6		
Erythrocyte flow (ml/100 g/min)								
HES	17.2 ± 1.1	19.1 ± 1.7	21.9 ± 1.4****		22.9 ± 1.2***		21.2 ± 1.8**	19.4 ± 1.8*
LMWD	15.5 ± 1.3	13.7 ± 1.4*	12.9 ± 1.4***		14.0 ± 1.5*		13.9 ± 1.5*	14.8 ± 1.4
	NS	$P < 0.05$	$P < 0.002$		$P < 0.001$		$P < 0.02$	NS
NaCl	15.5 ± 1.3	15.4 ± 1.4	15.1 ± 1.3	15.2 ± 1.4	15.5 ± 1.4	15.4 ± 1.4		

(*Continued on Page 521*)

Table 1. (*continued*)

	SS	30 min	60 min	2 h	3 h	4 h	5 h	7 h
Plasma viscosity (mPa s)								
HES	1.32 ± 0.04	1.29 ± 0.04*	1.26 ± 0.04*		1.28 ± 0.03		1.29 ± 0.03	1.31 ± 0.03
LMWD	1.28 ± 0.03	1.39 ± 0.04**	1.46 ± 0.02***		1.43 ± 0.02**		1.40 ± 0.02*	1.40 ± 0.02**
	NS	NS	$P < 0.005$		$P < 0.005$		$P < 0.05$	NS
NaCl	1.28 ± 0.03	1.26 ± 0.04*	1.25 ± 0.04*	1.27 ± 0.03	1.27 ± 0.03	1.28 ± 0.04		
Erythrocyte aggregation index								
HES	6.1 ± 1.3	4.8 ± 1.3*	4.2 ± 1.3**		5.1 ± 1.3		5.7 ± 1.5	6.8 ± 1.6
LMWD	5.9 ± 2.1	3.6 ± 1.4	2.8 ± 1.1*		3.6 ± 1.3		4.2 ± 1.2	5.1 ± 1.6
	NS	NS	NS		NS		NS	NS
NaCl	5.9 ± 2.1	5.6 ± 1.8	5.1 ± 1.6**	5.5 ± 1.9	6.1 ± 2.1	5.9 ± 2.1		

SS steady state
* $P < 0.05$, ** $P < 0.01$, *** $P < 0.005$, **** $P < 0.001$ from the steady state values
Values are expressed as means ± SEM

decreases were further observed after 5 h from the beginning of infusion of HES, as compared with the steady state levels. With an infusion of LMWD, however, the values of hematocrit showed a maximal decrease of up to 20% at 60 min and continued to show significantly low values even after 7 h. The hematocrit values with an infusion of LMWD were continuously lower than with an infusion of HES but a significant difference was observed only 5 h after the beginning of infusion.

The erythrocyte flow, a product of mean rCBF and hematocrit, significantly increased during and after the infusion of HES and reached a maximal increase of up to 33% 60 min after the beginning of infusion. The significant increase continued for 7 h after the beginning of infusion from the steady state level. Conversely, with an infusion of LMWD, the erythrocyte flow significantly decreased during and after the infusion and reached a maximal decrease of up to 16.8% 60 min after the beginning of infusion. The significant decrease continued for 5 h after the beginning of infusion from the steady state level. With infusions of HES and LMWD, the erythrocyte flow values showed significant differences at 30 min, 60 min, 3 h, and 5 h after the beginning of infusions.

With respect to the plasma viscosity changes during and after infusion of plasma substitutes, LMWD significantly increased the plasma viscosity after 30 min, reaching a maximal increase after 60 min. These high viscosities continued for 7 h. On the other hand, with infusions of HES and NaCl, the viscosity did not increase during or after infusion but decreased significantly during the infusion. The plasma viscosity with an infusion of LMWD continuously showed significantly higher values than with an infusion of HES for 5 h after the start of infusion.

The values of the erythrocyte aggregation index significantly decreased during the infusion of HES (at 30 min), LMWD (at 60 min), and NaCl (at 60 min) from the steady state levels. With an infusion of LMWD, a persistent decrease of the index was also observed after 3 h. The values of the erythrocyte aggregation index with an infusion of LMWD were continuously lower than with an infusion of HES. However, the differences were never significant during or after the infusion.

The correlation between the values of serum hematocrit and plasma viscosity showed no significant correlation during or after the infusion of HES ($r = -0.1269$, $n = 36$), while a significant negative correlation between them was observed both during and after the infusion of LMWD ($r = -0.5323$, $n = 36$, $P < 0.001$); i.e., with higher values of hematocrit the plasma viscosity stayed lower, while with lower values the plasma viscosity rose proportionally.

The correlation between the values of plasma viscosity and the inverse of erythrocyte flow (a product of CBF and hematocrit) showed no significant correlation with the infusion of HES ($r = 0.0157$, $n = 36$), but there was a significant positive correlation ($r = 0.5170$, $n = 36$, $P < 0.005$) with the infusion of LMWD.

Discussion

Our study with normal baboons showed that an infusion of HES decreased the hematocrit and increased CBF by up to 48% and the erythrocyte flow by up to

33% without an increase in plasma viscosity. While an infusion of LMWD also decreased the hematocrit by up to 20% and increased CBF by up to 9.6%, it resulted in a significant decrease of erythrocyte flow by up to 16.8% in normal baboons and increased plasma viscosity at the same time. Wood et al. [4] have observed an insignificant increase of cortical blood flow in nine healthy dogs following the administration of LMWD. Gottstein and Held [2] have observed an increase in hemispheric blood flow of up to 56% in patients with cerebral ischemia. Heiss et al. [3] observed that in patients with nonacute cerebrovascular disease, dextran administration resulted in a slight increase (5.9%) of CBF, which was significant compared with repeated studies in nontreated control patients. With regard to plasma viscosity and cerebral blood flow, significant lower values of CBF were found in patients with paraproteinemia with anemia [11], in whom the plasma viscosity was raised compared with patients without paraproteinemia but who were anemic. The results suggest that plasma viscosity could be one of the important factors regulating the CBF. Our results in normal baboons indicate that the reduction of hematocrit has less influence on blood flow than plasma viscosity with the infusion of LMWD. The negative effect of HES infusion on plasma viscosity could be attributed to the electric charge phenomena and might be substantiated by hydrophilic properties of the hydroxy-end groups of the starch molecules [6]. In contrast, the LMWD solution includes smaller and larger molecules. The smaller molecules are rapidly eliminated by the kidney, whereas the larger molecules cannot pass the kidney barrier and increase the relative concentration of the larger dextran molecules and thus the plasma viscosity [7], which might counteract the increase in CBF. The absence of a correlation between the values of hematocrit and plasma viscosity by an infusion of HES and a significant negative correlation between them by an infusion of LMWD might explain why CBF increased more with an infusion of HES than with LMWD, despite the similar decreases of hematocrit values. Between the plasma viscosity and the inverse of erythrocyte flow, a significant positive correlation was observed by infusion with LMWD, and no correlation was observed by infusion with HES, which indicates that the increase of plasma viscosity causes an inhibitory effect on the erythrocyte flow.

In summary, different rheological effects with infusions of HES and LMWD on the physiological conditions of normal baboons were observed. The tendency of LMWD infusion to increase the plasma viscosity despite a decrease of hematocrit, which may suppress the CBF increase, and of HES to increase the CBF with a decrease in hematocrit values without an increase in plasma viscosity have to be considered for the clinical use of these substances.

Acknowledgments. This study was partially supported by the Alexander von Humboldt Foundation, Federal Republic of Germany and by the Deutsche Forschungsgemeinschaft (Ha/965), Federal Republic of Germany.

References

1. Brown MM and Marshall J (1982) Effect of plasma exchange on blood viscosity and cerebral blood flow. Br Med J 284: 1733–1736

2. Gottstein U and Held K (1969) Effekt der Hämodilution nach intravenöser Infusion von niedermolekularen Dextranen auf die Hirnzirkulation des Menschen. Dtsch Med Wschr 94: 522–526
3. Heiss W-D, Prosenz P, Tschabitscher H, Lasek C, Herles HJ (1972) Effect of low molecular dextran on total cerebral blood flow and regional flow within ischemic brain regions. Eur Neurol 8: 129–133
4. Wood JH, Simeone FA, Kron RE, Litt M (1982) Rheological aspects of experimental hypervolemic hemodilution with low molecular weight dextran: Relationships of cortical blood flow, cardiac output, and intracranial pressure to fresh blood viscosity and plasma volume. Neurosurgery 11: 739–753
5. Wood JH, Polyzoidis KS, Epstein CM, Gibby GL, Tindall GT (1984) Quantitative EEG alterations after isovolemic-hemodilutional augmentation of cerebral perfusion in stroke patients. Neurology (Cleveland) 34: 764–768
6. Harke H, Pieper CH, Meredig J, Rüssler P (1980) Rheologische und gerinnungsphysiologische Untersuchungen nach Infusion von HÄS 200/0.5 und Dextran 40. Anaesthesist 29: 71–77
7. Ehrly AM and Landgraf H (1981) Analysis of the specific hemorheological effects of low molecular weight dextran (LMWD)—and saline—infusions in healthy volunteers. Clin Hemorheol 1: 99–109
8. Hartmann A, Menzel J, Lange D, Buttinger C (1982) An experimental stroke model to study cerebrovascular responses to chronic regional ischemia. Adv Biosci 43: 167–183
9. Agress H, Bacharach SL, Hammock MK, Green MV, Johnson GS, Di Chiro G (1977) Stochastic analysis of ^{133}Xe clearance for determining regional blood flow in a primate model. Stroke 8: 222–226
10. Veall N and Mallett BL (1965) The partition of trace amounts of xenon between human blood and brain tissues at 37°C. Phys Med Biol 10: 375–380
11. Humphrey PRD, Du Boulay GH, Marshall J, Pearson TC, Ross Russel RW, Slater NGP, Symon L, Wetherley-Mein G, Zilkha E (1980) Viscosity, cerebral blood flow and hematocrit in patients with paraproteinemia. Acta Neurol Scand 61: 201–209

Evaluation of Blood Flow Velocity Waveforms in Intramyocardial Artery and Vein by Laser Doppler Velocimeter with an Optical Fiber

Keiichiro Mito, Yasuo Ogasawara, Osamu Hiramatsu, Yoshifumi Wada, Katsuhiko Tsujioka, and Fumihiko Kajiya[1]

Introduction

It is well established that the part of the left ventricle at greatest risk to ischemia is the subendocardium. Both in myocardial infarction in humans and experimental myocardial infarction in dogs, the subendocardial muscle shows the most extensive necrosis and the subepicardium is spared. Thus, it is important to evaluate phasic blood flow in deeper intramyocardial layers. Measurements, however, have been restricted in the region of epimyocardium because of the methodological limitations [1–3].

In this study, we applied our laser Doppler blood velocimeter with an optical fiber to measurements of the blood flow velocities in the intramyocardial septal artery and intramyocardial small veins [4].

Method

Laser Doppler Velocimeter with Optical Fiber

Figure 1 is a schematic illustration of our laser Doppler velocimeter (LDV) for measuring the blood flow velocities in intramyocardial coronary vessels. The He-Ne laser beam (632.8 nm, 5.5 mW) was divided by a beam splitter (BS). Half of the initial beam passing through the BS was guided into the intramyocardial vessels through the optical fiber (graded-index, multimode fiber, external diameter—0.125 mm) and the laser beam was delivered directly from the termination of the fiber into the bloodstream. Part of the back-scattered beam by flowing erythrocytes was collected by the same fiber tip and transmitted back to its entrance. The signal of the back-scattered beam has a Doppler shift frequency Δf, which is proportional to the blood flow velocity. The other beam was used as a reference beam to distinguish the forward blood flow from the reverse flow. Optical heterodyne detection was performed by mixing the reference beam and the back-scattered beam at the avalanche photodiode (APD), and the current from the APD was fed into a spectrum analyzer at the Doppler shift frequency

[1]Department of Medical Engineering and Systems Cardiology, Kawasaki Medical School, 577 Matsushima, Kurashiki, Okayama, 701-01 Japan

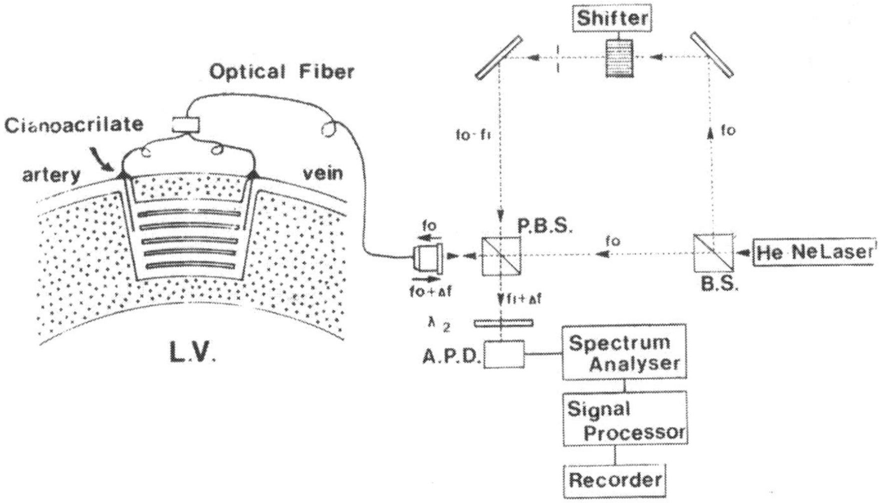

Fig. 1. Intramyocardial blood flow measurement using LDV with an optical fiber. *L.V.* left ventricle, *P.B.S.* polarized beam splitter, *B.S.* beam splitter, *A.P.D.* avalanche photodiode

Δf. The blood flow velocity is obtained from the shift frequency as follows:

$$V = \lambda \cdot \Delta f / 2n$$

where λ is the laser wavelength in free space—632.8 nm and n is the refractive index of blood—approximately 1.33.

The optical fiber tip was made into a convex shape by the heat of electric discharge so that the fiber tip did not injure the vascular wall. The convex shape was also beneficial in reducing the disturbance of the blood flow in the vicinity of the inserted fiber tip and stabilizing the tip in the center of the blood flow in the vessel.

Animal Preparation

Four mongrel dog (weight 15–25 kg) were anesthetized with sodium pentobarbital and the chest was opened. The heart was cradled in the open pericardium and the proximal of the septal artery and left anterior descending artery were dissected free. The veins penetrating the myocardium were investigated as to whether they were appropriate for velocity measurements.

The fine optical fiber was inserted carefully into the intramyocardial vessels (the septal artery and a small coronary vein) through a puncture in the surface vessel wall previously made by a puncher the same diameter as the fiber. The fiber was fixed at the epicardial surface with a drop of acrylate cement after confirmation of stable Doppler signals of blood flow.

The blood flow rate of the left anterior descending artery (LAD) was measured using the electromagnetic flowmeter. Pressure in the left ventricle, aorta, and great cardiac vein (GCV) and ECG were monitored. Interventricular and intramyocardial pressures were measured using a needle tip micromanometer (Millar PR230).

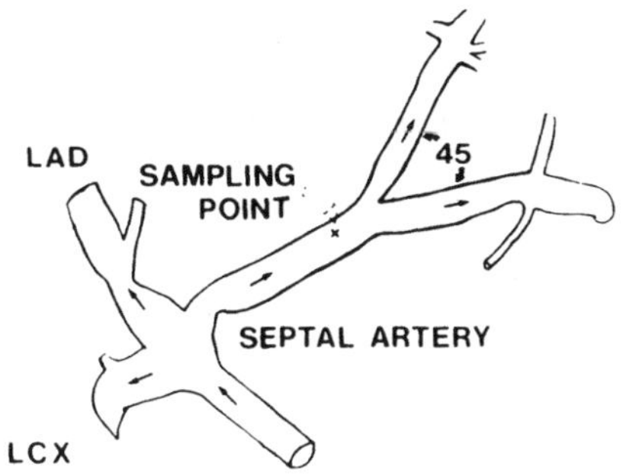

Fig. 2. Cast of the septal artery. The blood flow velocity was measured at a depth of about 18 mm from the orifice of the artery. *LAD* left anterior descending artery, *LCX* left circumflex artery

After finishing the blood flow velocity measurement, the heparinized saline was infused from the coronary main artery to the veins and then 40 ml casting elastomer (Mercox-CL, viscosity approximately 27 cP) was injected manually to verify the depth of the sampling point. After hardening, the heart was removed and suspended in 37°C buffer solution, which contained the enzyme papain, (0.07 g/ml/unit weight of heart) to corrode away the tissue. For 1 week, changes of the solution were frequently made until the elastomer cast was bare and clean. The cast was then completely cleaned using alcohol solution.

Results

Figure 2 shows an example of a cast of the septal artery. In this case, the blood flow velocity was measured at a depth of about 18 mm from the orifice of the artery. The velocity pattern of this case is shown in Fig. 3. The velocity waveform was almost exclusively diastolic and reverse flow was always observed during early systole.

Figure 4 illustrates a typical example of the blood flow velocity pattern of an intramyocardial vein. It was characterized by a prominent systolic flow pattern. The velocity increased abruptly in the isovolumic contraction phase and decreased rapidly after the beginning of diastole. The momentary reverse flow pattern was frequently repeated in the early diastolic phase.

Concluding Remarks

The major contribution of our study is that it is the first continuous measurement of phasic blood velocity patterns in the deeper vessels of the beating canine left ventricle. From our preliminary study, we observed the following: (a) In the septal artery, blood flow velocity is accelerated more abruptly during early diastole and the waveform is almost exclusively diastolic; the reverse flow was always observed during isovolumic contraction. (b) In the intramyocardial small vein, the blood flow was increased rapidly after the beginning of the isovolumic contraction phase and momentary reverse flow was observed during early diastole. (c) The velocity waveform in the deeper intramyocardial artery shows a reciprocal relation with that of the intramyocardial vein.

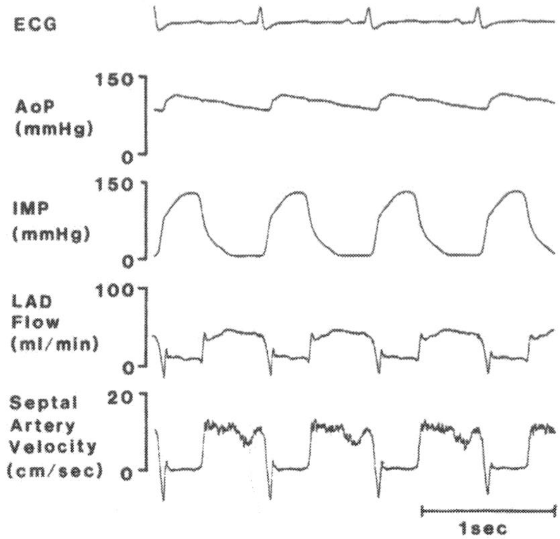

Fig. 3. Blood flow velocity waveform in septal artery. *ECG* electrocardiogram, *AoP* aortic pressure, *IMP* intramyocardial pressure, *LAD* left anterior descending artery

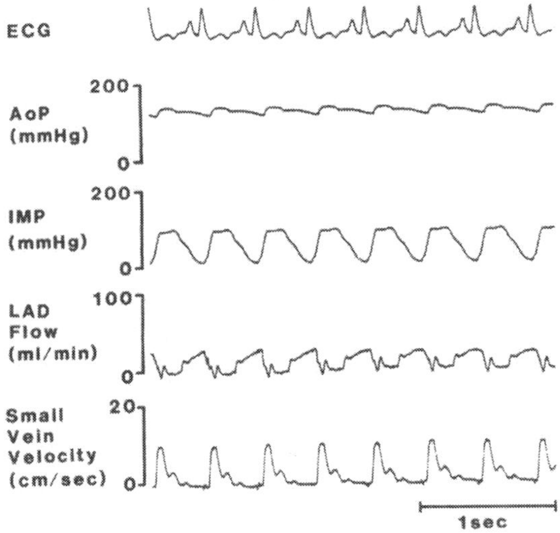

Fig. 4. Blood flow velocity waveform in intramyocardial small vein

References

1. Hellberg K, Wayland H, Rickart AL, Bing RJ (1972) Studies on the coronary microcirculation by direct visualization. Am J Cardiol 29: 593–597
2. Tillmanns H, Ikeda S, Hansen H (1974) Microcirculation in the ventricle of the dog and turtle. Circ Res 34: 561–569
3. Ashikawa K, Kanatsuka H, Suzuki T, Takishima T (1986) Phasic blood flow velocity pattern in epimyocardial microvessels in the beating canine left ventricle. Circ Res 59: 704–711
4. Mito K, Ogasawara Y, Hiramatsu O, Wada Y, Matsuoka S, Goto M, Kagiyama M, Tsujioka K, Kajiya F (1987) Evaluation of the velocity wave-form in intramyocardial small arterial and vein by laser Doppler velocimeter. Proceedings of the 26th Conference of the Japan Society of Medical Electronics and Biological Engineering, p 253

Determinants of Myocardial Oxygen Demand: Total Mechanical Energy and Contractility

HIROYUKI SUGA, YOSHIO YASUMURA, TAKASHI NOZAWA, SHIHO FUTAKI, NOBUAKI TANAKA, and MASAAKI UENISHI[1]

Introduction

Many determinants (indices or predictors) of myocardial oxygen consumption (VO_2) have been proposed over recent decades [1, 2]. They include peak or mean ventricular pressure, myocardial systolic force, time integrals of pressure and force, contractile element work, dP/dt, Vmax, and their various combinations including Bretschneider's total myocardial energy requirement E_t [1] and the Rooke and Feigl pressure-work index [2]. Some of them are empirical and others are theoretical. However, we do not feel satisfied with them because their correlations with VO_2 are not always good under a variety of loading, heart rate, and contractile conditions.

In a series of experimental studies over the past 10 years, we have found close and linear correlations between VO_2 and the total mechanical energy (TME) generated by contraction in the left ventricle of excised, cross-circulated dog left ventricles [3–6]. TME is determined by the area (PVA) circumscribed by the end-systolic pressure-volume (P-V) and end-diastolic P-V relation (ESPVR and EDPVR) curves and the systolic P-V trajectory in the P-V diagram [7], as shown in Fig. 1.

Methods

We always used the left ventricle of the excised, cross-circulated dog heart preparation that Suga and Sagawa developed [8]. In each experiment, two mongrel dogs were anesthetized either with pentobarbital sodium (30 mg/kg i.v.) or with a mixture of urethane (500 mg/kg i.v.) and α-chloralose (50 mg/kg i.v.). The heart was excised from one dog under cross circulation with the other dog. The left ventricle was filled with a water-filled balloon and connected to a volume servopump which enabled us to control precisely and measure accurately left ventricular volume [9]. By adjusting the left ventricular volume and its changes with a volume command signal generator, we varied left ventricular preload and

[1]Department of Cardiovascular Dynamics, National Cardiovascular Center Research Institute, 7-1, Fujishirodai 5-chome, Suita, Osaka, 565 Japan

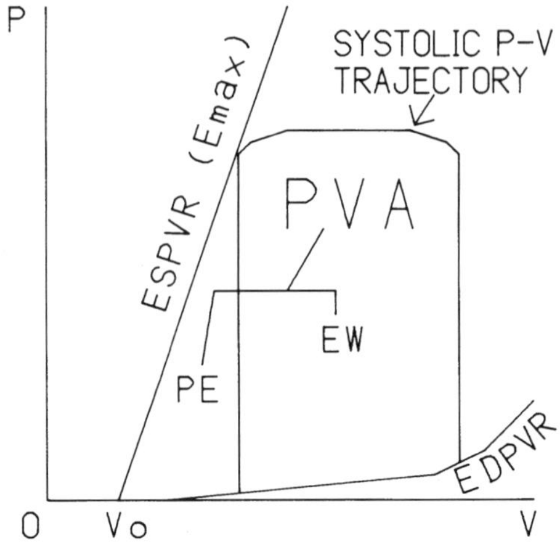

Fig. 1. Systolic pressure-volume area (*PVA*) and contractility index (*Emax*) drawn in the pressure-volume (*P-V*) diagram of the left ventricle. *ESPVR* end-systolic P-V relation, *EDPVR* end-diastolic P-V relation, *Emax* slope of ESPVR, *EW* external work, *PE* potential energy, *PVA* EW + PE

afterload over a wide range.

The total coronary flow was measured with an electromagnetic flowmeter in the coronary venous return tube. The coronary arteriovenous oxygen content difference was measured with an AVOX systems apparatus [10]. The total cardiac oxygen consumption was determined continuously as the product of coronary flow and arteriovenous oxygen content difference. It was divided by the heart rate in each steady state to obtain VO_2/beat. The right ventricular VO_2 was assumed to be a constant fraction of the total unloaded VO_2 because the right ventricle was kept unloaded by continuous hydrostatic drainage of coronary venous blood.

Emax, the slope of the end-systolic P-V relation line [5, 8], was determined as the slope of the line connecting the end-systolic P-V point and V_O, i.e., the left ventricular volume at which peak isovolumic pressure was zero, with a signal processor (NEC San-ei, 7T17).

PVA was also measured simultaneously with the same signal processor by using the same algorithm described before [5].

The details of the experimental protocols are to be found in the individual references [3–6, 11–14].

Results

The correlation between VO_2 and PVA was first studied in a given contractile state with a constant Emax [3]. We found that VO_2 closely and linearly correlated with PVA in both isovolumic and variously ejecting contractions in a given heart, as shown in Fig. 2a. This load-independent VO_2-PVA relation is unique as compared with the load-dependent VO_2 relation of systolic pressure, systolic force, and their time integrals [11, 12]. This was more specifically confirmed by

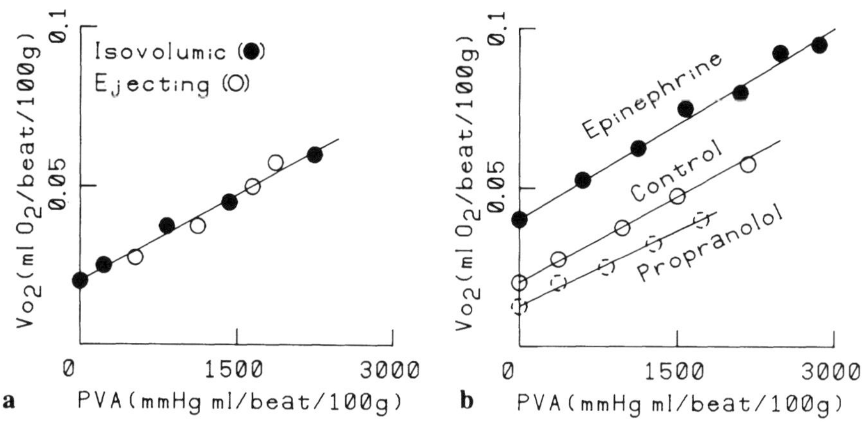

a b

Fig. 2a, b. Representative examples of the VO_2-PVA relation in the dog left ventricle. **a** Different loading conditions; **b** different contractile states

changing the shape of the contour of PVA while keeping the magnitude of PVA constant. As long as the magnitude of PVA remained the same, VO_2 remained unchanged despite marked changes in the shape of the contour of PVA [11, 12].

We also confirmed the load-independence of the VO_2-PVA relation by finding the most appropriate weight of the potential energy (PE) part of PVA relative to the external work (EW) part of PVA (Fig. 1) [13]. Statistical analyses indicated that the correlation between VO_2 and the variably weighted sum of PE and EW became highest when both PE and EW were weighted equally; the sum of PE and EW is PVA.

We then studied the effect of changes in Emax on the VO_2-PVA relation. When Emax was doubled in value by epinephrine administration, the VO_2-PVA relation was elevated in a virtually parallel fashion along the VO_2 axis [5], as shown in Fig. 2b. A similar elevation was observed with isoproterenol or dobutamine (unpublished data). $CaCl_2$ also caused a similar elevation [5]. When Emax was halved by propranolol, the VO_2-PVA relation was lowered in a virtually parallel manner [14], as shown in Fig. 2b.

When heart rate was varied between 80 and 220 beats/min, the VO_2-PVA relation on a per beat basis remained virtually unchanged [4].

When the heart was arrested with KCl, VO_2 decreased considerably from the level of unloaded contraction with zero PVA [5]. VO_2 of the arrested heart, corresponding to the basal metabolism, was of the order of 20 $J \cdot min^{-1} \cdot 100$ g. This basal VO_2 was not significantly increased with epinephrine or $CaCl_2$ [5]. Therefore, we assumed that the basal VO_2 was independent of Emax even under variously loaded contractions.

We also produced ejecting contractions against minimal afterload pressure from different end-diastolic volumes. These contractions had negligibly small PVAs as compared with PVAs of normally afterloaded ejecting contractions from comparable end-diastolic volumes. We found VO_2s of these ejecting contractions with minimal PVAs to be close to the VO_2 of unloaded isovolumic contractions at V_O despite widely varied end-diastolic volumes of ejecting contraction [6]. This result suggests that the length-dependent activation if any was negligible in the preparation used.

We varied widely the diastolic segment of the P-V trajectory without changing the systolic segment of the P-V trajectory. This method changed markedly the relative magnitudes of both EW and PE without changing PVA. We found that VO_2 remained unchanged as long as PVA remained unchanged [6]. This confirmed the uniqueness of PVA as a correlate of VO_2.

From these results, we considered that the VO_2-PVA relation could be formulated as $VO_2 = A \cdot PVA + B \cdot Emax + C$, where VO_2 and PVA are expressed in $J \cdot beat^{-1} \cdot 100\ g^{-1}$ and Emax in $mmHg \cdot ml^{-1} \cdot 100\ g$, A = 2.7 (dimensionless), B = $0.048\ J \cdot beat^{-1} \cdot 100\ g^{-1}/(mmHg \cdot ml^{-1} \cdot 100\ g)$, and C = $0.28\ J \cdot beat^{-1} \cdot 100\ g^{-1}$ on average. On a per minute basis, the above equation is modified to $VO_2\ (min^{-1}) = A \cdot HR \cdot PVA + B \cdot HR \cdot Emax + BM$, where BM = basal metabolic $VO_2/min = 20\ J \cdot min^{-1} \cdot 100\ g$.

Discussion

No other determinants and indices of VO_2 have been critically evaluated to the extent that PVA has been evaluated. PVA has been shown to correlate closely and linearly with VO_2 at a constant Emax and changes in Emax vary VO_2 proportionally at a constant PVA. The empirical equation shown above represents succinctly all our experimental findings. Therefore, we consider that TME assessed by PVA and contractile state assessed by Emax are the two major determinants of VO_2 in the dog left ventricle.

It may be considered that accurate measurement of ventricular volume is difficult and PVA is, therefore, impractical although the concept of PVA can be appreciated. However, we would emphasize that all other so far proposed determinants and indices of VO_2 have basic problems, although we admit that many of them, such as peak pressure, peak force, pressure time integral, force time integral, double product (pressure-rate product), triple product (pressure-rate-ejection time product), are practical and have a close correlation with VO_2 in ordinary ejecting contractions. However, if VO_2s of isovolumic contractions are included in the correlogram, the correlation decreases [11, 12].

Some may prefer Bretschneider's E_t [1] or the pressure-work index [2]. These are practical and correlate closely with VO_2. However, we can consider conditions under which these indices would not be so accurate. Bretschneider's second term E_2 is important for energy demand for maintenance of myocardial tension, but this term is reduced to zero in isovolumic contractions. This prediction does not match the fact that VO_2 of the isovolumic contraction is greater than that of an ejecting contraction starting from the same end-diastolic volume in the same contractile state. The pressure-work index has a constant ($1.43\ ml\ O_2 \cdot min^{-1} \cdot 100\ g^{-1}$) for basal metabolism. The index is equal to this constant in mechanically unloaded contractions. However, VO_2 of unloaded contractions increases from about 3 to $5\ ml\ O_2 \cdot min^{-1} \cdot 100\ g^{-1}$ with an enhancement of the contractile state by epinephrine. This increase in VO_2 cannot be predicted by the pressure-work index. Thus, even these two most recently proposed indices of VO_2 cannot be considered ideal from the basic point of view. PVA can predict reliably VO_2 even under these specific conditions.

We would reasonably expect that our present contention is applicable to the heart and myocardium in general. In fact, we recently found that VO_2 of the left ventricle of young dogs is also correlated practically linearly with PVA despite the nonlinear end-systolic P-V relation [14]. The systolic force-length area (FLA), the linear-muscular version of PVA, has also been shown to correlate linearly with VO_2 in ferret papillary muscles [15]. This correlation was shown to be better than the correlation of VO_2 with peak force or systolic force time integral. The dimensions of FLA are g·cm, which are convertible to J with 1 $g \cdot cm = 9.81 \times 10^{-5}$ J. Like PVA, FLA represents the total mechanical energy generated by a linear muscle.

The VO_2-PVA and VO_2-FLA relations suggest to us that if the total mechanical energy of a ventricular wall region were quantified, there would be a close and linear correlation between the regional VO_2 and regional TME. We know how to quantify regional TME. We have found that regional mechanical work can be quantified by the area within a loop relating regional tension (T) to regional area (S) [16]. Note the difference between the area in the T-S diagram and the area (S) of the region. This T is called surface tension or interfacial tension and is equal to the total circumferential force per unit circumference perpendicular to the force. The dimensions of this T-S loop area are $g \cdot cm^{-1} \cdot cm^2 = g \cdot cm$, which are dimensions of energy like those of PVA and FLA. If we add the T-S area corresponding to the potential energy to the T-S loop area, we obtain the area equivalent to TME generated by the region. We can term the total area "TSA" as an abbreviation of tension-surface area, where the first area represents S and the second area represents the T-S area. We have already devised a technique to assess TSA and demonstrated its feasibility [16].

Thus, it is quite likely that the concept of PVA will lead to the development of a determinant or index of regional VO_2, which could be coupled with regional VO_2 under a variety of coronary microcirculary disorders.

Summary

Disorders of the coronary microcirculation should be evaluated in terms of the balance between regional myocardial oxygen supply and demand. However, direct measurement of regional myocardial oxygen consumption is difficult at present. Therefore, the development of a reliable determinant of regional myocardial oxygen demand is needed. Toward this end, we reviewed the experimental results of our recent studies on the determinants of myocardial oxygen consumption (VO_2) under aerobic conditions.

Acknowledgments. Partly supported by grants-in-aid for Scientific Research (C59570047, B61480102) from the Ministry of Education, Science and Culture and Research grants for Cardiovascular Diseases (60A-1 and 60C-3) from the Ministry of Health and Welfare of Japan.

References

1. Baller D, Bretschneider HJ, Hellige G (1979) Validity of myocardial oxygen consumption parameters. Clin Cardiol 2: 317–327
2. Rooke GA, Feigl EO (1982) Work as a correlate of canine left ventricular oxygen consumption, and the problem of catecholamine oxygen wasting. Circ Res 50: 273–286
3. Suga H, Hayashi T, Shirahata M (1981) Ventricular systolic pressure volume area as a predictor of cardiac oxygen consumption. Am J Physiol 240: H39–H44
4. Suga H, Hisano R, Hirata S, Hayashi T, Yamada O, Ninomiya I (1983) Heart rate-independent energetics and systolic pressure-volume area in dog heart. Am J Physiol 244: H206–H214
5. Suga H, Hisano R, Goto Y, Yamada O, Igarashi Y (1983) Effect of positive inotropic agents on the relation between oxygen consumption and systolic pressure volume area in canine left ventricle. Circ Res 53: 306–318
6. Suga H, Igarashi Y, Yamada O, Goto Y (1986) Cardiac oxygen consumption and systolic pressure volume area. Bas Res Cardiol 81 (Suppl 1): 39–50
7. Suga H (1979) Total mechanical energy of a ventricle model and cardiac oxygen consumption. Am J Physiol 236: H498–H505
8. Suga H, Sagawa K (1974) Instantaneous pressure-volume relationships and their ratio in the excised, supported canine left ventricle. Circ Res 35: 117–126
9. Suga H, Sagawa K (1977) End-diastolic and end-systolic ventricular volume clamper for isolated canine heart. Am J Physiol 233: H718–H722
10. Shepherd AP, Burger CG (1977) A solid-state arteriovenous oxygen difference analyzer for flowing whole blood. Am J Physiol 232: H437–H440
11. Suga H, Hayashi T, Suehiro S, Hisano R, Shirahata M, Ninomiya I (1981) Equal oxygen consumption rates of isovolumic and ejecting contractions with equal systolic pressure volume areas in canine left ventricle. Circ Res 49: 1082–1091
12. Suga H, Goto Y, Nozawa T, Yasumura Y, Futaki S, Tanaka N (1987) Force-time integral decreases with ejection despite constant oxygen consumption and pressure-volume area in dog left ventricle. Circ Res 60: 797–803
13. Suga H, Hayashi T, Shirahata M, Ninomiya I (1980) Critical evaluation of left ventricular systolic pressure volume area as predictor of oxygen consumption. Jpn J Physiol 30: 907–919
14. Suga H, Yamada O, Goto Y, Igarashi Y, Yasumura Y, Nozawa T, Futaki S (1987) Left ventricular O_2 consumption and pressure-volume area in puppies. Am J Physiol 253: H770–H776
15. Hisano R, Cooper G IV (1987) Correlation of force-length area with oxygen consumption in ferret papillary muscle. Circ Res 61: 318–328
16. Goto Y, Suga H, Yamada O, Igarashi Y, Saito M. Hiramori K (1986) Left ventricular regional work from wall tension-area loop in the canine heart. Am J Physiol 250: H151–H158

Pathophysiology of Acute Embolization of Small Coronary Arteries: Detrimental Effects of Oxygen-Free Radicals

MASATSUGU HORI[1], KOICHI GOTO[1], KUNIMITSU IWAI[1], KATSUOMI IWAKURA[1], YUKIHIRO KORETSUNE[1], AKIRA KITABATAKE[1], MICHITOSHI INOUE[2], and TAKENOBU KAMADA[1]

Introduction

Recent studies have demonstrated that blood cell plugging occurs after reperfusion of the occluded coronary artery and may impede the perfusion after recanalization [1–4]. Despite the clinical significance of this microcirculatory disturbance, however, the pathophysiology of acute microembolization of coronary vessels is still unclear. We investigated the response of coronary blood flow and histological changes in the myocardium after coronary embolization in dogs and found that the myocardial ischemia induced by coronary embolization is a good ischemic model for assessment of interventions which may influence the ischemic injury. In this study, we attempted to evaluate the role of oxygen-free radicals as a cause of ischemic cell injury in this acute microcirculatory disturbance.

Hyperemic Response of Coronary Blood Flow in Microembolization

Figure 1 shows the coronary blood flow measured at the proximal site of the left anterior descending artery after the injection of 15-μm microspheres (5×10^4/g myocardium) into this artery. Within 1 min after embolization, the coronary blood flow increased after a transient decrease and went beyond the control level. The repetitive injection of microspheres further increased the coronary blood flow despite occlusion of the microvasculature. The maximal increase in the coronary blood flow was 175% $\pm$ 36% of the control flow, which was obtained when microspheres of $1.5–2.0 \times 10^5$/g myocardium were embolized. With a larger dose, however, the coronary blood flow was almost linearly decreased as the amount of microspheres increased (Fig. 2) [5]. In contrast to the biphasic change in coronary blood flow, the regional fractional shortening determined by paired ultrasonic dimension gauges and the lactate extraction ratio both linearly decreased with the dose of microspheres. These results indicate that the extent of myocardial ischemia is dependent on the degree of emboliza-

First Department of Medicine[1] and Department of Medical Information Science[2], Osaka University Medical School, 1–50, Fukushima 1-chome, Fukushima-ku, Osaka, 553 Japan

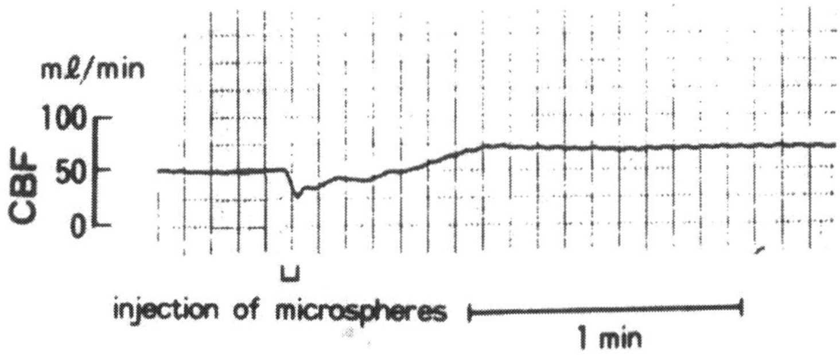

Fig. 1. Representative changes in coronary blood flow in the left anterior descending coronary artery after intracoronary injection of microspheres (15 μm in diameter, 5×10^4/g myocardium). Immediately after injection, coronary blood flow transiently decreased but subsequently increased. Note that coronary blood flow in steady state after injection was higher than in controls

tion, whereas coronary blood flow is not directly related to the dose of microspheres. It should be noted that hyperemic flow was associated with a decrease in the coronary arteriovenous oxygen difference. Thus, this hyperemic response may be attributed to the shunt flow, which does not contribute to the oxygen supply to the myocardium. Although previous studies also demonstrated an increase in coronary blood flow or a decrease in the coronary vascular resistance after coronary embolization [6, 7], the mechanism of this hyperemic response has not been clarified. We observed that a very large amount of adenosine was released after the embolization and the hyperemic response was markedly attenuated by adenosine receptor blockade [5, 8]. This evidence suggests that the hyperemic flow is due to vasodilation of coronary arteries in response to the released adenosine.

Characteristics of Myocardial Ischemia in Microembolization

Myocardial ischemia elicited after coronary embolization is substantially different from that induced by coronary artery occlusion. As described above, hyperemic flow observed after embolization could be attributed to the hyperemic response of the small coronary arteries in the nonischemic area to adenosine released from the ischemic myocardium. Thus, this paradoxical increase in coronary flow is primarily due to patchy distribution of ischemic foci in the myocardium. the succinic dehydrogenase staining of the embolized myocardium demonstrated that a solitary ischemic region was 100–200 μm (transverse) $\times$ 800–500 μm (longitudinal) in size [9]. Patchy ischemic regions were also observed 1 h after embolization in the sections stained with toluidine blue as a cluster of myocytes with severe intracellular edema. From these histological studies and the coronary flow response, we made a hypothetical model of capillary flow distribution in the embolized myocardium.

Figure 3 shows a two-dimensional model of the capillary distribution and re-

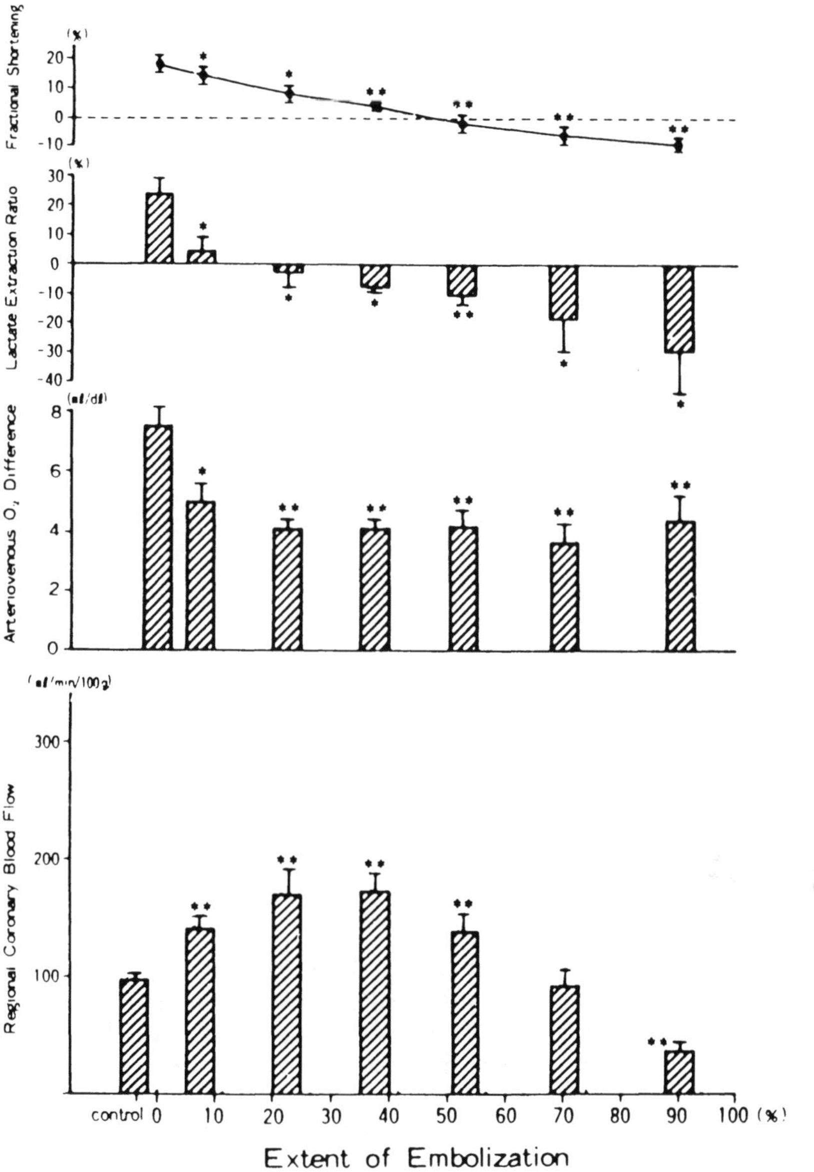

Fig. 2. Mean changes in fractional shortening in the regional segment length, lactate extraction ratio, coronary arteriovenous O_2 difference, and resting coronary blood flow following the intracoronary embolization with 15-μm microspheres. Of the maximal embolization, 100% was obtained from the intercept of the extrapolated downslope of the coronary blood flow. Values are means ± SE ($n = 8$). * $P < 0.05$, ** $P < 0.01$ compared with controls. Modified from Hori et al. [5]

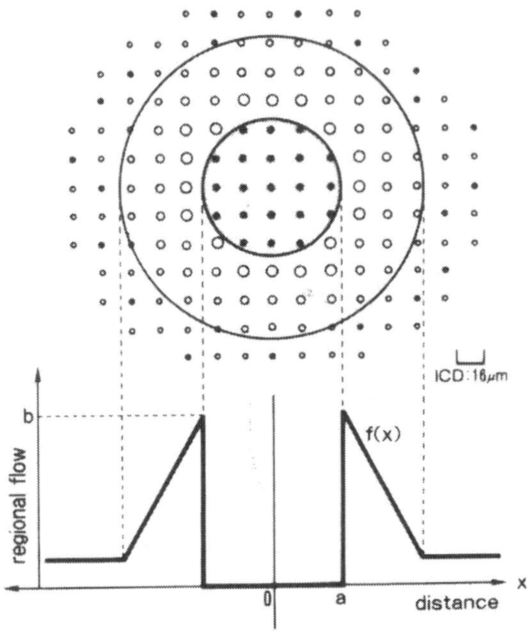

Fig. 3. Model of capillary distribution and regional coronary blood flow. *Upper panel* cross section of myocardium where capillaries are distributed in rectangular stacking pattern. The *central shadowed area* represents an occluded area by microsphere embolization in which capillary flow is zero. The ischemic area is surrounded by a hyperemic area, in which the hyperemic flow is symbolically depicted by the dilated capillaries. In the nonhyperemic area, a *closed circle* represents an unperfused capillary, and an *open circle* a perfused capillary. *Lower panel* flow distribution as a function of the distance—f(x)—from the center of the ischemic area. *a* size of ischemic area, *b* maximal flow, *ICD* intercapillary distance. After Hori et al. [9]

gional coronary blood flow. The central shadowed area represents an occluded area by microsphere embolization in which capillary flow is assumed to be zero. The ischemic area is surrounded by a hyperemic area with dilated capillaries, in which adenosine released from ischemic myocytes induces hyperemic flow. Out of these affected areas, the capillaries are normally distributed with an intercapillary distance of 19 μm (capillary density 2770/mm^2). In our model, we assumed that the maximal capacity of the vasodilation of the arterioles was 400% of the resting flow, and the flow in each capillary was determined by the regional concentration of adenosine, which decreased linearly with the distance from the ischemic boundary. With this theoretical model, we simulated the change in the coronary blood flow after embolization of various doses of microspheres, assuming that a plug of microsphere in the arteriole results in the obstruction of 21 capillaries, based on the histological study of embolized myocardium. In the simulation study, the embolization at a random site was repeated up to 2800 times, at which the total coronary blood flow was decreased almost to zero. Figure 4 shows the simulated coronary blood flow when the extent of embolization was increased with three different values for the diffusion distance

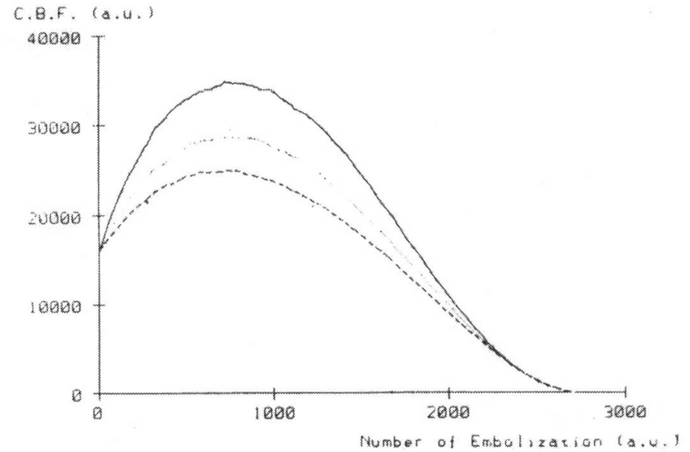

Fig. 4. Simulated coronary blood flow (*C.B.F.*) in relation to the number of embolizations when the diffusion distance of adenosine varied from 12 μm to 23 μm when the capillary recruitment was 60%. *Upper line* 12 μm, *middle line* 17μm, *low line* 23 μm. After Hori et al. [9]

of adenosine, i.e., 12, 17, and 23 μm. The biphasic flow change is compatible with our previous results depicted in Fig. 2. Although the diffusion distance of adenosine largely affected the maximal hyperemic response, the percentage embolization (the number of microspheres) for the maximal flow was minimally influenced by this parameter. The results obtained in this simulation study further strengthened our adenosine theory for regulation of coronary blood flow in microembolization [5, 9].

The patchy focal ischemia induced by microsphere embolization may be characteristic for its interrelation with the surrounding nonischemic area since hyperemic response in the surrounding area may have some feedback effects on the ischemia. The ischemic border zone of myocardial infarct is adjacent to the nonischemic surrounding area and, hence, may be under similar conditions to patchy ischemia in microembolization. It has been reported that the direct diffusion of oxygen from the endocardium may supply the necessary oxygen to the subendocardial layers even in acute myocardial infarction [10]. This evidence suggests that an ischemic area of 100–200 μm may be partially supplied with oxygen from the surrounding area. Thus, the myocardial ischemia in microembolization could be on the critical divide between reversible and irreversible ischemia and, therefore, may be sensitive to the metabolic alterations induced by the intervention. The embolization model has another advantage in that the metabolic changes in ischemia can be easily determined, since lactate metabolism and oxygen extraction can be determined by coronary venous blood sampling. Furthermore, in this model, the extent of ischemia can be controlled by the dose of microspheres: the linear relation between the fractional shortening and dose of microspheres (Fig. 2) suggests that the extent of ischemia is directly determined by the embolized microspheres. It should also be noticed that at a given a dose of microspheres, the individual variation in the extent of ischemia is relatively small and the ischemic condition is fairly stable for a few hours. These two factors may further support the capability of this ischemic model for the assessment of interventions.

Detrimental Effects of Oxygen-Free Radicals in Coronary Microembolization

In the previous studies, there has been no direct evidence that oxygen-tree radicals exert a detrimental effect on ischemic cell injury in sustained myocardial ischemia induced by coronary artery occlusion. In microembolization, however, the ischemic condition is different from that in coronary artery occlusion; the hyperemic flow surrounding the patchy ischemic area may supply oxygen and, hence, produce oxygen-free radicals. To test this hypothesis, dogs with acute coronary embolization were treated with human recombinant superoxide dismutase (SOD). SOD (25 mg) was given intravenously 10 min before embolization, and intravenous administration (25 mg/h) was continued until the end of the study. In the control study without SOD, coronary blood flow decreased to zero at embolization of 5×10^5/g myocardium. At this maximal embolization, ventricular wall motion demonstrated dyskinesis, as indicated by the negative value of fractional shortening, and marked lactate production was observed. In contrast to this, treatment with SOD improved ischemic changes at all doses of embolization, although SOD per se did not alter the baseline coronary blood flow, fractional shortening, and lactate extraction ratio; at 5×10^5/g myocardium, fractional shortening was still positive and lactate extraction was much less than that without SOD treatment. Moreover, the maximal dose of microspheres was greatly increased. This improvement in ischemia may be attributed to the attenuation of myocardial edema, which may compress the microvasculature and increase the impedance for coronary perfusion. Our results indicate that in sustained myocardial ischemia by coronary microembolization, oxygen-free radicals play an important role in ischemic injury, particularly by increasing the membrane permeability.

Conclusion

It is well recognized that after 25–50 min of ischemia, no-reflow occurs frequently in the subendocardial region associated with microvascular damage. We found that microsphere embolization of the coronary arteries induced hyperemic flow due to adenosine release. The simulation study based on the capillary distribution suggests that the affected area by released adenosine is small (15–23 μm), but hyperemic flow response in this nonischemic surrounding area is sufficient to explain the biphasic flow change in repetitive embolization by microspheres. This microembolization model is good for assessing interventions in myocardial ischemia, since the model is hemodynamically stable for a couple of hours and the individual variation in ischemia is small. In the present study, we applied this model to evaluate the role of oxygen-free radicals in microembolization. The treatment of human recombinant superoxide dismutase markedly attenuated the myocardial edema and, hence, ischemic changes. This indicates that oxygen-free radicals play an important role in ischemic injury, even in sustained myocardial ischemia, by coronary microembolization.

References

1. Engler RL, Schmid-Schonbein GW, Pavelec RS (1983) Leukocyte capillary plugging in myocardial ischemia and reperfusion in the dog. Am J Pathol 111: 98–111
2. Moschos CB, Lahiri K, Lyons M, Weisse AB, Oldewurtel Ha, Regan TJ (1973) Relation of microcirculatory thrombosis to thrombus in the proximal coronary artery: effect of aspirin, dipyridamole, and thrombolysis. Am Heart J 86: 61–68
3. Kloner RA, Ganote CE, Jennings RB (1974) The "no-reflow" phenomenon after temporary coronary occlusion in the dog. J Clin Invest 54: 1496–1508
4. Leinberger H, Suehiro GT, McNamara JJ (1979) Myocardial platelet trapping after coronary ligation in primates (*Papio anubis*), platelet trapping in infarct marginal zone. J Surg Research 27: 36–40
5. Hori M, Inoue M, Kitakaze M, Koretsune Y, Iwai K, Tamai J, Ito H, Kitabatake A, Sato T, Kamada T (1986) Role of adenosine in hyperemic response of coronary blood flow in microembolization. Am J Physiol 250: H509–H518
6. Bing RJ, Castellanos A, Gradel E, Lupton C, Siegel A (1956) Experimental myocardial infarction: circulatory, biochemical and pathologic changes. Am J Med Sci 232: 533–554
7. West JW, Kobayashi T, Anderson FS (1962) Effects of selective coronary embolization on coronary blood flow and coronary sinus venous blood oxygen saturation in dogs. Circ Res 10: 722–738
8. Kitakaze M, Hori M, Tamai J, Iwakura K, Koretsune Y, Kagiya T, Iwai K, Kitabatake A, Inoue M, Kamada T (1987) $Alpha_1$-adrenoceptor activity regulates release of adenosine from the ischemic myocardium in dogs. Circ Res 60: 631–639
9. Hori M, Inoue M, Iwai K, Kitakaze M, Orihashi Y, Kitabatake A, Kamada T (1986) Computer simulation of hyperemic flow in microembolization of coronary arteries. The role of adenosine in patchy myocardial ischemia. Automedica 7: 63–76
10. Gavin JB, Nevalainen TJ, Seelye RN, Webster V, Thomson RW (1978) An association between the onset of rigor and loss of vascular competence in early myocardial infarcts. Pathology 10: 219–225

Author Index

Subject Index

GPSR Compliance

The European Union's (EU) General Product Safety Regulation (GPSR) is a set of rules that requires consumer products to be safe and our obligations to ensure this.

If you have any concerns about our products, you can contact us on ProductSafety@springernature.com

In case Publisher is established outside the EU, the EU authorized representative is:

Springer Nature Customer Service Center GmbH
Europaplatz 3
69115 Heidelberg, Germany

FSC
www.fsc.org
MIX
Papier | Fördert gute Waldnutzung
FSC® C083411

Kolibri 360 GmbH
Ferdinand-Jühlke-Straße 7
99095 Erfurt, Deutschland
produktsicherheit@kolibri360.de